# Introduction to Biliary Atresia

Masaki Nio
Editor

# Introduction to Biliary Atresia

Springer

*Editor*
Masaki Nio
Department of Pediatric Surgery
Tohoku University Graduate School of Medicine
Sendai
Japan

ISBN 978-981-16-2159-8 ISBN 978-981-16-2160-4 (eBook)
https://doi.org/10.1007/978-981-16-2160-4



This Springer imprint is published by the registered company Springer Nature Singapore Pte Ltd.
The registered company address is: 152 Beach Road, #21-01/04 Gateway East, Singapore 189721, Singapore

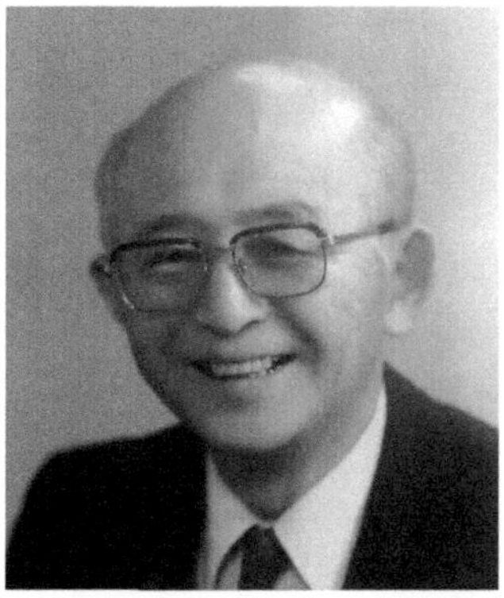

*This book is respectfully and affectionately dedicated to Morio Kasai, a pioneering surgeon who developed the world's first corrective surgery for biliary atresia, known as Kasai portoenterostomy.*

# Preface

Until Kasai portoenterostomy was developed by Professor Morio Kasai in 1957, biliary atresia (BA) was believed to be an incurable and fatal disease. Kasai portoenterostomy made surgical treatment possible for patients with BA; however, approximately one-third of patients in Japan (and more in many other parts of the world) still require liver transplantation before 1 year of age. BA is a rare disease, and its treatment is so complicated that the centralization of cases has progressed only to a limited number of highly specialized pediatric institutions in select European countries. While the surgical outcome has gradually improved, it is still not optimal. In Japan, the centralization of specialties is not considered important; thus, Kasai portoenterostomy has been performed in more than 100 facilities, most of which deal with one or two cases per year. Why, then, are the overall surgical results in Japan equivalent to or even greater than those in Western countries? This question is a major concern for medical professionals worldwide involved in the treatment of BA for which this book will hopefully provide some insights.

In 1975, an academic organization (the Japanese Society of Biliary Atresia, JBAS) was founded at the behest of Dr. Kasai and continues to study and discuss BA. Around 100 pediatric facilities in Japan, where Kasai portoenterostomy is predominantly performed, participate in the JBAS and share their experiences with the disease. In addition, in 1989, the National Registration System of BA [Japanese Biliary Atresia Registry (JBAR)] was launched under the leadership of Professor Ryoji Ohi. JBAR data on initial, liver transplantation, and follow-up registries are presented at the annual JBAS meeting. In other words, a sound understanding and standard BA treatment have been shared nationwide for over three decades. These efforts have led to improved outcomes for patients with BA. To date, data on over 3500 patients with BA have been compiled, an extraordinary number of cases given the rarity of this disease.

In this book, pediatric experts in fields such as hepatology, surgery, pathology, and liver transplantation familiar with BA describe our latest knowledge regarding standard medical procedures, surgical techniques, perioperative care, long-term follow-up, transitions, and social support systems for BA. I believe that this book will be extremely useful for medical professionals involved in BA worldwide, especially pediatric colleagues.

Sendai, Japan Masaki Nio

# Contents

# 1 Historical Overview of Biliary Atresia

Masaki Nio and Ryoji Ohi

**Abstract**

The non-correctable type of biliary atresia had been regarded as a fatal disease until Kasai portoenterostomy was developed in the 1950s. Since the early 1980s, liver transplantation has been widely adopted worldwide as a practical, surgical modality for biliary atresia. In Japan, liver transplantation from living donors progressed remarkably in the 1990s, whereas the system of deceased-donor transplantation was not readily adopted. Even today, despite the widespread adoption of liver transplantation, universal consensus maintains that Kasai portoenterostomy is the first-line surgical treatment modality for biliary atresia. In this chapter, the history, diagnostic and therapeutic development, current clinical issues, research directions, and future aspects of biliary atresia are addressed.

**Keywords**

Biliary atresia · Kasai portoenterostomy · Liver transplantation · History

## Abbreviations

| | |
|---|---|
| ISSBA | The International Sendai Symposium on Biliary Atresia |
| JBAR | The Japanese Biliary Atresia Registry |
| JBAS | The Japanese Biliary Atresia Society |

M. Nio (✉) · R. Ohi
Department of Pediatric Surgery, Tohoku University Graduate School of Medicine, Sendai, Japan
e-mail: mnio@ped-surg.med.tohoku.ac.jp

## 1.1 Before the Era of Kasai Portoenterostomy

In 1817, biliary atresia was first described in the textbook by J. Burns [1] of the University of Glasgow, as an "incurable state of the biliary apparatus." J. Thompson of Edinburgh systematically described biliary atresia for the first time [2]. He reported the details of his own case and a review of the autopsy results of 49 cases. In 1916, J.B. Holmes of Johns Hopkins University reviewed the cases of biliary atresia and concluded that about 16% of the cases were a correctable type of atresia, in which surgical treatment was theoretically possible [3].

W.E. Ladd of Boston Children's Hospital reported the first successful case of the correctable type of biliary atresia in 1928 [4]. For the non-correctable type of biliary atresia, various treatment attempts were made, including an anastomosis between the resected surface of the biliary remnant and the intestine [5], an artificial bile duct [6], second-look surgery [7], and thoracic duct–esophagus anastomosis [8]. However, none of them was successful. In 1968, Thaler and Gelis [9], pediatricians from the United States, reported that surgery for infants with obstructive jaundice should be postponed until 4 months of age, because the prognosis of neonatal hepatitis was worse when an exploratory laparotomy was performed. This report was accepted widely in Europe and in the United States; thus, achieving the appropriate timing for biliary atresia surgery was almost impossible.

## 1.2 Dawn of Surgery for Biliary Atresia

Kasai portoenterostomy was developed in Sendai, in the 1950s. Following this, treatment of the non-correctable type of biliary atresia started in Japan. Initially, we had introduced an episode that helped Morio Kasai conceive the idea of Kasai portoenterostomy. This story was told by Kasai himself in his retiring lecture at the auditorium of Tohoku University School of Medicine in 1986.


M. Nio (ed.), *Introduction to Biliary Atresia*, https://doi.org/10.1007/978-981-16-2160-4_1

In 1955, Professor Shigetsugu Katsura dissected porta hepatis and searched for the hepatic duct in a patient with obstructive jaundice, but he could not find any bile duct. He made a small incision in the duodenum and created several stiches between the porta hepatis and the duodenum. The patient passed cholic stools after a week or so.

One month later, another patient with biliary atresia was operated on. In this case, Professor Katsura created several stitches between the porta hepatis and the duodenum without incising the duodenum. After a while, this patient also passed cholic stools.

At that time, Kasai was an associate professor, and Katsura was his mentor.

Following such experiences, Kasai performed surgery on a 72-day-old boy with non-correctable type of biliary atresia in May 1957. Kasai removed the extrahepatic biliary remnant, created a Roux-en Y limb, and performed an anastomosis between the porta hepatis and the end of the Roux-en Y limb. This was the first case of an intentionally performed hepatic portoenterostomy, known as Kasai portoenterostomy [10].

In 1959, Kasai et al. published their experience with10 cases, including the one mentioned above, in "Shujutsu," a Japanese journal [11]. Of the 10 cases, bile flow was established in 6, and 2 survived.

Kasai portoenterostomy was published in Therapiewoche in German [12] and in the *Journal of Pediatric Surgery* (JPS) in English [13] in 1963 and in 1968, respectively.

In the JPS report in 1968, 89 cases were included and 69 of them underwent Kasai portoenterostomy. Among them, only 9 patients survived. Although the surgical outcome was not good, 3 patients had survived for 10 years or more until then, and these results were groundbreaking and unbelievable for pediatric surgeons around the world. The report was initially received with skepticism, considering the situation in the United States and Europe, where the non-correctable type of biliary atresia was believed to be a fatal disease at that time.

Another surgical modality that had a significant impact on the progress of treatment of biliary atresia was liver transplantation. T.E. Starzl [14] reported the first case of liver transplantation in 1963, the same year when Kasai portoenterostomy was reported in Germany. The recipient was a 3-year-old boy with biliary atresia, and the donor was a 3-year-old patient with brain tumor who had died following a brain surgery. The recipient died shortly after vascular reconstruction. Liver transplantation became a viable surgical treatment option after some time (described later).

Kasai portoenterostomy and liver transplantation, which are currently regarded as collaborative surgical modalities like the two wheels of a cart in the treatment of biliary atresia, started around the same time; however, the treatment of biliary atresia was mainly Kasai portoenterostomy until sometime later.

## 1.3 Kasai Portoenterostomy Spreading Around the World

In the 1970s, Kasai et al. [15, 16] repeatedly advocated the role of Kasai portoenterostomy and the significance of early surgery. In Japan, the usefulness of Kasai portoenterostomy was recognized early, and the surgical outcomes gradually improved. The 1st International Sendai Symposium on Biliary Atresia (ISSBA) was held in 1972, chaired by Kasai, and many pediatric surgeons from around the world visited Sendai (Fig. 1.1). They played a major role in spreading the understanding of Kasai portoenterostomy around the world. In 1975, Kasai called for a nationwide meeting to determine the classification of biliary atresia, which was the beginning of the Japanese Biliary Atresia Society (JBAS). The society meeting has been held annually since then and many researchers share their research results and discuss biliary atresia for an entire day, even until now.

In the 1970s, Kasai portoenterostomy gradually gained attention in the United States and Europe, and this trend was influenced by the study results of passionate pediatric surgeons, such as J. R. Lilly [17], R. P. Altman [18], D. M. Hays [19], C. E. Koop [20], and J. Valayer [21].

In the late 1970s, when there were long-term survivors in the Western countries following Kasai portoenterostomy [18], it was globally established as the practical treatment modality for biliary atresia.

## 1.4 Modifications of Kasai Portoenterostomy and Postoperative Management

While bile excretion following Kasai portoenterostomy was achieved in an increasing number of cases in many institutions, cholangitis was noticed as a significant complication. The prevention of cholangitis became a major challenge for pediatric surgeons. To prevent cholangitis, a variety of modifications was developed between the late 1960s and early 1990s. Surgical techniques to prevent cholangitis included Sawaguchi's temporary external biliary fistula method [22], Mikulicz type Roux-en Y jejunostomy method [23], Kasai's double Roux-en Y method [24], jejunal interposition hepatic portoduodenostomy with intestinal valve [25], SurugaII method [26], etc.

Besides modifications in the biliary reconstructive procedures, various postoperative management methods were also developed. Therapeutic and prophylactic usage of antibiotics,

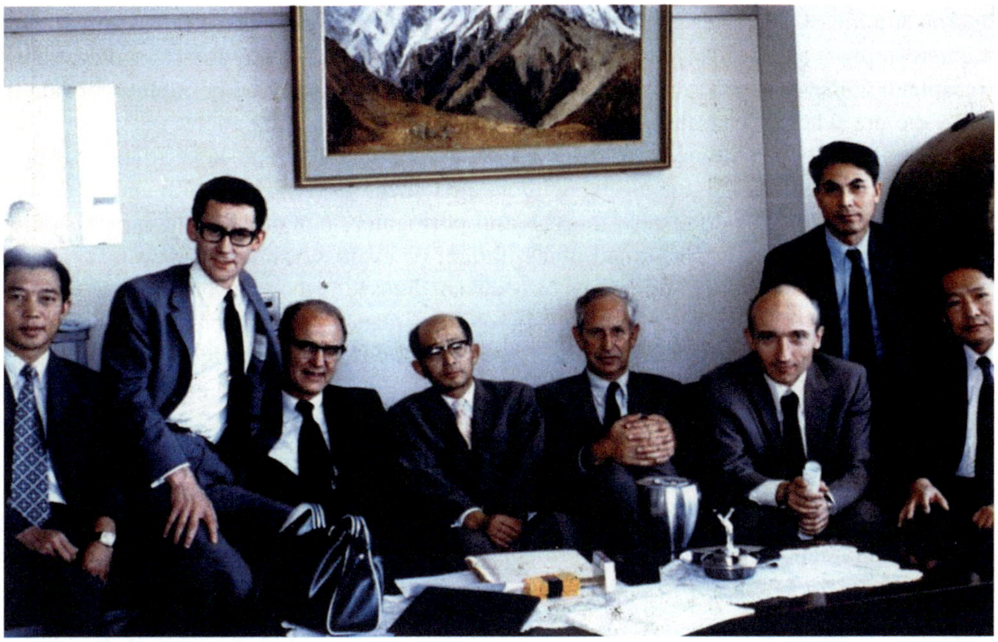

**Fig. 1.1** First International Sendai Symposium on Biliary Atresia (ISSBA). Pediatric surgeons from around the world met in Sendai and discussed biliary atresia in 1972. ISSBA played a significant role in spreading understanding of Kasai portoenterostomy across the world. From the left, Dr. Chen, Dr. Otte, Dr. Hays, Dr. Kasai, Dr. Bill, Dr. Valayer, Dr. Kimura, and Dr. Hung. (In Dr. Kasai's office in Sendai, June 19, 1972)

steroids aimed at preventing the formation of postoperative granulation and facilitating bile excretion, choleretic agents (ursodeoxycholic acid, dehydrocholic acid, prostaglandin E2, glucagon, etc.), intravenous administration of fat emulsion, and oral administration of medium chain fatty acids, fat-soluble vitamins, minerals, and branched chain amino acids were attempted or established during this period.

In 1989, JBAS launched the Japanese Biliary Atresia Registry (JBAR) under the leadership of Ohi of Tohoku University, aiming to elucidate the etiology of biliary atresia and improve the treatment results, and this is still ongoing [27].

## 1.5 Liver Transplantation and Its Impact on Kasai Portoenterostomy

While the outcome of Kasai portoenterostomy has greatly improved, a considerable number of patients could not be saved only by Kasai portoenterostomy. The last hope of survival for these patients was liver transplantation.

In the early 1980s, the outcome of liver transplantation showed dramatic improvement with the introduction of a new regimen of immunosuppression [28], and subsequently, deceased-donor liver transplantation increased rapidly in the United States, Europe, and other countries in the world. However, this trend did not pick up in Japan, because the concept of brain death was difficult to accept socially. The practical means of survival for patients requiring liver transplantation was to travel to other countries to undergo the transplantation.

Living-donor liver transplantation was performed in Brazil in 1988 [29] and in Australia in 1989 [30]. In 1989, the first living-donor liver transplantation was performed at Shimane Medical University (now Shimane University) in Japan as well [31]. The recipient was a 1-year-old boy with biliary atresia and the donor was his father. Although the recipient died 9 months after the surgery, these techniques quickly spread all over Japan.

In Japan, while the system of deceased-donor transplantation could not be established, liver transplantation from living donors progressed remarkably. The outcomes have also improved significantly [32, 33]. In 1997, the law was amended to promote deceased-donor transplantation, and organ donation from brain-dead donors has been gradually increasing. However, living-donor liver transplantation continues to play a central role in Japan [34].

Liver transplantation greatly improved the treatment outcomes of biliary atresia. At the same time, it had a great impact on Kasai portoenterostomy as well. Suruga II method, the procedure involving total diversion of bile excretion through an external fistula, was the common anti-cholangitis procedure between the 1980s and early 1990s in Japan. However, the Suruga II method was abandoned in the mid-1990s due to a report that the presence of external fistula adversely affected the outcomes of liver transplantation [35]. With this trend, various complex biliary reconstruction procedures were also abandoned. Currently, the original Kasai portoenterostomy method with long (40–60 cm) Roux-en Y limb is employed in 90% of the patients. The remaining 10% of the patients in Japan undergo Kasai portoenterostomy with an intestinal valve.

The attitude of pediatric surgeons toward redo-Kasai portoenterostomy also changed in the era of liver transplantation.

In the era when liver transplantation was not available, redo-Kasai portoenterostomy was a common procedure, because the patients could not survive without clearance of the jaundice by Kasai portoenterostomy. Kasai portoenterostomy was occasionally performed twice, thrice, or even more. Cases of redo-Kasai portoenterostomy also decreased in number due to the report that multiple laparotomies made liver transplantation more difficult, and repeated Kasai portoenterostomy was associated with higher morbidity [36]. The indications for redo-surgery have become limited since then. Currently, our consensus is that patients who develop sudden cessation of bile flow after achieving adequate bile drainage following the initial Kasai portoenterostomy are the best candidates for redo-Kasai portoenterostomy, and that redo-surgery is employed only once for this selective subset [37].

## 1.6 Significance of Early Diagnosis and Screening for Diagnosis

Even today, when liver transplantation is widely established, there is universal consensus that Kasai portoenterostomy is the first-line surgical treatment modality for biliary atresia. Thus, every effort for further improvement of Kasai portoenterostomy must be continued. However, as far as JBAR results are concerned, the improving tendency in jaundice clearance and native-liver survival following Kasai portoenterostomy is not as clear as before. While the improvement in the outcome of Kasai portoenterostomy might have reached optimal levels, we believe there is still room for improvement. Early diagnosis might be important for this. The age at surgery is believed to be an important prognostic factor, and early surgery is generally recommended [15, 16]. However, some studies did not show any advantage with early surgery [38]. The significance of early surgery is still a subject of debate [39]. However, according to JBAR data, the group of patients who underwent Kasai portoenterostomy during the neonatal period (<30 days of age) were associated with the best jaundice clearance and long-term native-liver survival rates. The results became significantly poorer in the group of patients who underwent Kasai portoenterostomy at 3 months of age or later [27]. Although the advantage of surgery during the neonatal period is clear, the number of cases that actually underwent surgery during this period is only 5 percent. Neonatal surgery must be encouraged as much as possible. However, some patients do not achieve jaundice clearance, even following neonatal surgery. Thus, better surgery timing needs to be further considered for such patients. Further investigations, including pathological assessment, may provide clues for better timing of the surgery in this particular subset of patients. Based on such experiences, it may be possible to decide the optimal timing of surgery for each patient.

The keys to increasing neonatal surgeries are prenatal diagnosis [40] and mass screening [41]. Currently, the target of prenatal diagnosis is only the cystic type of biliary atresia. Although the cystic type is less common and known to have more favorable outcomes than the ordinary type III biliary atresia, prenatal diagnosis for this special subset must be emphasized.

In the early 2000s, a nationwide mass screening system using stool color cards in Taiwan was quite successful [42]. The stool color card was originally developed by Matsui in the mid-1990s and utilized in few regions in Japan [41]. Since 2012, this card has been included nationwide in Japan in the Maternal and Child Health Handbook, and earlier diagnosis is expected.

Screening with the stool color card is a low-cost system, and everyone including the family members and medical staff can easily use the card. On the other hand, the evaluation is subjective, in which they determine the abnormality of the stool color referring to the color card with the naked eye; thus, over and under estimations are likely to happen. This maybe a limitation of the system. Screening systems were recently reported using objective criteria such as measurement of serum direct bilirubin [43] and urinary sulfated bile acid [44]. The establishment of an optimal screening system is anticipated, and the combination of the color card and other objective screening methods may be an option.

## 1.7 Recent Trends in Biliary Atresia in Japan

Since 2013, biliary atresia has become the target disease of the Research Project of the Ministry of Health, Labour and Welfare in Japan (research representative, Nio). Long-term survivors following Kasai portoenterostomy are increasing in number and many of them had various degrees of complications, including cholangitis, portal hypertension, and hepatic dysfunction. The transition from pediatric to adult medicine is becoming a major challenge for long-term survivors of biliary atresia, both for native-liver survivors and recipients of liver transplantation. Collaboration between pediatric surgeons, adult medical practitioners, and multi-occupational professions is important. Establishing an optimal transition system is a major objective of the research project, and various products supporting physicians and medical staff for both pediatric and adult medicine are required. Through this research project, the clinical practice guidelines were created [45]. While the medical expense for pediatric patients with biliary atresia has been covered by the government in Japan, that for adult patients was not. In 2016, biliary atresia was nominated as a nationally designated intractable disease, because of the progress of the national research project. Following this, the medical expenses for both pediatric and adult patients are now covered by the government, although it is based on a framework of severity.

## 1.8 Research Directions and Future Aspects

Improving the treatment outcome of biliary atresia currently means improving the outcomes of both Kasai portoenterostomy and liver transplantation. To achieve better clinical outcomes, it is important to refine the surgical techniques and perioperative management and overcome the problems of short and long-term complications. More importantly, a better way of combining these two modalities should be carefully considered.

In the JBAR 2019, the total number of patients who have undergone Kasai portoenterostomy is approaching 3,500, and the number of patients who have undergone liver transplant exceeds 1,400. Various data have been collected, and a big database of biliary atresia is now available. The number of adult registrations is also increasing, and the data of long-term survivors is gradually becoming clearer. However, the number of patients lost to follow-up is also increasing, as the follow-up period becomes longer. It is important to maintain the registration rate, capture the current state of survivors, and link the data of survivors to future treatment strategies.

As an innovative treatment modality, regenerative medicine utilizing iPS cells and others is being applied in many clinical areas. If the study of liver regeneration [46] proceeds, new treatment options for biliary atresia might become available.

The most important objective in the future of biliary atresia is the elucidation of the etiology. Only when the etiology is elucidated and prevention becomes possible, this intractable disease can be truly overcome.

The hypothesis that both external, environmental, or genetic factors and the host immune response may influence the disease process of biliary atresia has been put forth [47], and the details are yet to be substantiated.

Besides JBAR, research groups or consortiums have been organized in Europe [48], the United States/Canada/the United Kingdom [49], Netherlands [50], Switzerland [51], and other countries, and various other research projects may be ongoing. However, biliary atresia is basically a rare disease, and the rarity makes the research difficult. There are various phenotypes of this disease, and there are differences in the incidence of the disease and in the frequency of association of splenic malformations between geographical areas. Furthermore, it is assumed that different etiologies and disease processes exist. Thus, it is essential to work together under international and intercontinental collaborations to understand the entire spectrum of biliary atresia. With worldwide collaboration, early elucidation of the etiology of biliary atresia is expected with rapid accumulation of information, due to the recent developments in innovative research technologies.

## References


1. Burns J. Principals of midwifery, including the diseases of women and children. London: Longman; 1817.
2. Thomson J. On congenital obliteration of the bile ducts. Edinb Med J. 1891;37:523–31.
3. Holmes JB. Congenital obliteration of the bile ducts. Diagnosis and suggestions for treatment. Am J D Child. 1916;11:405.
4. Ladd WE. Congenital atresia and stenosis of the bile ducts. JAMA. 1928;91:1082–5.
5. Longmire WP Jr, Sanford MC. Intrahepatic-cholangiojejunostomy with partial hepatectomy for biliary obstruction. Surgery. 1948;24:264.
6. Sterling JA. Artificial bile ducts in the management of congenital biliary atresia, a clinical report. J Int Coll Surg. 1961;36:293.
7. Carson E. Salvage of the "noncorrectable" case of congenital extrahepatic biliary atresia. AMA Arch Surg. 1960;81:893.
8. Williams LF, Dooling JA. Thoracic duct-esophagus anastomosis for relief of congenital biliary atresia. Surg Forum. 1963;14:189.
9. Thaler MM, Gellis SS. Studies in neonatal hepatitis and biliary atresia. II. The effect of diagnostic laparotomy on long-term prognosis of neonatal hepatitis. Am J Dis Child. 1968;116:262.
10. Kasai M, Ohi R, Chiba T, et al. A patient with biliary atresia who died 28 years after hepatic portojejunostomy. J Pediatr Surg. 1988;23:430–1.
11. Kasai M, Suzuki M. A new operation for "non-correctable" biliary atresia: hepatic portoenterostomy. Shujutsu. 1959;13:733–9.
12. Kasai M. Die chirurgischen Behandlungen der angeborenen Missbildungen des Gallengangs. Die Therapiewoche. 1963;16:710–5.
13. Kasai M, Kimura S, Asakura Y, et al. Surgical treatment of biliary atresia. J Pediatr Surg. 1968;3:665–75.
14. Starzl TM, Marchioro TL, Von Kaulia KN, et al. Homotransplantation of the liver in humans. Surg Gynecol Obstet. 1963;117:659–76.
15. Kasai M, Watanabe I, Ohi R. Follow-up studies of long-term survivors after hepatic portoenterostomy for "noncorrectable" biliary atresia. J Pediatr Surg. 1975;10:173–82.
16. Kasai M. Hepatic portoenterostomy and its modifications. In: Japan Medical Research Foundation, editor. Cholestasis in infancy. Tokyo: University Tokyo Press; 1980. p. 337–44.
17. Lilly JR. Surgical jaundice in infancy. Ann Surg. 1977;186:549–58.
18. Altman RP. The portoenterostomy procedure for biliary atresia: a five-year experience. Ann Surg. 1978;188:351–62.
19. Hays DM. Differences in attitude toward the management of biliary atresia among surgeons in Japan and in North America. J Pediatr Surg. 1979;14:580–7.
20. Koop CE. Biliary atresia and the Kasai operation. Pediatrics. 1975;55:9–11.
21. Odiévre M, Valayer J, Razemon-Pinta M, et al. Hepatic portoenterostomy or cholecystostomy in the treatment of extrahepatic biliary atresia. A study of 49 cases. J Pediatr. 1976;88:774–9.
22. Sawaguchi S, Nakajo T, Hori T, et al. Surgical treatment of congenital biliary atresia by making a temporary external biliary fistula. J Jap Surg Soc. 1968;69:1317–20.

23. Lilly JR, Altman RP. Hepatic portoenterostomy (the Kasai operation) for biliary atresia. Surgery. 1975;78:76–86.
24. Ohi R, Chiba T, Hanamatsu M, et al. Modification of Hepatic portojejunostomy for prevention of postoperative cholangitis in biliary atresia– Evaluation of Double Roux—Y Procedure in 68 Patients. J Jpn Soc Pediatr Surg. 1985;22:22–229.
25. Tanaka K, Satomura K, Ohnishi S, et al. A new operation for treatment of biliary atresia -jejunal interposition hepatic portoduodenostomy with intestinal valve. J Jpn Soc Pediatr Surg. 1980;16(2):227–35.
26. Suruga K. Our operative procedures and operative results of biliary atresia. Jpn J Pediatr Surg. 1978;10:659–63.
27. Nio M. Japanese Biliary Atresia Registry. Pediatr Surg Int. 2017;33:1319–25.
28. Starzl TE, Klintmalm GB, Porter KA, et al. Liver transplantation with use of cyclosporin a and prednisone. N Engl J Med. 1981;305:266–9.
29. Raia S, Nery JR, Mies S. Liver transplantation from live donors. Lancet. 1989;2:497.
30. Strong RW, Lynch SV, Ong TH, et al. Successful liver transplantation from a living donor to her son. N Engl J Med. 1990;322:1505–7.
31. Nagasue N, Kohno H, Matsuo S, et al. Segmental (partial) liver transplantation from a living donor. Transplant Proc. 1992;24:1958–9.
32. Tanaka K, Yamada T. Living donor liver transplantation in Japan and Kyoto University: what can we learn? J Hepatol. 2005;42:25–8.
33. Kasahara M, Umeshita K, Sakamoto S, et al. Liver transplantation for biliary atresia: a systematic review. Pediatr Surg Int. 2017;33:1289–95.
34. Umeshita K, Eguchi S, Egawa H, et al. Liver transplantation in Japan: Registry by the Japanese Liver Transplantation Society. Hepatol Res. 2019;49:964–80.
35. Whitington PF. Advances in pediatric liver transplantation. Adv Pediatr Infect Dis. 1990;37:357–89.
36. Millis JM, Brems JJ, Hiatt JR, et al. Orthotopic liver transplantation for biliary atresia. Evolution of management. Arch Surg. 1988;123:1237–9.
37. Nio M, Sasaki H, Tanaka H, et al. Redo- surgery for biliary atresia. Pediatr Surg Int. 2013;29:989–93.
38. Volpert D, White F, Finegold M, Nio M, Sasaki H, Tanaka H. Outcome of early hepatic portoenterostomy for biliary atresia. J Pediatr Gastroenterol Nutr. 2001;32:265–9.
39. Nio M, Wada M, Sasaki H, Nio M, Sasaki H, Tanaka H. Effects of age at Kasai portoenterostomy on the surgical outcome: a review of the literature. Surg Today. 2015;4:813–8.
40. Tanaka H, Sasaki H, Wada M, et al. Postnatal management of prenatally diagnosed biliary cystic malformation. J Pediatr Surg. 2015;50:507–10.
41. Matsui A. Screening for biliary atresia. Pediatr Surg Int. 2017;33:1305–13.
42. Tseng JJ, Lai MS, Lin MC, et al. Stool color card screening for biliary atresia. Pediatrics. 2011;128(5):e1209–15.
43. Harpavat S, Garcia-Prats JA, Anaya C, et al. Diagnostic yield of newborn screening for biliary atresia using direct or conjugated bilirubin measurements. JAMA. 2020;323:1141–50.
44. Suzuki M, Muraji T, Obatake M, et al. Urinary sulfated bile acid analysis for the early detection of biliary atresia in infants. Pediatr Int. 2011;53:497–500.
45. Ando H, Inomata Y, Iwanaka T, et.al. Clinical practice guidelines for biliary atresia in Japan: A secondary publication of the abbreviated version translated into English. J Hepatobiliary Pancreat Sci. 2021;28:55–61.
46. Sekine K, Takebe T, Taniguchi H. Liver regeneration using cultured liver bud. Methods Mol Biol. 2017;1597:207–16.
47. Asai A, Miethke A, Bezerra JA. Pathogenesis of biliary atresia: defining biology to understand clinical phenotypes. Nat Rev Gastroenterol Hepatol. 2015;12:342–52.
48. Petersen C. Biliary atresia: unity in diversity. Pediatr Surg Int. 2017;33:1255–61.
49. Alonso EM, Ye W, Hawthorne K, et al. Impact of steroid therapy on early growth in infants with biliary atresia: the multicenter steroids in biliary atresia randomized trial. J Pediatr. 2018;202:179–85.
50. Witt M, van Wessel DBE, de Kleine RHJ, et al. Prognosis of biliary atresia after 2-year survival with native liver: a nationwide cohort analysis. J Pediatr Gastroenterol Nutr. 2018;67:689–94.
51. Calinescu AM, Wilde JCH, Korff S, et al. Perioperative complications after Kasai hepato portoenterostomy: data from the Swiss National Biliary Atresia Registry. Eur J Pediatr Surg. 2020;30:364–70.

# History and Current Status of The Japanese Biliary Atresia Society

2

Ryoji Ohi

**Abstract**

The Japanese Biliary Atresia Society (JBAS) was organized in Sendai, Japan, in 1975 at the behest of Dr. Morio Kasai. JBAS has played a significant role in achieving scientific and clinical progress in the treatment of biliary atresia. In this chapter, the history, achievements, award systems, and social contributions of JBAS are presented. JBAS's roles in the Japanese Nationwide Study Group and the International Sendai Symposium on Biliary Atresia (ISSBA) are also addressed.

**Keywords**

Biliary atresia · Japanese Biliary Atresia Society · Japanese Biliary Atresia Registry · History

## Abbreviations

| | |
|---|---|
| ISSBA | The International Sendai Symposium on Biliary Atresia |
| JBAR | The Japanese Biliary Atresia Registry |
| JBAS | The Japanese Biliary Atresia Society |
| MINDS | The Medical Information Network Distribution Service |
| UNICEF | United Nations Children's Fund |

R. Ohi (✉)
Department of Pediatric Surgery, Tohoku University Graduate School of Medicine, Sendai, Japan
e-mail: ryoji_oi@micjapan.or.jp

## 2.1 Purpose of The Japanese Biliary Atresia Society (JBAS)

JBAS has played a significant role for 45 years since 1975, offering a forum to present research outcomes on scientific issues related to every aspect of biliary atresia. The purpose of JBAS is to promote research on epidemiology and etiology and to improve the treatment outcomes of biliary atresia. Participants of JBAS mainly comprise pediatric surgeons, pediatricians, and researchers in basic medicine, including pathology and molecular biology.

## 2.2 History of JBAS

In 1975, representatives of nine facilities across Japan who had experienced a large number of cases of biliary atresia convened at Sendai at the behest of Dr. Morio Kasai, professor of the Second Department of Surgery, Tohoku University. They deliberated on the classification proposal put forth by Dr. Kasai and Ohi. The idea for the classification was that it was important to evaluate the treatment outcomes of biliary atresia more objectively by unifying the classification, although various classifications of biliary atresia were followed in facilities throughout Japan in those days. The classification review meeting was held twice in Sendai. The drafts were completed, summarized, and published as A Proposal of New Classification of Biliary Atresia [1]. These two review meetings were regarded as the first and second meetings of JBAS, and JBAS has since conducted annual scientific meetings where 40 to 50 basic or clinical research papers, including special works of prevalent themes requested by each chairperson, have been presented every year. A total of 47 meetings have been held until 2020 all over Japan (Table 2.1). JBAS is a unique society where a single disease is discussed. JBAS comprises institutional members who agree with the purpose of the society and is managed by board members nominated to the board of direc-


M. Nio (ed.), *Introduction to Biliary Atresia*, https://doi.org/10.1007/978-981-16-2160-4_2

**Table 2.1** JBAS annual meetings and secretariat

| No. | Year | Chairperson | Institution |
|---|---|---|---|
| 1 | 1975 | Morio Kasai | Tohoku University |
| 2 | 1975 | Morio Kasai | Tohoku University |
| 3 | 1976 | Eizo Okamoto | Hyogo College of Medicine |
| 4 | 1977 | Shigenori Sawaguchi | Tsukuba University |
| 5 | 1978 | Jiro Yura | Nagoya City University |
| 6 | 1979 | Sumio Saito | The University of Tokyo |
| 7 | 1980 | Shigeru Kimura | Ehime University |
| 8 | 1981 | Keijiro Suruga | Juntendo University |
| 9 | 1982 | Yoichi Kasai | Hokkaido University |
| 10 | 1983 | Makoto Iwafuchi | Niigata University |
| 11 | 1984 | Masayuki Sho | Ryukyu University |
| 12 | 1985 | Akio Tsunoda | Kanagawa Children's Medical Center |
| 13 | 1986 | Hiroshi Akiyama | Kagoshima University |
| 14 | 1987 | Takahiro Ito | Nagoya University |
| 15 | 1988 | Ryoji Ohi | Tohoku University |
| 16 | 1989 | Toshio Nakajo | The University of Tokyo |
| 17 | 1990 | Hiroshi Suzuki | Mie University |
| 18 | 1991 | Hideyo Takahashi | Chiba University |
| 19 | 1992 | Morihiro Saeki | National Children's Hospital |
| 20 | 1993 | Kazuo Shiraki | Tottori University |
| 21 | 1994 | Sachiyo Suita | Kyushu University |
| 22 | 1995 | Takeshi Miyano | Juntendo University |
| 23 | 1996 | Akira Okada | Osaka University |
| 24 | 1997 | Yoshihisa Sera | Kumamoto University |
| 25 | 1998 | Koichi Tanaka | Kyoto University |
| 26 | 1999 | Yoshiaki Tsuchida | Gunma Children's Medical Center |
| 27 | 2000 | Toshiji Nishi | Kanagawa Children's Medical Center |
| 28 | 2001 | Naomi Iwai | Kyoto Prefectural University of Medicine |
| 29 | 2002 | Yuichiro Yamashiro | Juntendo University |
| 30 | 2003 | Tetsuo Kato | Akita University |
| 31 | 2004 | Hideo Takamatsu | Kagoshima University |
| 32 | 2005 | Naomi Onuma | Chiba University |
| 33 | 2006 | Hiromichi Ikawa | Kanazawa Medical University |
| 34 | 2007 | Takashi Hashimoto | Fujita Health University |
| 35 | 2008 | Matsui Akira | Tsukuba University |
| 36 | 2009 | Yokatsu Ohama | Kanagawa Children's Medical Center |
| 37 | 2010 | Yasuhide Morikawa | Keio University |
| 38 | 2011 | Hisami Ando | Nagoya University |
| 39 | 2012 | Masahiro Fukuzawa | Osaka University |
| 40 | 2013 | Toshihiro Muraji | Ibaraki Children's Hospital |
| 41 | 2014 | Yukihiro Inomata | Kumamoto University |
| 42 | 2015 | Tadashi Iwanaka | Saitama Children's Medical Center |
| 43 | 2016 | Masayuki Kubota | Niigata University |
| 44 | 2017 | Tomoaki Taguchi | Kyushu University |
| 45 | 2018 | Minoru Yagi | Kurume University |
| 46 | 2019 | Takashi Akiyama | Chuden Hospital |
| 47 | 2020 | Masaki Nio | Tohoku University |
| Secretariat of JBAS: Department of Pediatric Surgery, Tohoku University | | | |
| Secretary General | | | |
| 1987–2003 | | Ryoji Ohi | |
| 2004–2008 | | Yutaka Hayashi | |
| 2008– | | Masaki Nio | |

tors and entrusted by the chairperson who presides over the annual meeting.

There was initially no formal society, and researchers participated in the meetings arbitrarily. In 1987, at the 14th JBAS meeting, the constitution was established, and a board meeting was held. It was also decided that the secretariat of JBAS will be in the Department of Pediatric Surgery, Tohoku University (Table 2.1). In 1992, at the 19th JBAS meeting, an institutional membership system was established. Currently, JBAS has 34 board members and 101 institutional members covering the entire country.

## 2.3 Achievements of JBAS

While JBAS achieved a lot more besides conducting the annual scientific meeting according to the purpose of the society, the details are presented in other chapters of this book; this chapter only enumerates the achievements. Among them, the classification of biliary atresia described above is widely used in Japan and in many other countries even today. Furthermore, the Japanese Biliary Atresia Registry (JBAR) [2–4], which was launched in 1989 and has continued for more than 30 years, is a notable achievement of JBAS. A multicenter randomized trial of postoperative corticosteroid therapy for biliary atresia was conducted using the framework of JBAS [5]. Moreover, with the aim to standardize the treatment of biliary atresia, the clinical practice guidelines on biliary atresia were recently published [6]. This was a significant effort by the members of JBAS. These guidelines were created according to the Medical Information Network Distribution Service (MINDS) Handbook for Clinical Practice Guideline Development 2014, and answers to 25 clinical questions essential for daily clinical practice were provided following a comprehensive systematic review process. It is hoped that the guidelines will lead to a dramatic improvement in the treatment outcomes.

## 2.4 Award System of JBAS

The award system by the Ryotaro-chan Fund based on donations from the bereaved family of a biliary atresia patient was established in JBAS in 2012. The best original paper and case report presented each year, and the best presentations of basic and clinical works as well as the best case presentation at each annual meeting are awarded during the JBAS meeting (Table 2.2), thus encouraging researchers in the field of biliary atresia.

## 2.5 Nationwide Study Group and JBAS

In addition, JBAS participated in the Scientific Research Group of the Ministry of Health, Labor, and Welfare of Japan for a nationwide research project on hepatobiliary and pancreatic diseases in children. As an outcome of this project, a mother and child handbook with a stool color card was published, which is useful for the early diagnosis of biliary atresia. A guide to the medical treatment of biliary atresia for specialized and non-specialized physicians was also created. Finally, biliary atresia was certified as an incurable disease, for which medical costs are supported by the Japanese government.

**Table 2.2** Recipients of JBAS Ryotaro-chan fund award

| Year | Recipients |
|---|---|
| 2012 | Paper: Yukihiro Sanada (Original) |
| | Presentation: Yusuke Yanagi (Basic), Hiroko Suda (Clinical) |
| 2013 | Paper: Atsushi Okamura (Original) |
| | Presentation: Yukihiro Sanada (Basic), Naoya Yamada (Clinical) |
| 2014 | Paper: Hirofumi Tomita (Original) |
| | Presentation: Mari Sonoda(Clinical), Hiromu Tanaka (Clinical) |
| 2015 | Paper: Sorahiko Fujisawa (Original) |
| | Presentation: Tatsuki Mizuochi (Basic), Daiki Yoshii (Clinical) |
| 2016 | Paper: Naoya Yamada (Original) |
| | Presentation: Yukihiro Sanada (Clinical) |
| 2017 | Paper: Masaki Nio (Original), Masahiro Zenitani (Case Report) |
| | Presentation: Hideyuki Sasaki (Basic), Yoshiaki Takahashi (Clinical), Shinya Yamoto (Case Presentation) |
| 2018 | Paper: Hirofumi Tomita (Original), Rei Matsuura (Case Report) |
| | Presentation: Daiki Yoshii (Basic), Yudai Nakajima (Clinical), Kenichiro Konishi (Case Presentation) |
| 2019 | Paper: Takeshi Saito (Original), Kosuke Endo (Case Report) |
| | Presentation: Masayuki Obatake (Basic), Hiromu Tanaka (Clinical), Kazuki Shirane (Case Presentation) |

## 2.6 JBAS and The International Sendai Symposium on Biliary Atresia (ISSBA)

ISSBA is also an indirect academic achievement of JBAS. In 1972, Dr. Kasai called on the world experts to play an important role for deeper international understanding of Kasai portoenterostomy. At ISSBA, they shared the current state of diagnosis and treatment of biliary atresia around the world. The ISSBA has since been taken over by Ohi and Nio of the Department of Pediatric Surgery, Tohoku University (Fig. 2.1). I believe that JBAS and ISSBA greatly contributed in expanding the role of Kasai portoenterostomy worldwide.

## 2.7 Social Contributions of JBAS

Social contributions of JBAS include support for the publication of the first edition of “Everything About Biliary Atresia,” published by the Society of the Children with Biliary Atresia and Their Families in 1986. All works of editing and writing of scientific chapters of this publication were contributed by members of JBAS. JBAS continued to support all revisions of this book until the current fourth edition.

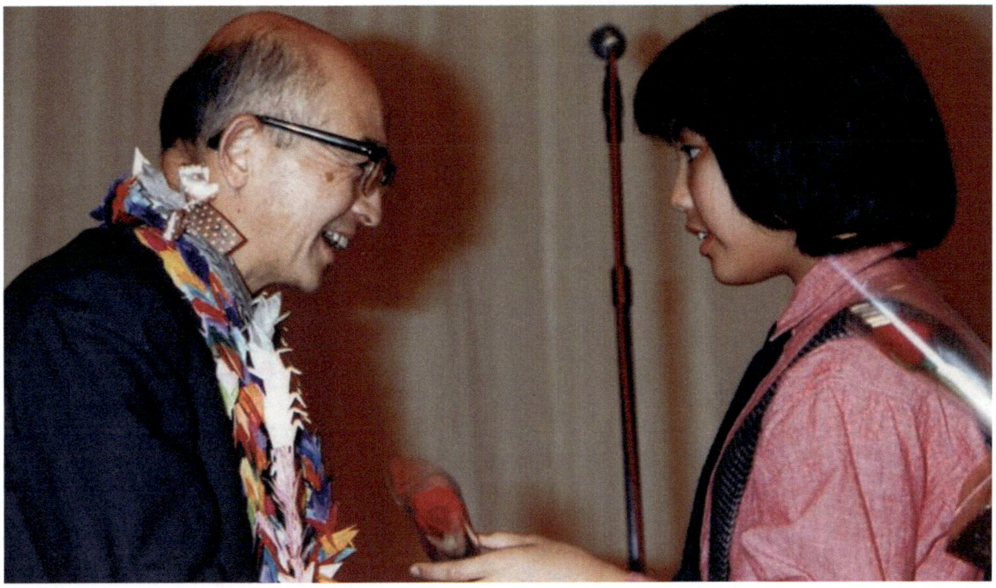

**Fig. 2.1** Dr. Morio Kasai at the fourth ISSBA. (Dr. Kasai was the honorary chairman of the fourth ISSBA in 1986. This symposium was held in honor of Dr. Kasai’s retirement from Tohoku University School of Medicine. In this picture, he was receiving flowers at the congress banquet from a patient of his with biliary atresia)

Participation in activities of "Nonprofit organization Himawari-no-kai" is another contribution of JBAS. The purpose of this organization is to support for pregnant women and babies. Board members of this organization include presidents of scientific societies for health care of mothers and babies, politicians, United Nations Children's Fund (UNICEF) officials, and celebrities in Japan. They distribute a "maternity passport," which includes medication notes of the baby, important parenting suggestions, and a stool color card to all pregnant women in Japan.

## 2.8 Future Aspects

As mentioned above, JBAS plays an important role in elucidating the etiology and disease process and improving the treatment outcomes of biliary atresia. Unfortunately, many issues remain to be solved. Continuing effort by JBAR, the establishment of an ideal mass-screening system for the early diagnosis, and further nationwide/international research collaborations are important to overcome the current challenges. It seems that the role of JBAS will be fulfilled when these challenges are resolved; hopefully, we do not have a very long way to go.

## References

1. Kasai M. A proposal of new classification of biliary atresia. J Jpn Soc Pediatr Surg. 1976;12:327–31. (in Japanese)
2. Ibrahim M, Miyano T, Ohi R, Saeki M, Shiraki K, Tanaka K, et al. Japanese biliary atresia registry, 1989 to 1994. Tohoku J Exp Med. 1997;181:85–95.
3. Nio M, Ohi R, Miyano T, Saeki M, Shiraki K. Tanaka K; Japanese biliary atresia registry. Five- and 10-year survival rates after surgery for biliary atresia: a report from the Japanese biliary atresia registry. J Pediatr Surg. 2003;38:997–1000.
4. Nio M. Japanese biliary atresia registry. Pediatr Surg Int. 2017;33:1319–25.
5. Japanese Biliary Atresia Society, Nio M, Muraji T. Multicenter randomized trial of postoperative corticosteroid therapy for biliary atresia. Pediatr Surg Int. 2013;29:1091–5.
6. Japanese Biliary Atresia Society. Clinical practice guidelines on biliary atresia. https://minds.jcqhc.or.jp/n/med/4/med0362/G0001073 (in Japanese).

# Definition and Classifications of Biliary Atresia

3

Hiroaki Kitagawa

**Abstract**

In the late 1950s, Professor Kasai from Tohoku University in Japan noted that bile flow from the porta hepatis was possible after excision of the entire fibrotic extrahepatic biliary tree. The prognosis of these patients is related to the differences in the site of obstruction and most classifications are based on these, using the macroscopic findings and a direct cholangiogram. There are many different types of classification for biliary atresia (BA) in the literature. There are five recent large-scale reports that refer to disease types, including those from Japan, the United States, the United Kingdom, the Netherlands, and France. We introduce these five large-scale reports using the Japanese Biliary Atresia Society (JBAS) classification and compare their long-term native liver outcomes.

The age at surgery is also important for BA. The overall average age at surgery in Japan was 66.5 days. The group of patients who underwent surgery less than 30 days of age (the neonatal period) showed the best jaundice clearance rate (71.9%). Finally, we introduce a severity classification because, in Japan, the cost of treatment is supported by publicly funded medical care.

**Keywords**

Biliary atresia · Classification of extrahepatic biliary atresia · Cholangiography · Prognosis · Long-term outcome

H. Kitagawa (✉)
Department of Pediatric Surgery, St. Marianna University School of Medicine, Kawasaki, Japan
e-mail: h2kita@marianna-u.ac.jp

## 3.1 Definition of Biliary Atresia

Biliary Atresia (BA) is a hepatobiliary tract disease occurring in neonates or early infancy, obstructing the extrahepatic bile ducts due to an unexplained sclerosing inflammation. This obstructs biliary excretion.

## 3.2 Classification of BA from Five Large-Scale Reports

There are two types of classification: one is based on clinical features and the other is based on the site of the occlusion.

The classification based on clinical features includes the polysplenia, asplenia, situs ambiguus, preduodenal portal vein, inferior vena cava defect, intestinal malrotation, the so-called biliary atresia splenic malformation syndrome (BASM): things that accompany biliary atresia, originally proposed by Davenport et al. [1]. Davenport later proposed four types of BA, based on their clinical features [2]. (1) Syndromic type (including BASM), (2) Cystic type [3], (3) Cytomegalovirus (CMV)-related type, and (4) Isolated BA. Balistreri et al. [4], in a report from an international symposium on BA, classified BA according to the timing of onset into two types: (1) the fetal type (Embryonic type or fetal type) and (2) the Perinatal type (acquired type). In the past, correctable (a patent proximal bile duct) and non-correctable (atresia of the hepatic radicles) were used mainly in Europe and America, but in Japan, the disease type classification was established by the Japan Biliary Atresia Study Group is widely used [5, 6]. There are five recent large-scale reports that refer to disease types, including those from Japan [7], the United States [8], the United Kingdom [9], the Netherlands [10], and France [11]. Table 3.1 shows four reports based on the Japanese disease classification. The French report has a different classification, which makes accurate comparison difficult. Table 3.2 shows the subtypes according to the patterns of the distal bile duct and Table 3.3 shows the subtypes according to the patterns of the hepatic


M. Nio (ed.), *Introduction to Biliary Atresia*, https://doi.org/10.1007/978-981-16-2160-4_3

**Table 3.1** There are five recent large-scale reports that refer to disease types, including those from Japan, the United States, the United Kingdom, the Netherlands, and France

| | | Type I | | | | |
|---|---|---|---|---|---|---|
| | Registration (*n*) | Type I | Type I Cyst | Type II | Type III | References |
| Japan | 3483 | 3.70% | 8% | 2% | 85.20% | [7] |
| United States | 244 | 10.20% | | 7.40% | 80.70% | [8] |
| United Kingdom | 424 | 2% | | 1.40% | 95.80% | [9] |
| Netherlands | 214 | 6.50% | | 12.60% | 80.40% | [10] |

This table shows four reports based on the Japanese disease classification of the Main Types. The percentages refer to the percentage of the total in each Type for each report

**Table 3.2** This table shows the subtypes according to the patterns of the distal bile ducts from Japan and the United States

| | a | | b | | c | | | |
|---|---|---|---|---|---|---|---|---|
| | a1 | a2 | b1 | b2 | c1 | c2 | d | References |
| Japan | 12.60% | 3.70% | 58.60% | 2.80% | 8.70% | 2.90% | 4.60% | [7] |
| United States | 20.10% | | 45.90% | | 24.60% | | 4.10% | [8] |

**Table 3.3** This table shows the subtypes according to the patterns of the hepatic radicles at the porta hepatis from Japan and the United States

| | α | β | γ | μ | ν | O | Unknown | References |
|---|---|---|---|---|---|---|---|---|
| Japan | 2.99% | 5.09% | 4.91% | 10.30% | 68.00% | 3.60% | 5.20% | [7] |
| United States | 0.00% | 2.90% | 2.50% | 7.40% | 78.70% | 7.00% | 0.00% | [8] |

radicles at the porta hepatis. The most common main type is Ohi Type III [5]. The most common subtype according to the patterns of distal bile ducts is b: fibrous common bile duct and the most common subtype according to the patterns at the porta hepatis is *ν*: fibrous mass.

The French classification is as follows: Type 1 (Atresia of the common bile duct), Type 2 (Cyst of the liver hilum communicating with dystrophic intra-hepatic bile ducts), Type 3 (Gallbladder, cystic duct, and common bile duct are patents), Type 4 (Atresia of all the extrahepatic bile ducts). These types make up 2.2%, 7.6%, 17.1%, and 73.0%, respectively, of the total cases [11]. The French Type 1 in this classification corresponds to the Japanese Biliary Atresia Society (JBAS) classification Type I. The French Type 2 is JBAS classification Type II, and the French Types 3 and 4 are JBAS classification Type III, patent common bile duct subtype (a), and fibrous common bile duct subtype (b), respectively.

## 3.3 Japanese Biliary Atresia Society (JBAS) Classification

In this classification, there are three basic types depending on the site of extrahepatic bile duct obstruction and do not include intrahepatic bile duct obstruction. In 1976, Kasai published a new classification of BA in the *Journal of Japanese Society of Pediatric Surgery* in Japanese with an English abstract [5]. He stated that most of the cases of BA are due to the obstruction of the extrahepatic bile ducts. Cholestasis and liver damage are secondary effects of extrahepatic bile duct obstruction. There are some cases that might have intrahepatic obstruction but since the JBAS did not have sufficient data to accurately identify this type of obstruction, they focused only on the extrahepatic bile duct obstruction at that time. In addition to the basic types, the detailed forms are classified according to the histological findings on examination of the lower bile duct and the hilar bile ducts [5, 6] (Fig. 3.1). Kasai mentioned that the above three factors (the state of the common bile duct, the state of the common hepatic duct, and the state of the ducts at the porta hepatis) can be combined into more than 80 types, but some of them include unlikely combinations. There are over 50 combinations that can be realized even if the unlikely combinations are excluded, but they can be easily expressed by combining the three factors, and, conversely, it is possible to easily imagine the morphology of the extrahepatic bile ducts from that simple expression. He states that this is an advantage of this classification.

### 3.3.1 The Main Types

The main types are defined according to the macroscopic findings of the extrahepatic bile ducts (EHBD).

**Type I**: Atresia of the common bile duct with no communication into the duodenum demonstrated on cholangiography. Cases in which the extrahepatic bile ducts are replaced by fibrous tissue at porta hepatis, are also diagnosed as type I, when direct cholangiography through the gallbladder reveals hepatic ducts and intrahepatic bile ducts. Cholangiography is absolutely necessary to make a correct diagnosis.

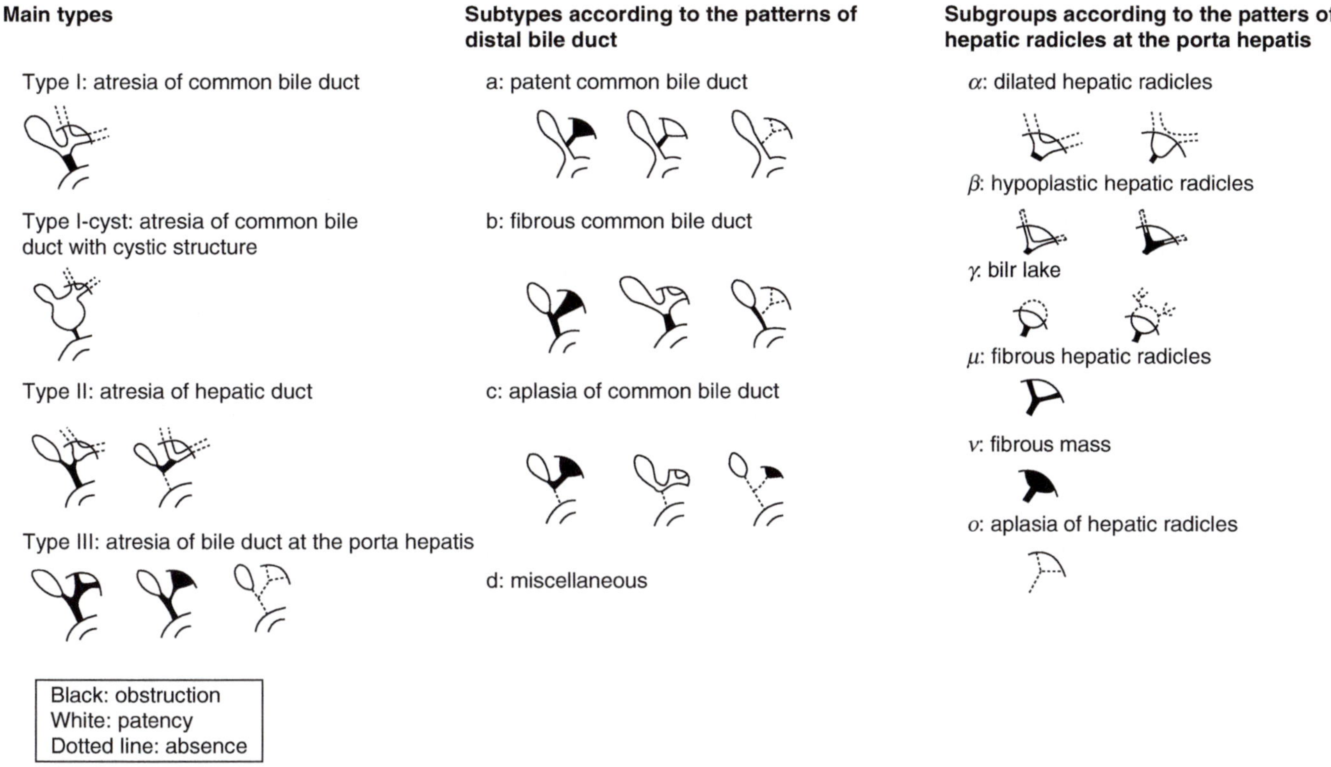


**Fig 3.1** The classification of the type of obstruction which was established by Kasai et al. is illustrated. The morphology of this disease can be classified by the macroscopic findings and direct cholangiogram in terms of three categories. The main types are classified according to the site of obstruction, the subtypes according to the patterns of distal bile ducts, and the subgroups according to the patterns of the hepatic radicles at the porta hepatis

Type I-cyst: Atresia of the common bile duct with a cystic structure that has macroscopic or microscopic communication with the intrahepatic bile ducts.

If there is normal stool color after birth till 2–3 months old, with cyst formation in the common bile duct, BA is excluded. Such cases are more likely to be diagnosed as choledochal cysts.

Cases of Type I / Type I cyst should still be classified into the relevant subtypes according to the pattern of distal bile ducts (either b or c) and into the relevant subgroups according to the patterns of hepatic radicles at the porta hepatis (either α or β).

**Type II:** Atresia of the common hepatic duct.

**Type III:** Atresia of the bile ducts at the porta hepatis.

### 3.3.2 The Subtypes

The subtypes are classified according to the patterns of the distal bile ducts, mainly according to the macroscopic findings of the common bile duct, and are subcategorized according to the existence of a common hepatic duct.

a: Patent common bile duct
- a1: Patent common bile duct and atretic hepatic duct
- a2: Patent common bile duct and aplastic hepatic duct

b: Fibrous common bile duct
- b1: Fibrous common bile duct and patent or atretic hepatic duct
- b2: Fibrous common bile duct and aplastic hepatic duct

c: Aplastic common bile duct
- c1: Aplastic common bile duct and patent or atretic hepatic duct
- c2: Aplastic common bile duct and hepatic duct

d: Miscellaneous (form that does not correspond to subtype a, b, or c)

Most cases of subtype d are associated with a solitary cyst, which does not communicate with the intrahepatic bile ducts, located in the extrahepatic biliary remnant.

### 3.3.3 The Subgroups

These are classified according to the patterns of hepatic radicles at the porta hepatis.

A case with hepatic radicles having a lumen at the porta hepatis is categorized into **α, β, or γ**. Alternatively, a case with hepatic radicles without a lumen at the porta hepatis is categorized into μ, **ν, or o**. Each subgroup is defined as follows:

**α:** Dilated hepatic radicles (internal diameter ≥1 mm) with communication to the intrahepatic biliary tree.
**β:** Hypoplastic hepatic radicles (internal diameter <l mm) with communication to the intrahepatic biliary tree.
**γ:** Bile lake (extravasated pool of bile at the porta hepatis that is mainly associated with Type III cases, including contrast media shift into the liver with minute mustache-like appearances as seen on direct cholangiography [equivalent to Type II]).
**μ:** Fibrous hepatic radicles (a strand-like bile duct without a lumen that divides into right and left sides).
**ν:** Fibrous mass (hard connective tissue mass that does not diverge and leads to the Glisson's capsule at the hepatic portal region).
**o:** Aplasia of the hepatic radicles.

## 3.4 Data Collection and Analysis of Japanese Biliary Atresia Registry

The Japanese Biliary Atresia Registry (JBAR) was launched in 1989 by the Japanese Biliary Atresia Society (JBAS). Entries into this registry have been performed annually to elucidate the epidemiology and etiology of BA and improve the therapeutic outcome [7]. In this study, we used data obtained from JBAR. Between 1989 and 2018, 3483 patients were registered on the JBAR database. Long-term survival data and Kaplan Meier survival curves were generated from the data from 2649 selected patients who underwent KP or hepatico-/cystoenterostomy initially between the ages of 31 and 90 days.

1. Main type (Tables 3.4 and 3.5)

   There was a significant difference in the jaundice clearance rate (JCR) between the main types of BA following the initial operation (Type I: 69%, Type I-cyst: 78.9%, Type II: 69.1%, and Type III: 59.3%;) (Table 3.4). The 10-year native liver survival rate (NLSRs) were Type I: 58%, Type I-cyst: 79.7%, Type II: 71.4%, and Type III: 47.0%. The 20-year NLSRs were Type I: 47.1%, Type I-cyst: 74.8%, Type II: 71.3%, and Type III: 38.8%. There was a significant difference between the main types ($p < 0.0001$) (Table 3.5).
2. Subtypes according to the patterns of the distal bile ducts (Table 3.6)

   More than half of the cases had the distal bile duct pattern b1: Fibrous common bile duct and patent or atretic hepatic duct. JCR following the initial operation were as follows: Type a1, 63.9%, a2:59.7%, Type b1, 60.4%, Type b2, 47.9%, Type c1, 66.1%, Type c2, 40%. If Type a1 and a2, Type b1 and b2, Types c1 and c2 are added to the analysis, there is no significant difference between these distal bile duct patterns ($p > 0.001$).
3. Subgroups according to the patterns of hepatic radicles at the porta hepatis (Table 3.7).

   Subgroups categorized into α, β, or γ are those with a lumen at the porta hepatis. There were 104 cases classified as α and this is the smallest number of cases in any subgroup. Subgroup α cases where the internal diameter of the hepatic ducts was more than 1 mm with communication to the intrahepatic biliary tree had the highest jaundice clearance rate of 90.4%. However, when the internal diameter was less than 1 mm (categorized as β), the jaundice clearance rate dropped to 74%. Of the patients categorized as γ, μ, ν, o (Type III), ν (fibrous mass) is the largest group with 2364 (68%) patients in this group. Jaundice clearance rates following the initial operation were: γ: 61.4%, μ: 59.0%, ν: 60.5%, and o: 35.9%. The worst jaundice clearance group is o: aplasia of hepatic radicles.

## 3.5 Age at Surgery and Jaundice Clearance Rate

The overall average age at surgery was 66.5 days. The average age at the surgery was 63.2 days in 2018 [12], which continues a slow downward trend over the years. While there was a peak between 46 and 60 days old in the distribution of the age at the surgery, many patients still underwent the surgery at 3 months old or later, showing a small

**Table 3.4** The main types of BA showing the jaundice clearance rate (JCR) and cholangitis rate. There was a significant difference between the main types in the JCR following the initial operation

| Basic type | Total number | Number of bile drainage surgeries | Jaundice disappearance | (%) | Cholangitis | (%) |
|---|---|---|---|---|---|---|
| I | 129 | 129 | 89 | 69 | 53 | 41.1 |
| I-cyst | 280 | 279 | 220 | 78.9 | 103 | 36.9 |
| II | 69 | 68 | 47 | 69.1 | 20 | 29.4 |
| III | 2968 | 2933 | 1738 | 59.3 | 1218 | 41.5 |
| Total | 3446 | 3409 | 2094 | 69.075 | 1394 | 37.225 |

**Table 3.5** The difference of long-term survival data and Kaplan Meier native liver survival curves for the main types of BA were generated from the data from 2649 selected patients

| Type | 1 year | 5 years | 10 years | 20 years | 25 years |
|---|---|---|---|---|---|
| I | 77.5% | 64.7% | 58.0% | 47.1% | 43.2% |
| I-cyst | 87.4% | 81.5% | 79.7% | 74.8% | 64.4% |
| II | 83.8% | 77.2% | 71.4% | 71.4% | 61.2% |
| III | 71.9% | 54.1% | 47.0% | 38.8% | 36.9% |

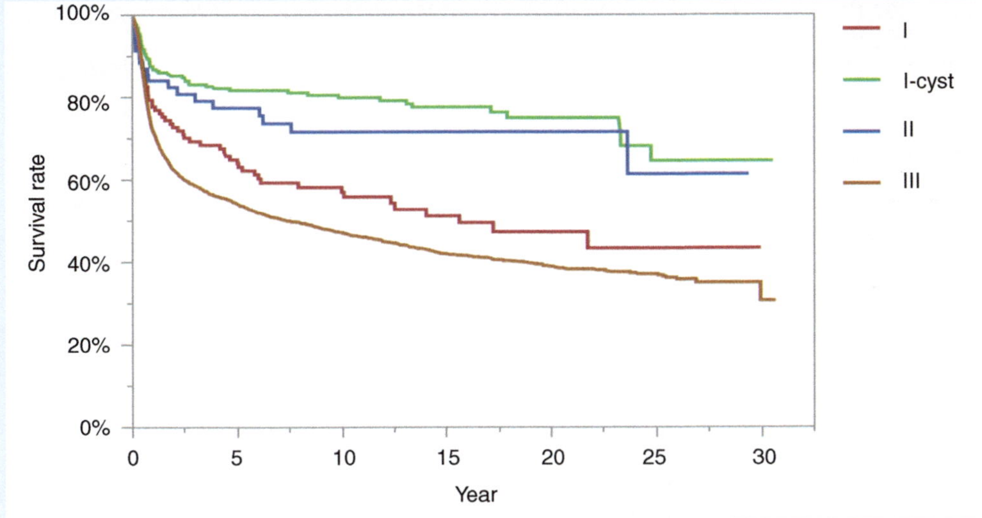


**Table 3.6** The subtypes of jaundice clearance rate between 1989 and 2018

| Subtypes | Total number | Number of bile drainage surgeries | Jaundice disappearance | (%) |
|---|---|---|---|---|
| a1 | 450 | 441 | 282 | 63.9 |
| a2 | 127 | 124 | 74 | 59.7 |
| b1 | 2039 | 2026 | 1224 | 60.4 |
| b2 | 97 | 96 | 46 | 47.9 |
| c1 | 304 | 304 | 201 | 66.1 |
| c2 | 101 | 95 | 38 | 40 |
| d | 159 | 158 | 118 | 74.7 |
| Unknown | 201 | 194 | 125 | 64.4 |
| Total | 3478 | 3438 | 2108 | 61.3 |

**Table 3.7** The jaundice clearance rate between subgroups according to the patterns of hepatic radicles at the porta hepatis

| Subtypes | Total number | Number of bile drainage surgery | Jaundice disappearance | (%) |
|---|---|---|---|---|
| α | 104 | 104 | 94 | 90.4 |
| β | 177 | 177 | 131 | 74 |
| γ | 169 | 166 | 102 | 61.4 |
| μ | 359 | 354 | 209 | 59 |
| ν | 2364 | 2348 | 1420 | 60.5 |
| o | 125 | 117 | 42 | 35.9 |
| Unknown | 180 | 172 | 110 | 64 |
| Total | 3478 | 3438 | 2108 | 61.3 |

peak of the distribution between 91 and 120 days [13]. The age at the surgery and the jaundice clearance rate was almost stable from 31 to 80 days at around 60%. The group of patients who underwent surgery at less than 30 days (the neonatal period) showed the best jaundice clearance rate, which was 71.9%. This was the only group that had a jaundice clearance rate greater than 70%. The jaundice clearance declined after 81 days and became even worse after 120 days (Table 3.8).

**Table 3.8** The age at surgery and jaundice clearance rate

| Age at Op. | Total number | Surgery | Jaundice disappearance | (%) |
|---|---|---|---|---|
| ~30 | 234 | 231 | 166 | 71.9 |
| 31–45 | 542 | 541 | 338 | 62.5 |
| 46–60 | 833 | 830 | 543 | 65.4 |
| 61–70 | 540 | 540 | 343 | 63.5 |
| 71–80 | 471 | 468 | 288 | 61.5 |
| 81–90 | 295 | 294 | 164 | 55.8 |
| 91–120 | 361 | 356 | 200 | 56.2 |
| 121–150 | 123 | 118 | 47 | 39.8 |
| 151~ | 67 | 48 | 11 | 22.9 |
| Unknown | 12 | 12 | 8 | 66.7 |
| Total | 3478 | 3438 | 2108 | 61.3 |

## 3.6 Age at Surgery and Native Liver Survival Rate

In the patients who underwent KP at less than 30 days, the native liver survival rate at 5 years and 10 years after KP remains more than 65% (Table 3.9). These patients showed the best native liver survival rate which was similar to the

**Table 3.9** Age at surgery and native liver survival rate

| Group | Age at Op. | 1 year | 5 years | 10 years | 20 years | 25 years |
|---|---|---|---|---|---|---|
| A | ~30 | 85.3% | 73.6% | 66.1% | 53.3% | 53.3% |
| B | 31–60 | 76.2% | 60.8% | 54.5% | 47.2% | 45.2% |
| C | 61–90 | 74.3% | 56.6% | 50.0% | 41.0% | 36.7% |
| D | 91–120 | 65.1% | 49.0% | 38.3% | 32.4% | 32.4% |
| E | 121–150 | 49.6% | 29.2% | 26.9% | 24.4% | 19.5% |
| F | 151~ | 46.8% | 27.4% | 24.3% | 20.3% | 20.3% |

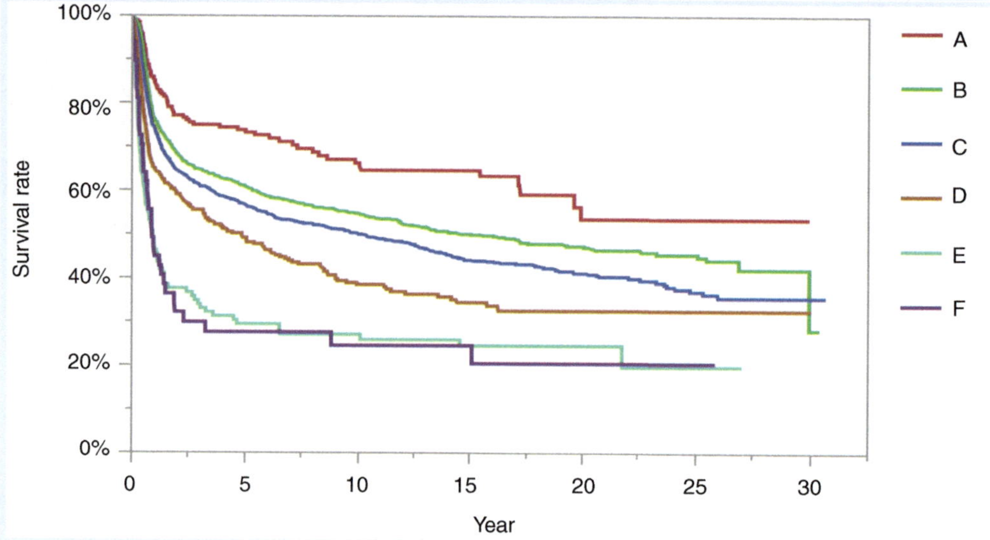


jaundice clearance rate shown in Table 3.8. In patients in whom the KP was performed later than 91 days, the native liver survival declined significantly, being below 50% at 5 years. However, in those undergoing KP after 121 days, there is still a native liver survival rate of 29.2% and 26.9% at 5 and 10 years after KP, suggesting that it is still worth trying a Kasai even in cases diagnosed that late.

In the group who underwent surgery is less than 30 days age at surgery, the native liver survival rate remained more than 65% at both 5 years and 10 years after KP (Table 3.9). This group of patients also showed the best native liver survival rate, similar to the jaundice clearance rate shown in Table 3.8. The long-term native liver survival rate at 10 years declined in those cases whose KP was performed after 91. The native liver survival rate at 10 years dropped to 26.9% in cases who underwent surgery after 121 days. There is still a native liver survival rate close to 24.3% even in cases undergoing KP after 150 days, suggesting that it is still worth trying a Kasai even late diagnosed cases.

## 3.7 Severity Classification

Biliary atresia is one of the diseases included in the Japanese Intractable Diseases classification and the cost of treatment is supported by publicly funded medical care. The severity classification is divided into 3 stages and patients classified as Stage 2 or higher are targeted for support.

1. The baseline classification is as follows:

   Relieved: No symptoms or findings due to biliary atresia and no treatment is required.
   Severity 1: Symptoms/findings caused by biliary atresia require medical treatment, but physical activity is not limited or nursing care is not required.
   Severity 2: Symptoms/findings caused by biliary atresia require medical treatment, resulting in limitation of physical activity, but the condition is reversible or its progression is gradual. There is no need for a liver transplant in the immediate future.
   Severity 3: Symptoms/findings due to biliary atresia, with life-threatening conditions due to sequelae that significantly reduce QOL, or a condition requiring early liver transplantation.

2. Severity classification is further refined by the following 6 severity assessment items.
   (a) Cholestasis.
   (b) Severity of biliary tract infection, including the frequency of episodes. (This score includes the frequency of infections and also the severity as reflected in the blood data.)
   (c) Severity of portal hypertension.
   (d) Presence or absence of related conditions caused by biliary atresia, such as pruritus or the severity of growth retardation.

(e) Evaluation of liver dysfunction including the Child-Pugh score.
(f) The performance status.

The overall severity classification is determined by the factor with the highest severity level.

## References


1. Davenport M, Savage M, Mowat AP, Howard ER. Biliary atresia splenic malformation syndrome: an etiologic and prognostic subgroup. Surgery. 1993 Jun;113(6):662–8.
2. Davenport M. Biliary atresia: clinical aspects. Semin Pediatr Surg. 2012 Aug;21(3):175–84. https://doi.org/10.1053/j.sempedsurg.2012.05.010. Review.
3. Redkar R, Davenport M, Howard ER. Antenatal diagnosis of congenital anomalies of the biliary tract. J Pediatr Surg. 1998 May;33(5):700–4.
4. Balistreri WF, Grand R, Hoofnagle JH, Suchy FJ, Ryckman FC, Perlmutter DH, Sokol RJ. Biliary atresia: current concepts and research directions. Summary of a symposium. Hepatology. 1996 Jun;23(6):1682–92. Review.
5. Kasai M, Sawaguchi S, Akiyama Y, Saito S, Suruga K, Yura J, Ueda T, Okamoto E, Kimura S, Ikeda K. A proposal of new classification of biliary atresia. J Jpn Soc Pediatr Surg. 1976;12(2):327–31. (in Japanese with English Abstract)
6. Ibrahim M, Miyano T, Ohi R, Saeki M, Shiraki K, Tanaka K, Kamiyama T, Nio M. Japanese Biliary Atresia Registry, 1989 to 1994. Tohoku J Exp Med. 1997;181:85–95.
7. Japanese Biliary Atresia Society National Register. Total Number. 2018. https://jbas.net/en/national-registration/
8. Superina R, Magee JC, Brandt ML, et al. The anatomic pattern of biliary atresia identified at time of Kasai hepato porto enterostomy and early postoperative clearance of jaundice are significant predictors of transplant-free survival. Ann Surg. 2011 Oct;254(4):577–85.
9. Davenport M, Ong E, Sharif K, et al. Biliary atresia in England and Wales: results of centralization and new benchmark. J Pediatr Surg. 2011 Sep;46(9):1689–94.
10. de Vries W, de Langen ZJ, Groen H, et al. Biliary atresia in the Netherlands: outcome of patients diagnosed between 1987 and 2008. J Pediatr. 2012;160(4):638–644.e2.
11. Chardot C, Buet C, Serinet MO, et al. Improving outcomes of biliary atresia: French national series 1986–2009. J Hepatol. 2013 Jun;58(6):1209–17.
12. Japanese Biliary Atresia Society. Japanese Biliary Atresia Registry 2020. J Jpn Soc Pediatr Surg. 2020;53:319–25. (in Japanese)
13. Nio M. Japanese Biliary Atresia Registry. Pediatr Surg Int. 2017;33:1319–25.

# Japanese Biliary Atresia Registry

4

Hideyuki Sasaki, Masaki Nio, Ryuji Okubo,
and Yoko Murai

**Abstract**

The Japanese Biliary Atresia Registry (JBAR) was launched in 1989 by the Japanese Biliary Atresia Society (JBAS). The Japanese Biliary Atresia Registry (JBAR) used an initial questionnaire, a questionnaire for liver transplantation, and a follow-up questionnaire. Each patient is to be followed up for 40 years. An annual report of the JBAR has been published in the *Journal of the Japanese Society of Pediatric Surgeons*. In addition, aggregation data can be browsed on the JBAS website (https://jbas.net/en/). Between 1989 and 2018, 3483 patients were registered in the JBAR. Among them, 1446 patients underwent liver transplantation. The 20-year overall and native-liver survival rates were 86.4% and 42.5%, respectively. The age at Kasai portoenterostomy had a significant impact on the long-term native liver survival rate ($p < 0.001$). Surgical outcomes of biliary atresia have markedly improved, owing to the cooperation of Kasai portoenterostomy and liver transplantation. JBAR also functions as a research infrastructure for biliary atresia. To date, several research projects have been conducted using this function.

**Keywords**

Biliary atresia · Registry · Prognosis · Kasai portoenterostomy · Liver transplantation

H. Sasaki (✉) · M. Nio · R. Okubo · Y. Murai
Department of Pediatric Surgery, Tohoku University Graduate School of Medicine, Sendai, Japan

Secretariat of The Japanese Biliary Atresia Society, Sendai, Japan
e-mail: h-sasaki@ped-surg.med.tohoku.ac.jp

## Abbreviations

| | |
|---|---|
| BA | Biliary atresia |
| JBAS | Japanese Biliary Atresia Society |
| JBAR | Japanese Biliary Atresia Registry |
| LTx | Liver transplantation |

## 4.1 The Japanese Biliary Atresia Registry

The JBAR, a nationwide registry of patients with biliary atresia (BA), was launched in 1989 by the Japanese Biliary Atresia Society (JBAS), comprising 101-member hospitals caring for patients with BA. The JBAR employed an initial questionnaire, a questionnaire for liver transplantation (LTx), and a follow-up questionnaire. Each patient is to be followed up for 40 years. Between 1989 and 2018, 3483 patients were registered in the JBAR. Pediatric surgeons who registered the initial questionnaire data were responsible for registering subsequent registries for the entire follow-up period of patients, including recipients of LTx. An annual report of the JBAR has been published in the *Journal of the Japanese Society of Pediatric Surgeons*. In addition, aggregation data can be browsed on the JBAS website (https://jbas.net/en/). In addition, four reports of JBAR data have been published in English [1–4].

## 4.2 The Initial Registry

### 4.2.1 Perinatal History

Collected data on family and perinatal history are summarized in Table 4.1. Regarding the family history of BA, three siblings and four other relatives were associated with BA. No parent of pediatric patients with BA was associated with BA. Approximately two-third of patients were women. Among patients whose stool color was confirmed, approxi-


M. Nio (ed.), *Introduction to Biliary Atresia*, https://doi.org/10.1007/978-981-16-2160-4_4

**Table 4.1** Summary of family and perinatal history

| | *N* | % |
|---|---|---|
| *Family history of biliary atresia* | | |
| Parents | 0 | 0 |
| Siblings | 3 | 0.09 |
| Others | 4 | 0.11 |
| *Perinatal history* | | |
| *Sex* | | |
| Male | 1290 | 37 |
| Female | 2190 | 62.9 |
| Unknown | 3 | 0.1 |
| *Color of meconium* | | |
| Normal | 1520 | 43.6 |
| Pale | 508 | 14.6 |
| Unknown | 1455 | 41.8 |
| *Yellow stools before the initial surgery* | | |
| Yes | 1962 | 56.3 |
| No | 752 | 21.6 |
| Unknown | 769 | 22.1 |

**Table 4.2** Birth weight and gestational age

| Birth weight (g) | |
|---|---|
| Mean (range, SD) | 2903.6 (824–4940, 452.1) |
| **Birth weight (g)** | ***N*** |
| <1499 | 32 |
| 1500–1999 | 72 |
| 2000–2499 | 413 |
| 2500–2999 | 1490 |
| 3000–3499 | 1161 |
| 3500–3999 | 229 |
| >4000 | 30 |
| Unknown | 56 |
| **Gestational age (weeks)** | |
| Mean (range, SD) | 38.6 (24–42, 1.8) |
| **Gestational age (weeks)** | ***N*** |
| <29 | 11 |
| 30–31 | 17 |
| 32–33 | 34 |
| 34–35 | 88 |
| 36–37 | 498 |
| 38–39 | 1622 |
| 40–41 | 1078 |
| >42 | 26 |
| Unknown | 109 |

*SD* standard deviation

mately three-fourth of patients passed normal color meconium and yellowish stools.

The mean birth weight and gestational age were 2903.6 g and 38.6 weeks, respectively (Table 4.2).

Pathological bleeding due to vitamin K deficiency is one of the most serious conditions preoperatively. In Japan, the incidence of this condition is approximately 9%. Intracranial hemorrhage accounted for approximately half of patients with pathological bleeding (Table 4.3). A total of 159 registrants had intracranial bleeding episodes between 1989 and 2017. The average age at intracranial bleeding was 61.4 days (2–108 days) (Fig. 4.1). These data suggest that the incidence of intracranial hemorrhage would be remarkably reduced by employing early surgery before 50 days of age in BA.

**Table 4.3** Pathological bleeding before the initial surgery

| | *N* | % |
|---|---|---|
| Yes | 317 | 9.1 |
| Intracranial | 162 | |
| Alimentary tract | 97 | |
| Subcutaneous | 30 | |
| Other | 53 | |
| No | 3024 | 86.8 |
| Unknown | 142 | 4.1 |

## 4.2.2 Diagnosis

### 4.2.2.1 Stool Color Card

Since 2012, the stool color card has been included nationwide in the Maternal and Child Health Handbook in Japan, aiming for the early diagnosis of BA (Fig. 4.2). If the stool color is similar to color numbers 1, 2, or 3, the infant's family is advised to visit a pediatrician or a pediatric surgeon in this system. Among 720 registrants, the color card number was obtained from 243 patients until 2018. Before 1 month of age, around 1 month of age, and after 1 month of age, 46%, 50%, and 78% of patients passed stools of color numbers 1, 2, or 3, respectively (Table 4.4). The remaining patients passed stools of color numbers 4, 5, 6, or 7. An earlier diagnosis of BA is expected to be achieved by universal utilization of the stool color card. However, it may be difficult to identify majority of patients with BA at around 1 month of age or before using this system.

### 4.2.2.2 Serum Bilirubin Level

The total and direct serum bilirubin levels preoperatively were 9.4 ± 3.8 mg/dL and 6.4 ± 2.8 mg/dL, respectively.

### 4.2.2.3 Diagnostic Modalities

Ultrasonography was the most common diagnostic modality of BA in the JBAR; 94% of patients underwent ultrasonography. Hepatobiliary scintigraphy, serum bile acid analysis, duodenal fluid sampling, and serum lipoprotein X were used in 66%, 63%, 55%, and 46% of patients, respectively.

### 4.2.2.4 Associated Anomalies

The incidence of associated anomalies is very low. Splenic malformation (polysplenia in 70 patients and asplenia in 4 patients), intestinal malrotation (62 patients), and preduodenal portal vein (46 patients) occurred in 3483 patients.

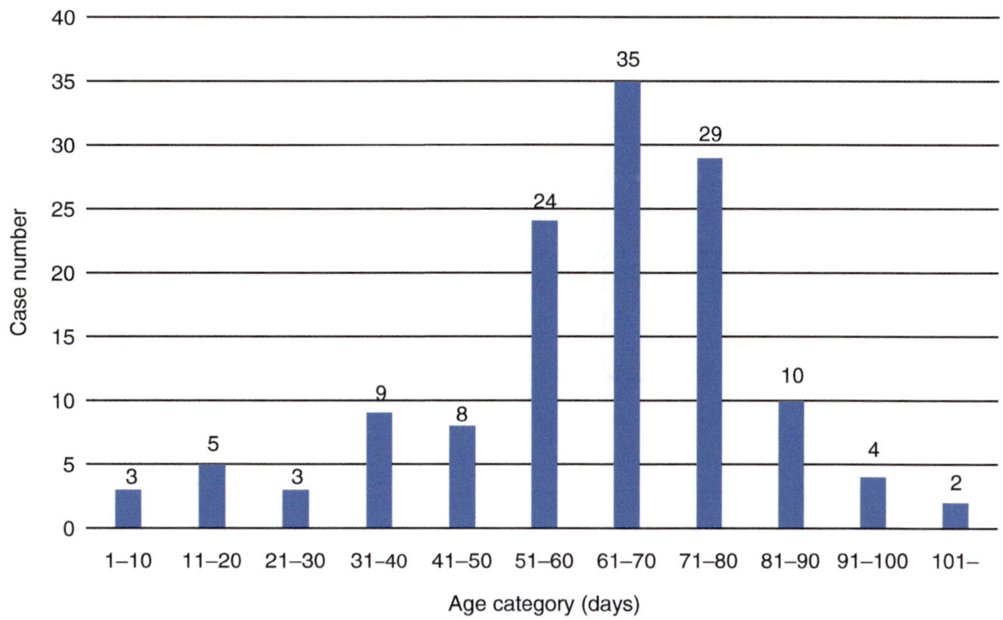


**Fig. 4.1** Distribution of the age at intracranial bleeding. The average age at intracranial bleeding was 61.4 (2–108 days)

| Average (days) | Standard deviation (days) | Maximum (days) | Minimum (days) |
|---|---|---|---|
| 61.4 | 19.9 | 108 | 2 |

The incidence of chromosomal abnormalities is approximately the same as the general incidence (13/2, 649, 0.5%).

### 4.2.3 Surgery

#### 4.2.3.1 Age at Surgery

The average age at surgery was 63.2 days. As a peak in the age distribution at the time of surgery occurred between aged 46 and 60 days, many patients still underwent surgery at aged ≥3 months, showing a small peak in the distribution between 91 and 120 days (Table 4.5). The group of patients who underwent surgery during the neonatal period showed the best jaundice clearance rate, i.e., >70%. The jaundice clearance was approximately stable until 80 days, approximately 60%, and then decreased with age at the time of surgery (Table 4.5). Recently, there has been a tendency to perform surgery earlier, presumably due to the introduction of the stool color card system (Fig. 4.3).

#### 4.2.3.2 Surgical Treatment

The employed surgical treatment was hepaticoenterostomy in 196 patients, Kasai portoenterostomy in 3212, primary LTx in 17, and exploratory laparotomy in 23 patients. Primary LTx is an available option in Japan; however, it is indicated for extremely selective cases.

#### 4.2.3.3 Reconstruction Procedure

Approximately 40% of registrants had cholangitis episodes within a year postoperatively. Regarding the reconstruction procedure aimed at preventing cholangitis, registrants underwent various types of reconstruction procedures, with the original Kasai, anti-reflux valve, and Suruga II procedures as the most common. The jaundice clearance rates of these three procedures were similar (Table 4.6).

In the original Kasai procedure, the most frequently used, a higher incidence of cholangitis was observed in the group of patients with limb length of <40 cm (Table 4.6).

Among the three reconstructions, the incidence of cholangitis was the highest in the Suruga II group and the lowest in the anti-reflux valve procedure (Table 4.6).

### 4.2.4 Anatomical Patterns of Obstruction

The JBAR employs the JBAS classification [5] consisting of three parts: the main type according to the obstruction site, subtype according to patterns of distal bile ducts, and subgroup according to patterns of hepatic radicles at the porta hepatis. A specific description is shown in Chap. 4 "Definition and Classifications of Biliary Atresia."

The incidences of type I/I cyst (atresia of the common bile duct; type II, atresia of the hepatic duct; and type III, atresia

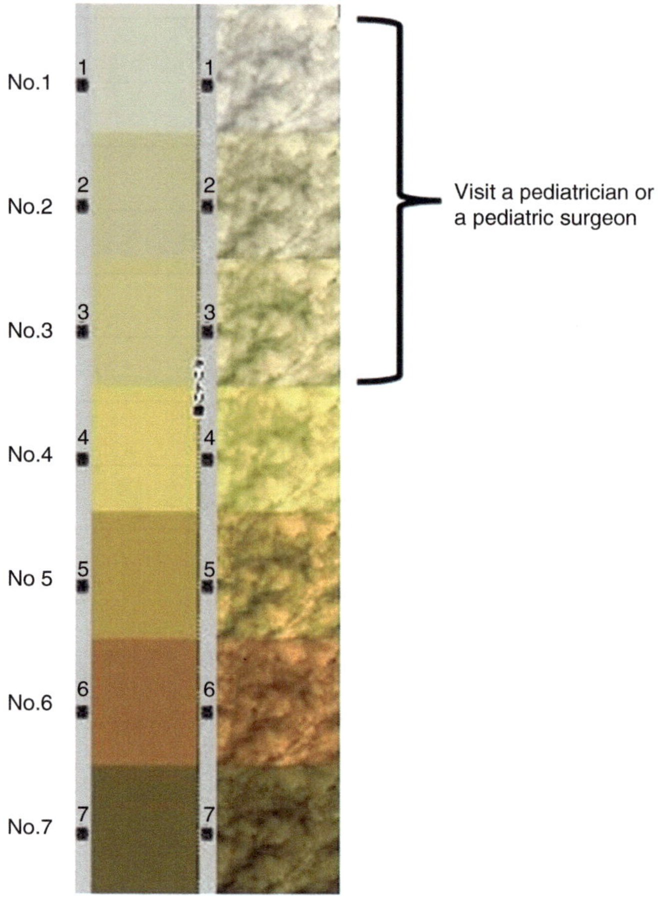


reference from https://www.jagat.or.jp/cat6-2/cat6-2-6

**Fig. 4.2** Color number of the stool color card. If the stool color is similar to the color numbers 1, 2, or 3, the family of the infant is advised to visit a pediatrician or a pediatric surgeon in this system

**Table 4.4** Stool color status before the initial surgery

| | Before 1 month | 1 month | After 1 month |
|---|---|---|---|
| #1–3 | 70 (54.7%) | 75 (58.6%) | 102 (85.7%) |
| #4 | 52 (40.6%) | 50 (39.1%) | 15 (12.6%) |
| #5–7 | 6 (4.7%) | 3 (2.3%) | 2 (1.7%) |

The color card number was obtained from 243 patients until 2018, and the data included duplications

at the hepatic hilum) were 11.8%, 2%, and 85.3%, respectively. The jaundice clearance rate was the highest in type I cyst (78.9%), followed by types II (69.1%) and I (69%), and was the worst in type III (59.3%) (Table 4.7).

## 4.3 The Follow-Up Registry

The follow-up registry consisted of two steps: annual confirmation of patient outcomes (dead or alive with/without LTx), comprising >95% of survivors registered, and the use of a case report form with a follow-up questionnaire, with approximately 70% of survivors registered (Table 4.8).

**Table 4.5** Age at the bile drainage surgery and jaundice clearance

| 3438 Registrants with bile drainage surgery | | |
|---|---|---|
| Age at surgery (days) | *N* | Jaundice clearance (number (%)) |
| <30 | 231 | 166 (71.9%) |
| 31–45 | 541 | 338 (62.5%) |
| 46–60 | 830 | 543 (65.4%) |
| 61–70 | 540 | 343 (63.5%) |
| 71–80 | 468 | 288 (61.5%) |
| 81–90 | 294 | 164 (55.8%) |
| 91–120 | 356 | 200 (56.2%) |
| 121–150 | 118 | 47 (39.8%) |
| >151 | 48 | 11 (22.9%) |
| Unknown | 12 | 8 (66.7%) |
| 2933 Registrants of type III with bile drainage surgery | | |
| Age at surgery (days) | *N* | Jaundice clearance (number (%)) |
| <30 | 154 | 105 (68.2%) |
| 31–45 | 448 | 270 (60.3%) |
| 46–60 | 722 | 465 (64.4%) |
| 61–70 | 462 | 280 (60.6%) |
| 71–80 | 428 | 257 (60%) |
| 81–90 | 262 | 142 (54.2%) |
| 91–120 | 315 | 170 (54%) |
| 121–150 | 98 | 35 (35.7%) |
| >151 | 34 | 7 (20.6%) |
| Unknown | 10 | 7 (70%) |

### 4.3.1 Liver Function Tests in Native-Liver Survivors

While these values appeared to be stable until the 15-year follow-up, they may fluctuate or become worse at the 20th and 25th years. As the number of long-term survivors in the JBAR remains limited, further follow-up is essential (Table 4.9).

### 4.3.2 Cholangitis

Cholangitis is one of the most common sequelae in native liver survivors of BA. The incidence of cholangitis was 18.4% in the 2nd year following the registration. It was ever higher in long-term survivors (24% and 29.6% in 20- and 25-year follow-ups, respectively) (Table 4.9).

### 4.3.3 Portal Hypertension and Developmental Status in Native-Liver Survivors

Approximately 30% of patients developed portal hypertension, such as esophageal varices and hypersplenism, during the follow-up period. The incidence of hepatopulmonary syndrome was approximately 1–2% at the 5- and 10-year follow-ups. The incidence of porto-pulmonary hypertension was similar to that of patients with hepatopulmonary syn-

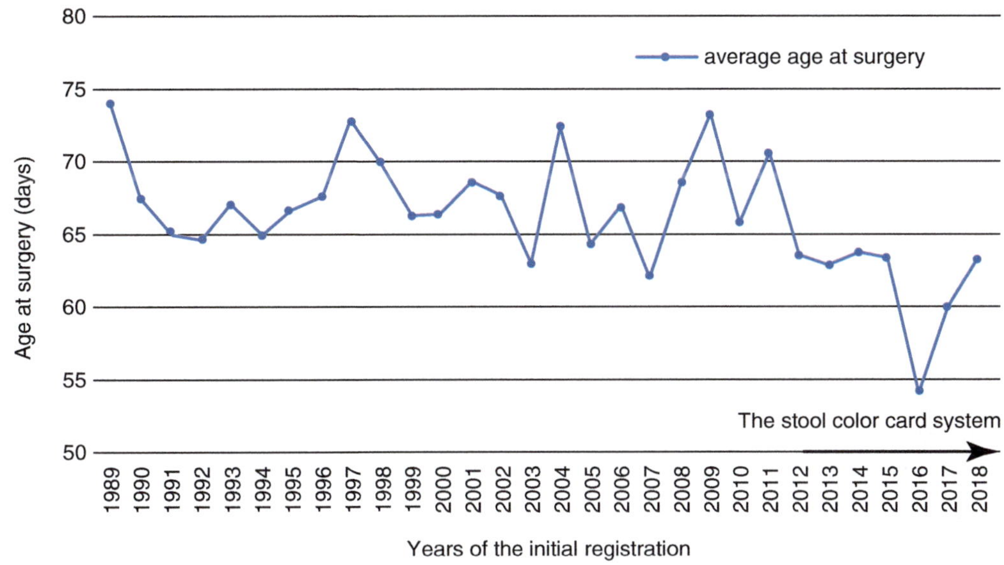


**Fig. 4.3** The trend of the age at initial surgery. There appeared to be the tendency to perform surgery earlier, presumably due to the introduction of the stool color card system in 2012

**Table 4.6** Procedure, jaundice clearance, and cholangitis

| | *N* | Jaundice clearance | Jaundice clearance rate | Cholangitis | Incidence of cholangitis |
|---|---|---|---|---|---|
| Original Kasai | 2473 | 1529 | 61.8% | 1049 | 42.4% |
| Length of Roux-Y | | | | | |
| <40 cm | 781 | 476 | 60.9% | 355 | 45.5% |
| 40–60 cm | 1402 | 885 | 63.1% | 575 | 41.0% |
| >60 | 257 | 152 | 59.1% | 108 | 42.0% |
| Others | 33 | | | | |
| Anti-reflux valve | 626 | 384 | 61.3% | 215 | 34.3% |
| Suruga II | 162 | 90 | 55.6% | 74 | 45.7% |

**Table 4.7** Main type, jaundice clearance, and cholangitis

| Basic Type | No. of Bile drainage surgery | Jaundice disappeared (%) | Cholangitis (%) |
|---|---|---|---|
| I | 129 | 89 (69) | 53 (41.1) |
| I-Cyst | 279 | 220 (78.9) | 103 (36.9) |
| II | 68 | 47 (69.1) | 20 (29.4) |
| III | 2933 | 1738 (59.3) | 1218 (41.5) |
| Unknown | 29 | 14 (48.3) | 11 (37.9) |
| Total | 3438 | 2108 (61.3) | 1405 (40.9) |

drome after the 15th year following the initial registration (Table 4.9). Physical growth and mental development were approximately within the normal range in native-liver survivors (Table 4.9).

## 4.4 LTx Registry

The LTx registry has been conducted for initial registrants in the JBAR since 1995, and 1446 patients underwent LTx up to 2018. In Japan, LTx has become widely available since the late 1990s. For this reason, the number of recipients increased during the early and mid-1990s. Approximately 40% of registrants required LTx for >25 years.

**Table 4.8** Status of follow-up registration using a case report form

| Year | 2nd | 5th | 10th | 15th | 20th | 25th |
|---|---|---|---|---|---|---|
| No. of NLS | 1666 | 1238 | 875 | 586 | 304 | 125 |
| No. of survival with LTx | 613 | 637 | 579 | 389 | 234 | 90 |
| No. of dead | 84 | 28 | 19 | 16 | 4 | 6 |
| Total | 2363 | 1903 | 1473 | 991 | 542 | 221 |

*LTx* liver transplantation, *NLS* native liver survival

### 4.4.1 Donor Source

Grafts from cadaveric donors were available in only 25 patients. In contrast, grafts from living donors were transplanted in 1393 (96.3%) patients. The donor source was extremely dependent on living donors, especially on parents of recipients (father: 557, mother: 740, relatives: 58, others: 3, unknown: 25) in Japan.

### 4.4.2 Patient Survival at LTx Registration

Of the 1446 recipients, 1338 (92.5%) survived at the initial LTx registration. However, the major donor source was living donors. Problems associated with living-donor LTx remain unresolved. The establishment of cadaveric-donor

**Table 4.9** Follow-up data of native-liver survivors

| Year | 2nd | 5th | 10th | 15th | 20th | 25th |
|---|---|---|---|---|---|---|
| No. of NLS | 1666 | 1238 | 875 | 586 | 304 | 125 |
| T-Bil (mg/dL) | 1.1 | 1 | 1.1 | 1.2 | 1.1 | 1.4 |
| ALT (IU/L) | 68.8 | 52.9 | 52.1 | 37.7 | 47.1 | 38.6 |
| GGTP (IU/L) | 170.7 | 104 | 92.1 | 81 | 102.1 | 126.4 |
| Normal Ch-E (%) | 721 (69%) | 661 (68%) | 590 (68%) | 394 (69%) | 195 (64%) | 65 (54%) |
| Cholangitis (%) | 306 (18.4%) | 214 (17.3%) | 105 (12%) | 108 (18.4%) | 73 (24%) | 37 (29.6%) |
| Intrahepatic cholelithiasis (%) | 3 (0.2%) | 5 (0.4%) | 2 (0.2%) | 5 (0.9%) | 4 (1.3%) | 6 (4.8%) |
| Esophageal Varices (%) | 300 (18%) | 352 (28.4%) | 238 (27.2%) | 151 (25.8%) | 75 (24.7%) | 26 (20.8%) |
| Hypersplenism (%) | 289 (17.3%) | 375 (30.3%) | 312 (35.7%) | 187 (31.9%) | 89 (29.3%) | 39 (31.2%) |
| Hepatopulmonary syndrome (%) | 4 (0.2%) | 20 (1.6%) | 20 (2.3%) | 11 (1.9%) | 2 (0.7%) | 2 (1.6%) |
| Pulmonary hypertension (%) | 0 (0%) | 4 (0.3%) | 4 (0.5%) | 7 (1.2%) | 3 (1%) | 3 (2.4%) |
| Mentally delayed (%) | 22 (1.3%) | 43 (3.5%) | 39 (4.5%) | 24 (4.1%) | 12 (3.9%) | 6 (4.8%) |
| Physically delayed (%) | 44 (2.6%) | 28 (2.3%) | 20 (2.3%) | 9 (1.5%) | 9 (3%) | 3 (2.4%) |

*ALT* alanine transferase, *GGTP* gamma-glutamyl transferase, *NLS* native liver survival, *T-Bil* total bilirubin

LTx is ongoing in Japan. Follow-up registration for recipients of LTx is also ongoing in the JBAR.

## 4.5 Current Status of JBAR Registrants

The outcome of registrants was well recognized by the annual confirmation of the follow-up registration, and the number of patients who were lost to follow-up was very small. In Japan, currently, most patients survive owing to the cooperation of constructive surgery, including the Kasai portoenterostomy, hepaticoenterostomy, and liver transplantation (Table 4.10).

The 20-year overall and native-liver survival rates were 86.4% and 42.5%, respectively (Fig. 4.4a).

The age at the time of surgery had a significant impact on the long-term native liver survival rate ($p < 0.001$) (Fig. 4.4b).

The best rates of jaundice clearance and long-term native-liver survival were achieved in patients who underwent surgery during the neonatal period.

## 4.6 JBAR as a Research Infrastructure in BA

The JBAR also functioned as a research infrastructure in BA. To date, several articles have been published using this function.

Recently, laparoscopic surgery has been implemented for BA. However, some studies have suggested that laparoscopic surgery is relatively harmful for BA [6]. In this situation, a nationwide survey was conducted based on the JBAR framework. This survey revealed that the difference in surgical approach was not a significant independent predictor of the postoperative jaundice clearance rate and 1-year native liver survival rate [7].

Primary LTx for patients with decompensated cirrhosis in early infancy is a critical issue. Regarding this matter, a nationwide survey was conducted based on the JBAR framework. This survey revealed that primary liver transplantation was implemented for very limited cases, and appropriate clinical practice guidelines are required based on further studies [8].

## 4.7 Current Problems and Future Tasks

Currently, approximately 90% of patients with BA in Japan and 70% of surviving initial registrants are registered in the initial and follow-up registries, respectively. Some problems with BA were unresolved, such as elucidating the etiology, improving treatment outcomes after Kasai portoenterostomy, adequate management for long-term sequelae, and establishment of a suitable long-term follow-up system including transitional care. Therefore, improving the completeness of JBAR is critical.

The JBAR has worked as research infrastructure in BA. It is important to continue multi-institutional collaborative research utilizing this framework and especially important to promote international collaborative research.

**Table 4.10** The current status of the registrants of the JBAR

| Year of registration | 1989 | 1990 | 1991 | 1992 | 1993 | 1994 | 1995 | 1996 | 1997 | 1998 | 1999 | 2000 | 2001 | 2002 | 2003 | 2004 | 2005 | 2006 | 2007 | 2008 | 2009 | 2010 | 2011 | 2012 | 2013 | 2014 | 2015 | 2016 | 2017 | 2018 |
|---|---|---|---|---|---|---|---|---|---|---|---|---|---|---|---|---|---|---|---|---|---|---|---|---|---|---|---|---|---|---|
| No. of NLS | 40 | 50 | 58 | 41 | 46 | 49 | 58 | 55 | 49 | 53 | 59 | 52 | 62 | 57 | 52 | 51 | 49 | 49 | 54 | 42 | 54 | 51 | 58 | 60 | 55 | 67 | 65 | 46 | 52 | 64 |
| No. of survival with LTx | 19 | 26 | 22 | 43 | 30 | 45 | 50 | 48 | 46 | 48 | 50 | 61 | 46 | 55 | 41 | 51 | 47 | 44 | 36 | 54 | 41 | 50 | 40 | 46 | 39 | 43 | 48 | 36 | 39 | 25 |
| No. of dead | 42 | 38 | 49 | 31 | 29 | 29 | 29 | 20 | 28 | 14 | 20 | 7 | 8 | 14 | 6 | 12 | 5 | 7 | 5 | 8 | 7 | 5 | 12 | 2 | 5 | 6 | 4 | 1 | 2 | 2 |
| No. of unknown status | 14 | 15 | 8 | 12 | 9 | 9 | 12 | 7 | 6 | 11 | 8 | 6 | 9 | 3 | 3 | 0 | 3 | 7 | 3 | 4 | 4 | 2 | 1 | 1 | 1 | 3 | 3 | 4 | 1 | 0 |
| No. of registrants | 115 | 129 | 137 | 127 | 114 | 132 | 149 | 130 | 129 | 126 | 137 | 126 | 125 | 129 | 102 | 114 | 104 | 107 | 98 | 108 | 106 | 108 | 111 | 109 | 100 | 119 | 120 | 87 | 94 | 91 |

*JBAR* Japanese Biliary Atresia Registry, *LTx* liver transplantation, *NLS* native liver survival

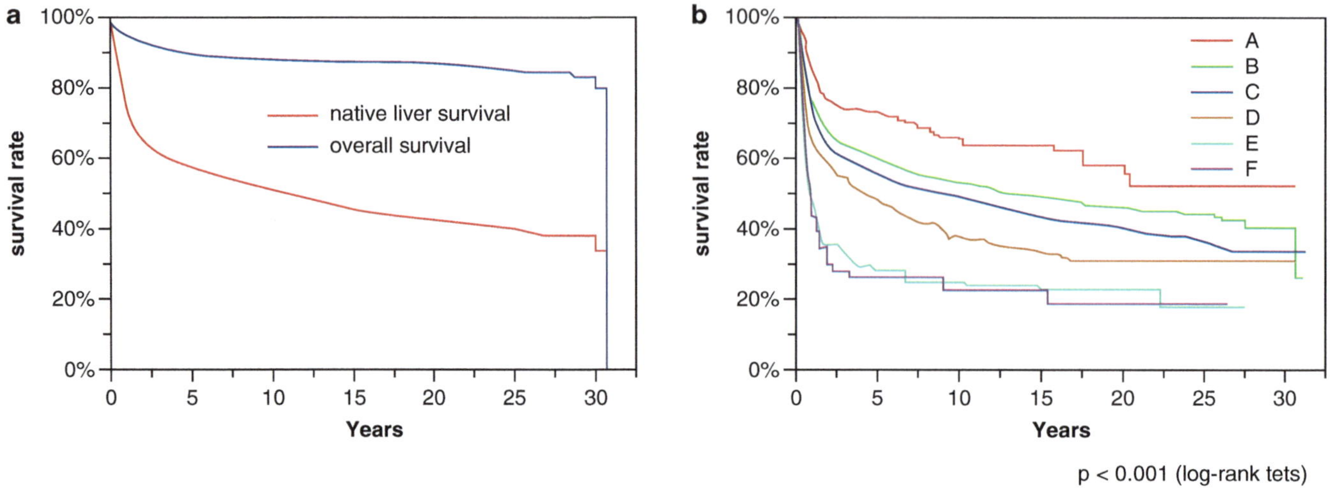


| | Overall survival (%) | Native liver survival (%) |
|---|---|---|
| 1-year | 93.9 | 73.6 |
| 5-years | 89.5 | 57.2 |
| 10-years | 88.3 | 50.4 |
| 20-years | 86.4 | 42.5 |
| 25-years | 85.3 | 39.7 |

| | age at surgery | 1-year (%) | 5-years (%) | 10-years (%) | 20-years (%) | 25-years (%) |
|---|---|---|---|---|---|---|
| A | ~30 | 85.3 | 73.6 | 66.1 | 53.3 | 53.3 |
| B | 31~60 | 76.2 | 60.8 | 54.5 | 47.2 | 45.2 |
| C | 61~90 | 74.3 | 56.6 | 50.0 | 41.0 | 36.7 |
| D | 91~120 | 65.1 | 49.0 | 38.3 | 32.4 | 32.4 |
| E | 121~150 | 49.6 | 29.2 | 26.9 | 24.4 | 19.3 |
| F | 151~ | 46.8 | 27.4 | 24.3 | 20.3 | 20.3 |

**Fig. 4.4** Kaplan–Meier survival curves. (**a**) Kaplan–Meier survival curves of registrants. The 20-year overall and native-liver survival rates were 86.4 and 42.5%, respectively. (**b**) Age at surgery and Kaplan–Meier survival curves of registrants. The age at Kasai portoenterostomy had a significant impact on the long-term native-liver survival rate

## References


1. Chiba T, Ohi R, Kamiyama T, Nio M, Ibrahim M. Japanese Biliary Atresia Registry. Biliary Atresia (1991) ICOM Associates Inc.
2. Ibrahim M, Miyano T, Ohi R, Saeki M, Shiraki K, Tanaka K, et al. Japanese Biliary Atresia Registry, 1989 to 1994. Tohoku J Exp Med. 1997 Jan;181(1):85–95. https://doi.org/10.1620/tjem.181.85.
3. Nio M, Ohi R, Miyano T, Saeki M, Shiraki K, Tanaka K. Japanese Biliary Atresia Registry. Five- and 10-year survival rates after surgery for biliary atresia: a report from the Japanese Biliary Atresia Registry. J Pediatr Surg. 2003 Jul;38(7):997–1000. https://doi.org/10.1016/s0022-3468(03)00178-7.
4. Nio M. Japanese Biliary Atresia Registry. Pediatr Surg Int. 2017 Dec;33(12):1319–25. https://doi.org/10.1007/s00383-017-4160-x.
5. Ohi R, Ibrahim M. Biliary atresia. Semin Pediatr Surg. 1992;1:115–24.
6. Lishuang M, Zhen C, Guoliang Q, Zhen Z, Chen W, Long L, et al. Laparoscopic portoenterostomy versus open portoenterostomy for the treatment of biliary atresia: a systematic review and meta-analysis of comparative studies. Pediatr Surg Int. 2015;31:261–9.
7. Murase N, Hinoki A, Shirota C, Tomita H, Shimojima N, Sasaki H, et al. Multicenter, retrospective, comparative study of laparoscopic and open Kasai portoenterostomy in children with biliary atresia from Japanese high-volume centers. J Hepatobiliary Pancreat Sci. 2019 Jan;26(1):43–50. https://doi.org/10.1002/jhbp.594.
8. Uto K, Inomata Y, Sakamoto S, Hibi T, Sasaki H, Nio M. A multicenter study of primary liver transplantation for biliary atresia in Japan. Pediatr Surg Int. 2019 Nov;35(11):1223–9. https://doi.org/10.1007/s00383-019-04553-7.

# Embryological and Anatomical Considerations in Biliary Atresia

5

Nobuyoshi Shiojiri, Ryosuke Yoshii, and Yotsuba Arai

**Abstract**

The developmental origins of intrahepatic bile ducts, and extrahepatic bile ducts with the gallbladder are different in mammalian embryos: the former is derived from the cranial part, and the latter from the caudal part of the liver primordium. Secondary joining of both extrahepatic and intrahepatic bile ducts occurs in a stochastic fashion during liver development. Embryologically their impaired development, including the failure of their joining, might result in biliary atresia (BA). Although portal mesenchyme induces adjacent hepatoblasts to give rise to epithelial cells of intrahepatic bile ducts during development, several signaling molecules may be involved in this inductive event, including Jag1, Wnt5a, and TGFβ. Maturation of hepatic tissue may be coupled to normal bile duct development. The development of an in vitro culture system is required to demonstrate molecular mechanisms of normal bile duct formation, and also the cause of BA.

**Keywords**

Bile ducts · Biliary atresia · C/EBPα · Jag1 · Notch2 · Organ culture

## 5.1 Introduction

Biliary atresia (BA) is a neonatal disease of the liver, in which extrahepatic bile ducts are abnormally narrow, blocked, or absent. The disease leads to fibrosis and end-stage liver disease by 2 years of age. Although the BA may be classified into congenital or acquired types, it still remains to be demonstrated what is the cause of the BA. To better understand the mechanism of BA and develop its medical treatment, it should be noted how bile ducts are formed at a molecular level in mammalian embryos. Several papers have been published on mouse models of BA [1–4]. They may shed a light on the cause of BA. In this chapter, important events of murine bile duct development will be reviewed with considering the possibility of BA development. Mutant mice with anomalous bile duct development will be introduced.

## 5.2 Normal Biliary Development

Liver primordium develops as a diverticulum in the ventral foregut of the anterior intestinal portal region at 8.5–9.0 days of gestation (E8.5-9.0) in mouse embryos, which corresponds to 3 weeks of gestation in human embryos [5]. The primordium becomes of two portions at E9.5; the cranial and caudal portions (Fig. 5.1a–c). The cranial portion gives rise to the liver parenchyma with intrahepatic bile ducts whereas the caudal part develops into the gallbladder and extrahepatic bile ducts in later development. At the early phase of development, the liver is a hemopoietic organ, and contains many hemopoietic cells. Hepatoblasts are scattered among hemopoietic cells as an endodermal component, but do not form intrahepatic bile ducts. From E13.5 on, which corresponds to 5 weeks of gestation in human embryos, periportal hepatoblasts are induced to form ductal plates (intrahepatic bile duct progenitors) by portal mesenchyme (Fig. 5.1d). The development of ductal plates proceeds from the hilum to the periphery region. When connections between each ductal plate are examined, they are first discontinuous and become confluent with development (Fig. 5.2b). Connections of intrahepatic ductal plates with extrahepatic bile ducts are also not confluent at the early phase. Various configurations of bile ducts are found in the hilum even in the syngeneic mouse liver (C3H/HeSlc strain) (Fig. 5.2a). Connection of intrahepatic bile ducts with extrahepatic bile ducts, and that between each ductal plate may occur in a stochastic fashion [6]. At E16.5 to

N. Shiojiri (✉) · R. Yoshii · Y. Arai
Department of Biology, Faculty of Science, Shizuoka University, Shizuoka, Japan
e-mail: shiojiri.nobuyoshi@shizuoka.ac.jp



M. Nio (ed.), *Introduction to Biliary Atresia*, https://doi.org/10.1007/978-981-16-2160-4_5

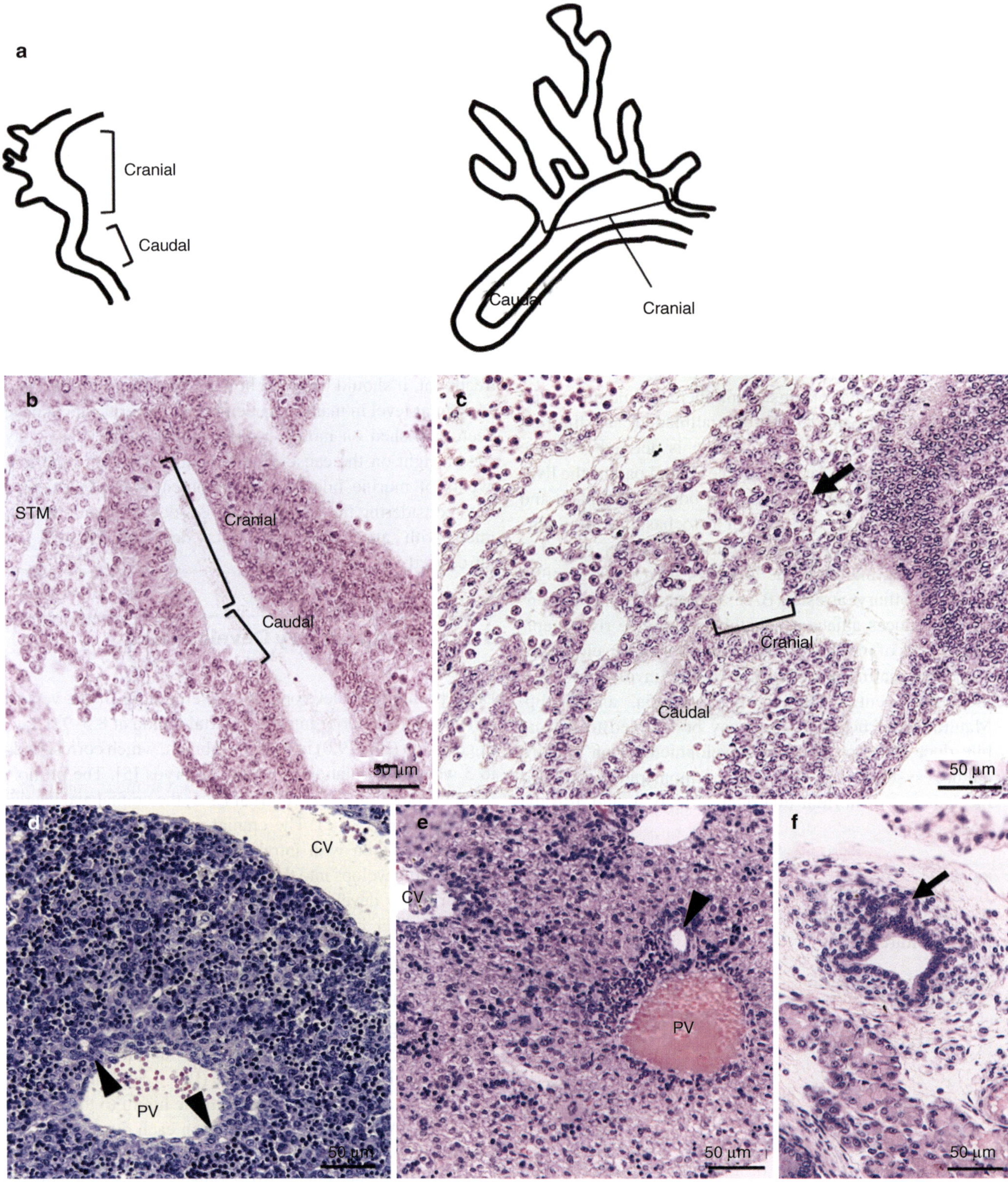


**Fig. 5.1** Normal biliary development in mouse embryos. (**a**) Line drawing of liver primordium development. The liver primordium at E9.5 consists of cranial and caudal portions (left). The cranial portion extends hepatic cords of hepatoblasts into the septum transversum mesenchyme, and gives rise to the liver proper (right). Caudal portion develops into the gallbladder and extrahepatic bile ducts. (**b**) Liver primordium at E9.5. It consists of cranial and caudal portions. The cranial portion starts to extend hepatic cords into the septum transversum mesenchyme (STM). (**c**) Liver primordium at E10.5. It is well vascularized. Arrow indicates hepatic cords. (**d**) Ductal plates (arrowheads) around portal veins at E15.5. Hemopoietic cells with heavily blue nuclei are abundant. (**e**) Intrahepatic bile duct (arrowhead) in neonatal liver. (**f**) Extrahepatic bile duct having the biliary gland (arrow) at neonatal stage. b-f, hematoxylin-eosin staining. *CV* central vein, *PV* portal vein

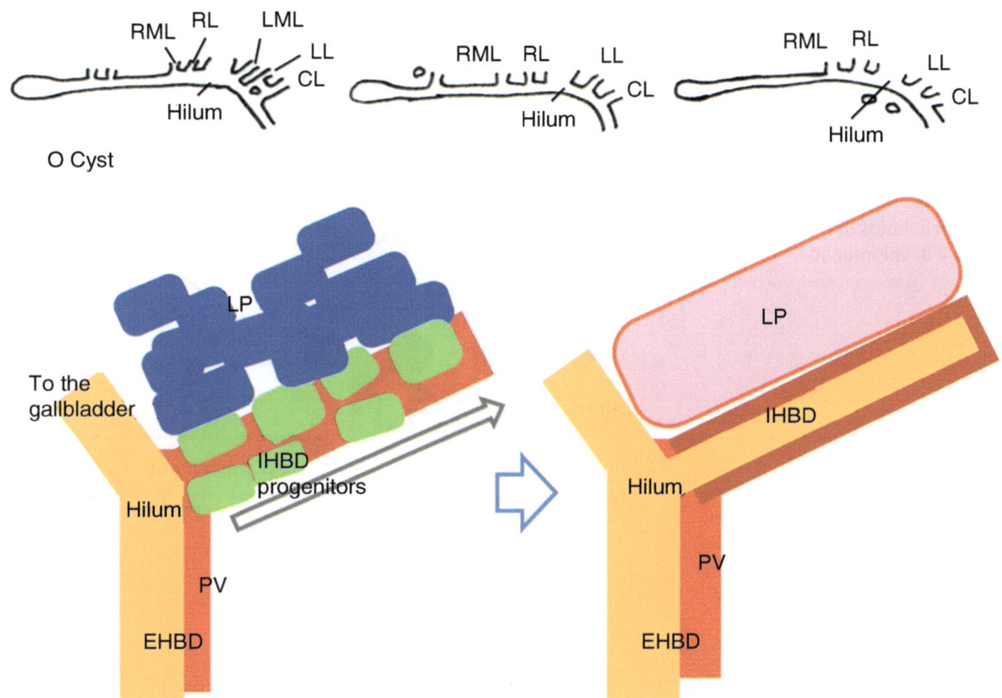


**Fig. 5.2** Secondary joining of extrahepatic bile ducts and intrahepatic bile progenitors (ductal plates). (**a**) Various connections of extrahepatic bile ducts with intrahepatic bile duct progenitors at E15.5 in syngeneic C3H/HeSlc strain mice. Cyst development in the hilum is noted in one of syngeneic mice. *CL* caudal lobe, *LL* left lobe, *LML* left medial lobe, *RL* right lobe, *RML* right medial lobe. (**b**) Discontinuous bile duct progenitors appearing around portal veins. They connect with one another with development. Bile duct formation proceeds from the hilum to the periphery. *EHBD* Extrahepatic bile duct, *IHBD* intrahepatic bile duct, *LP* liver parenchyma, *PV* portal vein

17.5, intrahepatic bile ducts having squamous epithelial cells and supported by connective tissue cells develop around portal veins (Fig. 5.1e). Hepatocyte maturation starts at E13.5, and hepatocytes become larger at E16.5.

Extrahepatic bile ducts appear earlier than, and is independent of intrahepatic bile ducts. At perinatal stages, the biliary gland develops in the cystic duct and common bile duct (Fig. 5.1f). Smooth muscle is well developed around the gallbladder. Both extrahepatic and intrahepatic bile ducts do not have smooth muscle tissues.

## 5.3 Mechanisms of Bile Duct Development

Although portal mesenchyme induces adjacent hepatoblasts to give rise to epithelial cells of intrahepatic bile ducts during liver development, several signaling molecules may be involved in this induction, including Jag1, Wnt5a, and TGFβ1-3 (Fig. 5.3) [7–10]. In addition to biliary cell differentiation, portal mesenchyme may play a key role in the secondary connection of extrahepatic bile ducts with intrahepatic ductal plates, and of each ductal plate. It may also regulate bile duct morphogenesis from ductal plates. Jag1 may control this morphogenetic step [11]. However, it is still unknown how these histogenetic events are regulated at a molecular level.

When molecular characterization of portal veins is performed during mouse liver development, they have a molecular signature, including expression of connexin37, connexin40, and Jag1 in their endothelial cells from E10.5 at the latest (Fig. 5.4a–c) [12]. Expression of Hes1, one of target genes for Jag1-Notch2 signaling, is immunohistologically detected in intrahepatic biliary progenitor cells, and endothelial cells and mesenchyme cells of portal veins from E13.5 on. However, not all biliary progenitor cells are positive for Hes1 (Fig. 5.4d). Thus, molecular mechanisms of intrahepatic bile duct development may be more complicated than expected. Nerve cells, which are acetylated tubulin-positive, are detected only in portal veins near the hilum in E15.5 and E17.5 livers (Fig. 5.4e), and enter the liver along portal veins after birth, suggesting that nerve cells are not directly involved in development of ductal plates along portal veins.

*Hes1* knockout mouse exhibits agenesis of extrahepatic bile ducts and their differentiation into the pancreatic tissue [13]. Notch signaling may suppress pancreatic development in extrahepatic bile ducts. Sox17 haploinsufficiency causes an impaired development of the smooth muscle tissue of the gallbladder, which results in embryonic cholecystitis [1].

## 5.4 Importance of Hepatocyte Maturation in Intrahepatic Bile Duct Morphogenesis

Inactivation of the gene coding for C/EBPα, which engages in transcriptional regulation of several liver-specific enzymes such as carbamoylphosphate synthase I and phosphoenolpyruvate carboxykinase, induces pseudoglandular

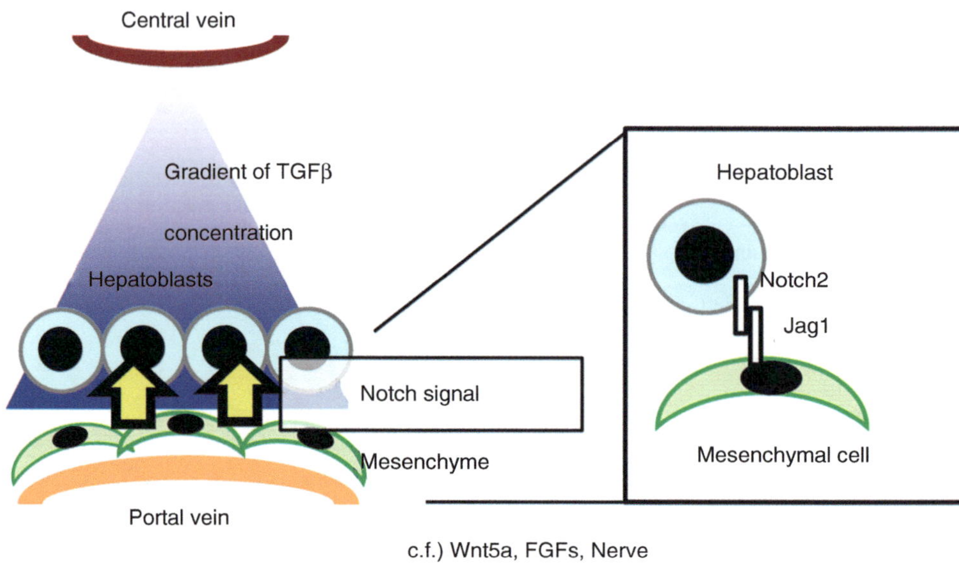


**Fig. 5.3** Molecular mechanism of intrahepatic bile duct formation. Portal mesenchyme may induce adjacent hepatoblasts to give rise to biliary epithelial cells through Jag1-Notch2 signaling. TGFβ concentration in liver lobules may involve biliary development

tissues in addition to the suppression of hepatic maturation (Fig. 5.5a, b) [14]. In its knockout liver, occasional (stochastic) expression of biliary markers (Spp1, Sox9, and cytokeratins) in the parenchyma also occurs (Fig. 5.5c, d) [15]. These data indicate that the loss of C/EBPα expression may be a prerequisite for biliary cell differentiation. The knockout bile ducts around portal veins are abnormal for *Spp1* and Sox9 expressions and are not segregated from the parenchyma. From these data, the maturation of liver parenchyma through C/EBPα expression may be required for normal bile duct morphogenesis (Fig. 5.5e) [15]. Several signaling molecules, including Jag1, TGFβ1, and FGFs, were upregulated in microarray data of the knockout livers, and they may be involved in normal intrahepatic bile duct development.

## 5.5 Bile Duct Development In Vitro

An in vitro culture system, in which normal bile duct development proceeds, is required to demonstrate molecular mechanisms of bile duct formation or to screen the effect of various factors, including growth factors, toxic chemicals, and viruses possibly causing the BA, on bile duct development. A recent paper has indicated that Sox17 haploinsufficiency causes the dysfunction of smooth muscle tissue in the gallbladder using organ culture of fetal liver fragments with the gallbladder, which may lead to BA [1]. When murine liver fragments at E12.5, which do not have intrahepatic bile duct development, are cultured in vitro using Trowell's organ culture technique, intrahepatic bile ducts are not constructed irrespective of the presence of the hilum part and extrahepatic bile ducts (Fig. 5.6a) [16]. When both proximal liver fragments containing the hilum part and extrahepatic bile ducts, and distal liver fragments at E12.5 are transplanted into the testis for 2 months, they similarly generate mature liver tissue accompanied by intrahepatic bile ducts around portal veins [17, 18]. The mature tissue has a hepatic zonation of ammonia metabolizing enzymes.

The importance of Notch signaling in intrahepatic bile duct development has been indicated in vitro. When inhibitors for Notch signaling is added to the culture medium of primary hepatoblasts, they inhibit biliary cell differentiation [19]. By contrast, when Notch intracytoplasmic domain (NICD) is overexpressed in primary hepatoblasts, it stimulates biliary differentiation in vitro. Other signaling molecules, including Wnt5a and vasoactive intestinal peptide, also stimulate biliary development in three-dimensional cultures of hepatoblasts in collagen gels [9, 20]. However, it should be noted that cyst structures were formed but no bile ducts were formed in these cultures.

When endodermal cells of the liver primordium are recombined and cultured with chick lung mesenchyme in vitro, they construct typical duct epithelial cells with mature hepatocytes [21]. Because these endodermal cells contain progenitors for epithelial cells of extrahepatic bile ducts and gallbladder, they may respond to the stimuli of lung mesenchyme to make duct structures. When hepatoblasts isolated from E12.5 mouse livers with a temperature-reversible gelation polymer were recombined and cultured with avian lung mesenchyme in vitro, they never formed ductular structures as seen in cultures of liver endodermal cells (Fig. 5.6b, c). Addition of Jag1 peptides promoted isolated hepatoblasts to express biliary markers (Fig. 5.6d).

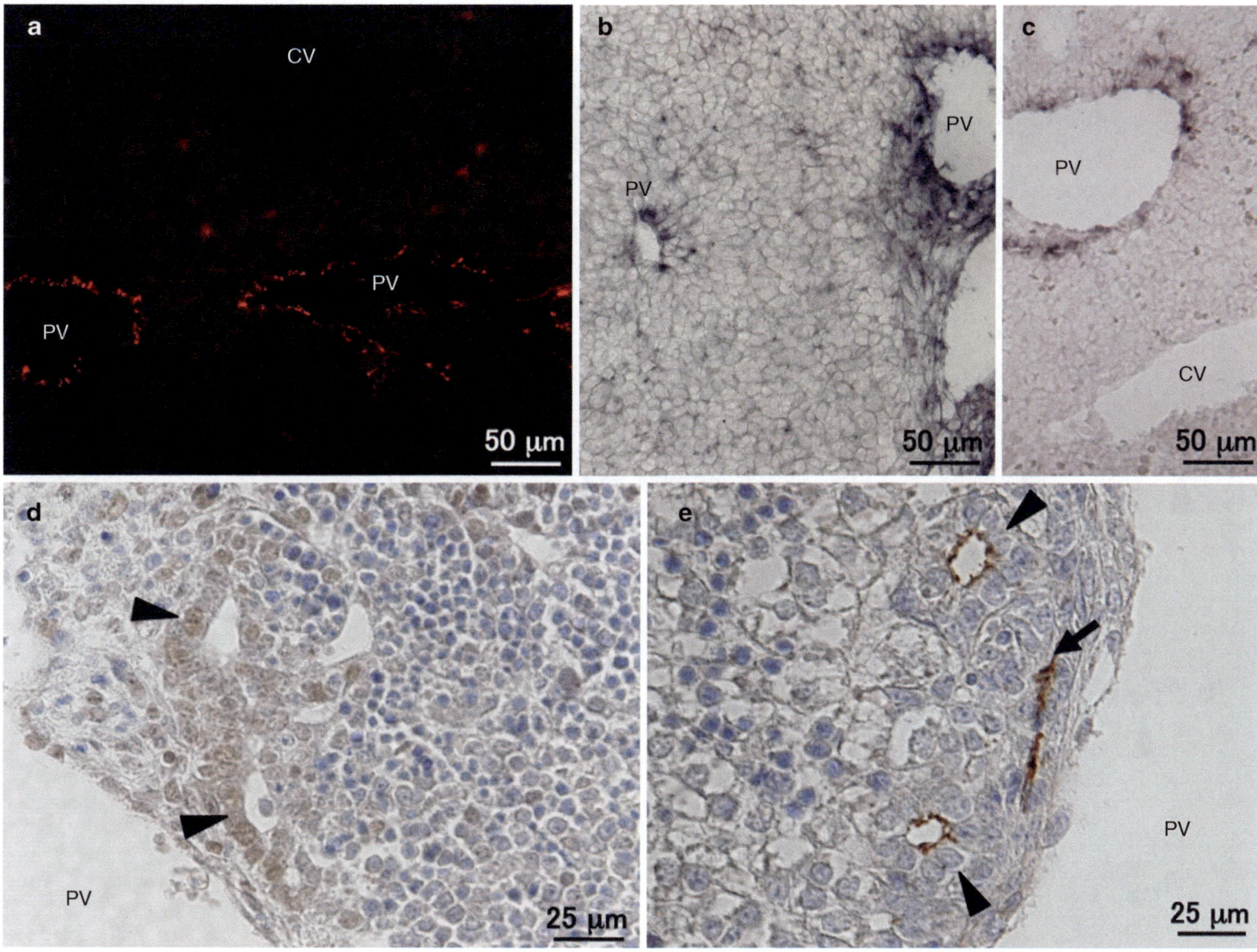


**Fig. 5.4** Immunohistochemical characterization of portal vein tissues in fetal mouse livers. (**a**) Immunohistochemical detection of connexin40 in endothelial cells of portal veins at E12.5. Those of central veins do not express connexin40. (**b**, **c**) in situ hybridization of *Jag1* mRNA in E12.5 and E15.5 mouse liver, respectively. Portal endothelial cells and mesenchyme cells express *Jag1*. (**d**) Hes1 expression in biliary progenitors, and endothelial cells and mesenchyme cells of portal veins at E15.5. Not all biliary progenitors (arrowheads) are positive. (**e**) Immunodetection of nerve cells with anti-acetylated tubulin. Nerve cells (arrow) are detected only in portal veins near the hilum in E17.5 liver. Apical staining of bile progenitors is derived from acetylated tubulin-positive cilia. Arrowheads indicate ductal plates. *CV* central vein, *PV* portal vein

Special mesenchyme expressing Jag1 in portal veins may be important for bile duct formation.

Our preliminary data indicated that several growth factors, which are upregulated in C/EBPα knockout livers having pseudoglandular structures in place of mature hepatic tissue, stimulated bile duct development in organ cultures of fetal liver fragments, especially of the proximal fragments containing the hilum part, but not the distal liver fragments. The data suggest that the hilum part may have a decisive center for bile duct formation.

## 5.6 Conclusion

Bile duct development may be a stochastic event for secondary joining of extrahepatic bile ducts and intrahepatic bile ducts. Several signaling molecules may be involved in bile duct development, including Jag1, Wnt5a, and TGFβ. An in vitro culture system having normal bile duct development should be developed to reveal molecular mechanisms of BA as well as those of bile duct development.

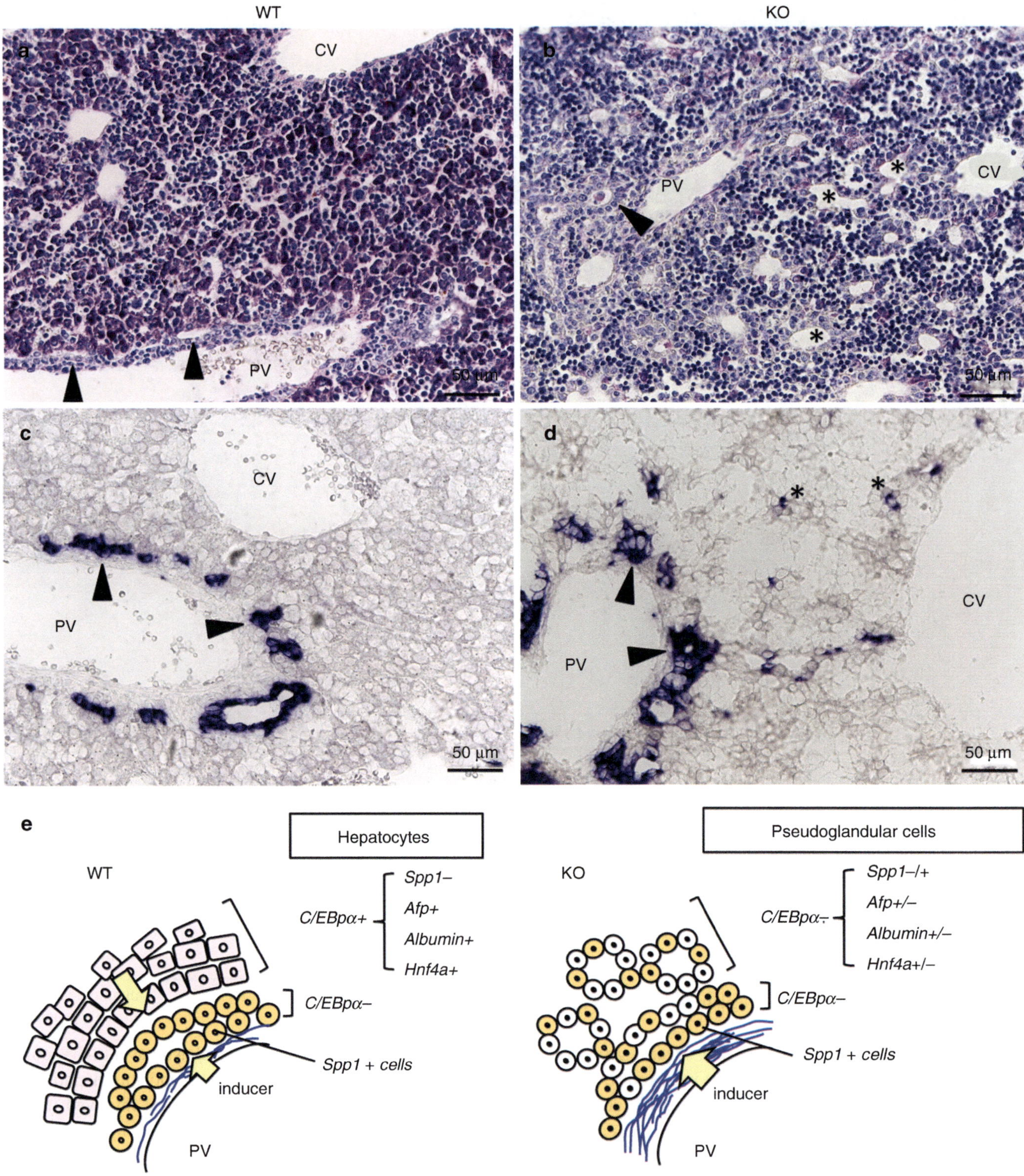


**Fig. 5.5** Impairment of hepatocyte maturation and abnormal biliary development in *C/EBPa*-knockout mouse liver at E17.5. (**a**, **b**) Periodic acid-Schiff (PAS)-hematoxylin staining of wild-type and knockout livers, respectively. Glycogen storage is impaired in the knockout liver, compared with that of the wild-type liver. Pseudoglandular cells (asterisks) are noted in the liver parenchyma, including those of pericentral regions. (**c**, **d**) in situ hybridization of *Spp1* in wild-type and knockout livers, respectively. *Spp1* expression in the wild-type liver is highly specific for periportal biliary epithelial cells. By contrast, *Spp1* expression in the knockout liver is heterogeneous and shows a mosaic pattern of positive cells and negative cells even in periportal bile duct progenitors. *Spp1*-positive cells are also detectable in the parenchymal regions. Arrowheads and asterisks indicate periportal biliary structures and parenchymal cells, respectively. (**e**) C/EBPα expression and bile duct formation. Normal biliary development may need maturation of the hepatic parenchyma. *CV* central vein, *PV* portal vein

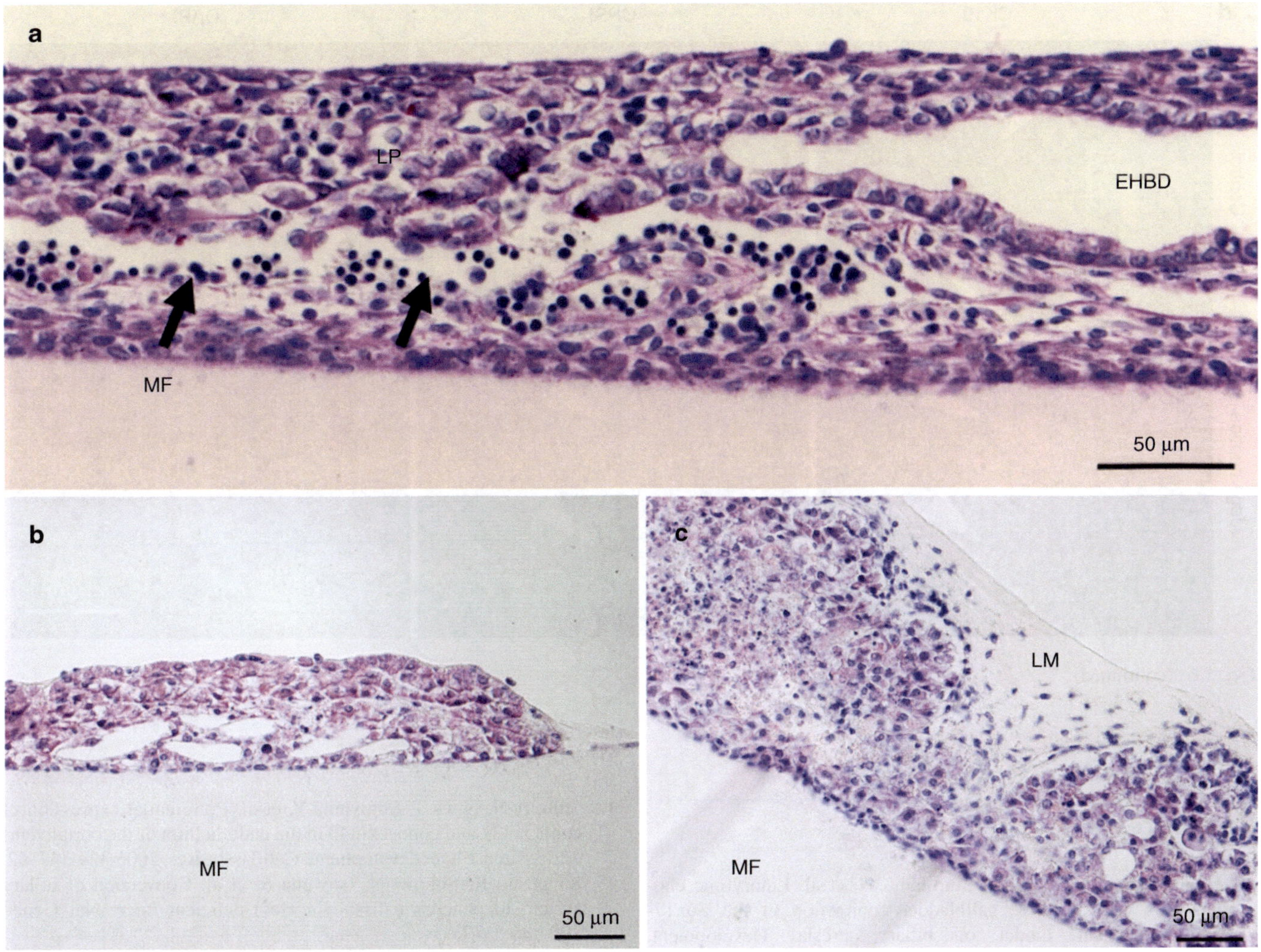


**Fig. 5.6** Bile duct development in organ culture of liver fragments of fetal mice. (**a**) Proximal liver fragments with extrahepatic bile duct in vitro for 5 days (PAS-hematoxylin staining). No intrahepatic bile duct develops around a portal vein-like structure (arrows). (**b**) Culture of E12.5 hepatoblasts isolated with a temperature-responsive gelation polymer for 5 days (hematoxylin-eosin staining). (**c**) Co-culture of purified E12.5 hepatoblasts with quail lung mesenchyme for 5 days (hematoxylin-eosin staining). The mesenchyme does not induce bile duct development. (**d**) Immunofluorescent analyses of hepatic cell aggregate cultured in a temperature-responsive gelation polymer for 5 days. Addition of Jag1 peptide (10 μg/ml) in the culture medium increases cytokeratin19-positive cells (yellow arrowheads), and decreases carbamoylphosphate synthase I-positive cells (white arrowheads). *EHBD* extrahepatic bile duct, *LM* lung mesenchyme, *LP* liver parenchyma, *MF* membrane filter

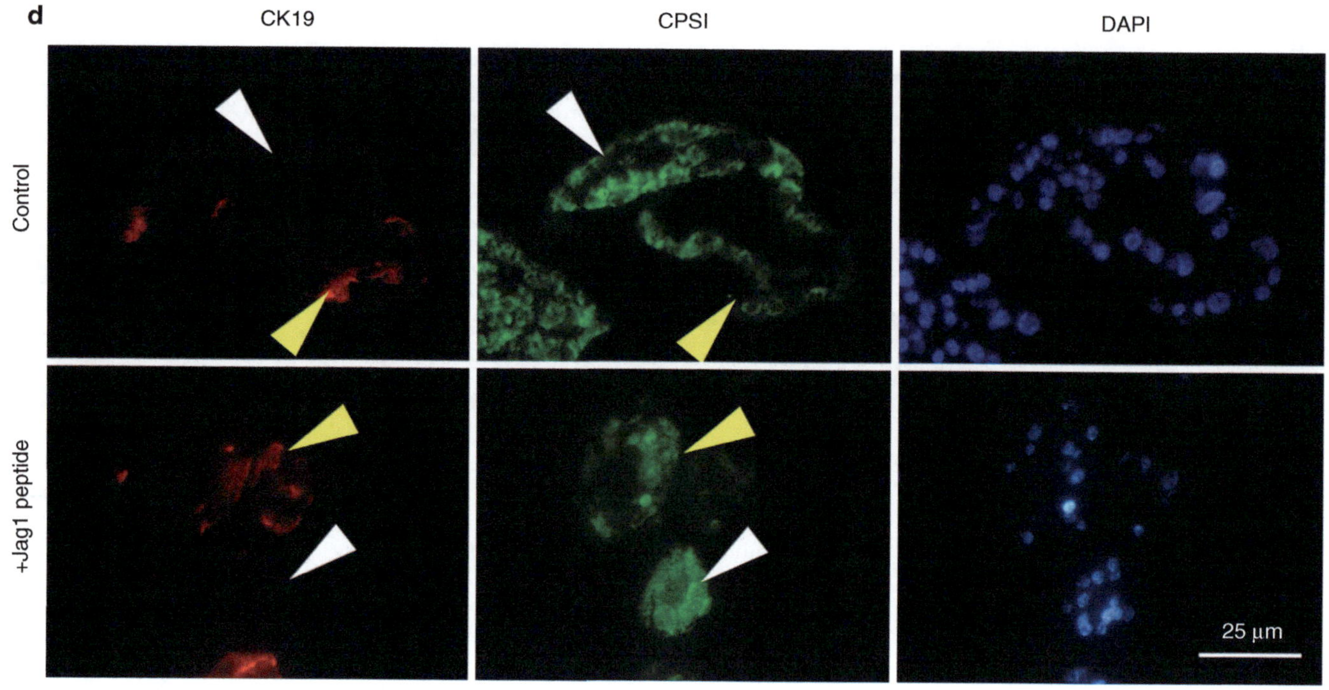


Fig. 5.6 (continued)

## References


1. Higashiyama H, Ozawa A, Sumitomo H, et al. Embryonic cholecystitis and defective gallbladder contraction in the Sox17-haploinsufficient model of biliary atresia. Development. 2017;144:1906–17.
2. Mazziotti MV, Willis LK, Heuckeroth RO, et al. Anomalous development of the hepatobiliary system in the inv mouse. Hepatology. 1999;30:372–8.
3. Mohanty SK, Lobeck I, Donnelly B, et al. Rotavirus reassortant-induced murine model of liver fibrosis parallels human biliary atresia. Hepatology. 2020;71:1316–30.
4. Shimadera S, Iwai N, Deguchi E, et al. The inv mouse as an experimental model of biliary atresia. J Pediatr Surg. 2007;42:1555–60.
5. Shiojiri N. Development and differentiation of bile ducts in the mammalian liver. Microsc Res Tech. 1997;39:328–35.
6. Shiojiri N, Katayama H. Secondary joining of the bile ducts during the hepatogenesis of the mouse embryo. Anat Embryol. 1987;177:153–63.
7. Antoniou A, Raynaud P, Cordi S, et al. Intrahepatic bile ducts develop according to a new mode of tubulogenesis regulated by the transcription factor SOX9. Gastroenterology. 2009;136:2325–33.
8. Clotman F, Jacquemin P, Plumb-Rudewiez N, et al. Control of liver cell fate decision by a gradient of TGFb signaling modulated by Onecut transcription factors. Genes Dev. 2005;19:1849–54.
9. Kiyohashi K, Kakinuma S, Kamiya A, et al. Wnt5a signaling mediates biliary differentiation of fetal hepatic stem/progenitor cells in mice. Hepatology. 2013;57:2502–13.
10. McCright B, Lozier J, Gridley T. A mouse model of Alagille syndrome: *Notch2* as a genetic modifier of *Jag1* haploinsufficiency. Development. 2002;129:1075–82.
11. Hofmann JJ, Zovein AC, Koh H, et al. Jagged1 in the portal vein mesenchyme regulates intrahepatic bile duct development: insights into Alagille syndrome. Development. 2010;137:4061–72.
12. Shiojiri N, Niwa T, Sugiyama Y, et al. Preferential expression of connexin37 and connecxin40 in the endothelium of the portal veins during mouse liver development. Cell Tissue Res. 2006;324:547–52.
13. Sumazaki R, Shiojiri N, Isoyama S, et al. Conversion of biliary system to pancreatic tissue in Hes1-deficient mice. Nat Genet. 2004;36:83–7.
14. Yamasaki H, Sada A, Iwata T, et al. Suppression of C/EBPα expression in periportal hepatoblasts may stimulate biliary cell differentiation through increased HNF6 and HNF1b expression. Development. 2006;133:4233–43.
15. Akai Y, Oitate T, Koike T, et al. Impaired hepatocyte maturation, abnormal expression of biliary transcription factors and liver fibrosis in *C/EBPα*(Cebpa)-knockout mice. Histol Histopathol. 2014;29:107–25.
16. Shiojiri N, Mizuno T. Differentiation of functional hepatocytes and biliary epithelial cells from immature hepatocytes of the fetal mouse *in vitro*. Anat Embryol. 1993;187:221–9.
17. Shiojiri N. The origin of intrahepatic bile duct cells in the mouse. J Embryol Exp Morphol. 1984;79:25–39.
18. Shiojiri N, Wada J, Gebhardt R. Heterogeneous carbamoylphosphate synthetase I expression in testicular transplants of fetal mouse liver. Eur J Cell Biol. 1998;75:389–92.
19. Tanimizu N, Miyajima A. Notch signaling controls hepatoblast differentiation by altering the expression of liver-enriched transcription factors. J Cell Sci. 2004;117:3165–74.
20. Sato A, Kakinuma S, Miyoshi M, et al. Vasoactive intestinal peptide derived from liver mesenchymal cells mediates tight junction assembly in mouse intrahepatic bile ducts. Hepatol Commun. 2020;4:235–54.
21. Shiojiri N, Koike T. Differentiation of biliary epithelial cells from the mouse hepatic endodermal cells cultured *in vitro*. Tohoku J Exp Med. 1997;181:1–8.

# Pathogenesis: Overview

# 6

A. Inui and T. Fujisawa

It is clear that biliary atresia (BA) is not a single disease with defined etiology and predictable response to treatment [1]. Rather it seems to a phenotype characterized by extrahepatic biliary obliteration or absence connected to an array of abnormal, intrahepatic ductules often lacking the usual branching pattern of mature ducts [1].

BA is a disease of the intrahepatic and extrahepatic biliary tree that causes liver injury as a result of extrahepatic obstruction. BA occurs in one in 8000 to 18,000 live births and appears to be more frequent in Asians and Africans than Europeans and more common in females than males. Epidemics of BA in humans have not been described and it rarely appears in clusters, temporal, or geographic. The clinical phenotype of BA is classified into several variants (Table 6.1) [2], these include isolated, typical BA (80%), BA with cystic dilatations of the biliary tree (5–10%), a variant attributed to cytomegalovirus (CMV) infection (5–10%), and several variants with associated congenital diseases which are generally grouped together as biliary atresia-splenic malformation syndrome (BASM: 5–15%). Whether these different variants have different causes is not clear, but their clinical course and response to Kasai hepatic portoenterostomy (HPE) may differ [2, 3].

Recently, inflammation of the extrahepatic bile duct irreversible fibrosis, which causes an abnormal immune response against some antigens.

**Table 6.1** Classification of biliary atresia (BA) phenotypes

| BA phenotype | Incidence and features |
|---|---|
| I. Isolated form | 80% of patients, variable jaundice-free period and after birth, absence of other major congenital malformations |
| CMV variant | Variable incidence based on geography and methodological detection, poor response to HPE |
| II. Congenital Malformation form | 10–20% of patients with at least one major congenital malformation, early onset of jaundice, poorer outcome after HPE |
| a. BASM variant | 1–10% of patients, associated, laterality defects (poly/asplenia, midline liver, interrupted IVC, intestinal malrotation, preduodenal portal vein, congenital heart disease), poor response to HPE |
| b. BA with major malformation variant (non-laterality defect) | 5–10% of patients, with major cardiovascular, gastrointestinal, and genitourinary malformation that are related to laterality |
| c. Cystic variant | 8% of patients, might co-exist with BASM, better response to HPE than over variants in this group |

## 6.1 Infectious Causes

The American pediatrician Landing suggested that there might be a common factor in the etiology of choledochal cyst, neonatal hepatitis, and BA in the 1970s invoking the influence of a hepatotropic virus capable of causing cholangiolar and actual structural bile damage [4].

Initially supporting evidence for this was provided by Moreki et al. showing higher titers of antibodies against reovirus type 3 compared to jaundiced infants without BA [5]. In a later study, Tyler et al. detected reovirus RNA in liver and/or biliary tissues by RT-PCR in 55% of infants with BA and almost 80% of patients with choledochal cysts [6]. However, Saito et al. could find no evidence of reovirus RNA in over 60 infants with BA, choledochal cyst, and a variety of other hepatobiliary pathologies using similar technology [7].

Candidates for causative viruses other than reovirus are rotavirus, and CMV have been proposed etiologies of BA. The *Rhesus* rotavirus (RRV)-induced BA mouse model has proved helpful in investigating the role of viruses and inflammation in pathogenesis of bile duct injury in BA. The largest body of literature supporting a viral infection as an

A. Inui (✉) · T. Fujisawa
Department of Pediatric Hepatology and Gastroenterology, Saiseikai Yokohamashi Tobu Hospital, Yokohama, Japan
e-mail: a_inui@tobu.saiseikai.or.jp; t_fujisawa@tobu.saiseikai.or.jp


M. Nio (ed.), *Introduction to Biliary Atresia*, https://doi.org/10.1007/978-981-16-2160-4_6

initiating event in BA pathogenesis pertains to CMV [2]. CMV DNA was identified in 60% of BA patients at the time of diagnosis in one study [8]. Xu et al. stained various DNAs with fluorescent antibodies using liver biopsy samples obtained at HPE in 85 Chinese BA patients [8]. CMV DNA was found in 51/85 and they proposed CMV is one of the important etiologies for BA in China. In this point of view, Brindley et al. reported that liver T cell responses to CMV were identified in the majority of BA patients at diagnosis, suggesting perinatal CMV infection as a plausible initiator of bile duct damage of regulatory T cells (Tregs) in BA implies decreased inhibition and autoreactivity allowing for exaggerated bile duct injury [9]. Zani et al. reported that a subgroup of BA patients with CMV-IgM positivity at diagnosis had higher rates of jaundice, liver inflammation, fibrosis, and need for transplant [10]. Regarding CMV and BA, Bezerra et al. suggested it is plausible that the infection is short lived, leading to an inability to identify the virus in some cases, and that viral infection of cholangiocytes sets the stage for an aberrant autoimmune response targeting cholangiocytes and leading to progressive biliary injury and cirrhosis [2].

The other causative virus is group C rotavirus looking promising. Riepenhoff-Talty et al. in a key paper published in 1996 identified, using RT-PCR, rotavirus DNA in half of 20 liver samples from infants with BA or choledochal cyst [11]. However, more recently negative reports have been made regarding the relation between group C rotavirus and BA.

As Bezerra et al. state [2], a search for the etiology of BA may require viral infection diagnosis, such as detection of universal virus in the liver tissue. The weakness of the viral hypothesis has to be that many viruses or at least parts of their genome can be found later in infants [12].

## 6.2 Environmental Toxins

Spontaneous outbreaks of a BA-like disease in neonatal livestock in Australia recently led to the identification of biliary toxin called biliatresone [12, 13]. However, humans are almost certainly not exposed to this toxin. Furthermore, the use of biliatresone in model systems has already yielded important insights into the disturbed cellular pathways involved in bile duct damage and repair [2].

## 6.3 Developmental Immaturity of the Neonatal Bile Ducts

BA occurs only in newborns, suggesting that the fetus and young neonate, by virtue of developmental stage, are particularly susceptible to injury and dysregulated repair (fibrosis) after an insult to the biliary tree [2]. The human and murine hepatobiliary systems follow the same general pattern of development, although in relative terms have different time courses [14].

Approximately 10% of children with BA in the Western world have associated BASM. These associations, which have been reported in 7.5% of 308 cases of BA treated between 1975 and 1991 in Kings College [15, 16]. The progress of BASM remains controversial [17].

The embryological development of the biliary tree and liver is complex. There are histological and immune-histochemical similarities between 11 and 13 week's gestation and the appearance of established BA. Bile is produced by hepatocytes from 12 week's gestation and coincident with this there are remodeling, selection, and deletion of bile ducts originating from the ductal plate membrane to form the definitive pattern of proximal intrahepatic bile ducts. Tan et al. [16] have suggested that BA without syndromic features may present an arrested development of these biliary radicals.

Cystic BA can be defined as cystic change in an otherwise obliterated biliary tract and is seen in about 5–10% of most large series [17]. The cyst itself may contain bile (–20%) implying onset after the establishment of continuity between intra- and extrahepatic ducts (10–12 weeks gestation) or mucus [17]. Around half of these are picked up antenatally on the maternal ultrasound scan and they have a good prognosis post HPE [18].

In 1992, Desmet reported morphological and immunohistological features of the developing bile duct in early pregnancy, and BA retained the fetal morphology due to the shared bile duct epithelium [19]. The ductal plate is a hepatic precursor cell that forms from about 7 to 8 weeks of gestation and is remolded into mature intrahepatic bile duct. Many studies have been conducted, the pathological diagnosis is difficult and the relation between DPM and BA has not been clarified. The association between mutation in biliary tract development-related genes and BA has been investigated, but the causal relationship is still unclear.

On the other hand, in animal experiments, Spence J et al. reported Sox 17 [20] and Sumazaki et al. [21] reported Hes 1 which is a gene that converts pancreatic tissue to the biliary system in mice, others include HNF6 [22], HNF-1β [23], and Hhex [24].

## 6.4 Genetics

BA shows little evidence of being genetic: familial cases are rarely found, and most twin studies discordance of the disease, even between identical twins [2].

In 2020, Garcia-Barecelo et al. reported BA sensitive genes using genome-wide association study (GWAS) [25]. Large-scale genetic screening studies in the Chinese population have shown that there were are two particular single nucleotide polymorphisms (SNPs) (rs17095355C/T and re10509906 G/C) in the *ADD3* gene, located in the 10q24.2 region which appears to be more frequent in infants with BA ($n = 134$) versus controls [26]. Further genetic probing of the region was performed in 171 Caucasian infants with BA confirming association outside of China and identified the strongest signal at re7099604 in intron 1 of the *ADD3* gene [27]. Another potential causative gene, glypican 1 (GPC1), has garnered attention through GWAS of DNA copy number variation that identified a potential region of susceptibility to BA on chromosome 2q37.353, which was replicated in an independent cohort of patients demonstrating heterozygous of deletion of GPC1 as the sole in this region [28].

As described above, there are some candidate genes that develop BA, but the definitive gene is not yet clear.

## 6.5 The Immune Dysregulation

During the 1990s, Dillon et al. identified abnormal expression of ICAM-1 and less commonly VCAM-1 in the livers of 7 infants with BA suggesting the triggering phase of an inflammatory reaction was occurring [29].

In this point of view, Davenport et al. followed this using a larger cohort of 28 Infants and confirmed significant abnormal expression of ICAM-1, VCAM, and E-selection on sinusoidal and biliary epithelium in 50%, 25%, and 10%, respectively [30]. And they have analyzed inflammatory response and noted that there was abnormal class II antigen HLA-DR expression particularly on Kupffer cells and proliferating bile ducts.

Thus, abnormalities in immune system are considered to play a central role in the pathogenesis of BA [31]. Activated immune cells have been identified in BA livers at diagnosis, and have been linked experimentally to autoimmunity, amplification of epithelial injury, and bile duct obstruction [31].

The Cincinnati group has been reporting the relation between cell-mediated immunity and various kind of cytokines.

In 2004, Shivakumar et al. addressed the hypothesis that production of IFN gamma is a key pathogenic mechanism of disease using a mouse model of rotavirus-induced biliary atresia [32]. Furthermore, they comprehensively analyzed gene expression in BA patients and liver tissue of neonatal intrahepatic cholestasis, and reported that IFN gamma was significantly elevated in BA patients.

In general, autoimmune diseases develop from either a primary breakdown in tolerance or secondary to a deficiency in immune regulation [2]. Regulatory T cells (Treg), characterized by the expression of the transcription factor FOXP3, are essential to control the low levels of autoreactivity that occur normally in humans [2]. In the RRV-induced model of BA and in human BA, defects in the number and function of Treg have been associated with autoreactive T cells targeting bile epithelia [33]. One mechanism to explain Treg deficits is hypermethylation of the FOX3 promoter region, resulting in decreased Treg function [34].

Analyses of human tissues have shown that CD4+ and CD8+ lymphocytes are activated in BA, populate the livers at diagnosis and express Th1 cytokines, such as IFN gamma interleukin (IL)-2, and tumor necrosis factor-alpha [31, 35]. More direct functional insight emerged from the report that CD4+ and CD8+ lymphocytes undergo oligoclonal expansion in the liver and bile duct remnants, and activate upon exposure to CMV [36].

In 2009, Shivakumar et al. revealed that in human liver tissue of BA, NK cells were significantly infiltrated in the portal area and cholangiocytes [36].

In 2011, Saxena et al. Showed that plasmacytoid dendritic cells (pDC) were significantly infiltrated in the liver tissue of BA patients. In experiments using pDC-deficient mice, pDC released IL-15 and released NK cells [37].

Thus, in BA, immune cells and various cytokines are considered to be involved in extrahepatic bile duct injury. It is clear that the innate immune system is important for BA.

Recently, it was reported that the relationship between microRNA (miRNA) and various diseases. MicroRNAs (miRNAs) are small noncoding RNAs that bind to target mRNAs and induce mRNA cleavage, destabilization, or translational repression [38]. It was reported that miR-29a/29b-1 are upregulated in the RRV-BALB/c model of BA. Consistent with this increase in miR-29 levels of DNA methyltransferase 3, a direct target of miR-29, are likewise decreased [39]. The reciprocal relation between miR-29 and methyltransferase gene expression in experimental BA is remarkable given the recent observation that DNA hypomethylation leads to bile defects in a zebrafish model and correlates with clinical BA [39, 40].

## 6.6 Maternal Microchimeris

Suskind et al. first showed that using fluorescent in situ hybridization (FISH) there was a consistent presence of double X chromosomes in male infant livers with BA but not in male livers with neonatal hepatitis used as controls [41]. The maternal cells appear to be CD8+ CD45+ and therefore stem cells with the potential to differentiate into progenitor lymphocytes, effector lymphocytes or differentiated biliary epithelial cell [42]. The maternal chimerism theory is interesting, but it is necessary to further analyze why only the bile duct is the target of immunity [43].

## References


1. Lakshminarayanan B, Davenport M. Biliary atresia: a comprehensive review. J Autoimmun. 2016;73:1–9.
2. Bezerra J, Welis RG, Mack CL, et al. Biliary atresia: clinical and research challenges for 21st century. Hepatology. 2018;68:1163–73.
3. Asai A, Miethke A, Bezerra JA. Pathogenesis of biliary atresia: defining biology to understand clinical phenotypes. Nat Rev Gastroenterol Hepatol. 2015;12:342–52.
4. Landing BH. Considerations of the pathogenesis of neonatal hepatitis, biliary atresia and choledochal cyst – the concept of infantile obstructive cholangiopathy. Prog Pediatr Surg. 1974;6:113–39.
5. Moreki R, Glaser JH, Cho S, Balisterei WB, Horwitz MS, et al. Biliary atresia and reovirus type 3 infection. NEJM. 1982;307:481–4.
6. Tyler KL, Sokol RJ, Oberhaus SM, et al. Detection of reovirus RNA in hepatobiliary tissues from patients with extrahepatic biliary atresia and choledochal cysts. Hepatology. 1998;27:1475–82.
7. Saito T, Shinozaki K, Matsunaga T, et al. Lack of evidence for reovirus infection in tissues from patients with biliary atresia and congenital dilatation of bile duct. J Hepatol. 2004;40:203–11.
8. Xu Y, Yu J, Zhang R, Yin Y, Ye J, Tan L, Xia H. The perinatal infection of cytomegalovirus is an important etiology of biliary atresia in China. Clin Pediatr (Phila). 2015;51:109–13.
9. Brindley SM, Lanham AM, Karrer FM, Tucker RM, Fontenot AP, Mack CL. Cytomegalovirus-specific T cell reactivity in biliary atresia at the time of diagnosis associated with deficits in regulatory cell. Hepatology. 2012;55:1130–8.
10. Zani A, Quaglia A, Hadzix N, Zuckerman M, Davenport M. Cytomegalovirus-associated biliary atresia: an aetiological and prognostic subgroup. J Pediatr Surg. 2015;50:1739–45.
11. Riepenhoff-Talty M, Gouvea V, Evans MJ, et al. Detection of group C rotavirus in infants with extrahepatic biliary atresia. J Infect Dis. 1996;174:8–5.
12. Lorent K, Gong W, Koo KA, Waisbourd-Zinman O, Karjoo S, Zhao X, Stealy I, et al. Identification of a plant isoflavonoid that causes biliary atresia. Sci Transl Med. 2015;7:286ra267.
13. Raynaud P, Carpenitier R, Antoniou A, et al. Biliary differentiation and bile duct morphogenesis in development and disease. Int J Biochem Cell Biol. 2011;43:245–56.
14. Davenport M, Kerkar N, Mieli-Vergani G, Mowat AP, Howard ER. Biliary atresia: King's College Hospital experience. J Pediatr Surg. 1997;32:479–85.
15. Davenport M, Savage M, Mowat AP, Howard ER. The biliary atresia splenic malformation syndrome. Surgery. 1993;113:662–8.
16. Tan CEL, Driver M, Howard ER, Moscoso GJ. Extrahepatic biliary atresia: a first trimester event? Clues from light microscopy and immunohistochemistry. J Pediatr Surg. 1994;29:808–14.
17. Nio M, Wada M, Sasaki H, et al. Long-term outcomes of biliary atresia with splenic malformation. J Pediatr Surg. 2015;50:2124–7.
18. Caponcelli E, Knisley AS, Davenpor M. Cystic biliary atresia: an etiologic and prognostic subgroup. J Pediatr Surg. 2008;43:1619–24.
19. Desmet VJ. Ludwig symposium on biliary disorders-part I. Pathogenesis of ductal plate malformations. Mayo Clin Proc. 1998;73:80–9.
20. Spence JR, Lange AW, Lin SC, Kaestner KH, Lowy AM, Kim I, Whitsett JA, Wells JM. Sox17 regulates organ linage segregation of vettral forgut progenitor cell. Dev Cell. 2009;17:62–74.
21. Sumazaki JR, Shiojiri N, Isoyama S, Masu M, Keino-Masu K, Osawa M, Nakauchi H, Kageyama R, Matsui A. Conversion of biliary system to pancreatic tissue in Hes1-deficient mice. Nat Genet. 2004;36:83–7.
22. Clotman F, Lannoy VJ, Reber M, Cereghini S, Cassiman D, Jaquemin P, Roskams T, Rousseau GG, Legaigre FP. The onecut transcription factor HNF 6 is required for normal development of biliary tract. Development. 2002;129:1819–20.
23. Coffiner C, Gresh L, Fiette L, Tronche F, Schutz G, Babinet C, Pontglio M, Yaniv M, Barra J. Bile system morphogenesis defects and liver dysfunction upon targeted deletion of HNF1beta. Development. 2002;129:1829–38.
24. Hunter MP, Wilson CM, Jiang X, Vong R, Vasavada H, Kaestner KH, Bogue CW. The homeobox gene Hhex is essential for proper hepatoblast differentiation and bile duct morphogenesis. Dev Biol. 2007;15:355–67.
25. Garcia-Barcelo MM, Yeng MY, Miano XP, Tang CS, Cheng G, et al. Genome-wide association study identifies a susceptibility locus for biliary atresia on 10q24.2. Hum Mol Genet. 2010;19:2917–25.
26. Zeng S, Sun P, Chen Z, Mao J, Wang J, Wang B. Association between single nucleotide polymorphisms in the ADD3 gene and susceptibility to biliary atresia. PLoS One. 2014;9:e107977.
27. Tsai EA, Grochowski CM, Loomes KM, Bessho K, Hakonarson H, Bezerra JA, et al. Relationship of a GWAS signal in a Caucasian population implicates ADD3 in susceptibility to biliary atresia. Hum Genet. 2014;133:235–42.
28. Cui S, Leyva-Vega M, Tsai EA, Eauclaire SF, Glessner JT, Hakonarson H, et al. Evidence from human and zebrafish that GPC1 is a biliary atresia susceptibility gene. Gastroenterology. 2013;5(144):1107–1115.e3.
29. Dillon P, Belchis D, Tracy T, Cilley R, Hafer L, Krummel T. Increased expression of intracellular adhesion molecules in biliary atresia. Am J Pathol. 1994;145:263–7.
30. Davenport M, Gonde C, Redkar R, Koukoulis G, Tredger M, Mieli-Vergani G, et al. Immunohistochemistry of the liver and biliary tree in extrahepatic biliary atresia. J Pediatr Surg. 2001;36:1017–25.
31. Shivakumar P, Campbell K, Sabia G, Mietheke A, Tiao G, MnNeal M, Ward R, Bezerra JA. Obstruction of extrahepatic bile ducts by lymphocytes is regulated by IFN gamma in experimental biliary atresia. J Clin Invest. 2004;114:322–9.
32. Mack CL. What causes biliary atresia? Unique aspects of the neonatal immune system provide clues to disease pathogenesis. Cell Mol Gastroenterol. 2015;1:267–74.
33. Lages CS, Simmons J, Chougnet CA, Miethke AG. Regulatory T cells control the CD8 adaptive immune response at the time of ductal obstruction in experimental biliary atresia. Hepatology. 2012;56:219–27.
34. Mack CL. The pathogenesis of biliary atresia: evidence for a virus-induced autoimmune disease. Semin Liver Dis. 2007;27:233–42.
35. Mack CL, Falta MT, Sullivan AK, Karrer F, Sokol RJ, Fontenot AP. Oligoclonal expansions of CD4; and CD8+ T-cells in the target organ of patients with biliary atresia. Gastroenterology. 2007;133:278–87.
36. Shivakumar P, Sabla G, Whitington P, Choignet CA, Bezerra JA. Neonatal NK cells target the mouse duct epithelium via Nkg2d and drive tissue-specific injury in experimental biliary atresia. J Clin Invest. 2009;119:2281–90.
37. Sexena V, Shivakumar P, Sabla G, Chougnet C, Bezerra JA. Dendritic cells regulate natural killer cell activation and epithelial injury in experimental biliary atresis. Sci Transl Med. 2011;28:102ra94.
38. Nakamura K, Tanoue A. Etiology of biliary atresias as a developmental anomaly: recent advances. J Hepatobiliary Pancreat Sci. 2013;20:459–64.
39. Hands NJ, Horner AM, Master ZR, Boateng LA, LeGuen C, Uvadova M, et al. MicroRNA profiling identifies miR-29 as a regulator of disease-associated pathways in experimental biliary atresia. JPGN. 2012;54:186–92.
40. Matthews RP, Eauclaire SF, Mugnier M, Lorent K, Cui R, Ross MM, et al. DNA hypomethylation causes bile duct defects in zebrafish and a distinguishing feature of infantile biliary atresia. Hepatology. 2011;53:905–14.

41. Suskind DL, Rosenthal P, Heyman MB, Kong D, Magrane G, Baxter-Lowe LA, et al. Maternal microchimerism in the livers of patients with biliary atresia. BMC Gastroenterol. 2004;4:14.
42. Muraji T. Maternal microchimerism in biliary atresia: are maternal cells effector cells, targets, or just bystander? Chimerism. 2015;5:1–5.
43. Schwarz KB, Haber BH, Rosenthal P, Mack CL, Moore J, Bove K, Bezzera JA, et al. Extrahepatic anomalies in infants with biliary atresia: results of large prospective North American multicenter study. Hepatology. 2013;58:1724–31.

# Genetics and Epigenetics in the Pathogenesis of Biliary Atresia

7

Kazuhiko Bessho and Yoshinori Satomura

**Abstract**

Biliary atresia (BA) is a progressive fibroinflammatory obstruction affecting both the intra- and extrahepatic bile ducts, and 25%–30% of neonatal cholestasis cases are caused by BA. Despite intensive research, the precise pathogenesis of BA remains elusive. Abnormal biliary development has been cited as a potential trigger of BA along with viral infection, immune disorder, and toxins.

As supported by several studies, genetic susceptibility factors predispose an individual to BA. The incidence of BA differs in terms of ethnic and racial backgrounds. In addition, 10%–20% of patients manifest non-hepatic anomalies associated with laterality defects. There are genetically modified animal models of BA that exhibit abnormal bile duct development with/without non-hepatic anomalies. Furthermore, several copy number studies and genome-wide association studies complementary to animal models suggest that *GPC1* copy number and polymorphism in the region of *ADD3* gene are susceptibility factors for BA. However, some studies demonstrate contradictory findings for each observation.

In this chapter, we discuss recent progress in the understanding of genetic and epigenetic contributions in the pathogenesis of BA according to patient-based studies and complementary studies using animal models of bile duct development and injury.

**Keywords**

Multifactorial · Isolated form · BASM syndrome · Laterality defects · Ductal plate malformation · Genome-wide association study (GWAS) · Epigenetic regulation · Disease-specific induced pluripotent stem cells

K. Bessho (✉) · Y. Satomura
Department of Pediatrics, Graduate School of Medicine, Osaka University, Osaka, Japan
e-mail: bessho@ped.med.osaka-u.ac.jp

## 7.1 Introduction

Biliary atresia (BA) is a progressive fibrosing obstructive cholangiopathy of the intra- and extrahepatic biliary system, causing bile flow obstruction and neonatal cholestasis. BA is the most common cause of neonatal cholestasis, accounting for 25%–30% of cases, and it is a primary indication for liver transplantation in children.

Recently, it has been gradually accepted that BA is not a single disease entity; it is the end result of a progressive process affecting the bile duct, leading to partial or complete duct obliteration [1]. However, its precise mechanisms remain undefined. Nonetheless, intensive patient-based studies coupled with experimental animal models of BA suggest that the pathogenesis of this disease is multifactorial. The mechanisms of BA are thought to involve an interplay between genetic susceptibility and environmental factors that are currently undefined, causing a proinflammatory response that targets the biliary epithelium and generates the clinical spectrum of BA.

The survival of patients with BA has been dramatically improved by Kasai operation (hepatoportoenterostomy) and liver transplantation, but to develop new medical therapies, a greater understanding of its pathogenesis is indispensable. In this chapter, we present an overview of the prevailing hypothesis for BA pathogenesis, mainly focusing on genetic susceptibility.

## 7.2 Ethnics

The incidence of BA varies in terms of patients' ethnic and racial backgrounds, and it is higher in the Asian and Pacific regions than in other regions. The reported incidence was highest in French Polynesian (1 per 3000 live births) [2], followed by Taiwan (1 per 5000) [3], Japan (1 per 10,000) [4]; the United States (1 per 15,000) [5]; and the United Kingdom and France (1 per 17,000–19,000) [6, 7]. Conversely, the


M. Nio (ed.), *Introduction to Biliary Atresia*, https://doi.org/10.1007/978-981-16-2160-4_7

lowest incidence is in the Netherlands, with 1 per 19,000 [8]. These data suggest an inherited predisposition to BA.

## 7.3 Familial Recurrence and Twin Studies

While BA incidence varies among ethnic groups, BA rarely occurs within families [9, 10], and twins are discordant for the disease. Xu et al. conducted a systematic review and meta-analysis to analyze the characteristics and patterns of BA in twins [11]. They found 12 articles investigating 35 twin pairs. Out of 70 twin subjects, 36 had BA, with only one pair of dizygotic twins demonstrating concordance for the disease and having one affected family member. Hence, BA does not demonstrate strict Mendelian inheritance.

## 7.4 Clinical Variants

Several clinical variants of BA have been described according to the time of onset, anatomical features of the extrahepatic bile duct, and presence of non-hepatic malformations and cytomegalovirus infection [12]. On the basis of these variants, cholestasis occurs in approximately 10%–35% of infants soon after birth, without jaundice-free interval, indicating an embryonic (fatal) form. Furthermore, 10%–20% of patients with an embryonic form have extrahepatic malformations, such as the biliary atresia splenic malformation syndrome (BASM), which includes cardiovascular defects, polysplenia, abdominal situs inversus, intestinal malrotation, intestinal lumen obstruction (from the esophagus to jejunum), annular pancreas, and preduodenal portal vein [13, 14]. This type of BA complicated with extrahepatic malformations suggests the involvement of genetic factors in the pathogenesis of the disease in affected patients.

## 7.5 Abnormal Morphogenesis of Biliary Tree

The presence of ductal plate malformation (DPM) in some livers from infants with BA suggests abnormal morphogenesis of biliary tree contributes to the pathogenesis of BA. During the development of the intrahepatic bile ducts, primitive hepatic precursor cells form bilayer structure in the mesenchyme surrounding the portal vein approximately 8 weeks of fetal life, indicating the "ductal plate" [15]. Around 12 weeks of gestational age, the ductal plate is remodeled to form mature tubular ducts, with DPM as the abnormality of this remodeling. Considering DPM is also one of the characteristic features detected in ciliopathies that are often associated with abnormal left–right axis determination, and some of the infants with BA, especially in the embryonic form, have extrahepatic abnormalities related to visceral organ symmetry, such as polysplenia, abdominal situs inversus, intestinal malrotation, and cardiovascular defects, it is suggested that mutations or polymorphisms in genes that are implicated in the development of DCM and determination of left–right axis could act as susceptibility factors or modifier genes in the pathogenesis of BA.

Such genes include *INVS*, which participates in normal kidney development and left–right axis determination, *CFC1*, which is a cofactor of NODAL signaling, and *ZIC3*, which is a transcription factor in the early stages of left–right body axis formation. Deletion of the mouse *Invs* gene mostly results in visceral inversion and hepatobiliary defects [16]. In addition, *Invs* transgenic mice manifest obstructive jaundice and intrahepatic DPM [17], suggesting that mutations in the human *INVS* gene are closely related to BA. However, a study of the *INVS* gene in seven patients with BA showed no mutations [18]. Meanwhile, some cases of BA patients with laterality defects displayed heterozygous variants in *CFC1* gene [19, 20], and two cases of BA associated with congenital heart disease harbored mutations in *ZIC3* gene [21], suggesting that these gene mutations are associated with BA.

Overexpression or inactivation of various transcription factors (e.g., *Hes1*, *Hnf6*, *Hnf1b*, and *Foxa1/2*) also leads to abnormal biliary development including DPM-like lesions in mice [22]. However, mutational analyses in patients with BA associated with laterality defects failed to identify mutations in these genes [18]. Thus, further investigation is needed to clarify the role of mutations in these genes in the pathogenesis of human BA.

## 7.6 Copy Number Study and Genome-Wide Association Studies

Leyva-Vega et al. conducted a Genome-Wide Association Studies (GWAS) to screen 35 North American patients with BA for genomic deletions and duplications that might confer susceptibility to BA [23]. They identified two unrelated patients with BA with overlapping heterozygous deletions spanning 30 genes of 2q37.3, which constituted the critical region for susceptibility to BA.

From the same group, Ciu et al. extended the study by examining copy number variations in 61 patients with BA and 5088 healthy controls [24]. They found that the region at 2q27.3 was heterozygously deleted in 4 additional patients (6 patients in total, 9.84%) and 4 controls (0.08%) ($P = 4.4 \times 10^{-10}$). The region contained only one gene, that is, *GPC1*, which encodes GPC-1 protein, located in the apical membrane of cholangiocytes. GPC-1 is a heparan sulfate proteoglycan that regulates Hedgehog signaling and inflammation. Knockdown of *Gpc1* in zebrafish with morpholino resulted in developmental biliary defects [24]. *The*

*Gpc1* morphant larvae had decreased number and complexity of bile duct and less uptake of dye in gallbladder than control morphants. Interestingly, when the Hedgehog antagonist cyclopamine was administered in *Gpc1* morphant, these phenotypes were partially rescued, and the zebrafish injected with recombinant Sonic Hedgehog had similar biliary defects to *Gpc1* morphant. Along with the reduced GPC1 expression in the apical membrane of cholangiocytes in the liver of patients with BA, GPC1, and the Hedgehog pathway may have potential roles in BA pathogenesis. However, *GPC1* deletion alone is insufficient to develop BA because the father of one of the two patients in the study by Leyva-Vega et al. bared the deletion but did not manifest any liver diseases.

Several other GWASs have been conducted, and the loci on chromosome 10q24 have the strongest association. Using a genome-wide SNP array, Garcia-Barcelo et al. compared 181 Chinese patients with BA and 481 healthy controls [25]. They found that several SNPs, including rs17095355 that is located in an intergenic locus on chromosome 10q24.2 were strongly associated with BA. The association between rs17095355 and BA was validated with 124 independent Chinese patients with BA and 90 controls. This intergenic SNP is located at downstream of *XPNPEP1* and upstream of *ADD3* gene, which encodes F-actin-binding protein adducin 3 and regulates *ADD3* expression. Moreover, Tsai et al. examined whether this association is also present in a North American cohort by evaluating genotypes at 550,000 SNP loci in 171 patients with BA and 1630 controls. They used an SNP array that did not contain SNP rs17095355 itself. The most significant association was identified at rs7906904, which was located in the first intron of *ADD3*. They also examined the expression level of *XPNPEP1* and *ADD3* mRNAs in the liver tissue from infants with BA obtained during hepatoportoenterostomy. They found that *ADD3* expression, but not the *XPNPEP1* expression was significantly reduced. In a Thai cohort of 124 patients and 114 controls, rs17095355, which is the SNP locus associated with BA in Chinese populations, was also significantly associated with BA [26].

*ADD3* is expressed in the liver and biliary epithelial cells, especially in fetal livers. It participates in cytoskeleton remodeling, but no functional role has been assigned to the rs17095355 SNP. However, Tang et al. reported that the loss of the zebrafish ortholog *Add3a*, not *Xpnpep1*, leads to biliary structure defects and impaired biliary function [27]. *Add3a* morphants also showed upregulation of hedgehog pathway target genes, and inhibition of hedgehog rescued the phenotype. Furthermore, the combined knockdown of *Add3a* and *Gpc1* resulted in a more severe phenotype; hence, these genes might act within the same Hedgehog pathway.

Another group from Pittsburgh and Philadelphia conducted GWAS to identify potential susceptibility loci in 80 Caucasian patients with BA and 2818 controls. They found rs3126184 and rs10140366 in the 3′-flanking region (a putative enhancer region) of the *ARF6* gene on chromosome 14q21.3, and patients with BA had higher minor allele frequencies than the controls [28]. *ARF6* is activated in the EGF signaling pathway and regulates lever development. In zebrafish, *Arf6* knockdown upregulated the expression of *EGFR* and Hedgehog signaling genes; as a result, the intrahepatic biliary system was poorly developed. These results imply *GPC1*, *ADD3*, *AFP6* might serve as a susceptibility factor or disease modifier of BA.

Extraneous factors such as toxins and viral infections have been putative triggers of biliary injury in the pathogenesis of BA. In the 1990s, lambs in Australia had two BA-like endemics, suggesting that the grazing plants contained some toxins. A Philadelphian team screened and purified the chemical extracts of the plants by using a zebrafish bile excretion assay and identified a compound, which they named biliatresone, as the causative toxic molecule [29]. Biliatresone caused the obliteration of developed gallbladders and bile ducts in zebrafish, and in mouse cholangiocyte culture, it induced lumen obstruction and loss of polarity. Interestingly, the team found that the zebrafish mutant *ductbend* showed heightened sensitivity to biliatresone and that the *ductbend* locus was located on chromosome 22, which is a region that has synteny to human chromosome 10q24.2, the BA-susceptible loci in GWAS. Furthermore, the group found that biliatresone exerted its toxicity by decreasing intrahepatic levels of glutathione, and loss-of-function mutation in genes involved in glutathione synthesis and metabolism markedly increased susceptibility to biliatresone in zebrafish [30]. These views are good examples of linking an environmental toxin to genetic susceptibility factors in the pathogenesis of BA.

Other genes whose polymorphisms are linked to BA pathogenesis include *CD14* [31], *ICAM1* [32], *VEGF* [33], adiponectin [34], and *ITBG2* [35]. However, their biological relevance remains unknown.

## 7.7 Human Leukocyte Antigen

Based on the findings, that inflammation causes epithelial injury in BA and an ethnic variation exists in BA incidence, some studies explored the association of Human Leukocyte Antigen (HLA) with BA pathogenesis. A study from Brazil demonstrated that patients without associated malformations had significantly higher frequencies of HLA-B12, haplotypes A9-B5 and A28-B35, and their disequilibrium values than the controls [36]. In another study, the relationship between HLA and susceptibility to BA was investigated by retrospectively analyzing 392 Japanese patients with BA without extrahepatic anomalies and 828 healthy Japanese volunteers; a significantly positive association was observed between patients and HLA-DR2 [37]. DR2 was not independently associated with BA in two locus analyses, but a linkage disequilibrium between -A24, -B52, and -DR2 and a significantly higher frequency of the haplotype HLA-A24-B52-DR2 were found in such patients.

Meanwhile, studies from Europe [38] and the United States [39] did not detect statistically significant differences in the distribution of any HLA allele frequency.

Although results from human studies are contradictory, the susceptibility to biliary injury in the rotavirus-induced murine model varies among mouse strains as well as in the time of infection and the amount of virus administered; the highest susceptibility was found in Balb/c mice [40]. This finding may support the existence of some non-HLA-linked genetic predisposition to BA.

## 7.8 Epigenetic Regulations

### 7.8.1 Methylation

The importance of epigenetic influences on various disorders has been increasingly elucidated. DNA methylation is an epigenetic DNA modification process involved in the regulation of many biological processes, such as gene transcription, chromatin modification, genomic imprinting, and X-chromosome inactivation.

A study comparing gene expression patterns between livers with embryonic and perinatal BA reported that the expression of chromatin-modifying genes, such as *SMARCA-1*, *RYBP*, and *HDAC3*, and imprinting genes, such as *IGF2*, *PEG3*, *PEG10*, *MEG3*, and *IPW*, were upregulated in the embryonic form of BA [41].

Dong et al. demonstrated that genomic DNA isolated from $CD4^+$ T cells in infants with BA was hypomethylated compared with that in healthy controls. The expression level of *IFN-γ* mRNA in patients was significantly increased, with hypomethylation of the promoter region of the *IFN-γ* gene in $CD4^+$ T cells [42].

Recently, another group from Philadelphia examined the methylation status of specific genes in human livers affected with BA by using methylation microarray technology [43, 44]. They found that BA samples had DNA hypomethylation at specific genetic loci including Hedgehog pathway members *SHH* and *GLI2* and a region near the *PDGFA* locus compared with the healthy controls. Validation assays confirmed the increased transcriptional and protein expression of PDGFA in BA livers. In a complementary study, the injection of PDGF-AA protein dimer into zebrafish larvae caused biliary developmental and functional defects, and the activation of the Hedgehog pathway increased PDGF-A expression. These studies support that DNA methylation potentially contributes to BA pathogenesis.

### 7.8.2 MicroRNA

MiRNAs (miRNAs) are small noncoding RNA molecules that represent another epigenetic mechanism of DNA modification. Their roles in the pathogenesis of diseases have recently attracted considerable attention. MiRNAs are small single-stranded RNAs with 18–25 nucleotides long. They target mRNAs with a complementary sequence, causing degradation or repression of their translation, and also suppress the expression of target genes.

Bessho et al. examined biliary transcriptomes from the rotavirus-induced murine model of BA to identify miRNAs that have potential roles in the pathogenesis of bile duct obstruction [45]. They identified 14 miRNAs whose expression was suppressed during duct obstruction. They also detected 26 potential target genes with coordinate expression by the 14 miRNAs, which were related to organogenesis and immune response. Hence, these miRNAs may play a regulatory role in the pathogenesis of experimental BA.

## 7.9 Genes Responsible for Other Causes of Intrahepatic Cholestasis as Modifiers of BA

In infancy, BA shares clinical features with other causes of neonatal intrahepatic cholestasis, such as Alagille syndrome and progressive familial intrahepatic cholestasis (PFIC).

Kohsaka et al. investigated mutations in *JAG1* gene, which is responsible for Alagille syndrome, in 102 patients with BA and found inhibition of missense mutation in 9 patients [46], without showing extrahepatic manifestation of Alagille syndrome. The *JAG1* gene mutations were generally found in severely ill patients undergoing liver transplantation at less than 5 years of age.

Furthermore, Sangkhathat et al. identified mutations in genes responsible for other infantile intrahepatic cholestatic syndromes by conducting whole-exome sequencing on the DNA obtained from 20 patients with BA, which was diagnosed by operative findings and histopathology [47]. They detected 13 rare variants in the following nine genes: 4 in *JAG1* (Alagille syndrome), 2 in *MYO5B* (PFIC type 6), and 1 each in *ABCC2* (Dubin–Johnson syndrome), *ABCB11* (PFIC type 2), *UGT1A1* (Crigler–Najjar syndrome), *MLL2* (Kabuki syndrome), *RFX6* (Mitchell–Riley syndrome), *ERCC4* (Fanconi anemia), and *KCNH1* (Zimmermann–Laband syndrome). Therefore, mutations in genes previously annotated in various infantile cholestatic syndromes may be one of the factors that increase the risk of developing BA or at least severe biliary injury triggered by some factors.

## 7.10 Disease-Specific Induced Pluripotent Stem Cells

Recently, Tian et al. generated disease-specific induced pluripotent stem cells (iPSCs) from six patients with BA, and by applying a genome-editing approach to healthy iPSCs to create iPSCs with defined mutations in the GWAS BA loci for *GPC1* and *ADD3* [48]. These two iPSCs were studied for their in vitro biliary differentiation potential. Both of them showed reduced biliary differentiation with increased fibrosis, which was lowered by antifibrotic drug treatment. Thus, BA-iPSCs can provide human-relevant models/assays to elucidate the pathogenesis of BA and to determine the corresponding therapeutic drugs.

## 7.11 Conclusion

Currently available studies cannot identify definitive causal genes or genetic models that can clearly explain the pathogenesis of BA. Future studies using novel technologies, such as disease-specific iPSC-based models of bile duct epithelial development, and in-depth analyses of the data from GWAS with a larger sample size will provide a better understanding of the genetic basis of BA pathogenesis and insights to stratify patients according to key mechanisms. Such studies will aid in designing innovative strategies for tailor-made treatment.

## References


1. Balistreri WF, Grand R, Hoofnagle JH, Suchy FJ, Ryckman FC, Perlmutter DH, et al. Biliary atresia: current concepts and research directions. Summary of a symposium. Hepatology. 1996;23(6):1682–92.
2. Vic P, Gestas P, Mallet EC, Arnaud JP. Biliary atresia in French Polynesia. Retrospective study of 10 years. Arch Pediatr. 1994;1(7):646–51.
3. Chiu CY, Chen PH, Chan CF, Chang MH, Wu TC, Taiwan Infant Stool Color Card Study Group. Biliary atresia in preterm infants in Taiwan: a nationwide survey. J Pediatr. 2013;163(1):100-3.e1.
4. Ando H, Inomata Y, Iwanaka T, Kuroda T, Nio M, Matsui A, et al. Clinical practice guidelines for biliary atresia in Japan: a secondary publication of the abbreviated version translated into English. J Hepatobiliary Pancreat Sci. 2021;28(1):55–61.
5. Hopkins PC, Yazigi N, Nylund CM. Incidence of biliary atresia and timing of hepatoportoenterostomy in the United States. J Pediatr. 2017;187:253–7.
6. McKiernan PJ, Baker AJ, Kelly DA. The frequency and outcome of biliary atresia in the UK and Ireland. Lancet. 2000;355(9197):25–9.
7. Chardot C, Carton M, Spire-Bendelac N, Le Pommelet C, Golmard JL, Auvert B. Epidemiology of biliary atresia in France: a national study 1986–96. J Hepatol. 1999;31(6):1006–13.
8. van Wessel DBE, Boere T, Hulzebos CV, de Kleine RHJ, Verkade HJ, Hulscher JBF, et al. Preterm infants with biliary atresia: a nationwide cohort analysis from the Netherlands. J Pediatr Gastroenterol Nutr. 2017;65(4):370–4.
9. Lachaux A, Descos B, Plauchu H, Wright C, Louis D, Raveau J, et al. Familial extrahepatic biliary atresia. J Pediatr Gastroenterol Nutr. 1988;7(2):280–3.
10. Smith BM, Laberge JM, Schreiber R, Weber AM, Blanchard H. Familial biliary atresia in three siblings including twins. J Pediatr Surg. 1991;26(11):1331–3.
11. Xu X, Zhan J. Biliary atresia in twins: a systematic review and meta-analysis. Pediatr Surg Int. 2020;36(8):953–8.
12. Asai A, Miethke A, Bezerra JA. Pathogenesis of biliary atresia: defining biology to understand clinical phenotypes. Nat Rev Gastroenterol Hepatol. 2015;12(6):342–52.
13. Davenport M, Savage M, Mowat AP, Howard ER. Biliary atresia splenic malformation syndrome: an etiologic and prognostic subgroup. Surgery. 1993;113(6):662–8.
14. Schwarz KB, Haber BH, Rosenthal P, Mack CL, Moore J, Bove K, et al. Extrahepatic anomalies in infants with biliary atresia: results of a large prospective North American multicenter study. Hepatology. 2013;58(5):1724–31.
15. Desmet VJ. Congenital diseases of intrahepatic bile ducts: variations on the theme "ductal plate malformation". Hepatology. 1992;16(4):1069–83.
16. Mazziotti MV, Willis LK, Heuckeroth RO, LaRegina MC, Swanson PE, Overbeek PA, et al. Anomalous development of the hepatobiliary system in the Inv mouse. Hepatology. 1999;30(2):372–8.
17. Shimadera S, Iwai N, Deguchi E, Kimura O, Fumino S, Yokoyama T. The Inv mouse as an experimental model of biliary atresia. J Pediatr Surg. 2007;42(9):1555–60.
18. Schon P, Tsuchiya K, Lenoir D, Mochizuki T, Guichard C, Takai S, et al. Identification, genomic organization, chromosomal mapping and mutation analysis of the human INV gene, the ortholog of a murine gene implicated in left-right axis development and biliary atresia. Hum Genet. 2002;110(2):157–65.
19. Davit-Spraul A, Baussan C, Hermeziu B, Bernard O, Jacquemin E. CFC1 gene involvement in biliary atresia with polysplenia syndrome. J Pediatr Gastroenterol Nutr. 2008;46(1):111–2.
20. Jacquemin E, Cresteil D, Raynaud N, Hadchouel M. CFCI gene mutation and biliary atresia with polysplenia syndrome. J Pediatr Gastroenterol Nutr. 2002;34(3):326–7.
21. Ware SM, Peng J, Zhu L, Fernbach S, Colicos S, Casey B, et al. Identification and functional analysis of ZIC3 mutations in heterotaxy and related congenital heart defects. Am J Hum Genet. 2004;74(1):93–105.
22. Bessho K, Bezerra JA. Biliary atresia: will blocking inflammation tame the disease? Annu Rev Med. 2011;62:171–85.
23. Leyva-Vega M, Gerfen J, Thiel BD, Jurkiewicz D, Rand EB, Pawlowska J, et al. Genomic alterations in biliary atresia suggest region of potential disease susceptibility in 2q37.3. Am J Med Genet A. 2010;152A(4):886–95.
24. Cui S, Leyva-Vega M, Tsai EA, EauClaire SF, Glessner JT, Hakonarson H, et al. Evidence from human and zebrafish that GPC1 is a biliary atresia susceptibility gene. Gastroenterology. 2013;144(5):1107–15.e3.
25. Garcia-Barcelo MM, Yeung MY, Miao XP, Tang CS, Cheng G, So MT, et al. Genome-wide association study identifies a susceptibility locus for biliary atresia on 10q24.2. Hum Mol Genet. 2010;19(14):2917–25.
26. Kaewkiattiyot S, Honsawek S, Vejchapipat P, Chongsrisawat V, Poovorawan Y. Association of X-prolyl aminopeptidase 1 rs17095355 polymorphism with biliary atresia in Thai children. Hepatol Res. 2011;41(12):1249–52.
27. Tang V, Cofer ZC, Cui S, Sapp V, Loomes KM, Matthews RP. Loss of a candidate biliary atresia susceptibility gene, add3a, causes

biliary developmental defects in Zebrafish. J Pediatr Gastroenterol Nutr. 2016;63(5):524–30.
28. Ningappa M, So J, Glessner J, Ashokkumar C, Ranganathan S, Min J, et al. The role of ARF6 in biliary atresia. PLoS One. 2015;10(9):e0138381.
29. Lorent K, Gong W, Koo KA, Waisbourd-Zinman O, Karjoo S, Zhao X, et al. Identification of a plant isoflavonoid that causes biliary atresia. Sci Transl Med. 2015;7(286):286ra67.
30. Zhao X, Lorent K, Wilkins BJ, Marchione DM, Gillespie K, Waisbourd-Zinman O, et al. Glutathione antioxidant pathway activity and reserve determine toxicity and specificity of the biliary toxin biliatresone in zebrafish. Hepatology. 2016;64(3):894–907.
31. Shih HH, Lin TM, Chuang JH, Eng HL, Juo SH, Huang FC, et al. Promoter polymorphism of the CD14 endotoxin receptor gene is associated with biliary atresia and idiopathic neonatal cholestasis. Pediatrics. 2005;116(2):437–41.
32. Arikan C, Berdeli A, Kilic M, Tumgor G, Yagci RV, Aydogdu S. Polymorphisms of the ICAM-1 gene are associated with biliary atresia. Dig Dis Sci. 2008;53(7):2000–4.
33. Lee HC, Chang TY, Yeung CY, Chan WT, Jiang CB, Chen WF, et al. Genetic variation in the vascular endothelial growth factor gene is associated with biliary atresia. J Clin Gastroenterol. 2010;44(2):135–9.
34. Udomsinprasert W, Tencomnao T, Honsawek S, Anomasiri W, Vejchapipat P, Chongsrisawat V, et al. +276 G/T single nucleotide polymorphism of the adiponectin gene is associated with the susceptibility to biliary atresia. World J Pediatr. 2012;8(4): 328–34.
35. Zhao R, Song Z, Dong R, Li H, Shen C, Zheng S. Polymorphism of ITGB2 gene 3′-UTR+145C/A is associated with biliary atresia. Digestion. 2013;88(2):65–71.
36. Silveira TR, Salzano FM, Donaldson PT, Mieli-Vergani G, Howard ER, Mowat AP. Association between HLA and extrahepatic biliary atresia. J Pediatr Gastroenterol Nutr. 1993;16(2):114–7.
37. Yuasa T, Tsuji H, Kimura S, Niwa N, Yurugi K, Egawa H, et al. Human leukocyte antigens in Japanese patients with biliary atresia: retrospective analysis of patients who underwent living donor liver transplantation. Hum Immunol. 2005;66(3):295–300.
38. Donaldson PT, Clare M, Constantini PK, Hadzic N, Mieli-Vergani G, Howard E, et al. HLA and cytokine gene polymorphisms in biliary atresia. Liver. 2002;22(3):213–9.
39. Mack CL, Anderson KM, Aubrey MT, Rosenthal P, Sokol RJ, Freed BM. Lack of HLA predominance and HLA shared epitopes in biliary Atresia. Springerplus. 2013;2(1):42.
40. Petersen C, Davenport M. Aetiology of biliary atresia: what is actually known? Orphanet J Rare Dis. 2013;8:128.
41. Zhang DY, Sabla G, Shivakumar P, Tiao G, Sokol RJ, Mack C, et al. Coordinate expression of regulatory genes differentiates embryonic and perinatal forms of biliary atresia. Hepatology. 2004;39(4):954–62.
42. Dong R, Zhao R, Zheng S. Changes in epigenetic regulation of CD4+ T lymphocytesin biliary atresia. Pediatr Res. 2011;70(6):555–9.
43. Matthews RP, Eauclaire SF, Mugnier M, Lorent K, Cui S, Ross MM, et al. DNA hypomethylation causes bile duct defects in zebrafish and is a distinguishing feature of infantile biliary atresia. Hepatology. 2011;53(3):905–14.
44. Cofer ZC, Cui S, EauClaire SF, Kim C, Tobias JW, Hakonarson H, et al. Methylation microarray studies highlight PDGFA expression as a factor in biliary atresia. PLoS One. 2016;11(3):e0151521.
45. Bessho K, Shanmukhappa K, Sheridan R, Shivakumar P, Mourya R, Walters S, et al. Integrative genomics identifies candidate microRNAs for pathogenesis of experimental biliary atresia. BMC Syst Biol. 2013;7:104.
46. Kohsaka T, Yuan ZR, Guo SX, Tagawa M, Nakamura A, Nakano M, et al. The significance of human jagged 1 mutations detected in severe cases of extrahepatic biliary atresia. Hepatology. 2002;36(4 Pt 1):904–12.
47. Sangkhathat S, Laochareonsuk W, Maneechay W, Kayasut K, Chiengkriwate P. Variants associated with infantile cholestatic syndromes detected in extrahepatic biliary atresia by whole exome studies: a 20-case series from Thailand. J Pediatr Genet. 2018;7(2):67–73.
48. Tian L, Ye Z, Kafka K, Stewart D, Anders R, Schwarz KB, et al. Biliary atresia relevant human induced pluripotent stem cells recapitulate key disease features in a dish. J Pediatr Gastroenterol Nutr. 2019;68(1):56–63.

# 8 Pathogenesis: Viral Infection

Kenichi Harada

**Abstract**

In biliary atresia (BA), extrahepatic bile ducts are initially affected and extrahepatic biliary obstruction causes cholestasis, a decrease in bile flow, leading to subsequent liver damage and a progressive loss of intrahepatic bile ducts. As speculated etiology of BA, although several viruses have been detected in the liver and biliary remnants in human BA samples, the virus' presence may not be necessary for the subsequent development of acquired immune-mediated bile duct injury. Lastly, recent BA studies have demonstrated a shift from innate to acquired immunity during the immune response to viral infections.

**Keywords**

Biliary atresia · Pathogenesis · CMV · Rotavirus
Reovirus · Innate immunity

## 8.1 Introduction

Biliary atresia (BA) is one of the most severe neonatal liver diseases. Initially, extrahepatic bile ducts are affected. Extrahepatic biliary obstruction will cause cholestasis, a decrease in bile flow, leading to subsequent liver damage and a progressive loss of intrahepatic bile ducts. Damaged intrahepatic bile ducts lead to obstructive outcomes, such as the profound loss of small intrahepatic bile ducts and recurrent cholestasis due to bile ducts paucity. Eventually, BA will progress to biliary cirrhosis and liver failure in the absence of treatment.

Usually, a Kasai portoenterostomy will successfully increase an infant's chance of survival. Since BA is not specific to the extrahepatic or intrahepatic bile ducts and that intrahepatic biliary lesions are considered secondary to extrahepatic bile duct obstruction, the treatment strategy should be different between extrahepatic and intrahepatic biliary lesions.

Other congenital biliary diseases, such as congenital biliary dilatation and paucity of intrahepatic bile ducts, have unknown etiology. However, BA's etiology is considered multifactorial, including genetic, environmental, and autoimmune. While the hepatitis virus is well-known to infect hepatocytes easily, cholangiocyte-tropic viruses have not been identified. Since a virus infection model of BA-like biliary lesion has been established, the role of viruses in the BA's etiopathogenesis has been under investigation.

In this chapter, the histogenesis of BA, the detection of viruses in clinical samples, and the experimental BA models are reviewed from the aspect of viral etiology in BA.

## 8.2 Histology

Perinatal BA in the newborn is histologically characterized by fibrosclerosing cholangitis, or the progressive fibro-obliterative lesions in the extrahepatic bile duct, which is associated with periductal and mucosal erosive inflammation and periductal fibrosis. These changes eventually result in the obliteration of the biliary lumen, replacement by fibrous scar, and the formation of lesion characteristic of BA (Figs. 8.1a, b). During the histogenesis of this ductopenic cholangiopathy, there is a concomitant increase in cell proliferation and the apoptosis of cholangiocytes in the affected bile ducts, suggesting that bile duct loss is caused by the imbalanced cell dynamics (1–3).

However, biliary remnants resected via the Kasai procedure shows that cholangitis does not occur uniformly throughout the extrahepatic biliary tree; most of the fibrous remnant completely lack biliary lumen and have been replaced by fibrous scar. On the other hand, cholangitis is found in the margins of both the duodenal and hepatic sides

K. Harada (✉)
Department of Human Pathology, Kanazawa University Graduate School of Medical Sciences, Kanazawa, Japan
e-mail: kenichih@med.kanazawa-u.ac.jp


M. Nio (ed.), *Introduction to Biliary Atresia*, https://doi.org/10.1007/978-981-16-2160-4_8

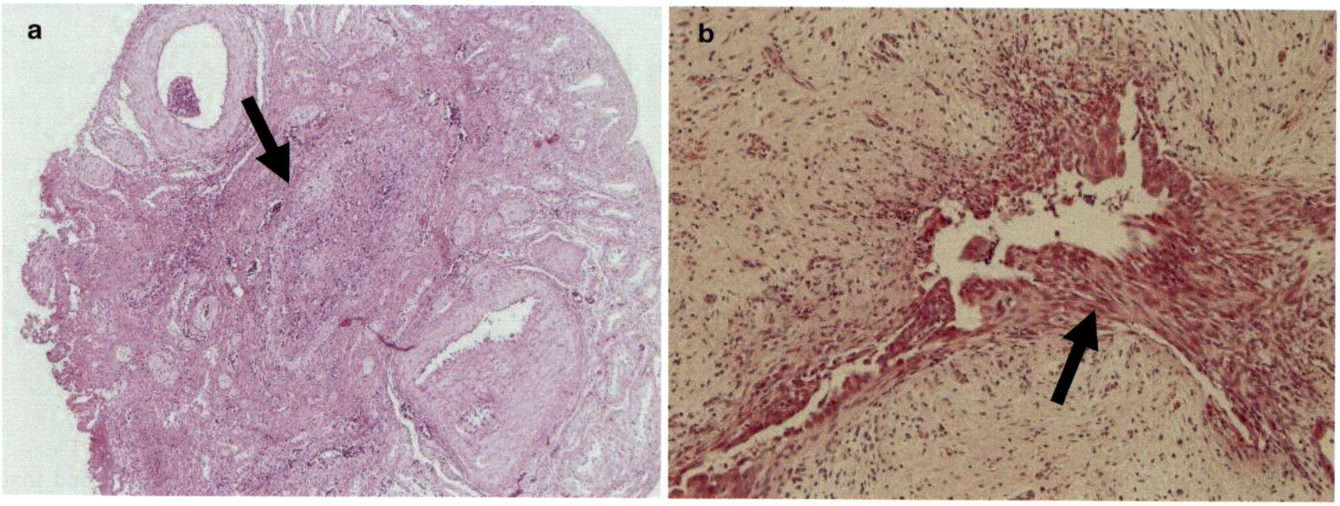


**Fig. 8.1** Cross sections of extrahepatic bile ducts (biliary remnant) in biliary atresia obtained by Kasai procedure. (**a**) Arrow denotes obliterative bile duct showing luminal occlusion and being replaced with fibrous tissue. (**b**) Bile duct shows erosive changes, a lack of epithelial lining, and signs of periductal inflammation. Mesenchymal components consisting of spindle-shaped cells (arrow) are found in the surface of the bile duct

of the extrahepatic bile duct. In the liver, biliary obstruction-related changes, such as ductular proliferation with irregular anastomosis resembling ductal plate malformation, variable portal edema, lobular cholestasis, and Mallory-Denk body, are visible within and around the fibrously expanded portal tracts. Also, there is periportal fibrosis in the portal-to-portal bridging. But these changes are due to extrahepatic biliary obstruction and may not be associated with the original etiology of BA. If without operation, the portal fibrosis progresses in the patient, further subdividing the hepatic lobule and resulting in biliary cirrhosis (4).

## 8.3 Virus Infection

Epidemiological studies implicate environmental and host factors, including viral, toxic, genetic abnormalities, and aberrant neonatal immune responses (5, 6) at the onset of BA.

In 1974, Landing et al. (7) first proposed that BA and other infant obstructive cholangiopathies were caused by a viral infection of the liver and hepatobiliary tree. Moreover, the BA's disease progression already starts in utero (8)—that is, the initial bile duct injury of BA occurs before birth—suggesting that the fetal bile duct is susceptible to causal agents such as viruses. Rotavirus, reovirus, cytomegalovirus (CMV), Epstein-Barr virus (EBV), and human herpesvirus (HHV)-6 have been identified in the clinical samples of BA (9–13); these viruses are also detected in neonatal hepatitis (10, 11). Therefore, multiple common virus species have been proposed to be viral factors of BA, but as shown in Table 8.1 (10–12, 14–26), Reoviridae (rotavirus and reovirus) and CMV have been identified as strong candidates of BA etiology.

### 8.3.1 Reoviridae

#### 8.3.1.1 The Mouse Model of Reovirus-Induced BA

Reoviridae is a family of double-strand RNA (dsRNA), epithelia-tropic viruses that include reovirus type 1 to 3, and rotavirus A to F groups. In particular, rotavirus type A is the most common etiological agent of acute diarrhea in young children.

Since the 1980s, several animal models of neonatal hepatitis and cholangitis have been established to study reovirus infections. In particular, the model of neonatal mice infected by reoviruses such as type A rhesus rotavirus (RRV) and type 3 reovirus (Abney) is a well-established study BA that is characterized by cholestasis due to bile duct obstruction (27–30). Several studies from abroad have modeled BA in mice by the intraperitoneal administration of rotavirus; however, such BA modeling has not been confirmed in Japan.

Rotavirus (RRV) has been shown to infect human and murine cholangiocytes similarly (31). Although RRV proteins are detected in the subepithelial cells in the RRV-infected BA model (32), RRV likely causes biliary diseases directly by targeting the cholangiocytes. RRV VP4 surface protein determines the epithelial tropism, and BA's onset is mediated by the VP4-specific activation of mononuclear cells (33). In the mouse models, RRV replication's influence on cholangiocytes was shown to be temporal; the robustness of RRV replication correlates with the severity of cholangi-

**Table 8.1** Summary of the published data on the incidence of viral DNA/RNA in hepatobiliary samples of children with biliary atresia

| Author | Year | Patient Cases | Detected Virus | Method | Positive/Total cases | Range of Age | Reference |
|---|---|---|---|---|---|---|---|
| Chang et al. | 1992 | 26 | CMV | PCR | 2/26 | 0.7–5 M | 11 |
| Steele et al. | 1995 | 14 | Reovirus type 3, M3 gene | Nested RT-PCR (hepatic tissue) | 0/14 | 3 W-3.5 M | 14 |
| | | 8 | Reovirus type 3, M3 gene | Nested RT-PCR (biliary tissue) | 0/8 | 21–105 D | |
| Riepenhoff-Talty et al. | 1996 | 19 | Rotavirus C, gene 5 | Nested RT-PCR | 10/20 | 24–103 D | 15 |
| | | 10 | Rotavirus A, gene 9 | Nested RT-PCR | 0/12 | 24–103 D | |
| | | 9 | Reovirus type 3, S3 gene | Nested RT-PCR | 0/9 | 24–103 D | |
| Bobo et al. | 1997 | 10 | Rotavirus A, B, C | Nested RT-PCR | 0/10 | 1 M-10 Y | 16 |
| Tyler et al. | 1998 | 20 | Reovirus, L1 | Nested RT-PCR | 11/20 | 1.5–6 M | 17 |
| Fischler et al. | 1998 | 18 | CMV | PCR | 9/18 | 1–21 W | 18 |
| Jevon et al. | 1999 | 12 | CMV | PCR; in situ hybridization | 0/12 | 44–200 D | 19 |
| Domiati-Saad et al. | 2000 | 9 | CMV | PCR | 1/9 | 1 M–4 Y | 10 |
| Saito et al. | 2004 | 26 | Reovirus, L3 | Nested RT-PCR | 0/26 | 0.7–46.6 M | 20 |
| De Tomasso et al. | 2005 | 32 | CMV | Nested PCR + antibody assay | 20/32 | 25–239 D | 21 |
| Fjær et al. | 2005 | 10 | CMV | Real-time PCR | 2/10 | 48–110 D | 12 |
| Rauschenfels et al. | 2008 | 74 | CMV | Real-time PCR | 8/74 | 19–149 D | 22 |
| | | 64 | Reovirus, L3 gene | Nested RT-PCR | 21/64 | 19–149 D | |
| | | 64 | Rotavirus, VP4 | Nested RT-PCR | 0/64 | 19–149 D | |
| Yaghobi et al. | 2011 | 34 | CMV | Nested PCR | 0/34 | 20–70 D | 23 |
| Soomro et al. | 2011 | 33 | CMV | PCR | 14/33 | 1–5 M | 24 |
| Xu et al. | 2012 | 85 | CMV | PCR | 51/85 | 12–180 D | 25 |
| Goel et al. | 2018 | 15 | CMV | Nested PCR | 8/15 | Not mentioned | 26 |

opathy (34). Lastly, RRV replication is regulated by IFN-α produced by cholangiocytes (34).

#### 8.3.1.2 The Detection of Reoviruses

Attempts to identify reoviruses in clinical samples from infants with BA, such as serum and liver tissue, have yielded varying and conflicting results. The detection rate of reoviruses in fresh samples using RT-PCR is 0–55% (14–17, 20). PCR, particularly nested PCR, is most sensitive; however, the detection rate is heavily influenced by the age of the infant with BA. Also, the PCR amplification efficiency is dependent on the targeted gene, primer sequences, and primer specificity. In addition, since Reoviridae are RNA viruses, the viral genome's degradation may affect its amplification; this is a problem that DNA viruses such as CMV do not have.

On the other hand, immunohistochemistry with anti-virus antibodies could detect reoviruses in the cholangiocytes in BA mice (35–37); the detection level was specific to certain antibodies.

The immunostaining of the Mx protein, which is known to mediate early innate immune response and a very sensitive marker for type I IFN activity against viral infection, is positive in hepatocytes and cholangiocytes. Mx's presence in hepatocytes and cholangiocytes suggests previous as well as present viral infection in BA (38). While the viral infection is necessary to initiate biliary lesion (in utero?), the virus' presence may be unnecessary in the progression of the bile duct injury mediated by acquired immunity. In fact, in RRV-infected mouse models, biliary injury is progressing after the disappearance of RRV.

#### 8.3.1.3 The Innate Immunity Against Reoviridae

While rotavirus type A is a well-known cause of acute infantile diarrhea, its role in causing damage to the bile duct is unclear; the keys to resolving this question may lie in the biliary innate immunity.

Human cholangiocytes express some of the Toll-like receptors (TLRs 1–6), which play a role in the biliary innate immunity (39, 40). In human cholangiocytes, TLR3 recognizes dsRNA (Fig. 8.2); therefore, cholangiocytes could mount a direct innate immune response against dsRNA viruses such as rotavirus and reovirus (39, 41).

Tolerance mechanisms such as TLR4-related endotoxin tolerance play a role in avoiding cytokine shock during the infection and maintaining mucosal homeostasis. Unlike other TLRs such as TLR4, the tolerance against TLR3 ligand is not present in human cholangiocytes (41, 42). Therefore, the tolerance against dsRNA viruses does not exist. The biliary innate immune response likely continues until the com-

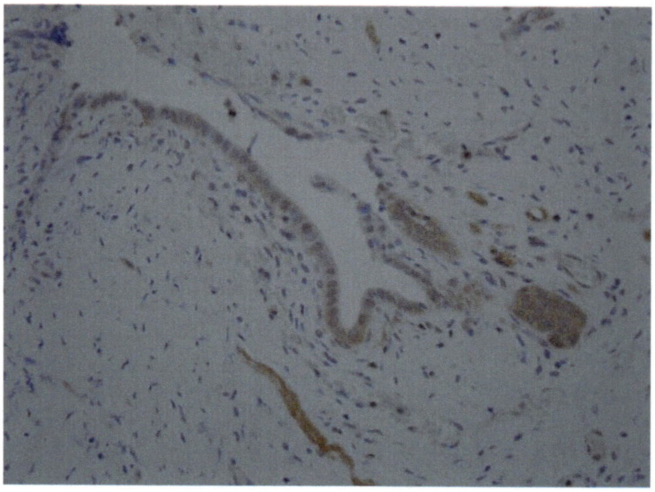

Fig. 8.2 Immunohistochemical staining for TLR3. TLR3 expression is found in cholangiocytes of extrahepatic bile ducts

plete elimination of dsRNA viruses; during this time, the overproduction of inflammatory cytokines likely leads to bile duct damage (39, 41).

On the other hand, the Reoviridae family (rotavirus and reovirus) shows an epitheliotropism and induces apoptosis in intestinal epithelial cells (43). Reovirus-induced apoptosis is mediated by the TNF-related apoptosis-inducing ligand (TRAIL) via the activation of NF-κB (44–46). These findings suggest that innate immune response against the virus could directly cause epithelial injury and cell death.

BA is characterized by the obstruction of extrahepatic bile ducts, the replacement with fibrous scars, and the epithelial-mesenchymal transition (EMT) of cholangiocytes during fibrosclerosis (3, 47, 48). Our *in vitro* study (3) revealed that approximately 30% of the human cultured cholangiocytes were affected by apoptosis on treatment with TLR3 ligand, poly(I:C), while the remaining 70% cells avoided cell death. By its continuous stimulation in the absence of TLR3-related tolerance, however, the survived cholangiocytes undergo EMT, suggesting the dual presence of biliary apoptosis and EMT in the TLR3-related biliary innate immunity. As a result, biliary innate immune response and the concomitant induction of apoptosis and EMT persisted until the complete elimination of dsRNA viruses.

The demonstrated presence of RRV in human BA samples supports the virus's role in BA. In addition, biliary innate immunity against viral infection has been shown to exist. However, the virus-induced histogenesis of BA biliary lesion and innate immunity cannot explain BA fully; therefore, acquired immunity should also be involved.

#### 8.3.1.4 The Acquired Immunity Against Reoviridae

In addition to the first line of defense in biliary innate immunity, the consequently acquired immunity is also involved in BA's histopathogenesis, at least after the clinical onset. CD4+ Th1 cell-mediated immunity and the involvement of Th1-dominant cytokines in BA's pathogenesis have been demonstrated (49–53). The γδ T cells, a unique subset of T cells common to innate and adaptive immune response, downregulates the immune function by inhibiting $Foxp3^+$ Treg cells. In liver tissues of patients with BA, the increased number of γδ T cells and the inhibition of Treg cell proliferation exacerbate the inflammatory-induced injury of bile ducts (54).

In animal models, much data associated with acquired immunity has been reported. The hepatic T cells from RRV-infected mice lead to a bile duct-specific inflammatory reaction in the recipient mice with severe combined immunodeficiency disease (55). Moreover, the presence of cholangiocyte-specific T cells and both cellular and humoral components of autoimmunity-mediated immune response were demonstrated in RRV-infected mice (55). Especially, the IFN-γ-producing T cell response in response to cholangiocytic autoantigens, the type I IFN-linked deregulation, and the dysregulation of Treg cells are involved in the cholangiopathy of RRV-infected experimental BA (53, 56, 57). These findings imply that infections of the biliary tree and subsequent cellular autoimmunity are important for progressive bile duct damage and loss in RRV-infected BA mice models (55, 58, 59).

In summary, the BA model, in which early postnatal RRV-infected mice lead to BA-like lesions in the extrahepatic bile duct, has become widely accepted. However, the universal implementation of rotavirus vaccination in the United States has not significantly altered the prevalence of BA (60). Therefore, the direct involvement of RRV in the pathogenesis of human BA remains to be fully delineated.

### 8.3.2 Cytomegalovirus

Cytomegalovirus (CMV), also known as human herpes virus-5, is a double-stranded DNA (dsDNA) virus of the Herpesviridae family. CMV infection is asymptomatic in healthy persons, including infants, but congenital CMV infection contributes to the development of disabilities such as hearing loss, vision loss, cerebral palsy, or cognitive impairment (61). Both BA and CMV infections are known to cause cholestatic jaundice in children (62). Therefore, it is important to discern whether a patient had liver disease with associated BA in the setting of congenital CMV infection or if he acquired the infection perinatally and subsequently developed pathology (63).

#### 8.3.2.1 The Molecular Detection of CMV

In addition to Reoviridae, CMV has been considered a cause in BA's etiopathogenesis; however, it is unknown whether the pathogenic infection process occurs in the intrauterine (congenital) or neonatal period. Rauschenfels et al. (22) investigated the presence of human hepatotropic viruses, including DNA viruses, such as HHV, EBV, varicella-zoster virus, CMV, adenovirus, and parvovirus B19, and RNA viruses, such as enteroviruses, rotavirus, and reovirus, in children with BA using nested RT-PCR and real-time PCR. It was revealed that reovirus and CMV are most frequently detected in the hepatobiliary samples from children with BA; nested RT-PCR detected 21 cases out of a total of 64, and real-time PCR detected 8 cases out of a total of 74, respectively (22).

Chang et al. (11) demonstrated the frequent presence of CMV, at 23 out of a total of 50 samples (46%), in liver specimens from the patients with neonatal hepatitis. In contrast, BA is only present in 2 out of 26 cases (7.6%) in patients with the same condition. Thus, neonatal hepatitis is more associated with CMV infection than with BA. Finally, the detection of CMV in BA clinical samples varies in frequency from 0 to 50% (18, 19). The different detection rates could be due to the detection methods, such as PCR or Nested PCR, the amplified regions, or primer design.

Moreover, irrespective of Reoviridae or CMV, because the causal virus infection in cholangiocytes may set the stage for an aberrant immune response targeting cholangiocytes (64), it could be unnecessary to confirm the continuous presence of these viruses in BA. Therefore, the detection of CMV DNA is not enough to conclude CMV's involvement in BA's etiopathogenesis; but additional immunological data is needed. For example, in 1998, Fischler et al. (18, 65) demonstrated the presence of CMV DNA in liver biopsy samples, the increased level of anti-CMV IgM in serum from cholestatic infants with BA, and the interaction between the IgM and the canalicular membrane of hepatocytes from patients with BA and also infected with CMV. Also, the presence of CMV-related antigens in BA patients' bile ducts, the cytopathic effect, and the apoptosis of CMV-infected human cholangiocytes have been demonstrated (25).

Clinically, a subgroup of BA patients who have CMV-related IgM has a higher rate of jaundice, liver inflammation, and fibrosis; they have a diminished response to the Kasai procedure and a greater need for liver transplant (66). The study by Xu et al. (25), in addition to detecting CMV DNA in 51 out of 85 (60%) of BA patients, identified CMV-related antigen pp65 in hepatocytes and bile ducts. Further, as BA progresses to late stages, a combined IgM positivity, an indicator of acute or persistent infection, and a pp65 negativity may mean that the patient had a recent infection that has subsequently cleared (63). Differing from IgG, IgM positivity generally indicates acute or persistent infection, and PCR/pp65 values are not likely to be false negatives (63).

#### 8.3.2.2 The Acquired Immunity Against CMV

Brindley et al. (67) identified the significant increase in the number of IFN-γ-producing liver T cells in response to CMV in 56% of infants. Also, CMV IgM in the plasma of BA samples and liver T cells' reactivity against CMV are correlated, indicating the CMV-related immunoreaction has already occurred at the diagnosis. In CMV-associated BA, Th1-1 cells predominate (68), and Tregs suffer a marked deficit (67). The presence of liver T cell response to CMV suggests that perinatal CMV infection is a plausible initiator of bile duct damage. Moreover, in Treg-depleted neonatal mouse, a low-dose CMV infection exhibited obstructive inflammation that mimicked human BA in both the intrahepatic and extrahepatic bile ducts; also, Th1-related cellular and humoral autoimmune responses were involved in the presence of serum autoantibodies reactive to proteins in cholangiocyte, such as the autoantigen α-enolase (69). These data support the possibility that after CMV infection, autoimmunologic mechanisms are important in the BA's pathogenesis.

## 8.4 Conclusion

The infection of several viruses may contribute to the etiology or pathogenesis of BA. These viruses have been detected in the liver and biliary remnants in human BA samples with molecular methods. This hypothesis has also been supported by the successful development of animal disease models and experiments that involve injecting the animals with reovirus, rotavirus, or CMV. The virus's presence may not be necessary for the subsequent development of acquired immune-mediated bile duct injury. Lastly, recent BA studies have demonstrated a shift from innate to acquired immunity during the immune response to viral infections.

## References

1. Funaki N, Sasano H, Shizawa S, Nio M, Iwami D, Ohi R, et al. Apoptosis and cell proliferation in biliary atresia. J Pathol. 1998;186(4):429–33.
2. Sasaki H, Nio M, Iwami D, Funaki N, Sano N, Ohi R, et al. E-cadherin, alpha-catenin and beta-catenin in biliary atresia: correlation with apoptosis and cell cycle. Pathol Int. 2001;51(12):923–32.
3. Harada K, Sato Y, Itatsu K, Isse K, Ikeda H, Yasoshima M, et al. Innate immune response to double-stranded RNA in biliary epithelial cells is associated with the pathogenesis of biliary atresia. Hepatology. 2007;46(4):1146–54.
4. Raweily EA, Gibson AA, Burt AD. Abnormalities of intrahepatic bile ducts in extrahepatic biliary atresia. Histopathology. 1990;17(6):521–7.

5. Nakamura K, Tanoue A. Etiology of biliary atresia as a developmental anomaly: recent advances. J Hepatobiliary Pancreat Sci. 2013;20(5):459–64.
6. Miethke AG, Huppert SS. Fishing for biliary atresia susceptibility genes. Gastroenterology. 2013;144(5):878–81.
7. Landing BH. Considerations of the pathogenesis of neonatal hepatitis, biliary atresia and choledochal cyst – the concept of infantile obstructive cholangiopathy. Prog Pediatr Surg. 1974;6:113–39.
8. Wehrman A, Waisbourd-Zinman O, Wells RG. Recent advances in understanding biliary atresia. F1000Res. 2019;8:218.
9. Weaver LT, Nelson R, Bell TM. The association of extrahepatic bile duct atresia and neonatal Epstein-Barr virus infection. Acta Paediatr Scand. 1984;73(1):155–7.
10. Domiati-Saad R, Dawson DB, Margraf LR, Finegold MJ, Weinberg AG, Rogers BB. Cytomegalovirus and human herpesvirus 6, but not human papillomavirus, are present in neonatal giant cell hepatitis and extrahepatic biliary atresia. Pediatr Develop Patholo. 2000;3(4):367–73.
11. Chang MH, Huang HH, Huang ES, Kao CL, Hsu HY, Lee CY. Polymerase chain reaction to detect human cytomegalovirus in livers of infants with neonatal hepatitis. Gastroenterology. 1992;103(3):1022–5.
12. Fjaer RB, Bruu AL, Nordbo SA. Extrahepatic bile duct atresia and viral involvement. Pediatr Transplant. 2005;9(1):68–73.
13. Mahjoub F, Shahsiah R, Ardalan FA, Iravanloo G, Sani MN, Zarei A, et al. Detection of Epstein Barr virus by chromogenic in situ hybridization in cases of extra-hepatic biliary atresia. Diagn Pathol. 2008;3:19.
14. Steele MI, Marshall CM, Lloyd RE, Randolph VE. Reovirus 3 not detected by reverse transcriptase-mediated polymerase chain reaction analysis of preserved tissue from infants with cholestatic liver disease. Hepatology. 1995;21(3):697–702.
15. Riepenhoff-Talty M, Gouvea V, Evans MJ, Svensson L, Hoffenberg E, Sokol RJ, et al. Detection of group C rotavirus in infants with extrahepatic biliary atresia. J Infect Dis. 1996;174(1):8–15.
16. Bobo L, Ojeh C, Chiu D, Machado A, Colombani P, Schwarz K. Lack of evidence for rotavirus by polymerase chain reaction/enzyme immunoassay of hepatobiliary samples from children with biliary atresia. Pediatr Res. 1997;41(2):229–34.
17. Tyler KL, Sokol RJ, Oberhaus SM, Le M, Karrer FM, Narkewicz MR, et al. Detection of reovirus RNA in hepatobiliary tissues from patients with extrahepatic biliary atresia and choledochal cysts. Hepatology. 1998;27(6):1475–82.
18. Fischler B, Ehrnst A, Forsgren M, Orvell C, Nemeth A. The viral association of neonatal cholestasis in Sweden: a possible link between cytomegalovirus infection and extrahepatic biliary atresia. J Pediatr Gastroenterol Nutr. 1998;27(1):57–64.
19. Jevon GP, Dimmick JE. Biliary atresia and cytomegalovirus infection: a DNA study. Pediatr Develop Pathol. 1999;2(1):11–4.
20. Saito T, Shinozaki K, Matsunaga T, Ogawa T, Etoh T, Muramatsu T, et al. Lack of evidence for reovirus infection in tissues from patients with biliary atresia and congenital dilatation of the bile duct. J Hepatol. 2004;40(2):203–11.
21. De Tommaso AM, Andrade PD, Costa SC, Escanhoela CA, Hessel G. High frequency of human cytomegalovirus DNA in the liver of infants with extrahepatic neonatal cholestasis. BMC Infect Dis. 2005;5:108.
22. Rauschenfels S, Krassmann M, Al-Masri AN, Verhagen W, Leonhardt J, Kuebler JF, et al. Incidence of hepatotropic viruses in biliary atresia. Eur J Pediatr. 2009;168(4):469–76.
23. Yaghobi R, Didari M, Gramizadeh B, Rahsaz M, Heidari T, Banihashemi M, et al. Study of viral infections in infants with biliary atresia. Indian J Pediatr. 2011;78(4):478–81.
24. Soomro GB, Abbas Z, Hassan M, Luck N, Memon Y, Khan AW. Is there any association of extra hepatic biliary atresia with cytomegalovirus or other infections? J Pak Med Assoc. 2011;61(3):281–3.
25. Xu Y, Yu J, Zhang R, Yin Y, Ye J, Tan L, et al. The perinatal infection of cytomegalovirus is an important etiology for biliary atresia in China. Clin Pediatr (Phila). 2012;51(2):109–13.
26. Goel A, Chaudhari S, Sutar J, Bhonde G, Bhatnagar S, Patel V, et al. Detection of cytomegalovirus in liver tissue by polymerase chain reaction in infants with neonatal cholestasis. Pediatr Infect Dis J. 2018;37(7):632–6.
27. Riepenhoff-Talty M, Schaekel K, Clark HF, Mueller W, Uhnoo I, Rossi T, et al. Group a rotaviruses produce extrahepatic biliary obstruction in orally inoculated newborn mice. Pediatr Res. 1993;33(4 Pt 1):394–9.
28. Szavay PO, Leonhardt J, Czech-Schmidt G, Petersen C. The role of reovirus type 3 infection in an established murine model for biliary atresia. Eur J Pediatr Surg. 2002;12(4):248–50.
29. Bangaru B, Morecki R, Glaser JH, Gartner LM, Horwitz MS. Comparative studies of biliary atresia in the human newborn and reovirus-induced cholangitis in weanling mice. Lab Invest J Tech Method Pathol. 1980;43(5):456–62.
30. Nakashima T, Hayashi T, Tomoeda S, Yoshino M, Mizuno T. Reovirus type-2-triggered autoimmune cholangitis in extrahepatic bile ducts of weanling DBA/1J mice. Pediatr Res. 2014;75(1–1):29–37.
31. Coots A, Donnelly B, Mohanty SK, McNeal M, Sestak K, Tiao G. Rotavirus infection of human cholangiocytes parallels the murine model of biliary atresia. J Surg Res. 2012;177(2):275–81.
32. Oetzmann von Sochaczewski C, Pintelon I, Brouns I, Dreier A, Klemann C, Timmermans JP, et al. Rotavirus particles in the extrahepatic bile duct in experimental biliary atresia. J Pediatr Surg. 2014;49(4):520–4.
33. Walther A, Mohanty SK, Donnelly B, Coots A, Lages CS, Lobeck I, et al. Rhesus rotavirus VP4 sequence-specific activation of mononuclear cells is associated with cholangiopathy in murine biliary atresia. Am J Physiol. 2015;309(6):G466–74.
34. Mohanty SK, Donnelly B, Bondoc A, Jafri M, Walther A, Coots A, et al. Rotavirus replication in the cholangiocyte mediates the temporal dependence of murine biliary atresia. PLoS One. 2013;8(7):e69069.
35. Morecki R, Glaser JH, Johnson AB, Kress Y. Detection of reovirus type 3 in the porta hepatis of an infant with extrahepatic biliary atresia: ultrastructural and immunocytochemical study. Hepatology. 1984;4(6):1137–42.
36. Brown WR, Sokol RJ, Levin MJ, Silverman A, Tamaru T, Lilly JR, et al. Lack of correlation between infection with reovirus 3 and extrahepatic biliary atresia or neonatal hepatitis. J Pediatr. 1988;113(4):670–6.
37. Qiao H, Zhaori G, Jiang Z, Chen Y, Chen Y, Hou D. Detection of group C rotavirus antigen in bile duct and liver tissues of an infant with extrahepatic biliary atresia. Chin Med J. 1999;112(1):93–5.
38. Al-Masri AN, Flemming P, Rodeck B, Melter M, Leonhardt J, Petersen C. Expression of the interferon-induced mx proteins in biliary atresia. J Pediatr Surg. 2006;41(6):1139–43.
39. Harada K, Nakanuma Y. Cholangiopathy with respect to biliary innate immunity. Int J Hepatolo. 2012;2012:793569.
40. Benias PC, Gopal K, Bodenheimer H Jr, Theise ND. Hepatic expression of toll-like receptors 3, 4, and 9 in primary biliary cirrhosis and chronic hepatitis C. Clin Res Hepatol Gastroenterol. 2012;36(5):448–54.
41. Harada K, Sato Y, Isse K, Ikeda H, Nakanuma Y. Induction of innate immune response and absence of subsequent tolerance to dsRNA in biliary epithelial cells relate to the pathogenesis of biliary atresia. Liver Int. 2008;28(5):614–21.
42. Harada K, Isse K, Sato Y, Ozaki S, Nakanuma Y. Endotoxin tolerance in human intrahepatic biliary epithelial cells is induced by upregulation of IRAK-M. Liver Int. 2006;26(8):935–42.

43. Sato A, Iizuka M, Nakagomi O, Suzuki M, Horie Y, Konno S, et al. Rotavirus double-stranded RNA induces apoptosis and diminishes wound repair in rat intestinal epithelial cells. J Gastroenterol Hepatol. 2006;21(3):521–30.
44. Clarke P, Tyler KL. Reovirus-induced apoptosis: a minireview. Apoptosis. 2003;8(2):141–50.
45. Connolly JL, Rodgers SE, Clarke P, Ballard DW, Kerr LD, Tyler KL, et al. Reovirus-induced apoptosis requires activation of transcription factor NF-kappaB. J Virol. 2000;74(7):2981–9.
46. Clarke P, Meintzer SM, Gibson S, Widmann C, Garrington TP, Johnson GL, et al. Reovirus-induced apoptosis is mediated by TRAIL. J Virol. 2000;74(17):8135–9.
47. Diaz R, Kim JW, Hui JJ, Li Z, Swain GP, Fong KS, et al. Evidence for the epithelial to mesenchymal transition in biliary atresia fibrosis. Hum Pathol. 2008;39(1):102–15.
48. Xiao Y, Zhou Y, Chen Y, Zhou K, Wen J, Wang Y, et al. The expression of epithelial-mesenchymal transition-related proteins in biliary epithelial cells is associated with liver fibrosis in biliary atresia. Pediatr Res. 2015;77(2):310–5.
49. Baba H, Ohtsuka Y, Fujii T, Haruna H, Nagata S, Kobayashi H, et al. Immunological investigation of the hepatic tissue from infants with biliary atresia. Pediatr Surg Int. 2009;25(2):157–62.
50. Mack CL, Tucker RM, Sokol RJ, Karrer FM, Kotzin BL, Whitington PF, et al. Biliary atresia is associated with CD4+ Th1 cell-mediated portal tract inflammation. Pediatr Res. 2004;56(1):79–87.
51. Shinkai M, Shinkai T, Puri P, Stringer MD. Elevated expression of IL2 is associated with increased infiltration of CD8+ T cells in biliary atresia. J Pediatr Surg. 2006;41(2):300–5.
52. Shinkai M, Shinkai T, Puri P, Stringer MD. Increased CXCR3 expression associated with CD3-positive lymphocytes in the liver and biliary remnant in biliary atresia. J Pediatr Surg. 2006;41(5):950–4.
53. Tucker RM, Feldman AG, Fenner EK, Mack CL. Regulatory T cells inhibit Th1 cell-mediated bile duct injury in murine biliary atresia. J Hepatol. 2013;59(4):790–6.
54. Li K, Zhang X, Tang ST, Yang L, Cao GQ, Li S, et al. Gammadelta T cells and Foxp3(+) Treg cells infiltration in children with biliary atresia and its significance. Int J Clin Exp Med. 2015;8(10):18512–7.
55. Mack CL, Tucker RM, Lu BR, Sokol RJ, Fontenot AP, Ueno Y, et al. Cellular and humoral autoimmunity directed at bile duct epithelia in murine biliary atresia. Hepatology. 2006;44(5):1231–9.
56. Shivakumar P, Campbell KM, Sabla GE, Miethke A, Tiao G, McNeal MM, et al. Obstruction of extrahepatic bile ducts by lymphocytes is regulated by IFN-gamma in experimental biliary atresia. J Clin Invest. 2004;114(3):322–9.
57. Kuebler JF, Czech-Schmidt G, Leonhardt J, Ure BM, Petersen C. Type-I but not type-II interferon receptor knockout mice are susceptible to biliary atresia. Pediatr Res. 2006;59(6):790–4.
58. Mack CL. The pathogenesis of biliary atresia: evidence for a virus-induced autoimmune disease. Semin Liver Dis. 2007;27(3):233–42.
59. Lages CS, Simmons J, Chougnet CA, Miethke AG. Regulatory T cells control the CD8 adaptive immune response at the time of ductal obstruction in experimental biliary atresia. Hepatology. 2012;56(1):219–27.
60. Danial E, Fleck-Derderian S, Rosenthal P. Has rotavirus vaccination decreased the prevalence of biliary atresia? J Clin Gastroenterol. 2019;53(8):e348–e51.
61. Fowler KB, Boppana SB. Congenital cytomegalovirus infection. Semin Perinatol. 2018;42(3):149–54.
62. Liberek A, Gora-Gebka M, Bako W, Rytlewska M, Kozielska E, Korzon M. Various types of cholestatic jaundice in infants – causes and diagnostic problems. Med Sci Monit. 2000;6(3):548–54.
63. Averbukh LD, Wu GY. Evidence for viral induction of biliary atresia: a review. J Clin Transl Hepatol. 2018;6(4):410–9.
64. Kilgore A, Mack CL. Update on investigations pertaining to the pathogenesis of biliary atresia. Pediatr Surg Int. 2017;33(12):1233–41.
65. Fischler B, Woxenius S, Nemeth A, Papadogiannakis N. Immunoglobulin deposits in liver tissue from infants with biliary atresia and the correlation to cytomegalovirus infection. J Pediatr Surg. 2005;40(3):541–6.
66. Zani A, Quaglia A, Hadzic N, Zuckerman M, Davenport M. Cytomegalovirus-associated biliary atresia: an aetiological and prognostic subgroup. J Pediatr Surg. 2015;50(10):1739–45.
67. Brindley SM, Lanham AM, Karrer FM, Tucker RM, Fontenot AP, Mack CL. Cytomegalovirus-specific T-cell reactivity in biliary atresia at the time of diagnosis is associated with deficits in regulatory T cells. Hepatology. 2012;55(4):1130–8.
68. Hill R, Quaglia A, Hussain M, Hadzic N, Mieli-Vergani G, Vergani D, et al. Th-17 cells infiltrate the liver in human biliary atresia and are related to surgical outcome. J Pediatr Surg. 2015;50(8):1297–303.
69. Wen J, Xiao Y, Wang J, Pan W, Zhou Y, Zhang X, et al. Low doses of CMV induce autoimmune-mediated and inflammatory responses in bile duct epithelia of regulatory T cell-depleted neonatal mice. Lab Invest J Tech Method Pathol. 2015;95(2):180–92.

# 9 Pathogenesis of Maternal Microchimerism

Toshihiro Muraji and Toshio Harumatsu

**Abstract**

Maternal microchimerism (MMC) is a common feature in patients with biliary atresia (BA). Although the role of maternal chimeric cells continues to be elusive, unique epidemiological and clinical observations and alloreactive responses between the mother and patient are consistent with the recent concept that BA begins before birth, possibly before the second trimester. The target tissues of the maternal effector lymphocytes in a fetus may be not only the bile duct epithelium but also the portal vein endothelium, resulting in mutually independent obstructive cholangiopathy and portal hypertension. The prognosis of the patients with BA is plausibly influenced by the balance of immune/tolerance between the patients with BA and their mothers, depending on the quantity of the maternal effector lymphocytes sensitized with the patient's antigen and the timing of their transplacental trafficking during an early phase of pregnancy. Further research on the immunological events occurring at the maternal–fetal interface is warranted in order to clarify the disease mechanism.

To this day, the etiopathogenesis of biliary atresia (BA) has remained unknown. BA is largely thought to be an immune-mediated disease associated with various mysterious characteristics, including ethnic/regional differences in incidence, discordance between human leukocyte antigen (HLA) identical twins, remarkable swelling of lymph nodes at the porta hepatis, and unique clinical courses, such as the development of portal hypertension despite earlier bile drainage achieved by Kasai operation or progression of portal hypertension even in jaundice-free patients as well as segmental atrophy of the liver. These unique clinical observations provide clues as to the disease mechanism. Conversely, any pathogenetic hypothesis is expected to fit such unique characteristics without contradiction.

The hypothesis of graft-versus-host reaction (GVHR) as a pathogenetic mechanism for BA is a relatively recently proposed theory because of the presence of maternal cells in the liver of patients with BA [1–4], which is known as maternal microchimerism (MMC). Although the causative relationship remains speculative, this hypothesis is promising. In this chapter, the author will describe the MMC theory in light of recent understanding of transplant immunology and the maternofetal immune/tolerance to test whether the MMC hypothesis displays compatibility with these unique findings without contradiction.

## 9.1 Historical Overview of GVHR and Tolerance

### 9.1.1 Actively Acquired Tolerance

Modern research for understanding the immune system has evolved following GVHR experiments conducted by Billingham, Brent, and Medawar in 1953 [5]. They demonstrated tolerance through a successful skin graft in mice that received adult splenic allogeneic lymphoid cells during their immunologically immature newborn period. This report was entitled "Actively Acquired Tolerance." While tolerance was induced in the recipients, some of the donor/recipient combi-

T. Muraji (✉)
Department of Pediatric Surgery, Kirishima Medical Center, Kirishima, Japan

Department of Pediatric Surgery, Research Field in Medical and Health Sciences, Medical and Dental Area, Research and Education Assembly, Kagoshima University, Kagoshima, Japan
e-mail: t-muraji@hayato-mc.jp

T. Harumatsu
Department of Pediatric Surgery, Research Field in Medical and Health Sciences, Medical and Dental Area, Research and Education Assembly, Kagoshima University, Kagoshima, Japan


M. Nio (ed.), *Introduction to Biliary Atresia*, https://doi.org/10.1007/978-981-16-2160-4_9

nations of those mice developed emaciation, abnormal sparse fur, and diarrhea with atrophy of the lymphoid tissue in recipients, which the researchers termed "runting syndrome." The induction of tolerance to maternal antigens or the initiation of runt disease in the fetus is not mutually exclusive possibilities.

In 1968 the successful engraftment of sibling bone marrow was described in one infant with severe combined immunodeficiency disease (SCID) [6], in which HLA identity and mixed lymphocyte culture (MLC) negativity were observed. However, mild self-limited graft-versus-host disease (GVHD) developed, which was considered the human equivalent of runt disease. GVHD is principally a reaction of donor effector Tlymphocytes against host cells presenting the host self-histocompatibility antigen. In 1966, Billingham [7] formulated the requirements for the development of GVHD: 1) the graft must contain immunologically competent cells, 2) the recipient must express tissue antigens that are not present in the transplant donor, and 3) the recipient must be incapable of mounting an effective response to destroy the transplanted cells. On this basis, GVHD may develop in HLA heterozygous patients who received a fresh whole blood transfusion from an HLA homozygous parent even though the patients are not immunocompromised [8]. Further clinical insights can be acquired from patients with SCID. Children with SCID have an increased occurrence of MMC, which can cause GvHD-like symptoms in their skin and liver [9].

GVHR may also induce a thymic atrophy characterized by fibrosis, the absence of Hassall's corpuscles, and focal calcifications. This involution was independent of the stress-mediated hypercorticoid condition and was experimentally reproduced and negated by prior adrenalectomy in mice [10]. In 1976, a symposium entitled "Immunodeficiency: Its nature and etiological significance in human diseases" was held in Tokyo. Interestingly, Landing [11] included BA in this symposium, reporting the progressive loss of thymic epithelium (Hassall's corpuscles) over 18 months of age in his autopsy series. Given that we presently have few opportunities to perform autopsies on BA patients due to the advent of liver transplantation, this information should be noted for a chain of knowledge.

### 9.1.2 Regulatory T Cells and Tolerance

In 1995, Sakuguchi [12] demonstrated a molecule called CD25 as a reliable marker for previously recognized suppressor T cells, which plays an important role in tolerance. CD25 is a high-affinity receptor for interleukin-2(IL-2), which suppresses autoreactive helper T cells. It is now known that naturally-occurring, thymus-derived T-regs (nT-regs) are defined by transcription factor FOXP3, providing essential control of autoimmunity through absorption of IL-2, CTLA-4-mediated masking of CD-80/86 costimulatory ligands on antigen presenting cells (APCs): expression of IL-10, IL-35, transforming growth factor-beta 1(TGF-β1) (immune inhibitory molecules); and granzyme-mediated killing of APCs. Patients with chronic GVHD had significantly lower expression levels of FOXP3, implying thymic function is substantially impaired following allogeneic hematopoietic stem cell transplant (HST) [13].

Peripheral T-regs (pT-reg) developed in the periphery upon engagement are defined by antigen exposure to target epitopes in a TGF-β1-rich environment. Though T-regs may exhibit non-antigen-specific suppressor functions, more potent inhibition occurs upon engagement of the T cell receptor. T-regs are also divided into two subsets based on inducible co-stimulator (ICOS) expression. $ICOS^+$ T-regs preferentially secrete high amounts of IL-10 and moderate levels of TGF-β1, while $ICOS^-$ T-regs exert a suppressive function primarily through the secretion of TGF-β1. $ICOS^-$ T-regs are mainly of the $CD45RA^{high}CD45RO^{low}$ phenotype identified by flow cytometry analysis.

In 2008, Mold et al. [14] showed that antigen-specific tolerance in humans is induced in utero and is probably active in regulating immune responses after birth. In mixed lymphocyte reactions (MLRs) to maternal antigens as the stimulator using lymphocytes from the spleen or lymph nodes of 18 human fetuses at 18 to 22 gestational weeks as responders, substantial proliferative responses were observed for both $CD4^+$ and $CD8^+$ fetal T cells. When regulatory T cells were depleted from these fetal immune cells, they showed substantial proliferative response against maternal antigens, indicating fetal immune system, including T-regs is already functional at this gestational age.

### 9.1.3 Organ Transplantation and Tolerance

In the 1980s and onward, during the era of liver transplantation, it is recognized that APC (dendritic cells) included in donated organs known as "passenger leukocytes" migrate widely, systemically leading to mixed allogeneic chimerism and tolerance. This was a natural consequence of organ transplantation under immunosuppression.

Living-related liver transplantation has become a widespread modality for end-stage liver disease because of the scarcity of deceased donor organs, providing a serendipitous opportunity to shed light on maternal tolerance of BA patients, at least in a cohort of BA patients with poor prognosis. Nijagal et al. [15] reviewed the national database of pediatric split liver transplants performed in the USA from 1996 to 2010 for any outcome differences according to the parental donor and reported BA patients receiving a maternal graft had a lower rate of graft failure than those receiving a paternal graft (3.7% versus 10.5%, $p = 0.02$). These differences were not seen among non-BA patients or among

BA patients who received female deceased donor grafts. As patients with BA have increased maternal cells in the liver represented by a better outcome of subsequent maternal donor liver transplant, it is plausible that this tolerance is promoted by the thymus-derived central mechanism against the non-inherited maternal antigen (NIMA) in the patients in utero.

## 9.2 Maternal–Fetal Interface

### 9.2.1 Successful Pregnancy

The immune tolerance in mothers occurs during pregnancy to accommodate foreign paternal antigens. $FOXP3^+CD4^+$Treg cells play an important role in the success of implantation and early pregnancy [16]. This occurs even before implantation. It was demonstrated in mice that fetus-specific Treg cells are primed by seminal fluid and accumulate locally in uterine-draining lymph nodes [17, 18]. After fertilization and implantation, maternal immune cells contact the extravillous trophoblasts (EVTs) that invade the decidua of the placenta. EVTs only express HLA-C and non-polymorphic HLA-E, G, and F. HLA-G positive EVTs regulate T cell activation through the induction of tolerogenic dendritic cells.

HLA-C is a ligand for natural killer (NK) cells. In the decidua, 70% of leucocytes are $CD3^-CD16^-CD56^{bright}$ NK cells, which play important roles in the maintenance of maternal–fetal tolerance by carrying killer cell Ig-like receptors (KIRs), CD94/NKG2A, and immunoglobulin-like transcript, all of which inhibit NK cell activity. Combinations of maternal KIRs and fetal HLA-C genes influence the risk of preeclampsia and reproductive success [19].

### 9.2.2 Villitis of Unknown Etiology (VUE)

VUE is an inflammatory condition of EVTs at the maternal–fetal interface due to an unknown cause. However, it is known that the origin and phenotypes of inflammatory cells involved include maternal $CD4^+$ and $CD8^+$ T cells and hyperplastic fetal macrophages, suggesting that it is analogous to allograft rejection or GVHD [20]. A breakthrough case was recently reported from Ibaraki Children's Hospital (unpublished) that described a discordant set of monozygotic twins, of which the placenta was dichorionic-diamniotic. An MLR disclosed that the mother became sensitized by the patient's antigens. The placenta of the BA twin was smaller and associated with segmental focuses of the VUE. This case clearly indicates the existence of a maternal–fetal interface disorder, which likely allowed more maternal cells to transfer to the twin with BA. It is plausible that immunological events occurring at the maternal–fetal interface are what occurs in the fetal liver. Thus, VUE may be the result of inadequate tolerance at the interface, thereby sensitizing maternal $CD8^+$ T cells.

## 9.3 Overview of Naturally Acquired Microchimerism

The bidirectional transplacental trafficking of cells was first recognized in the 1970s. Fetal cells pass into the mother, persisting for decades after the pregnancy and leading to fetal microchimerism (FMC), while maternal cells also pass into the fetus and persist long after birth into adulthood, resulting in MMC.

### 9.3.1 FMC

Fetal cells are present in maternal peripheral blood mononuclear cells at a frequency of 1 in $10^3$ cells by 14–15 weeks of gestation [21], and fetal cells retain in the long-term postpartum period [22]. However, since these fetal cells are foreign to mothers, maternal tissue seeding of fetal microchimeric cells can also be a target of maternal alloimmunity, causing low-grade inflammation, such as scleroderma [23]. Although the semi-allogeneic compatibility may cause maternal susceptibility to immune-mediated tissue injury, this pregnancy-induced immunological interaction intriguingly improves the severity of preexisting autoimmune disorders, such as rheumatoid arthritis and multiple sclerosis, during pregnancy. These beneficial effects of pregnancy are most apparent during the last trimester, at which point the level of FMC is highest. In turn, the remission of multiple sclerosis and rheumatoid arthritis is often reversed shortly after parturition, which parallels the sharp numerical decline in fetal microchimeric cells [24]. However, the pregnancy-induced symptomatic change varies from autoimmune diseases to diseases and its mechanism of each condition is still elusive.

### 9.3.2 MMC: Migration Occurs During Initial Immunological Development in a Fetus

#### 9.3.2.1 Ontogeny of the Immune Response

The stem cell population in the liver shows a proliferative response in MLRs at 5 weeks of gestation. At 8 to 9 weeks, fetal stem cells migrate to the thymus undergoing ontogenetic maturation and leading a cell-mediated immune response. Over the course of several weeks, nodal and splenic lymphocyte functional development follow, and by 16 weeks, fetuses have proliferative responses with foreign antigenic stimulation. Bone marrow develops an immune response at the last site at 16 to 18 weeks [25].

#### 9.3.2.2 Maternal Cell Migration

Maternal DNA is in the fetal circulation as early as 13 weeks of gestation [26]. Although fetomaternal microchimeric cells are seeded in an immunologically mature mother, the inherent difference in MMC is that mature maternal cells are transferred to the fetus before or during key milestones in immunological development. Since persistent chimeric cells are semi-allogeneic, microchimerism can induce GvHD as seen in hematopoietic stem cell transplantation (HST), which manifests as autoimmune diseases, such as juvenile idiopathic inflammatory myopathies (JDM) [27], neonatal lupus syndrome [28], and type 1 diabetes mellitus [29], in a pediatric population. It remains unclear whether these transferring maternal cells are previously primed with fetal antigens. In JDM, Reed [30] showed high frequencies of maternally transferred chimeric T cells secrete IFN-$\gamma$ when stimulated with T cells of JDM patients. In this respect, there is an intriguing observation of a higher incidence of positive autoantibodies in the mothers of offspring suffering from liver diseases, including BA [31]. Thus, patients with BA may sensitize the mother early during certain stages of pregnancy.

## 9.4 MMC in BA

### 9.4.1 Existence of Maternal Cells in BA Patients

In 2004, Suskind first proposed a hypothesis that MMC may trigger a series of immunological abnormalities in the bile duct epithelia [1]. Using fluorescence in situ hybridization (FISH) for X and Y chromosome and kinetic PCR for maternal HLAs, he demonstrated a higher presence of maternal cells in the livers of patients with BA than in the livers of patients with neonatal hepatitis. The MMC in BA was confirmed by three other researchers [2, 3], including the author of this chapter [4]. We quantitatively demonstrated significantly larger numbers of $XX^+$ cells, which are presumably maternal, in the portal area and sinusoids of male offspring with BA. Phenotypes of these cells included $CD8^+$ cytolytic T cells or cytokeratin$^+$ differentiated biliary epithelial cells. This observation implicates four possibilities of pathogenetic mechanisms [32]: (1) GVHD-like allo-response: Chimeric effector lymphocytes may damage biliary epithelial cells and portal vein endothelial cells in a graft-versus-host direction, (2) HVGD-like allo-response: autologous effector lymphocytes may damage biliary epithelial cells that are fused with chimeric cells or have acquired chimeric major histocompatibility complex antigens in a semi-direct pathway of presentation through dendritic cells in a host-versus-graft reaction (HGVR) direction, (3) defective host Treg cells: The BA patients do not effectively limit effector T cell responses or (4) simply innocent bystanders.

### 9.4.2 Allo-Reactivity Between the Patient and the Mother

Living-related liver transplant provides a unique opportunity for natural experiment on maternal tolerance in BA. As described previously (see Sect. 9.1.2), Nijagal's report on a favorable outcome of patients with BA after maternal donor liver transplant means that these patients with BA do not tend to reject their maternal donor graft, so the HGVR-type of allo-response is unlikely. Based on this observation, it is tempting to speculate that liver failure is progressive because of their tolerance, which allows one-way allo-reactivity of maternal effector T lymphocytes to the patients, at least in the cohort of liver failure, which is why they required liver transplantation. This finding suggests that maternal cells are actively involved in maternofetal immune reaction rather than being innocent bystanders.

Allo-reactivity between the patient and the mother were classically tested with an MLR, which reflects the disparity of HLAs between responders and stimulators. The responder lymphocytes were cultured for 5 days with stimulator lymphocytes, which are irradiated. [$^3$H] Thymidine uptake incorporated into the responder cells was measured, and responses were compared to those stimulated by unrelated third-party controls.

The ideal control for detecting allo-reactivity in BA patients with their mothers is a set of monozygotic twins with discordance in BA occurrence. According to a recent study from China [33] that collected 19 cases of BA twins, 8 sets were monozygotic twins, and all of them were discordant. Although the MMC hypothesis is rather unlikely if discordance exists in such a scenario as the same number of maternal cells migrating to twins with identical HLAs through the monochorionic placenta, one recently reported case identified dizygotic discordant twins with dichorionic and diamniotic placenta (unpublished). The placenta of the BA twin was smaller and associated with VUE (see Sect. 9.2.2). This case suggests that BA is likely to be an alloimmune disease, not an autoimmune disease triggered by a viral infection of toxins.

## 9.5 New Aspects of Unique Pathological Findings in BA

### 9.5.1 Hepatocellular Injury in BA

Clinically, patients with GVHD undergoing HST present with dermatitis, diarrhea, hepatitis with splenomegaly, and lymphadenopathy, whereas dermatitis and diarrhea are rare in BA. Why and how allo-stimulated effector T cells find their way to target organs in HST are now thought to be the homing of effector cells to target organs in modulated inflammatory conditions. For the skin lesion, endothelial activation of microvascular plexus in the superficial dermis slows migration of the effector cells, resulting from their localized accumulation. For intestinal injury, lipopolysaccharide (LPS), a major structural component of gram-negative bacteria in gut flora elicits inflammatory responses. In both target organs, the SCT conditioning regimen causes cytokine storm, which is probably the cause of this modulated inflammation. In maternofetal transplacental trafficking, on the other hand, a fetus is in the aseptic condition in utero without any preconditioning regimen, which is why GVHD associated with MMC does not damage the skin and gut [34].

The hepatic pathology in GVHD shows features homologous to those of BA, such as portal tract involvement with lymphocyte infiltration, bile duct disruption with cholangiolar proliferation as well as hepatocellular necrosis, acidophilic degeneration (possible apoptosis), and multi-nucleic giant cells in the parenchyma, which are a manifestation of cellular reactions similar to immunologically mediated hepatitis [35]. The semi-quantitated histological severity of hepatocellular injury affects liver function in the early postoperative period in BA but not in a long-term outcome [36].

### 9.5.2 NK Cells in BA

NK cells in the peripheral blood are $CD3^{-}CD16^{+}CD56^{dim}$ and alloreactive. NK cells carry KIRs, which comprise two groups of epitope C1 (ligands: KIR2DL2 and KIR2DL3) and C2 (ligands: KIR2DL1 and KIR2DS1). HLA-C carries a ligand for NK cells. Missing expression of the KIR ligand on mismatched allogeneic cells can trigger NK cell alloreactivity. This missing ligand model is known as the graft-versus-leukemia (GVL) effect reported in haploidentical HST for acute myeloid leukemia [37].

We had an opportunity to analyze HLA in the members of a family in which both the mother and her daughter were affected with BA [38]. Based on an MLR, the mother showed an intense proliferative response to her BA offspring antigen. There was an intriguing relationship in the HLA-C genotype of the BA mother and daughter. The genotype of the daughter was 03:03/14:03, both belonging to the C1 group, while HLA-C of the mother was 03:03, which is homozygous for the C1 group. According to recent findings regarding KIR-HLA interactions in NK function based on HST, their HLA-C groups are so compatible that the NK cells of the BA daughter could not eliminate maternal cells. Comparatively, the non-BA sibling had 03:03/0401 Cw genotypes (C1/C2 group), which are alloreactive to maternal graft cells (homozygous for C1 group), and therefore imply the rejection of maternal chimeric cells.

### 9.5.3 Treg Cells in BA

In BA patients, a decreased percentage of Treg cells in their peripheral blood [39] was reported, and patients with a favorable outcome showed a high infiltration of $ICOS^{-}$ T-regs (see 9.1.2) in the portal area of the liver. Lymphatic capillaries are minute and proliferate in the portal tract of the BA liver. Lymph nodes in the porta hepatis are often remarkably swollen, which has drawn attention from the pathogenetic point of view. We visualized the $XX^{+}$ cells, presumably maternal cells in the parafollicular region of the porta hepatis lymph nodes of a male patient with BA, using chromogenic in situ hybridization with a Y-chromosome-specific probe and immunohistochemistry (Fig. 9.1). Sakamoto [40] showed that active Treg ($CD45RA^{high}CD45RO^{low}$ phenotype) cells are decreased

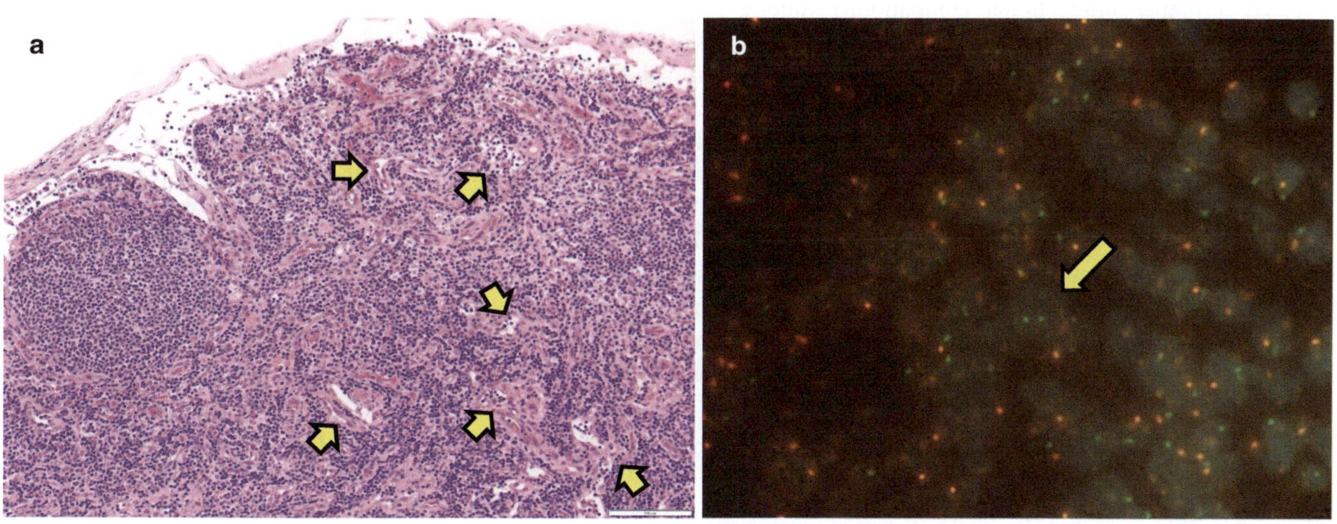


Fig. 9.1 (a) Lymph node of the porta hepatis (hematoxylin and eosin staining). Paracortical expansion (T cell zone) with the proliferation of high endothelial venules is observed (arrows). (b) An XX cell (arrow) is observed in the middle of the picture in the parafollicular region of the porta hepatis lymph node of a male patient with BA (fluorescence in situ hybridization; X chromosome: green, Y chromosome: red)

in the peripheral blood while they increased in the draining lymph nodes of the porta hepatis on BA patients. However, a recent report from Germany showed that there was no maternal genetic material in the lymph nodes investigated by short tandem repeat and single nucleotide polymorphism analysis in six consecutive patients with BA [41]. This discrepancy with our observation might be due to some confounding factors. Further investigation of the immunological significance of porta hepatis lymph node swelling is warranted.

## 9.6 Compatibilities of Unique Findings in the BA to MMC Hypothesis

### 9.6.1 Ethnic/Regional Differences in the Incidence of BA

In 1965, Shim, Kasai and Spence [42]. reported a significant difference in the incidence of BA among people in Hawaii of different ancestral origins. This ethnic/geographical diversity in the incidence of BA implicates a certain genetic susceptibility to BA. The strong genetic associations with autoimmunity are in HLA genes or shared epitopes. However, the possibility of common alleles in the HLAs or other candidate gene across ethnicities were negated [43].

In the era of liver transplantation, academic opportunities to reveal the features of HLAs were provided for BA patients when they received liver transplants, compared to non-BA patients who received liver transplants. Japanese patients with BA often have the most prevalent haplotype among the Japanese population known as HLA-A24-B52-DR2 [44]. Increased opportunities for living-related liver transplantation further allowed us to analyze the compatibility of HLAs between the patients and their mothers. Statistical analysis revealed a higher bidirectional compatibility among BA patients compared with patients who underwent liver transplants for diseases other than BA [45]. The extent of maternal–fetal histocompatibility has been shown to influence MMC through a mechanism related to major histocompatibility complex zygosity of the progeny in mice models [46]. Our recent analysis on the ethnicity-dependent incidence of BA further uncovered the fact that frequency of the most common HLA haplotype correlates with the incidence of BA across the countries [47] (Fig. 9.2), which intriguingly reflects global human colonization. Given these findings, the MMC hypothesis most closely fits the pathogenetic mechanism of BA from an epidemiological genetic susceptibility perspective.

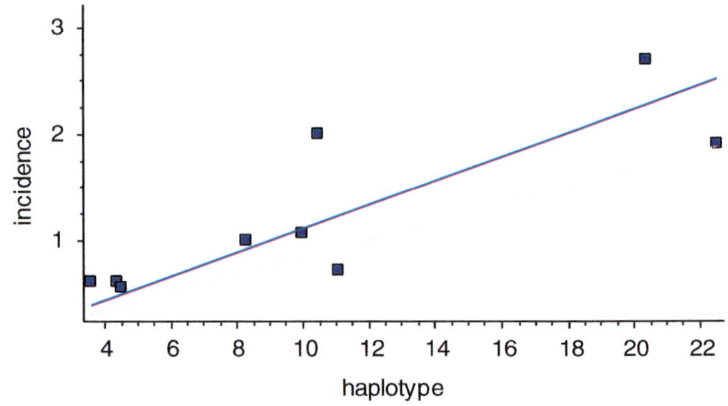


**Fig. 9.2** Linear regression analysis of the correlation between the frequency of the most prevalent haplotype (X-axis) and the incidence of BA (Y-axis) in nine countries: France, Japan, New Zealand (Maori population), Norway, Philippines, Sweden, South Korea, Taiwan, and the UK, (nonparametric Spearman's tow-tailed test. P = 0.0172, r = 0.7782)

### 9.6.2 Segmental Atrophy of the Liver Due to Possible Portal Vein Vasculopathy

In BA liver, cirrhotic atrophy occurs segmentally and most severely in the left lateral segment (LLS) [48, 49]. Inadequate bile drainage was intuitively thought to be responsible for the progression of the segmental fibrosis and atrophy. However, the intrahepatic bile ducts are not dilated, and microscopic bile plugs are not remarkable in these atrophic segments [50].

An alternative explanation for this segmental atrophy may be decreased portal flow associated with portal vein vasculopathy. The sinusoidal and portal vein endothelia in BA were previously known to be positive for HLA-DR [51] and CX3CL1 (Fractalkine) [52]. Antibodies also contribute to the acute rejection of the vascular component along with complement activation (humoral immunity). Complements (C4d) is involved in the endothelium in BA [53], which is also the case in GVHD [54]. Lymphocytic attachments to the endothelium are present in BA (Fig. 9.3), which is also the case in GVHD [34]. Endothelial injury is also known to occur in chronic GVHD and acute graft rejection; it is tempting to speculate that portal vein branches in the portal tract themselves are the alloreactive target tissue of maternal chimeric T and B cells. These findings led us to speculate that the immune-mediated endothelialitis of the portal vein branches is responsible for the diminution of portal vein vasculature and subsequent portal hypertension.

The intrahepatic portal vein branches are already hypoplastic at the time of Kasai portoenterostomy [55, 56], and the degree of hypoplasia correlated with patient prognosis [57]. The sclerotic extrahepatic portal vein was also evaluated recently, and intimal thickening was found, which may not be due to progressive cholestasis but rather primary obliterative portal venopathy [58]. It is now recognized that alloimmunologic targets in BA not only include the biliary epithelium but also may be the portal vein endothelium, which explains the occurrence of unique clinical courses such as the development of portal hypertension despite earlier Kasai operation or progressive portal hypertension even in jaundice-free patients.

We visualized and quantified the maternally-derived chimeric cells using FISH technique to compare the frequency of $XX^+$ cells in the LLS and right anterior segment (RAS) on the liver biopsy specimens taken from the male patients at the time of Kasai operation. There were more $XX^+$ cells in the RAS than in the LLS (Fig. 9.4). These fewer $XX^+$ cells in LLS are perhaps a reflection of lower portal perfusion at the time of Kasai operation.

This dominant atrophy of LLS can be embryologically explained. The two umbilical veins are initially present. The right vein diminishes around week 7 of gestation, while the left vein runs into the left branch of the portal vein. Half of the flow bypasses the liver through the ductus venosus, and the remaining half mainly perfuses the left lateral and partly medial segments of the liver. The right lobe is perfused by the portal vein. Thus, the maternal chimeric cells are anatomically prone to engrafting in the LLS. Therefore, it is plausible to speculate that maternal chimeric cells harboring in the LLS may cause more injury, leading to the atrophy of the segment. By sampling liver biopsy specimens from both the right and left lateral segments, we encountered a case in which there was no portal vein vascularity in the LLS, whereas the normal portal vein branches were seen in the portal tract in the right lobe [59].

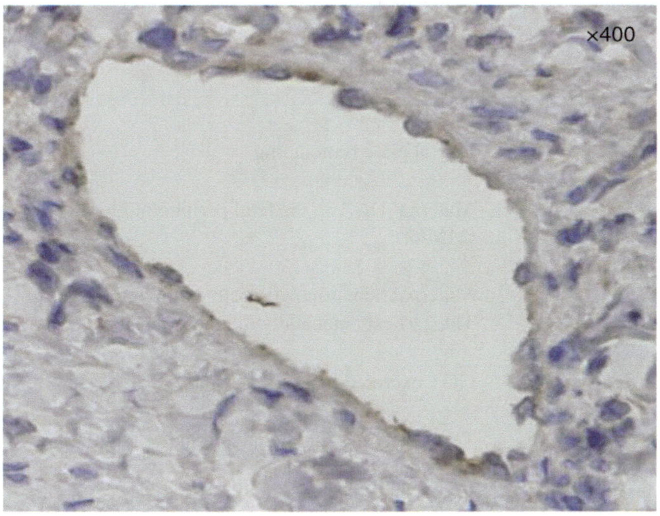


Fig. 9.3 The liver biopsy specimen of a male patient with BA who was sampled at the time of Kasai operation at the age of 111 days old was positive for C4d. (Immunohistochemistry; x400):Lymphocytic attachments to the endothelium of the portal vein branch are also observed

## 9.7 BA Begins Before Birth: Plausible Timing in Utero from the Perspective of the MMC Hypothesis

### 9.7.1 Consistency with Ductal Plate Malformation Theory

Around the 8th week of gestation, the liver precursor cells located around the largest portal vein branches become more strongly immunoreactive to the cytokeratins 8, 18, and 19, which are referred to as the ductal plate. In 1988, Desmet [60] proposed the ductal plate malformation theory, reporting that 20 ~ 25% of BA patients retain these morphological structures in their livers. Tan [61] reviewed series of 205 patients at King's College Hospital and found that the extrahepatic bile ducts in BA have a morphological structure that is identical to weeks 11 ~ 13 of gestation, resulting in speculation that the porta hepatis morphology in BA is a result of fibrosclerosing inflammation due to bile leakage, although the morphology does not influence survival [62].

The earliest antenatally diagnosed cystic BA was reported at 16 weeks of gestation [63]. This type of BA is often connected to the intrahepatic biliary tree, permitting intraoperative cholangiography via the gallbladder. It typically visualizes the intrahepatic biliary tree as brush-like structure

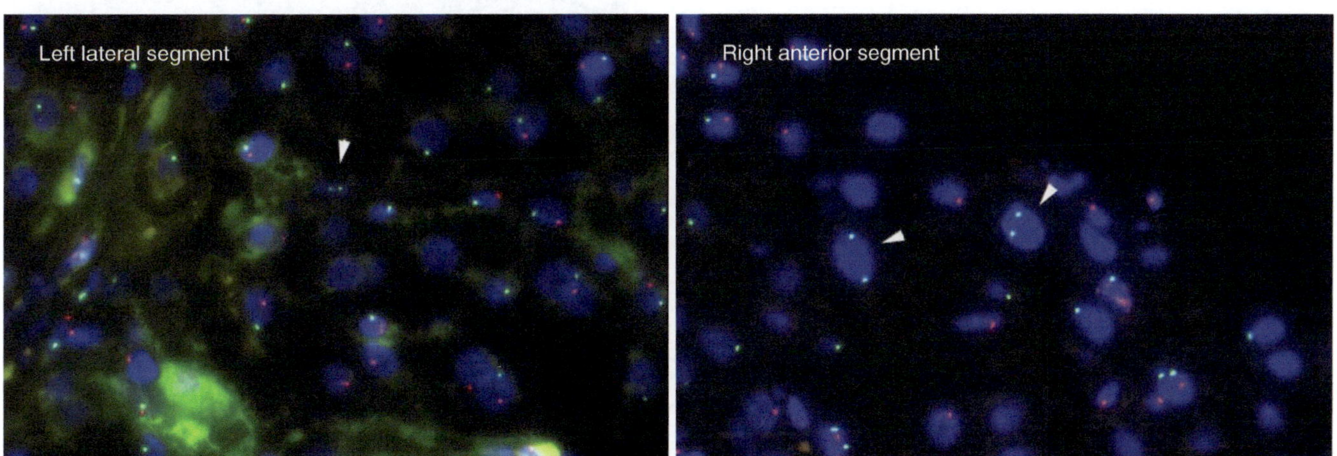


Fig. 9.4 Quantitative analysis of XX cells (arrows) in the liver specimens of male patients with BA from the right anterior segment (RAS) versus left lateral segment (LLS). (fluorescence in situ hybridization; X chromosome: green, Y chromosome: red). We counted 13 XX cells versus 987 XY cells in the RAS and 8 XX cells versus 992 XY cells in the LLS

with morphologically disorganized branching patterns as if the development of intrahepatic biliary trees is arrested during the early ductal plate period, which reminds us of the "pollard willow" that Desmet described in his publication (Fig. 9.5).

### 9.7.2 Gamma-Glutamyl Transferase (GGT) in Amniotic Fluid

While a fetus with normal biliary development is known to pass GGT from the liver into the amniotic fluid during weeks 18 to19 of gestation, there has been a report of a fetus with low amniotic fluid GGT levels at that particular gestational age in infants who turned out to suffer from BA [64]. All of these observations suggest that BA begins before birth, presumably during the end of the first trimester to the early second trimester [65].

### 9.7.3 The Timing of BA Development

The aforementioned observations and circumstantial evidences are summarized in the following sequence of embryological events (Table 9.1):

1. During week 7 of gestation, HLA class II⁺ cells appear in the liver.
2. At 8–9 weeks, fetal stem cells migrate to the thymus.
3. The anlage of bile ducts, called the ductal plate, occurs during weeks 11–13 of gestation.
4. As early as 13 weeks of gestation, maternal DNA is present in fetal circulation.
5. The earliest antenatally diagnosed cystic type of BA (type I) was observed at 16 weeks of gestation.
6. The absence of GGT in amniotic fluid, which should be present during 18–19 weeks of gestation, suggests that obstructive cholangiopathy has already begun.
7. Treg was shown to be functional during weeks 18–22 of gestation.

Given this sequence, we hypothesize that BA starts during weeks 11–17 of gestation. The initial immunological event of priming the mother with her offspring's antigens

**Table 9.1** Sequence of developmental events in fetus. BA plausibly develops during the period between weeks 9–17 of gestation, which is green-shaded

| Gestational weeks | Events in fetus |
|---|---|
| 7 | HLA class $II^+$ cells appear in the liver |
| 8 | Fetal stem cells migrate to the thymus |
| 9 | |
| 10 | |
| 11 | Ductal plate remodeling |
| 12 | |
| 13 | Maternal DNA in the fetal peripheral blood (MMC) |
| 14 | |
| 15 | Maternal hematopoietic cells in the fetal organs |
| 16 | The earliest antenatally diagnosed cyst-type BA |
| 17 | |
| 18 | GGT excreted in amniotic fluid |
| 19 | |
| 20 | T-regs become functional and maternal tolerance formed |
| 21 | |
| 22 | |

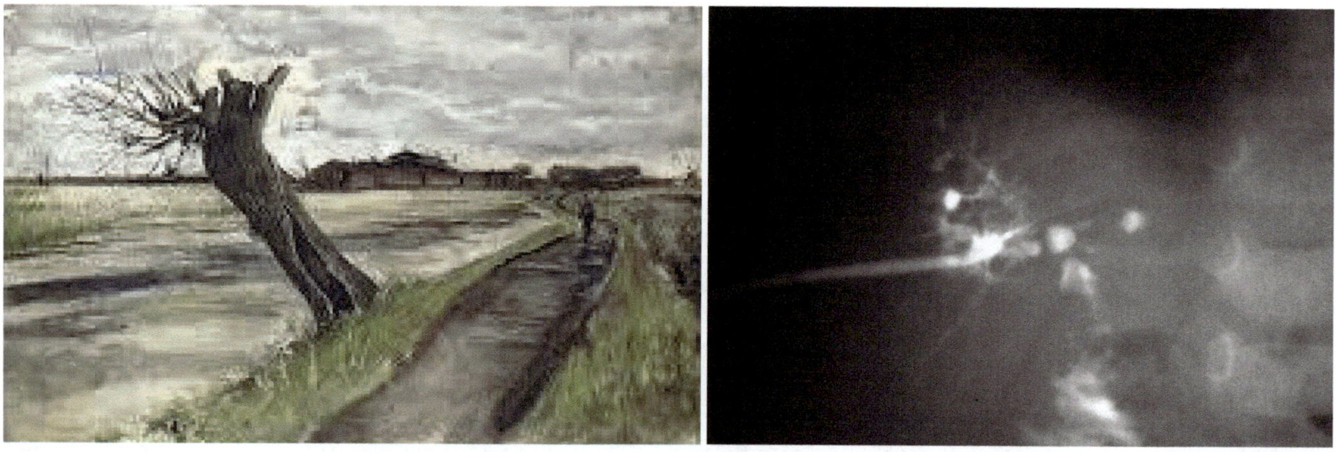

**Fig. 9.5** Left: "Pollard willow" by Vincent van Gogh (watercolor, Netherland, 1882). Right: Percutaneous intrahepatic cholangiogram, brush-like twig branching of intrahepatic bile ducts. This cholangiogram was obtained several months after the Kasai operation for type III BA at the time of the management for cholangitis. Adapted from Muraji et al., reprinted with permission from 2020;32(1):11–16. J Jap Soc for Neonatal Health and Development

may occur at the interface of the EVT. As previously discussed in 9.2, HLA-C expression by EVT has a unique and dual role in maternal–fetal immune tolerance and immunity. The expression of paternal HLA-C by EVT provides a target for maternal NK cells and cytotoxic T lymphocytes in pregnancy at the maternal–fetal interface. The first hit made by the primed maternal effector T lymphocytes transplacentally passed to the fetus is a damage of the developing bile ducts and portal vein endothelium of the offspring, presumably during the first trimester from week 11 or later of gestation. The severity of the disease presumably depends on when and how many maternal effector cells transfer to the offspring, affecting the balance of immune/tolerance between the BA patients and their mothers during the early phase of pregnancy. However, it is plausible that immune/tolerance may be well balanced during the rest of gestational weeks. The second hit would come after birth when the newborns are exposed to new antigens, such as maternal breastfeeding or postnatal exposure of viral antigens, leading to a flare-up of alloimmunity. The prognosis of patients with BA may very well depend on a balance between tolerance and persistent GVHD-type alloimmune responses.

## 9.8 Epilogue: BA as a Maternofetal Immune Disease (MFID)

Schreiber and Kleinman [66] described "genetic predisposition" and "environmental precipitating factors" in the etiopathogenesis of BA nearly 30 years ago. They thought that BA was an acquired disease. Borrowing their phrases, we now know the disease mechanisms that mediate BA are MMC with maternal–fetal histocompatibility as the "genetic predisposition" and fetal GVHD by maternal cell transplacental migration as the "environmental precipitating factors." The maternal effector lymphocyte priming may occur at the maternal–fetal interface of the placenta.

Future research of maternal–fetal interface focused on maternal–patient tolerance and immunity is warranted to clarify the etiopathogenesis of BA. We continue our quest for pathogenesis-based management, which may enable more effective anti-cholangitis therapies. All of these efforts will eventually help to achieve better native liver survival in BA patients.

## References


1. Suskind DL, Rosentahl P, Heyman MB, Kong D, Magrane G, Baxter-Lowe LA, Muench MO. Maternal microchimerism in the livers of patients with biliary atresia. BMC Gastroenterol. 2004;4:14.
2. Kobayashi H, Tamatani T, Tamura T, Kusafuka J, Yamataka A, Lane GJ, Kawasaki S, Ishizaki Y, Mizuta K, Kawarasaki H, et al. Maternal microchimerism in biliary atresia. J Pediatr Surg. 2007;42:987–91.
3. Hayashida M, Nishimoto Y, Matsuura T, Takahashi Y, Kohashi K, Taguchi T, et al. Evidence of maternal microchimerism in biliary atresia using in situ hybridization. J Pediatr Surg. 2007;42:2097–101.
4. Muraji T, Hosaka N, Irie N, Yoshida M, Imai Y, Tanaka K, Takada Y, Sakamoto S, Haga H, Ikehara S. Maternal microchimerism in underlying pathogenesis of biliary atresia: quantification and phenotypes of maternal cells in the liver. Pediatrics. 2008;121:517–21.
5. Bilingham RE, Brent L, Medawar PB. Actively acquired tolerance of foreign cells. Nature. 1953;172:603–6.
6. Gatti RA, Meuwissen HJ, Allen HD, et al. Immunological reconstitution of sex-linked lymphopenic immunological deficiency. Lancet. 1968;2:1366.
7. Billingham RE. Biology graft-versus-host reactions. Harvey Lect. 1966–67;62:21–78.
8. Hathaway WE, Fulginiti VA, Pierce CW, et al. Graft-versus-host reaction following a single blood transfusion. JAMA. 1967;201:1015–20.
9. Susanna M, Ege M, Pottharst A, et al. Transplacentally acquired maternal T lymphocytes in severe combined immunodeficiency: a study of 121 patients. Blood. 2001;98:1847–51.
10. Seemayor TA, Lapp WS, Bolande RP. Thymic epithelial injury in graft-versus-host reactions following adrenalectomy. Amer J Pathol. 1978;93:325–32.
11. Landing BH, Yutuc IL, Swanson VL. Clinicopathological correlations in immunologic deficiency diseases in children, with emphasis on athymic histologic patterns. Proceedings of the International Symposium on Immunodeficiency. Japan Medical Research Foundation. 1976;15–7.
12. Sakaguchi S, Sakaguchi N, Asano M, et al. Immunologic self-tolerance was maintained by activated T cells expressing IL-2 receptor alpha chains (CD25). Breakdown of a single mechanism of self-tolerance causes various autoimmune diseases. J Immunol. 1995;155:1151–64.
13. Zorn E, Kim HT, Lee SJ, et al. Reduced frequency of FOXP3+CD4+CD25+ regulatory T cells in patients with chronic GVHD. Blood. 2005;106:2903–11.
14. Mold JE, Michaelsson J, Burt TD, et al. Maternal alloantigens promote the development of tolerogenic fetal regulatory T cells in utero. Science. 2008;322:1562–5.
15. Nijagal A, Fleck S, Hills NK, et al. Decreased risk of graft failure with maternal liver transplantation in patients with biliary atresia. Ameri J Transplant. 2012;12:409–19.
16. Saito S, Shima T, Nakashima A, et al. What is the role of regulatory T cells in the success of implantation and early pregnancy? J Assist Reprod Genet. 2007;24:379–86.
17. Shima T, Inada K, Nakashima A, et al. Paternal antigen-specific proliferating regulatory T cells are increased in uterine-draining lymph nodes just before implantation and in the pregnant uterus just after implantation by seminal plasma priming in allogeneic mouse pregnancy. J Repro Immunol. 2015;108:72–82.
18. Tsuda S, Nakashima A, Shima T, et al. New paradigm in the role of regulatory T cells during pregnancy. Frontiers in Immunol. 2019;10:1–11.
19. Hiby SE, Walker JJ, O'Sahughnessy KM, et al. Combinations of maternal KIR and fetal HLA-C genes influence the risk of pre-eclampsia and reproductive success. J Exp Med. 2004;200:957–65.
20. Kim JS, Romero R, Kim MR, et al. Involvement of Hofbauer cells and maternal T cells in villitis of unknown etiology. Histopathology. 2008;52:457–64.
21. Herzenberg LA, Bianchi DW, Schroder J, et al. Fetal cells in the blood of pregnant women: detection and enrichment by

fluorescence-activated cell sorting. Pro Nat Acad Sci USA. 1979;76:1453–5.
22. Schroeder J. Fetal leukocytes in the maternal circulation after delivery. Transplantation. 1974;17:346–54.
23. Nelson JL, Furst DE, Maloney S, Gooley T, Evans PC, Smith A, Bean MA, Ober C, Bianchi DW. Microchimerism and HLA-compatibility relationships of pregnancy in scleroderma. Lancet. 1998;351:559–62.
24. Ostensen M, Villiger PM. The remission of rheumatoid arthritis during pregnancy. Semin Immunopathol. 2007;29:185–91.
25. Parkman R. Treatment of immunodeficiency diseases by organ transplantation. Prog Clin Immunol. 1977;3:85–102.
26. Lo YM, Lo ES, Watson N, et al. Two-way cell traffic between mother and fetus: biologic and clinical implications. Blood. 1996;88:4390–5.
27. Reed AM, Picomell YJ, Harwood A, et al. Chimerism in children with juvenile dermatomyositis. Lancet. 2000;362:1617–23.
28. Stevens AM, Hermes HM, Rutledge JC, et al. Myocardial-tissue-specific phenotype of maternal microchimerism in neonatal lupus congenital heart block. Lancet. 2003;362:1617–23.
29. Nelson JL, Gillespie KM, Lamert NC, et al. Maternal microchimerism in peripheral blood in type 1 diabetes and pancreatic islet beta cell microchimerism. PNAS. 2007;104:1637–42.
30. Reed AM, McNallan K, Wettstein P, et al. Does HLA-dependent chimerism underlie the pathogenesis of juvenile dermatomyositis? J Immunol. 2004;172:5041–6.
31. Burch JM, Sokol RJ, Narkewicz MR, et al. Autoantibodies in mothers of children with neonatal liver disease. J Ped Gastroenterol Nutri. 2003;37:262–7.
32. Muraji T, Suskind D, Irie N. Biliary atresia: a new immunological insight into etiopathogenesis. Expert Rev Gastroenterol Hepatol. 2009;3:599–606.
33. Gou Q, Chen Y, Yu C, Jia J, Feng J, Gao W, et al. Biliary atresia in twins' population: a retrospective multicenter study in mainland China. Pediatr Surg Int. 2020;36(6):711–8.
34. Ferrara JL, Cooke KR, Deeg HJ. Graft-versus-Host Disease. 3rd ed. Marcel Dekker; 2005. p. 195–328.
35. Haas JE. Bile duct and liver pathology in biliary atresia. World J Surg. 1978;2:561–9.
36. Suda K, Muraji T, Ohtani H, et al. Histological significance of hepatitis-like findings in biliary atresia: an analysis of 34 Japanese cases. Pediatr Int 2019;0:1–5.
37. Ruggeri L, Mancusi A, Capanni M, et al. Donor natural killer cell allorecognition of missing self in haploidentical hematopoietic transplantation for acute myeloid leukemia: challenging its predictive value. Blood. 2007;110:433–40.
38. Muraji T. Maternal microchimerism in biliary atresia: are maternal cells effector cells, targets, or just bystanders? Chimerism. 2014;5:1–5.
39. Zhang S, Goswami S, Ma J, et al. $CD4^+$ T cell subset profiling in biliary atresia reveals $ICOS^-$ regulatory T cells as a favorable prognostic factor. Front Immunol. 2019;7:1–13.
40. Sakamoto N, Muraji T, Ohtani H, et al. The accumulation of regulatory T cells in the hepatic hilar lymph nodes in biliary atresia. Surg Today. 2017;47:1282–6.
41. Engelmann CE, Maelzer M, Kreyenberg H. Absence of maternal microchimerism in regional lymph nodes of children with biliary atresia. JPGN. 2016;62:804–7.
42. Shim WK, Kasai M, Spence MA, et al. Racial influence on the incidence of biliary atresia. Prog Pediatr Surg. 1974;6:53–62.
43. Mack CL, Anderson KM, Aubrey MT, et al. Lack of HLA predominance and HLA shared epitopes in biliary atresia. Springerplus. 2013;2:42.
44. Yuasa T, Tsuji H, Kimura S, et al. Human leukocyte antigens in Japanese patients with biliary atresia: retrospective analysis of patients who underwent living donor liver transplantation. Hum Immunol. 2005;66:295–300.
45. Irie N, Muraji T, Hosaka N, et al. Maternal HLA class I compatibility in patients with biliary atresia. JPGN. 2009;49:488–92.
46. Kaplan J, Land S. Influence of maternal-fetal histocompatibility and MHC zygosity on maternal microchimerism. J Immunol. 2005;174:7123–8.
47. Muraji T, Tanaka H, Ieiri S. Ethnic variation in the incidence of biliary atresia correlates with the frequency of the most prevalent haplotype in its population. Human Immunol. 2018;79:668–71.
48. Takahashi A, Masuda N, Suzuki M, et al. Evidence for segmental bile drainage by hepatic portoenterostomy for biliary atresia: cholangiographic, hepatic venographic and histological evaluation of the liver taken at liver transplantation. J Pediatr Surg. 2004;39:1–5.
49. Matsuura T, et al. A morphological study of the removed livers from patients receiving living donor liver transplantation for adult biliary atresia. Pediatr Surg Int. 2012;28:1171–5.
50. Davenport M, Redkar GR, Koukoulis G, et al. Immunohistochemistry of the liver and biliary tree in extrahepatic biliary atresia. J Pediatr Surg. 2001;36:1017–25.
51. Santo K, Nakano N, Kasahara M, et al. Segmental atrophy of explanted livers in biliary atresia: pathological data from 63 cases of failed portoenterostomy. JPGN. 2021;72:8894.
52. Okamura A, Harada K, Nio M, et al. Participation of natural killer cells in the pathogenesis of bile duct lesions in biliary atresia. J Clin Pathol. 2013;66:99–108.
53. Fujisawa S, Muraji T, Sakamoto N, et al. Positive C4d staining of the portal vein endothelium in the liver of patients with biliary atresia: a role of humoral immunity in ongoing liver fibrosis. Pediatr Surg Int. 2014;30:877–81.
54. Sharif A, Shah V, McKinnon R, et al. Frequent expression of C4d in hepatic graft-versus-host disease: potential clue for diagnosis and distinguishing acute and chronic form. Transpl Immunol. 2010;23:77–80.
55. Ohuchi N, Ohi R, Takahashi T, et al. Postoperative changes of intrahepatic portal veins biliary atresia – a 3-D reconstruction study. J Pediatr Surg. 1986;21:10–4.
56. Masuya R, Muraji T, Ohtani H, et al. Morphometric demonstration of portal vein stenosis and hepatic arterial medial hypertrophy in patients with biliary atresia. Pediatr Surg Int. 2019;35:529–37.
57. Harumatsu T, Muraji T, Masuya R, et al. Microvascular proliferation of the portal vein branches in the liver of biliary atresia patients at Kasai operation is associated with a better long-term clinical outcome. Pediatr Surg Int. 2019;35:1437–41.
58. Patel K, Harpavat S, Khan Z, et al. Biliary atresia patients with successful Kasai portoenterostomy can present with features of obliterative portal venopathy. JPGN. 2020;71:91–8.
59. Muraji T, Ohtani H, Ieiri S. Unique manifestations of biliary atresia provide new immunological insight into its etiopathogenesis. Pediatr Surg Int. 2017;33:1249–53.
60. Desmet VJ. Congenital diseases of intrahepatic bile ducts: variations on the theme "ductal plate malformation". Hepatology. 1992;16:1069–83.
61. Tan CE, Driver M, Howard E, et al. Extrahepatic biliary atresia: a first-trimester event? Clues from light microscopy and immunohistochemistry. J Pediatr Surg. 1994;29:808–14.
62. Tan CE, Davenport M, Driver M, et al. Does the morphology of the extrahepatic biliary remnants in biliary atresia influence survival? A review of 205 cases. J Pediatr Surg. 1994;29:1459–64.
63. Redkar R, Davenport M, Howard ER. Antenatal diagnosis of congenital anomalies of the biliary tract. J Pediatr Surg. 1998;33:700–4.
64. Muller F, Gauthier F, Laurent J, et al. Amniotic fluid GGT and congenital extrahepatic biliary damage. Lancet. 1991;337:232–3.
65. MacGillivray TE, Adzick NS. Biliary atresia begins before birth. Ped Surg Int. 1994;9:116–7.
66. Schreiber RA, Kelinman R. Genetic, immunology, and biliary atresia: an opening or a diversion? JPGN. 1993;16:113–6.

# Epidemiology: Incidence, Gender Ratio, and Ethnic Variations

# 10

Satoshi Ieiri, Toshio Harumatsu, and Toshihiro Muraji

## 10.1 Incidence and Ethnic Variations

Biliary atresia (BA) is a rare pediatric liver disease characterized by fibrosclerosing obliteration of the extrahepatic bile ducts, leading to cholestasis, fibrosis, cirrhosis, and eventual liver failure [1]. BA is also the most devastating liver disease developing in neonates and early infancy, and the incidence has been generally reported as between one in 8000–15,000 live births.

In 1974, Shim et al. first reported a significant difference in the incidence of BA among people in Hawaii of different ancestral origins [2]. This ethnic/geographical diversity in the incidence of BA supported possible genetic susceptibility in the etiopathogenetic background of BA. Recent study from the USA also supported this ethnic diversity [3]. Hopkins et al. used the triennial Health Cost and Utilization Project-Kids' Inpatient Database for 1997–2012 and performed a retrospective analysis of BA in the USA. Infants aged <1 year of age with a diagnosis of BA who underwent a Kasai portoenterostomy were included. Nationwide infant population data were used to calculate incidence and evaluate trends. The sample size was 1057, and the overall incidence of BA in the USA was 0.45 per 10, 000 live births. The incidence of Caucasian and Hispanic were 0.4 and 0.44 per 10, 000 live births, respectively. On the other hand, the incidences of BA in Black (0.518 per 10,000 live birth) and Asian/Pacific Islander (0.755 per 10,000 live birth) were higher than those of Caucasian and Hispanic, respectively. The incidence BA in Native American (0.17 per 10,000 live births) was lower than those of white and Hispanic. The racial distribution was 62% Caucasian, 20% Black, 11% Hispanic, 4.2% Asian, and 1.5% Native American.

Table 10.1 showed the summary of collected incidence and ethnic variations in BA. It is more common in eastern countries, especially in Asia, than in western countries [1, 4, 5]. Regarding the newest data from the Japanese Biliary Atresia Registry (JBAR), the estimated incidence of BA in Japan is based on the registered number of cases (91) divided by the annual number of the newborn (918,400) was 1/10,092 live birth on 2018 [6].

In general, isolated BA occurs most frequently in the Eastern world, e.g., in one in 5000 newborn in Taiwan versus one in 15,000–19,000 births in Europe and North America [7–9]. In Taiwan, after the establishment of a universal screening system using an infant stool color card to promote the early diagnosis and treatment of BA, the annual incidence of BA was reported to be per 10,000 live births in 2004 and 2005 was 1.85 (40/216,419) and 1.70 (35/205,854) [5].

Muraji et al. reported ethnic variation in the incidence of biliary atresia correlates with the frequency of the most prevalent haplotype in its population [10]. The incidence of BA among Japanese ancestry in Hawaii was 0.8 ± 0.3 per 10,000 live births, whereas recent Japanese registry data in Japan shows 1.0 [1, 6]. The incidence of BA in South Korea (1.06 per 10,000 live births) is similar to that in Japan [4]. The incidence in Caucasians living in Hawaii was 0.6 ± 0.2 per 10,000 live births, which is also similar to that of recent reports, ranging from 0.5 to 0.6 per 10,000 live births in the UK [7], France [8], Germany [13], Netherland [12], Norway [14] Sweden [15] and Croatia [15] shows a higher incidence of 0.7. The incidence of BA in the Filipino population in Hawaii was 2.0 ± 0.9 per 10,000 live births, which is slightly lower than that of French Polynesians (3.2 per 10,000 live births) [11], whereas, in the Maori population in New Zealand [16], the incidence is 1.9 per 10,000 live births, similar to the Filipino population in Hawaii. The incidence of BA in black South African infants may be among the highest in the world; preliminary data estimated the local incidence to be between 1 in 2500 and 1 in 8000 live births [17].

S. Ieiri (✉) · T. Harumatsu
Department of Pediatric Surgery, Research Field in Medical and Health Sciences, Medical and Dental Area, Research and Education Assembly, Kagoshima University, Kagoshima, Japan
e-mail: sieiri@m.kufm.kagoshima-u.ac.jp

T. Muraji
Department of Pediatric Surgery, Kirishima Medical Center, Kirishima, Japan

Department of Pediatric Surgery, Research Field in Medical and Health Sciences, Medical and Dental Area, Research and Education Assembly, Kagoshima University, Kagoshima, Japan



M. Nio (ed.), *Introduction to Biliary Atresia*, https://doi.org/10.1007/978-981-16-2160-4_10

**Table 10.1** Summary of incidence and ethnic variations

| Population | Sample size (n) | Incidence of BA/10,000 live birth |
|---|---|---|
| Japanese [1, 6] | 18,604 | 1.0 |
| South Korea [4] | 7096 | 1.06 |
| Taiwan [5] | 40/35 | 1.85/1.70 |
| England [7] | 519 | 0.6 |
| France [8] | 100 | 0.6 |
| Germany [11] | 13,386 | 0.51 |
| Netherland [12] | | 0.5 |
| Norway [13] | 4510 | 0.55 |
| Sweden [14] | 154 | 0.71 |
| Croatia [15] | 29 | 0.42 |
| Philippine [8] | 50 | 2.0 |
| New Zealand [17] | 46 | 1.08 |
| Maori | | 1.89 |
| European | | 0.61 |
| United States [4] | 1057 | 0.447 |
| Caucasian | 403 | 0.4 |
| Black | 131 | 0.518 |
| Hispanic | 174 | 0.443 |
| Asian/Pacific Islander | 612 | 0.755 |
| Native American | 2 | 0.167 |
| Other | 79 | 0.772 |
| Unreported race | 207 | 0.425 |
| French Polynesians | 14 | 3.2 |
| South African (Black) | 70 | 1.25–4.0 |

Recently, Girard reported that the incidence of BA across various ethnicities was 0.5 per 10,000 live births in Caucasians, 1.0 in Japanese, and between 2.2 and 3.3 in Polynesians, which is as high as reported in Native Americans and Inuit's [18].

Assuming the hypothesis that against a background of a hereditary predisposition, BA is probably an (auto) immunological process, it is not surprising that the worldwide incidence of this disease differs.

## 10.2 Gender Ratio and Ethnic Variations

Theoretically, congenital anomalies arising from an organ that develops similarly in males and females should occur at a similar rate in both genders. However, a discrepancy between the prevalence of congenital anomalies in males versus females has long been reported. Black's study indicates that males have higher prevalence rates of most congenital anomalies [19]. However, bile duct diseases such as BA and choledochal cyst show higher prevalence rates. Table 10.2 showed the male/female ratio of representative pediatric surgery disease as references, which was modified from Black's report.

Black AJ et al. collected 8202 patients and conducted 0.7: 1 in male/female ratio in their report. Females had a higher prevalence of BA (0.70; 0.68–0.73) [19]. Nio et al. reported male/female ratio was 0.59: 1 data from 1990 to 2015 in Japan [1]. Barshes et al. reported male/female ratio was 0.67: 1 in the USA [20]. Townsend et al. 0.75: 1 in the USA [21].

**Table 10.2** Summary of gender ratio in pediatric surgery disease

| Disease | Sample size | Male: female (95% CI) |
|---|---|---|
| Biliary atresia | 8202 | 0.70 (0.68–0.73) |
| Nio et al. (Japan) | 3153 | 0.59 |
| Barshes et al. (USA) | 1976 | 0.67 |
| Townsend et al (USA) | 1243 | 0.75 |
| Anderson et al. (International) | 926 | 0.63 |
| Karrer et al. (International) | 904 | 1.40 |
| Choledochal cyst | 2229 | 0.37 (0.35–0.39) |
| Duodenal atresia | 787 | 0.94 (0.80–1.19) |
| Gastroschisis | 39,324 | 1.10 (1.07–1.13) |
| Omphalocele | 6702 | 1.16 (1.12–1.20) |
| Intestinal atresia | 4638 | 1.25 (1.20–1.30) |
| Congenital pulmonary airway malformation | 1691 | 1.21 (1.10–1.28) |
| Esophageal atresia | 11,755 | 1.22 (1.16–1.28) |
| Anorectal malformation | 3996 | 1.34 (1.27–1.39) |
| Congenital diaphragmatic hernia | 9246 | 1.44 (1.36–1.53) |
| Hirschprung's disease | 10,180 | 2.83 (2.65–3.03) |

Anderson et al. male/female ratio was 0.63: 1 [22]. Karrer et al. collected the BA registry data from Section of the American Academy of Pediatrics in the USA (from 1976 to 1989) and reported male/female ratio was 0.71: 1[23]. Further investigations are required to illuminate the embryology of BA underlying this gender distribution and whether gender influences outcomes.

## References


1. Nio M. Japanese Biliary Atresia Registry. Pediatr Surg Int. 2017 Dec;33(12):1319-1325. https://doi.org/10.1007/s00383-017-4160-x. Epub 2017 Oct 16
2. Shim WK, Kasai M, Spence MA. Racial influence on the incidence of biliary atresia. Prog Pediatr Surg. 1974;6:53–62.
3. Hopkins PC, Yazigi N, Nylund CM. Incidence of Biliary Atresia and Timing of Hepatoportoenterostomy in the United States. J Pediatr. 2017;187:253–7. https://doi.org/10.1016/j.jpeds.2017.05.006. Epub 2017 Jun 1
4. Lee KJ, Kim JW, Moon JS, Jung K. Epidemiology of Biliary Atresia in Korea. J Korean Med Sci. 2017;32(4):656–60. https://doi.org/10.3346/jkms.2017.32.4.656.
5. Hsiao CH, Chang MH, Chen HL, Lee HC, Wu TC, Lin CC, Yang YJ, Chen AC, Tiao MM, Lau BH, et al. Universal screening for biliary atresia using an infant stool color card in Taiwan. Hepatology. 2008;47(4):1233–40.
6. Japanese Biliary Atresia Society. Japanese Biliary Atresia Registry 2018. J Jpn Soc Pediatr Surg. 2020;56:219–25. (in Japanese)
7. Livesey E, Cortina Borja M, Sharif K, et al. Epidemiology of biliary atresia in England and Wales (1999–2006). Archives of disease in childhood. Fetal Neonatal Ed. 2009;94:F451–5.
8. Chardot C, Carton M, Spire-Bendelac N, Le Pommelet C, Golmard JL, Auvert B. Epidemiology of biliary atresia in France: a national study 1986–96. J Hepatol. 1999;31(6):1006–13.
9. Petersen C, Davenport M. Aetiology of biliary atresia: what is actually known? Orphanet J Rare Dis. 2013;8:128.
10. Muraji T, Tanaka H, Ieiri S: Ethnic variation in the incidence of biliary atresia correlates with the frequency of the most prevalent haplotype in its population. Hum Immunol. 2018 Sep;79(9):668-671. https://doi.org/10.1016/j.humimm.2018.07.001. Epub 2018 Jul 11.

11. Leonhardt J, Kuebler JF, Leute PJ, Turowski C, Becker T, Pfister ED, Ure B, Petersen C. Biliary atresia: lessons learned from the voluntary German registry. Eur J Pediatr Surg. 2011;21(2):82–7.
12. Houwen RH, Kerremans II, van Steensel-Moll HA, van Romunde LK, Bijleveld CM, Schweizer P. Time-space distribution of extrahepatic biliary atresia in The Netherlands and West Germany. Z Kinderchir. 1988 Apr;43(2):68–71. https://doi.org/10.1055/s-2008-1043419.
13. Henriksen NT, Drablos PA, Aagenaes O. Cholestatic jaundice in infancy. The importance of familial and genetic factors in etiology and prognosis. Arch. Dis. Child. 1981;56:622.
14. Fischler B, Haglund B, Hjern A. A population-based study on the incidence and possible pre-and perinatal etiologic risk factors of biliary atresia J. Pediatr. 2002;141:217.
15. Grizelj R, Vuković J, Novak M, Batinica S. Biliary atresia: the Croatian experience 1992–2006. European Journal of Pediatrics. 2010;169:1529–34.
16. Evans HM, Asher MI, Cameron-Christie S, Farthing S, McCall J, Robertson SP, Wong H, Morreau PN. Ethnic Disparity in the Incidence and Outcome of Biliary Atresia in New Zealand. J Pediatr Gastroenterol Nutr. 2018 Feb;66(2):218–21. https://doi.org/10.1097/MPG.0000000000001781.
17. Girard M, Besnard M, Jacquemin E, et al. Biliary atresia: does ethnicity matter? J. Hepatol. 2012;57:699.
18. De Maayer T, Lala SG, Loveland J, et al. Outcomes of Kasai hepatoportoenterostomy in children with biliary atresia in Johannesburg. South Africa S. Afr. Med. J. 2017;107:Article s7.
19. Black AJ, Lu DY, Yefet LS, Baird R. Sex differences in surgically correctable congenital anomalies: A systematic review. J Pediatr Surg. 2020;55(5):811–20. https://doi.org/10.1016/j.jpedsurg.2020.01.016. Epub 2020 Feb 12
20. Barshes NR, Lee TC, Balkrishnan R, et al. Orthotopic liver transplantation for biliary atresia: the U.S. experience. Liver Transpl. 2005;11(10):1193–200. https://doi.org/10.1002/lt.20509
21. Townsend MR, Jaber A, Nader HA, et al. Factors associated with timing and adverse outcomes in patients with biliary atresia undergoing Kasai hepatoportoenterostomy. J Pediatr Elsevier Inc. 2018;199:237–42. https://doi.org/10.1016/j.jpeds.2018.04.001.
22. Anderson CD, Turmelle YP, Lowell JA, et al. The effect of recipient-specific surgical issues on outcome of liver transplantation in biliary atresia. Am J Transplant. 2008 Jun;8(6):1197–204. https://doi.org/10.1111/j.1600-6143.2008.02223.x.
23. Karrer FM, Lilly JR, Stewart BA, et al. Biliary atresia registry, 1976 to 1989. J Pediatr Surg. 1990 Oct;25(10):1076–81. https://doi.org/10.1016/0022-3468(90)90222-U.

# 11 Epidemiology: Seasonality, Family History, and Heredity

Masayuki Kubota

**Abstract**

In this chapter, clinical characteristics of BA are reviewed from the viewpoints of seasonality, family history, and heredity, the results of which are summarized into two sections of seasonal and regional clustering and family history. Seasonal clustering was mainly found in some studies from the USA, Japan, and French Polynesia using institutional or regional databases, while reports favoring seasonal clustering have not been published from the European countries using nationwide survey data. Even though seasonal clustering of BA seemed to be more common from autumn to winter, actually all seasons and months of the year showed periods of seasonal clustering due to marked variations among studies. Regional clustering was also found in some of the studies that examined seasonal clustering but was less frequent. The presence of regional clustering does not support the presence of seasonal clustering. It is hypothesized that seasonal and regional clustering might be a local phenomenon that becomes more apparent in regional studies than in nationwide studies. Reports of BA occurring in siblings are also rare and were found in case reports published in the twentieth centuries but not in the twenty-first century. The occurrence of BA was not even concordant in monozygotic twins. The vertical penetrance of BA from parents with BA to their children was only reported in one family. The precise meaning of the seasonal and regional clustering and familial occurrence of BA is still unclear; however, but the present results are useful for understanding the epidemiological characteristics of BA, the pathophysiology of which still remains unknown.

**Keywords**

Biliary atresia · Seasonal clustering · Regional clustering Family history · Heredity

M. Kubota (✉)
Kokuraminami Medical Care Hospital, Kitakyushu City, Japan

## 11.1 Introduction

Biliary atresia (BA) is a devastating clinical condition where obstruction of the extrahepatic biliary tract occurs in the neonatal and/or early infantile period, leading to liver cirrhosis as a result of ongoing liver fibrosis and cellular destruction. Ongoing fibro-inflammatory changes are a prominent pathological feature of the biliary tree; however, the precise pathogenesis remains unknown. Davenport et al. [1] reported that 10.2% of BA patients in King's College Hospital were diagnosed with biliary atresia splenic malformation (BASM) with situs inversus (37%) and cardiac anomalies (45%). Based on data from the North American Childhood Liver Disease Research and Education, Schwartz et al. [2] further divided BA patients into three groups according to the types of associated malformations: Group 1 (84%), nonsyndromic, isolated BA without major malformation; Group 2 (6%), syndromic BA with at least one major malformation but without laterality defects; and Group 3 (10%), BA with laterality defects and spleen anomalies. In these two reports, the incidence rates of BASM and Group 3 BA were both approximately 10%. However, in a study in Taiwan, Yang et al. [3] reported that major anomalies were found in 15.4% of BA patients, while only one patient (0.7%) was diagnosed with BASM. Therefore, developmental anomalies are considered to be associated with the disease process in BA patients; however, racial or regional differences seem to exist in the occurrence of laterality defects in BA.

BA is found worldwide, and racial or regional differences are also noted in its incidence. In a systematic review of the reported incidence of BA in different nations, the incidence ranged widely, and the incidence in Asian countries was higher in comparison to European countries [4]. The Pacific region was also regarded as an area of high incidence due to a high prevalence in Hawaii [5] and French Polynesia [6].

The presence of such racial and/or regional differences in associated anomalies, as well as the incidence of BA, indicates that the epidemiological studies of BA will become important clues to elucidate the underlying pathophysiology


M. Nio (ed.), *Introduction to Biliary Atresia*, https://doi.org/10.1007/978-981-16-2160-4_11

of BA. In this chapter, the relevant literature on seasonal and regional clustering and the familial occurrence of BA are reviewed and discussed for this purpose.

## 11.2 Seasonal and Regional Clustering

### 11.2.1 Seasonal Clustering (SC)

Table 11.1 shows a list of 16 (English language) studies that examined the seasonal and/or regional clustering of BA [6–21]. The presence of SC of BA patients was reported in seven studies: four studies from the USA [7, 10, 13, 16], and one each from Niigata, Japan [14], French Polynesia [20], and Korea [21]. Thus, SC of BA is not a universal phenomenon. Interestingly, a regional difference in SC was reported in a study from New York State in the USA [13]. A period of SC was found from March to May in New York City and from September to November elsewhere in New York State [13]. Figure 11.1 illustrates the seasonal and monthly distribution of SC from seven studies [7, 10, 13, 16, 14, 20, 21]. Even though SC seems to be frequently found in autumn [7, 13, 20] and winter [10, 14, 16], all season and months of the year were actually involved in the period of SC. It was also shown that the season of SC varied among countries as well as regions within the same country [13]. It is not clear why such regional variance is observed in SC. A relationship with the spread of viral infection from autumn to winter is often discussed; however, this might not be conclusive, because SC is also observed in spring [13] and summer [21]. French Polynesia only has two seasons (dry and wet), and the period of SC, which lasts for 5 months from July to November, overlaps perfectly with the dry season of this area, which occurs from June to November [20]. French Polynesia is also famous for its high incidence of BA [6]. Therefore, SC might also be influenced by environmental factors, such as the weather or the atmospheric temperature.

On the other hand, SC of BA was not reported in the other nine studies from the Netherlands and West Germany [8], Michigan in the USA [9], south England [11], France [6], Sweden [12], Hyogo, Japan [15], Taiwan [17], Switzerland [18], and England and Wales [19]. Thus, the presence of SC has not been documented in studies from European countries. The representative incidence of BA per 10,000 live births in European countries was 0.5 in the Netherlands, 0.59 in West Germany, 0.5 in the UK, 0.51 in France, 0.71 in Sweden, and 0.56 in Switzerland [4]. The relatively low incidence of BA in these countries might be a causative factor for the absence of SC. However, the incidence of BA in Taiwan (1.46) was higher than that in the USA (0.85) and Japan (1.1). Thus, in addition to the prevalence of BA, domestic conditions might be involved in an occurrence of SC.

According to the database examined, nationwide survey data [6, 8, 12, 18, 19] or large institutional data [11] were used in studies from European countries, while the seven studies that revealed SC used an institutional database or registry data obtained in each State program [7, 10, 13, 14, 16, 20], with the exception of one study from South Korea using national health insurance data [21]. Therefore, SC may be an event more apparently revealed in the limited-size regional study. The accumulation of the regional data in a nationwide survey may result in obscuring the regional variance in certain areas with SC, as the study areas expand.

There are two institutional studies from Japan [14, 15]. One study from Niigata [14] showed SC in winter, while seasonal and geographical clustering was denied in Hyogo [15]. The background socioeconomic conditions differ considerably between Niigata and Hyogo. Niigata is an agricultural district with vast farmland and one major river, while Hyogo is a center of commercial activities and is densely populated. The climate in winter differs considerably between two areas; heavy snow in Niigata versus warmer weather with little snow in Hyogo; however, the incidence of BA is in Niigata (1.07) and Hyogo (1.1) is quite similar. The study from Niigata alluded SC in winter might be related to a low atmospheric temperature in the winter season [14]. However, in a study [15] from Hyogo, a comparison between the northernmost and southernmost islands in Japan (Hokkaido and Kyushu, respectively; difference of latitude, 10 degrees) was also conducted without revealing SC. Furthermore, an analysis of nationwide registry data conducted by the Japanese Biliary Atresia Society failed to show SC, even though a small peak in the incidence was found in February and March, and a slight reduction of incidence was observed in June and October (data shown in the Clinical Guidelines of Biliary Atresia, published in Japanese and downloaded from https://minds.jcqhc.or.jp/n/med/4/med0362/G0001073). It is therefore suggested that SC of BA may exist in some local regions, but further studies with proper statistical analyses focused on local SC are necessary to understand the precise background of SC among different regions or nations. Walter and Elwood [22] pointed out that seasonality tests with sample sizes of <50 should be interpreted with caution.

According to SC in syndromic or isolated BA cases, two studies from the USA [10, 16] examined only isolated cases, and SC was found in these studies. In contrast, two other studies from the same institute in England [11, 19] examined both syndromic and isolated cases without demonstrating significant SC in either type.

### 11.2.2 Regional Clustering (RC)

The relationship between RC and SC is interesting. Only two studies reported the presence of RC [7, 19]. In north Texas, the incidence of BA was significantly higher in rural areas, and the presence of SC was also reported [7]. In contrast, in

**Table 11.1** A list of 16 studies that examined seasonal clustering and/or regional clustering of BA

| No | Author (Reference no) | Year of Publication | Study period | Area | Database | Number of patients | Seasonal clustering | Regional clustering |
|---|---|---|---|---|---|---|---|---|
| 1 | Strickland [7] | 1982 | 1972–1980 | North Texas, USA | Institutional survey | 31 | August to October | Rural area |
| 2 | Houwen [8] | 1988 | 1977–1987<br>1969–1986 | Netherlands<br>West Germany | Nationwide survey | 89<br>130 | Not found | Not found |
| 3 | Ayas [9] | 1996 | 18-year | Michigan, USA | Institutional survey | 65 | Not found | Not examined |
| 4 | Yoon [10] | 1997 | 1968–1993 | Metropolitan Atlanta, USA | Metropolitan Atlanta Congenital Defects Program | Isolated 49 | December to March | Not found |
| 5 | Davenport [11] | 1998 | 1973– | Predominantly south England | Institutional survey | Nonsyndromic 346<br>Syndromic 34 | Not found | Not examined |
| 6 | Chardot [6] | 1999 | 1986–1996 | France | Nationwide survey | 461 | Not found | Not found |
| 7 | Fischler [12] | 2002 | 1987–1997 | Sweden | Swedish national health database | 85 | Not found | Not found |
| 8 | Caton [13] | 2004 | 1983–1898 | New York State, USA | New York State Congenital Malformation Registry data | 369 | March to May in New York City<br>September to November in other New York State | Not found |
| 9 | Nakamizo [14] | 2006 | 1974–2002 | Niigata, Japan | Institutional survey | 87 | December to March | Not examined |
| 10 | Wada [15] | 2007 | 1985–2004 | Hyogo, Japan | Institutional survey | 119 | Not found | Not found |
| 11 | The [16] | 2007 | 1997–2002 | Eight states (Arkansas, California, Georgia, Iowa, Massachusetts, New Jersey, New York, and Texas), USA | National Birth Defects Prevention Study | Isolated 62 | December to February | Not examined |
| 12 | Tiao [17] | 2008 | 1996–2003 | Taiwan | National Health Insurance database | 327 | Not found | Not examined |
| 13 | Wildhaber [18] | 2008 | 1994–2004 | Switzerland | Nationwide survey | 48 | Not found | Not found |
| 14 | Livesey [19] | 2009 | 1999–2006 | England and Wales | A national data registry | Nonsyndromic 219<br>Syndromic 76 | Not found | Regional differences along a north-west/south-east axis |
| 15 | Girard [20] | 2011 | 1979–2009 | French Polynesia | Institutional survey | 40 | July to November | Not examined |
| 16 | Lee [21] | 2017 | 2011–2015 | South Korea | Health Insurance Review and Assessment Service | 240 | June to August | Not examined |

England and Wales, marked regional differences along a north-west/south-east axis existed, ranging from 0.38 (north-west England) to 0.78 (south-east England) per 10,000 live births, which amounted to a statistically significant difference, without revealing SC [19]. RC was denied in seven other studies [6, 8, 10, 12, 13, 15, 18]. Two of these studies, which were from the USA [10, 13], showed the presence of SC. Thus, the presence of RC is much less frequently found in comparison to SC, and there seems to be no relationship between RC and SC.

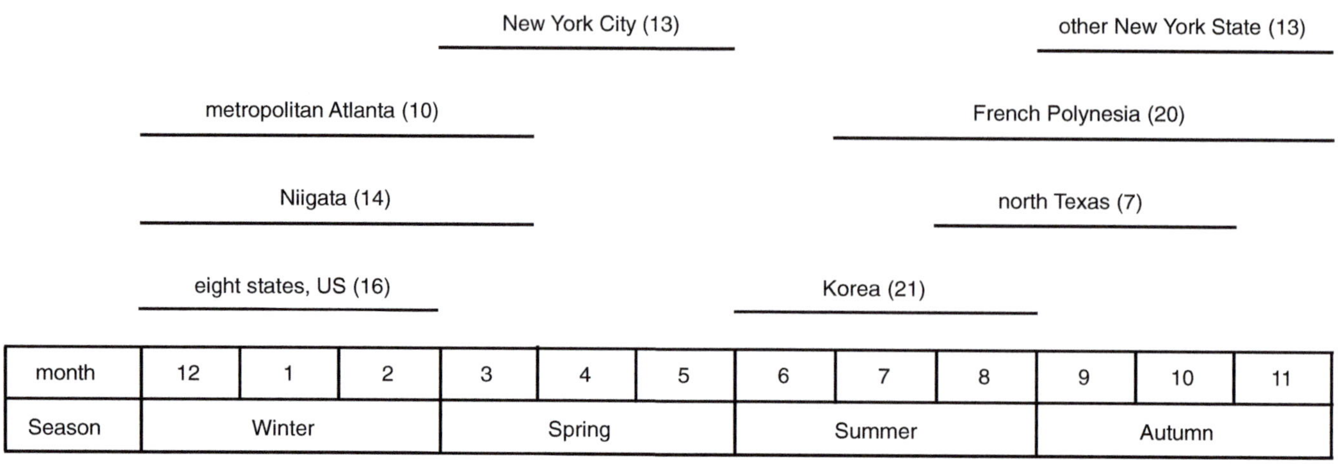


**Fig. 11.1** The seasonal and monthly distribution of SC from seven studies. Horizontal lines indicate the season or months of SC shown in each study, and the examined area and reference number are shown above the horizontal lines. Two different periods of SC were reported in one study from New York State

It would be interesting to know whether RC varies with time or not. We analyzed this issue in Niigata, Japan [23] using the same database in a study by Nakamizo et al. [14]. Ninety-six BA patients born in Niigata prefecture from 1972 to 2001 were analyzed. The prefecture was divided into 14 areas governed by local health centers, and the study period was divided into 10-year intervals. As shown in Fig. 11.2a–c, the patients seemed to be more frequently located along coastal areas in the 1970s, while in the 1980s and 1990s, the distribution was spread widely along the largest river, which runs from south to north. Based on the cumulative data of the 30-year study period, the population-based incidence of BA per 10,000 live births from 1972 to 2001 in areas 1, 2, 3, and 4 as shown in Fig. 11.2d, was 2.54, 1.58, 1.82, and 0.51, respectively. The incidence of BA was significantly higher in areas 1, 2, and 3 in comparison to that in area 4. Thus, RC might be a dynamic event related to time, which is probably influenced by local socioeconomic conditions.

## 11.3 Family History

### 11.3.1 Occurrence in Siblings

The familial occurrence of BA in siblings is quite rare. Table 11.2 summarizes a list of 11 case studies identified by a survey of the relevant literature in English [24–34]. The years of publication range from 1932 to 1998. Interestingly, no new familial cases have been published in the twenty-first century. A paucity of recent papers indicates that the accuracy of the diagnosis of BA should be taken into consideration in old reports. As additional information, four sibling cases from two families were reported by Cunningham et al. [30]. Parental consanguinity was found in one report by Lachaux et al. [31], and Gunasekaran et al. [33] reported the cases of two half-siblings with a common father. The sibling cases reported by Anneren et al. [34] were considered to be peculiar lethal syndromic cases associated with intrauterine growth retardation, intra- and extrahepatic biliary atresia, and esophageal and duodenal atresia, with autosomal recessive inheritance. The absence of laterality defects in these cases may suggest that they did not fit the definition of biliary atresia splenic malformation (BASM). Danesino et al. [35] also found sibling cases with similar phenotypic abnormalities. Even though they reported the case as familial biliary atresia, patient 2 showed intrahepatic atresia without obliteration of extrahepatic duct. Thus, these cases were not included in Table 11.2. As far as examined, the syndromic case associated with cardiac anomalies involved one of BA concordant twins [32], two of three sibling cases [24], and one of two sibling cases [27, 34], respectively.

As a result, 27 sibling cases from 12 families, including two cases from Anneren, were accumulated. These patients consisted of 15 boys and 12 girls, which was contradictory to the well-known tendency of a slight female preponderance in BA. There was one family with the concordance of BA in twins [32], and these cases involved boys. It is not clear whether a male preponderance in BA sibling cases reflects a true character of familial occurrence or is based on sampling bias of rare BA siblings. Recently, a systematic review of biliary atresia in twins was conducted [36]. With the exception of the cases of the concordance of BA in twins reported by Smith et al. [32], BA was discordant in the remaining 97.1% of twins, 55.9% of which were monozygotic twins sets, and the gender of 36 BA patients was evenly split. In a report of a New Zealand Maori family with a 50-fold increase in the risk of BA in comparison to unrelated Maori families, no cases of BA in siblings were found [37]. Furthermore, a genetic analysis of the members of this family did not reveal any conclusive underlying genetic factors.

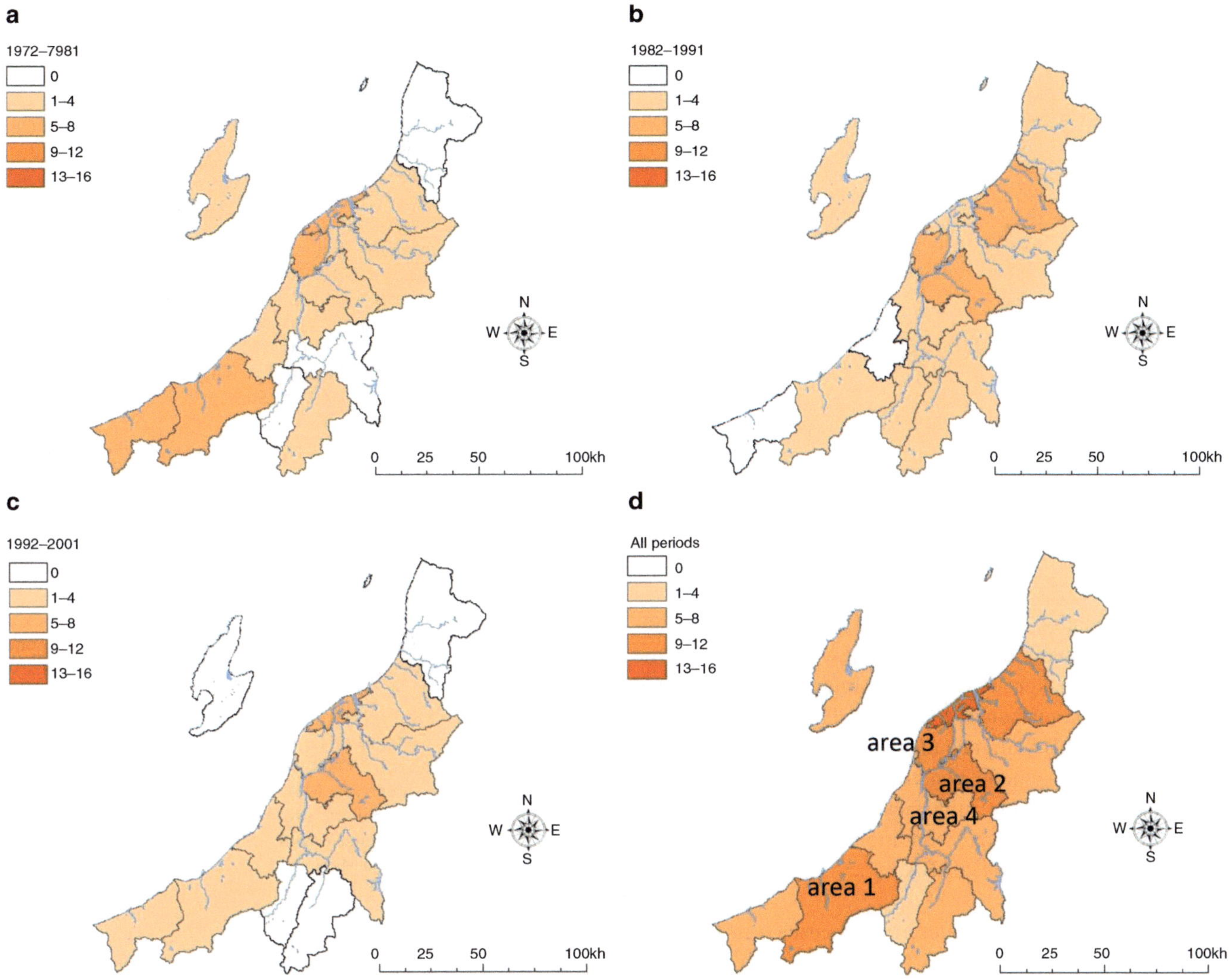


**Fig. 11.2** Regional clustering of BA patients in three 10-year periods in Niigata, Japan. Niigata prefecture is divided into 14 areas governed by local health centers, and the number of BA patients during each 10-year period in each area is shown in five shades from white (null incidence) to the darkest shade (13 to 16 patients). Niigata faces the Japan sea, and the area includes a large island. The running of rivers is shown in blue. **a**, **b**, and **c** are the results from the periods of 1972 to 1981, 1982 to 1991, and 1992 to 2001, respectively. (**d**) indicates the cumulative data from the three periods. Permission to use these data was obtained from the Department of Pediatric Surgery, Niigata University

### 11.3.2 Mother-to-Daughter Occurrence

Vertical penetrance of BA from BA parents to their children is much less frequent than the occurrence of BA in siblings. Thus far, one family has been reported, in the form of mother-to-daughter occurrence, in Niigata, Japan [38]. The mother with type III BA had a daughter with type I cyst BA. Both patients were successfully treated with Kasai hepatic porto-enterostomy. According to a recent analysis of 3160 patients in the Japanese Biliary Atresia Registry, who were registered from 1989 to 2015 [39], the 20-year overall and native-liver survival rates were 89% and 49%, respectively. Even though the survival rate of BA patients has increased, many BA patients do not bear children. Thus, future studies on familial occurrence will be necessary to understand the heredity of BA better.

## 11.4 Conclusions

Even though the results of seasonal and regional clustering of BA are not consistent among studies, these interesting topics should be kept examined in future studies. The seasonal and regional clustering of BA might be a result of complex multifactorial events, which could be more easily explored in a limited regional study with relatively little

**Table 11.2** A list of 11 case studies that examined the occurrence of BA in siblings

| No | Author (Reference no) | Year of publication | Numbers of patients | Number of boy | Number of girl |
|---|---|---|---|---|---|
| 1 | Sweet [24] | 1932 | 3 | 2 | 1 |
| 2 | Hopkins [25] | 1941 | 3 | 1 | 2 |
| 3 | Whitten [26] | 1952 | 2 | 2 | 0 |
| 4 | Krauss [27] | 1964 | 2 | 2 | 0 |
| 5 | Nevin [28] | 1969 | 2 | 2 | 0 |
| 6 | Sommer [29] | 1976 | 2 | 2 | 0 |
| 7 | Cunningham [30] | 1988 | 2 | 0 | 2 |
| | | | 2 | 0 | 2 |
| 8 | Lachaux [31] | 1988 | 2 | 2 | 0 |
| 9 | Smith [32] | 1991 | 3 | 0 | 3 |
| 10 | Gunasekaran [33] | 1992 | 2 | 1 | 1 |
| 11 | Anneren [34] | 1998 | 2 | 1 | 1 |
| | | Total | 27 | 15 | 12 |

variation in social background conditions. However, careful statistical validation is, of course, important in regional studies. The accumulation of such studies may facilitate the exploration of background socioeconomic or other regional conditions that contribute to SC or RC. The paucity of familial occurrence of BA might suggest that occurrence of BA is partly caused by genetic penetrance, but that teratogenic, infectious, and other multifactorial causes, including socioeconomic and weather conditions, play a more significant role in the prevalence of BA.

**Conflict of Interest** The author declares no conflicts of interest in association with the present study.

## References


1. Davenport M, Tizzard SA, Underhill J, Mieli-Vergani G, Portmann B, Hadzic N. The biliary atresia splenic malformation syndrome: a 28-year single-center retrospective study. J Pediatr. 2006;149(3):393–400.
2. Schwarz KB, Haber BH, Rosenthal P, Mack CL, Moore J, Bove K, et al. Extrahepatic anomalies in infants with biliary atresia: results of a large prospective North American multicenter study. Hepatology. 2013;58(5):1724–31.
3. Yang MC, Chang MH, Chiu SN, Peng SF, Wu JF, Ni YH, et al. Implication of early-onset biliary atresia and extrahepatic congenital anomalies. Pediatr Int. 2010;52(4):569–72.
4. Jimenez-Rivera C, Jolin-Dahel KS, Fortinsky KJ, Gozdyra P, Benchimol EI. International incidence and outcomes of biliary atresia. J Pediatr Gastroenterol Nutr. 2013;56(4):344–54.
5. Shim WK, Kasai M, Spence MA. Racial influence on the incidence of biliary atresia. Prog Pediatr Surg. 1974;6:53–62.
6. Chardot C, Carton M, Spire-Bendelac N, Le Pommelet C, Golmard JL, Auvert B. Epidemiology of biliary atresia in France: a national study 1986-96. J Hepatol. 1999;31(6):1006–13.
7. Strickland AD, Shannon K. Studies in the etiology of extrahepatic biliary atresia: time-space clustering. J Pediatr. 1982;100(5):749–53.
8. Houwen RH, Kerremans II, van Steensel-Moll HA, van Romunde LK, Bijleveld CM, Schweizer P. Time-space distribution of extrahepatic biliary atresia in The Netherlands and West Germany. Z Kinderchir. 1988;43(2):68–71.
9. Ayas MF, Hillemeier AC, Olson AD. Lack of evidence for seasonal variation in extrahepatic biliary atresia during infancy. J Clin Gastroenterol. 1996;22(4):292–4.
10. Yoon PW, Bresee JS, Olney RS, James LM, Khoury MJ. Epidemiology of biliary atresia: a population-based study. Pediatrics. 1997;99(3):376–82.
11. Davenport M, Dhawan A. Epidemiologic study of infants with biliary atresia. Pediatrics. 1998;101(4 Pt 1):729–30.
12. Fischler B, Haglund B, Hjern A. A population-based study on the incidence and possible pre- and perinatal etiologic risk factors of biliary atresia. J Pediatr. 2002;141(2):217–22.
13. Caton AR, Druschel CM, McNutt LA. The epidemiology of extrahepatic biliary atresia in New York State, 1983-98. Paediatr Perinat Epidemiol. 2004;18(2):97–105.
14. Nakamizo M, Toyabe S, Kubota M, Komata O, Suzuki H, Akazawa K. Seasonality in the incidence of biliary atresia in Japan. Acta Paediatr. 2006;95(4):509–10.
15. Wada H, Muraji T, Yokoi A, Okamoto T, Sato S, Takamizawa S, et al. Insignificant seasonal and geographical variation in incidence of biliary atresia in Japan: a regional survey of over 20 years. J Pediatr Surg. 2007;42(12):2090–2.
16. The NS, Honein MA, Caton AR, Moore CA, Siega-Riz AM, Druschel CM, et al. Risk factors for isolated biliary atresia, National Birth Defects Prevention Study, 1997–2002. Am J Med Genet A. 2007;143A(19):2274–84.
17. Tiao MM, Tsai SS, Kuo HW, Chen CL, Yang CY. Epidemiological features of biliary atresia in Taiwan, a national study 1996–2003. J Gastroenterol Hepatol. 2008;23(1):62–6.
18. Wildhaber BE, Majno P, Mayr J, Zachariou Z, Hohlfeld J, Schwoebel M, et al. Biliary atresia: Swiss national study, 1994–2004. J Pediatr Gastroenterol Nutr. 2008;46(3):299–307.
19. Livesey E, Cortina Borja M, Sharif K, Alizai N, McClean P, Kelly D, et al. Epidemiology of biliary atresia in England and Wales (1999–2006). Arch Dis Child Fetal Neonatal Ed. 2009;94(6):F451–5.
20. Girard M, Jannot AS, Besnard M, Leutenegger AL, Jacquemin E, Lyonnet S, et al. Polynesian ecology determines seasonality of biliary atresia. Hepatology. 2011;54(5):1893–4.
21. Lee KJ, Kim JW, Moon JS, Ko JS. Epidemiology of Biliary Atresia in Korea. J Korean Med Sci. 2017;32(4):656–60.
22. Walter SD, Elwood JM. A test for seasonality of events with a variable population at risk. Br J Prev Soc Med. 1975;29(1):18–21.
23. Kubota M. An evaluation of spatial clustering of patients with biliary atresia. Jpn J Pediatr Surg. 2008;40(1):35–40.
24. Sweet L. Congenital malformation of the bile ducts: A report of three cases in one family. J Pediatr. 1932;1:496–510.
25. Hopkins N. Congenital absence of the common duct – three cases in one family. Lancet. 1941;61:90–1.
26. Whitten WW, Adie GC. Congenital biliary atresia; report of three cases; two occurring in one family. J Pediatr. 1952;40(5):539–48.
27. Krauss AN. Familial Extrahepatic Biliary Atresia. J Pediatr. 1964;65:933–7.
28. Nevin NC, Bell M, Frazer MJ, Froggatt P. Congenital extrahepatic biliary atresia in two brothers. J Med Genet. 1969;6(4):379–81.
29. Sommer A, Moody PE Jr, Reiner CB. Familial extrahepatic biliary atresia. Report of a case situation. Clin Pediatr (Phila). 1976;15(7):627–9.
30. Cunningham ML, Sybert VP. Idiopathic extrahepatic biliary atresia: recurrence in sibs in two families. Am J Med Genet. 1988;31(2):421–6.
31. Lachaux A, Descos B, Plauchu H, Wright C, Louis D, Raveau J, et al. Familial extrahepatic biliary atresia. J Pediatr Gastroenterol Nutr. 1988;7(2):280–3.

32. Smith BM, Laberge JM, Schreiber R, Weber AM, Blanchard H. Familial biliary atresia in three siblings including twins. J Pediatr Surg. 1991;26(11):1331–3.
33. Gunasekaran TS, Hassall EG, Steinbrecher UP, Yong SL. Recurrence of extrahepatic biliary atresia in two half sibs. Am J Med Genet. 1992;43(3):592–4.
34. Anneren G, Meurling S, Lilja H, Wallander J, von Dobeln U. Lethal autosomal recessive syndrome with intrauterine growth retardation, intra- and extrahepatic biliary atresia, and esophageal and duodenal atresia. Am J Med Genet. 1998;78(3):306–7.
35. Danesino C, Spadoni E, Buzzi A. Familial biliary atresia. Am J Med Genet. 1999;85(2):195.
36. Xu X, Zhan J. Biliary atresia in twins: a systematic review and meta-analysis. Pediatr Surg Int. 2020;36(8):953–8.
37. Cameron-Christie SR, Wilde J, Gray A, Tankard R, Bahlo M, Markie D, et al. Genetic investigation into an increased susceptibility to biliary atresia in an extended New Zealand Maori family. BMC Med Genet. 2018;11(1):121.
38. Kobayashi K, Kubota M, Okuyama N, Hirayama Y, Watanabe M, Sato K. Mother-to-daughter occurrence of biliary atresia: a case report. J Pediatr Surg. 2008;43(8):1566–8.
39. Nio M. Japanese Biliary Atresia Registry. Pediatr Surg Int. 2017;33(12):1319–25.

# Epidemiology of Gestational Age, Birth Weight, and Associated Anomalies in Biliary Atresia

12

Takashi Akiyama

**Abstract**

This chapter shows the epidemiology of gestational age, birth weight, and associated anomalies in patients with biliary atresia (BA) (The Japanese Biliary Atresia Registry, JBAR). In Japan, 3478 cases of BA had been registered in the JBAR for the duration of 30 years from 1989 to 2018. The mean gestational age of infants with BA was 38.6 [standard deviation (SD) 1.8 wk. The records in the JBAR show that during the period 2009–2018, the incidence of BA was the highest in infants with a birth weight of 1500 g–1999 g. The incidence of BA in infants was significantly higher in infants with low birth weight (<2500 g) than in those with normal birth weight (> or = 2500 g) [1.86 vs. 0.94 per 10,000 live births, respectively ($p < 0.05$)]. Total 721 associated congenital anomalies had been recorded in the JBAR. In Japan, the latest registry data report a prevalence of 2.59% for BA splenic malformation (BASM). Further, the incidence of BASM in North America and Europe is higher than that in Asian countries, including Japan.

**Keywords**

Biliary atresia · Gestational age · Birth weight · Associated anomalies · Biliary atresia splenic malformation (BASM)

## 12.1 Introduction

Biliary atresia (BA) is characterized by obliterative cholangiopathy that may affect the extrahepatic and intrahepatic bile ducts. The Japanese Biliary Atresia Society was founded in 1980 to investigate all aspects of BA; the society started a nationwide registry of patients with BA (The Japanese Biliary Atresia Registry, JBAR) in 1989 (Chiba 1991). This chapter presents the epidemic data of BA in Japan. In particular, the epidemiological data on gestational age, birth weight, and associated anomalies were collected from the JBAR. Datasheets were collected from institutions throughout Japan for each year during the 30-year period from 1989 to 2018 (1). Moreover, we compared the data from Japan with the data from Western and Asian countries in terms of gestational age, birth weight, and associated anomalies of BA. We extracted the following information from the JBAR (1). We retrieved information about the patient's gestational age, birth weight, and associated anomalies during the period 1989–2018. The overall incidence was calculated with reference to the data on live births published by the Ministry of Health, Labor, and Welfare for the previous 10yeras (2009–2018). The birth weight of infants with BA was assessed using $\chi^2$ test. Significance was assumed at $p = 0.05$.

In Japan, 3478 BA cases were recorded and registered in the JBAR during the 30-year period (1989–2018) (1). Considering the population of Japan as well as the incidence of BA, about 99% of patients were registered each year.

T. Akiyama (✉)
Department of Pediatric Surgery, Chuden Hospital, The Chugoku Electric Power Co., Inc, Hiroshima, Japan

## 12.2 Gestational Age in BA

Regarding the gestational age, most patients were in the age range of 36–41 weeks. The majority of patients were within the age range 38–39 weeks. The maximum and the minimum gestational ages were 42 and 24 weeks, respectively, as per the JABR. The average gestational age of infants was 38.6 [standard deviation (SD) 1.8] weeks. A total 648 patients (18.6%) were < 37 weeks old (Table 12.1, Fig. 12.1).

## 12.3 Birth Weight in BA

Birth weight ranged from 2500–4000 g, and 515 (14.8%) patients weighed<2500 g at birth. The majority of patients were within the birth weight range of 2500–2999 g. The


M. Nio (ed.), *Introduction to Biliary Atresia*, https://doi.org/10.1007/978-981-16-2160-4_12

maximum and minimum birth weights were 4940 and 824 g, respectively, as per the JBAR. The average birth weight of infants was 2903.6 [SD 452.2] g (Table 12.2, Fig. 12.2).

The incidence of BA was significantly higher in the low birth weight group (those with birth weight of <2500 g) than in the normal birth weight group (those with birth weight of > or = 2500 g): 1.86 vs. 0.94 per 10,000 live births, respectively: Table 12.3: $p < 0.05$). During the period from 2009 to 2018, the incidence of BA was the highest in the group of infants with a birth weight of 1500–1999 g (Fig. 12.3).

This chapter describes the epidemiological characteristics of BA using a population-based approach. The incidence of BA in low birth weight infants (birth weight of <2500 g) was higher than that in normal birth weight infants (birth weight of > or = 2500 g). Similar a high incidence of BA is reported for low birth weight infants (birth weight of <2500 g) in the United States (2, 3), Taiwan (4), and the Netherlands (5).

## 12.4 Associated Anomaly in BA

Overall, 721 associated congenital anomalies were reported, including cardiac anomalies in 184 (5.29%), splenic anomalies in 90 (polysplenia, 70; asplenia, 4: accessory spleen, 16: 2.59%), vascular anomalies in 86 (preduodenal portal vein, 46; other vascular anomalies, 40: 2.47%), situs inversus in 41, and gastrointestinal anomalies in 176 (5.06%) patients (Table 12.4).

Situs inversus, polysplenia, portal vein anomaly, absent inferior vena cava, or cardiac defect are results of defective organogenesis at around 3–6 weeks of gestation. The extrahepatic bile duct system begins to grow from the primordial bud of the gut at around 5 weeks. Normal rotation and fixation of the gut develop at around 9–12 weeks. Davenport et al. suggested that the bile duct insult in infants who have a combination of splenic malformation and BA must occur

**Table 12.1** Epidemiology of gestational age (1989–2018)

| Gestational age (weeks) | Number of cases |
|---|---|
| ~29 | 11 |
| 30~31 | 17 |
| 32~33 | 34 |
| 34~35 | 88 |
| 36~37 | 498 |
| 38~39 | 1676 |
| 40~41 | 1076 |
| 42~ | 26 |
| Unknown | 109 |
| Total | 3478 |

Max 42 Weeks Min 24 Weeks
38.6 ± 1.8 Weeks (Mean ± SD)

**Table 12.2** Epidemiology of birth weight (1989–2018)

| Birth weight (g) | Number of cases |
|---|---|
| ~1499 | 32 |
| 1500–1999 | 72 |
| 2000~2499 | 411 |
| 2500~2999 | 1488 |
| 3000~3499 | 1160 |
| 3500~3999 | 229 |
| 4000~ | 30 |
| Unknown | 56 |
| Total | 3478 |

Max 4940 g Min 824 g
2903.6 ± 452.2 g (Mean ± SD)

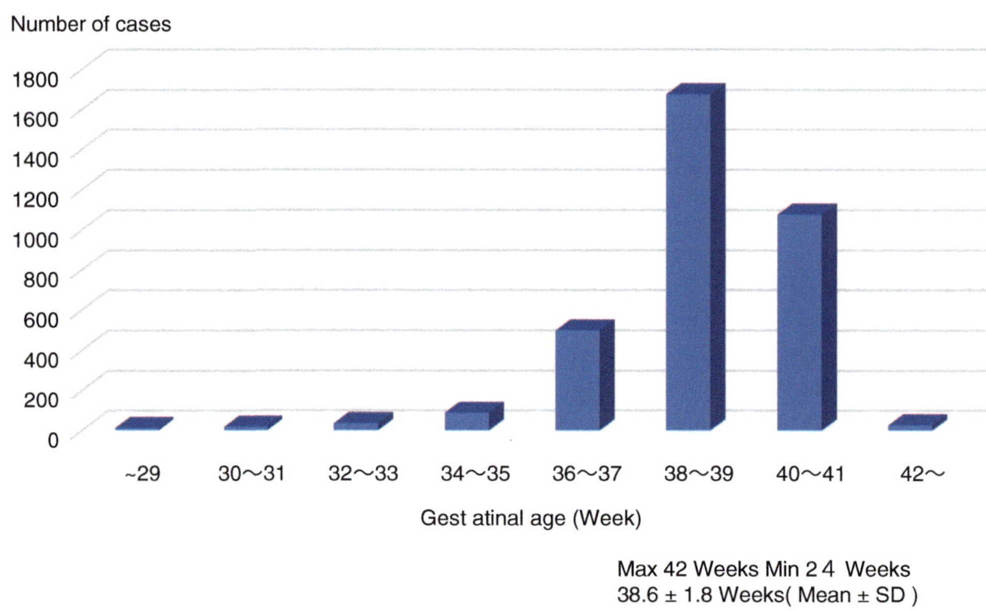


**Fig. 12.1** Epidemiology of gestational age (1989–2018)

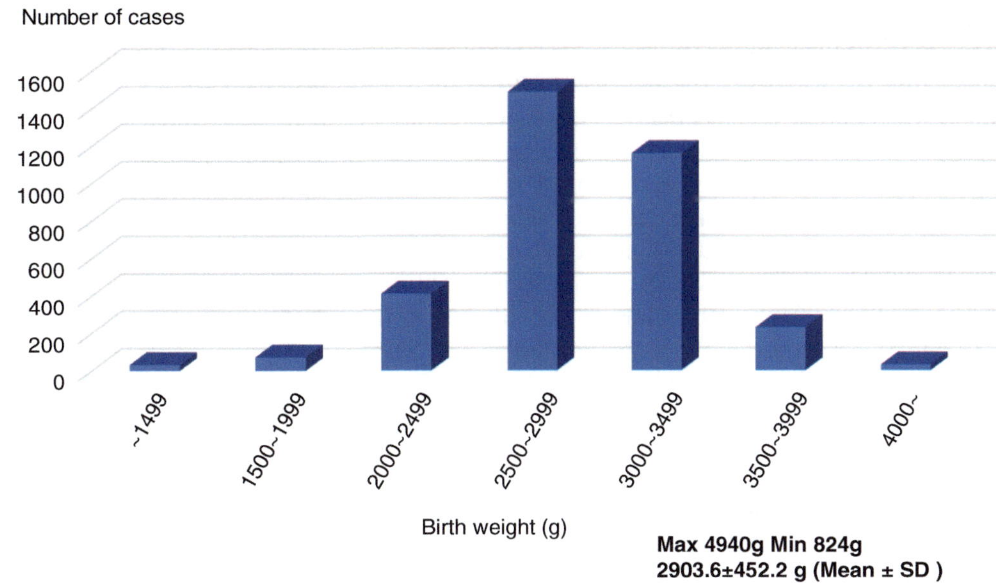


**Fig. 12.2** Epidemiology of Birth weight (1989–2018)

**Table 12.3** Incidence of BA by the total live infant, premature infant and, term infant in Japan (2009–2018), USA, Taiwan, and the Netherlands

| Country | Incidence of BA per 10,000 live births | Incidence of BA per 10,000 live births | Incidence of BA per 10,000 live births |
|---|---|---|---|
| | Total | 2500 g≧ | >2500 g |
| Japan (2018–2009) | 1.05 | 0.94 | 1.86 |
| USA (Atlanta) (2) | 0.73 | 0.75 | 2.62 |
| USA (New York State) (3) | 0.85 | | 3.24 |
| Taiwan (4) | 1.51 | 1.43 | 2.37 |
| Netherlands (5) | 0.54 | | 1.06 |

very early in embryogenesis (possibly, around 5 weeks) to coincide with the critical periods in the development of the spleen, rotation, and fixation of the gut, development of bile duct system, etc. (6). The coexistence of BA and anomalies has been widely reported and involves both single and multiple organ systems. BA-associated anomalies have been reported in North America (7), the United Kingdom (8), Canada (9), Taiwan (10), China (11), India (12), and Korea (13). The incidence and category of BA-associated anomalies are listed in Table 12.5. Davenport et al. reported that BA accompanied with spleen dysplasia syndrome was the most common deformity, and they proposed the term "biliary atresia splenic malformation" (BASM) syndrome (6). The incidence of BASM in North America (7), the UK (8), and

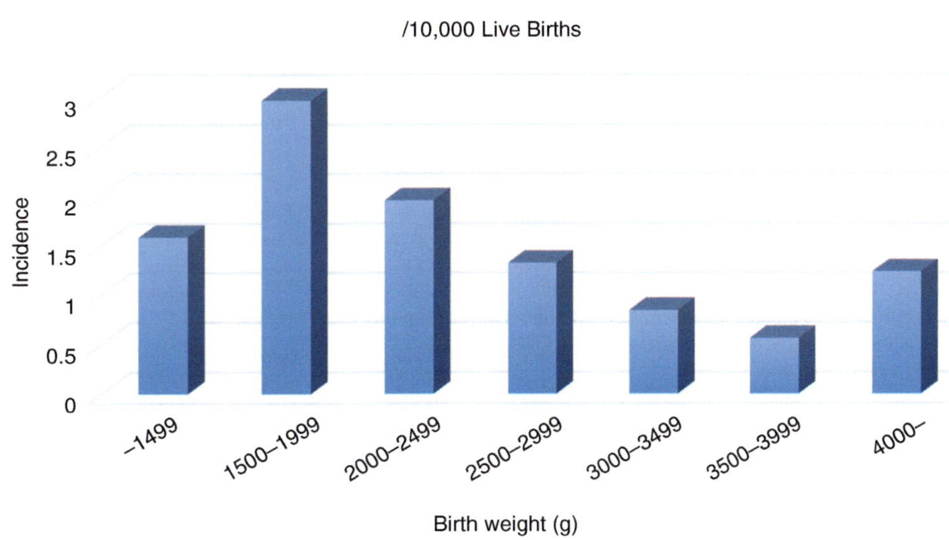


**Fig. 12.3** Incidence of BA by Birth weight in Japan (2009–2018)

Canada (9) ranged from 6.5% to 10.2%. Moreover, the incidence of BASM in Taiwan (10), China (11), and Korea (13) ranged from 0.5% to 0.8%. The incidence of BASM in North America and Europe is higher than that in Asian countries. In Japan, the latest registry data showed that the incidence of BASM was 2.59%. The incidence of BASM in India is similar to that in Japan (1, 12). The reason for this difference in the BASM incidence between South Asia and the western countries can be explained by the higher incidence of BA without BASM in Taiwan (10), China (11), India (12), Korea (13), and Japan (1) compared to that in Europe and North America.

**Table 12.4** Associated anomalies (JBAR, 1989–2018)

| Congenital anomaly | Number of cases | Congenital anomaly | Number of cases |
|---|---|---|---|
| ① Cardiac anomaly | | ④ Splenic anomaly | |
| Ventricular septal defect | 34 | Polysplenia | 70 |
| Atrial septal defect | 26 | Accessory spleen | 16 |
| Patent ductus arteriosus | 19 | Asplenia | 4 |
| Pulmonary stenosis | 22 | ⑤ Urogenital anomaly | 49 |
| Dextrocardia | 7 | ⑥ Respiratory anomaly | 11 |
| Tetralogy of Fallot | 6 | ⑦ Others | 84 |
| Others | 70 | | |
| ② Vascular anomaly | | | |
| Preduodenal portal vein | 46 | | |
| Absent inferior vena cava | 21 | | |
| Others | 19 | | |
| ③ Gastrointestinal anomaly | | | |
| Malrotation | 62 | | |
| Situs inversus | 41 | | |
| Meckel's diverticulum | 16 | | |
| Anorectal malformation | 15 | | |
| Meconium peritonitis | 13 | | |
| Intestinal atresia | 13 | | |
| Others | 57 | | |

Some BA cases include patients with associated congenital anomalies that develop during the same period owing to the relationship with the organogenesis of the bile duct system. Most anomalies are associated with spleen dysplasia syndrome and are termed as BASM syndrome. The incidence of BASM in North America and Europe is higher than that in Asian countries, including Japan (1, 7–13).

## References


1. The Japanese Biliary Atresia Society. Japanese biliary atresia registry, 1989 to 2018. Jpn J Pediatr Surg. 2020;56(2):219–25.
2. Yoon PW, Bresee JS, Olney RS, et al. Epidemiology of biliary atresia: a population-based study. Pediatrics. 1997;99(3):376–82.
3. Caton AR, Druschel CM, McNutt LA. The epidemiology of extrahepatic biliary atresia in New York state, 1983–98. Paediatr Perinat Epidemiol. 2004;18(2):97–105.
4. Chin CY, Chen PH, Chan CF, et al. Biliary atresia in preterm infants in Taiwan: a nationwide survey. J Pediatr. 2013;163(1):100–3.
5. Dean B. E van Wessel, Thomas Boere, C V Hulzebos, et al: preterm infants with biliary atresia: a Nationwide cohort analysis from the Netherlands. J Pediatr Gastroenterol Nutr. 2017;65(4):370–4.
6. Davenport M, Savage M, Mowat AP, et al. Biliary atresia splenic malformation syndrome: an etiologic and prognostic subgroup. Surgery. 1993;113:662–8.
7. Schwarz KB, Haber BH, Rosenthal P, et al. Extrahepatic anomalies in infants with biliary atresia: results of a large prospective North America multicenter study. Hepatology. 2013;58:1724–31.
8. Davenport M, Tizzard SA, Underhill J, et al. The biliary atresia splenic malformation syndrome: a 28-year single-center retrospective study. J Pediatr. 2006;149:393–400.
9. Guttman OR, Roberts EA, Schreider RA, et al. Biliary atresia with associated structural malformations in Canadian infants. Liver Int. 2011;31:1485–93.
10. Yang MC, Chang MH, Chiu SN, et al. Implication of early-onset biliary atresia and extrahepatic congenital anomalies. Pediatr Int. 2010;52:569–72.
11. Zhan J, Feng J, Chen Y, et al. Incidence of biliary atresia associated congenital malformations: a retrospective multicenter study in China. Asi J Surg. 2017;40:429–33.
12. Gupta L, Bhatnagar V. A study of associated congenital anomalies with biliary atresia. J Indian Assoc Pediatr Surg. 2016;21:10–3.
13. Kyung JL, Kim JW, Moon JS, et al. Epidemiology of biliary atresia in Korea. J Korean Med Sci. 2017;32:656–60.


**Table 12.5** Incidence and category of BA-associated malformations in different areas N (%)

| Country | Total of BA | Cardiac | Vascular | Splenic malformation | Situs inversus | Gastrointestinal |
|---|---|---|---|---|---|---|
| United Kingdom (8) | 548 | 25(4.6) | 22(4) | 56(10.2) | 21(3.8) | 34(6.2) |
| Taiwan (10) | 130 | 9(6.9) | | 1(0.7) | | 10(7.7) |
| Canada (9) | 328 | 26(7.9) | 25(7.6) | 25(6.5) | 9(2.7) | 19(5.8) |
| North America (7) | 289 | 47(16.3) | | 21(7.3) | | 40(13.8) |
| China (11) | 851 | 42(4.94) | 1(0.1) | 4(0.5) | 2(0.2) | 4(0.5) |
| India (12) | 137 | 4(6.89) | | 2(3.4) | 2(3.4) | 13(22.41) |
| Korea (13) | 240 | 15(6.3) | | 2(0.8) | 1(0.4) | 8(3.3) |
| Japan(JBAR) (1) | 3478 | 184(5.29) | 86(2.47) | 90(2.59) | 41(1.18) | 176(5.06) |

# Screening and Stool Color Card System of Biliary Atresia

# 13

Masayuki Obatake

**Abstract**

Biliary atresia (BA) is a rare disease of unknown etiology and a leading cause of liver failure and liver transplantation. Early Kasai portoenterostomy (KP) by early diagnosis is the only way to improve survival in the native liver. Several screenings for early diagnosis of BA have been proposed, and a stool color card screening is now expanding worldwide. While a stool color card screening has certainly contributed to earlier overall KP date, it has not led to an increase in early KP. No outstanding screening method has yet been discovered, and further studies are needed to assess the feasibility and cost-effectiveness of BA screening.

**Keywords**

Biliary atresia (BA) · Kasai portoenterostomy (KP) Screening · Stool color card · Direct bilirubin Conjugated bilirubin · Serum bile acid · Urinary sulfated bile acid · Modified stool color card

Biliary atresia (BA) is a rare disease of unknown etiology that causes gradual closure of extrahepatic and intrahepatic bile ducts, resulting in severe liver cirrhosis. If untreated, BA progress to liver failure leading to death within 1 to 2 years of age. Drainage of bile into the jejunal loop by Kasai portoenterostomy (KP) is the only way to improve survival in the native liver. According to the analysis of the age at the time of KP and prognosis of 3483 BA patients registered by the Japan Biliary Atresia Registry (JBAR) between 1989 and 2018 (Table 13.1) revealed that the patients who underwent KP before 30 days of age showed jaundice disappearance rate 71.9%, and even before 80 days group showed over 60% [1]. Native liver survival rate at the 25 years after KP is 63.9% patients underwent KP before 30 days of age and 50.8% before 60 days of age. For these reasons, the prognosis of BA depends on the time of KP and the structure of the remaining intrahepatic bile duct, but it is generally important to perform earlier KP, especially no later than 60 days of life, resulting in good prognosis with the native liver.

**Table 13.1** The number of jaundice-cleared and cholangitis developed patients after Kasai operation (KP)

| Age at KP (days) | Individulas | Patients with KP | Postoperative jaundice disappearance (n) | (%) | Patients with postoperative cholangitis (n) | (%) |
|---|---|---|---|---|---|---|
| <30 | 234 | 231 | 166 | 71.9 | 81 | 35.1 |
| 31–45 | 542 | 541 | 338 | 62.5 | 208 | 38.4 |
| 46–60 | 833 | 830 | 543 | 65.4 | 349 | 42.0 |
| 61–70 | 540 | 540 | 343 | 63.5 | 216 | 40.0 |
| 71–80 | 471 | 468 | 288 | 61.5 | 202 | 43.2 |
| 81–90 | 295 | 294 | 164 | 55.8 | 123 | 41.8 |
| 91–120 | 361 | 356 | 200 | 56.2 | 152 | 42.7 |
| 121–150 | 123 | 118 | 47 | 39.8 | 47 | 39.8 |
| >151 | 67 | 48 | 11 | 22.9 | 24 | 50.0 |

The jaundice disappearance rate is calculated within two years following KP. Cumulative data of Japanese Biliary Atresia Registry (JBAR) between 1989 and 2018

In order not to delay the time of KP, it is necessary to make a diagnosis as early as possible, and neonatal / infant "screening" for BA has been proposed. According to the World Health Organization (WHO), screening is defined as the presumptive identification of unrecognized disease in an apparently healthy, asymptomatic population by means of tests, examinations, or other procedures that can be applied rapidly and easily to the target population [2].

At the present time, no specific biomarkers exist for the diagnosis of BA. The screenings mainly use clinical features, such as pale-pigmented stool and product materials generated from pathophysiologies, such as high serum bilirubin and bile acid levels. However, these symptoms and laboratory findings are not specific to BA but are also found in cholestatic liver

M. Obatake (✉)
Kochi University, Kochi, Japan
e-mail: mobatake@kochi-u.ac.jp


M. Nio (ed.), *Introduction to Biliary Atresia*, https://doi.org/10.1007/978-981-16-2160-4_13

diseases. Thus, early detection screening for BA is only possible for cholestatic liver diseases, including BA.

The remainder of this chapter describes the characteristics, feasibility, and potentiality of screenings that are currently conducted, previously reported, and under investigation.

## 13.1 Stool Color Card Screening

First stool color card screening was launched in the Tochigi Prefecture in Japan in 1994 [3]. The stool color card has seven scales of stool color to help caregivers evaluate their children's stool color. As stool color gets darker, the number of stool color increases as well. Stool colors number 1 to 3 are defined as abnormal, indicating acholic stool. Colors 4 to 7 are defined as normal. After the 1-month health checkup, the completed card with stool color number by caregivers was mailed to the public health center. Cases with the suspected acholic stool were referred for further examination. During 12 years between 1994 and 2011, a total of 313,230 infants were screened, and 34 patients were diagnosed with BA [4]. Twenty-six out of 34 patients were identified by screening. The sensitivity and specificity at the 1-month checkup were 76.5% (95% CI 62.2–90.7) and 99.9% (95% CI 99.9–100). The mean age at the time of KP was 59.7 ± 19.4 days, which was earlier than that before the introduction of stool color card screening (70.3 days, 1987–1992). At the same period, JBAR reported that the percentage of age at the time of KP after 80 days was 25.3%, even though Tochigi's data was 11.8% ($P < 0.05$). The survival rate with native liver for the 34 patients was 87.6%, 76.9%, and 48.5% (at 5, 10, and 15 years after KP, respectively) and was better than that of historical controls. Stool color card screening, thereafter, expanded to 16 other administrative districts in Japan. In 2012, new stool color cards were attached to the maternity handbook for the nationwide screening method [5]. Recognition of color is based on the self-inspection by the caregivers. In the case of acholic stool, the caregivers should take the infants to the pediatrician for further evaluation. Two new observation times have been added, including at 2 weeks of age and 1–4 months after birth. Stool color survey at 2 weeks of age is designed to receive early KP within 30 days of age, but so far, JBAR's data after the introduction of the new stool color card reveals no apparent increase KP within 30 days of life (Fig. 13.1).

In 2002 in Taiwan, the pilot study of stool color card screening was started and in 2004 the first universal national wide screening program was implemented [6]. This stool color card also has 6 photographs of different colored stool samples from Taiwanese infants. Stool color was checked before discharged from the hospital at 3–5 days of age and at the 1-month health checkup. Lin et al. analyzed the 15 years outcomes of BA before and after implementation [7]. The patients were divided into three cohorts. The patients in cohort (1) ($n$ = 208) were born before the stool color card screening program from 1997 to 2001; the patients in cohort (2) ($n$ = 200) were received regional or universal screening program from 2002 to 2006; the patients in cohort (3) ($n$ = 132) were screened with universal screening program from 2007 to 2011. Age at KP was 58.2 ± 42.0 in cohort (1), 50.5 ± 30.8 in cohort (2), and 46.0 ± 23.8 days in cohort (3), respectively. The average proportion of patients who underwent KP at less than 60 days of age was 76.6, 88.5, and

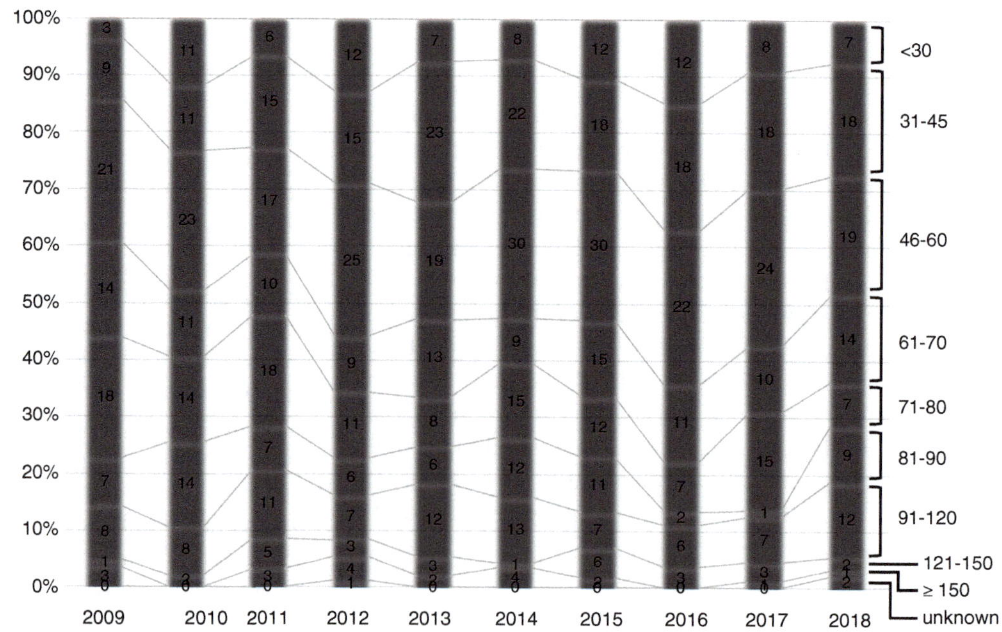


**Fig. 13.1** Annual age proportions at KP from 2009 to 2018. (The left axis represents the proportion of the age of the day at KP. The right axis is the age of the day at KP. The numbers in the graph are the number of KP in each age group)

81.1%, respectively, but this difference was not statistically significant. Authors found the reducing trend of the age of BA diagnosis has been started before this program launching in 2004. They concluded that earlier diagnosis and operation for BA were not entirely due to the stool color card screening alone; however, the stool color card has the potential benefit of increasing BA awareness in both caregivers and physicians. The liver transplant rate in three year-ranges was 32.7, 41.0, and 29.6%, respectively, and were 25.6% among those patients who received KP within 60 days of age and 32.3% over 60 days of age.

In reference to Taiwan's good results using stool color card screening for BA, Argentina [8], Switzerland [9], and other countries implemented similar regional or nationwide stool color card screening programs. Swiss stool color card screening pilot study was started in 2009. Seven different colors of photographs (4 normal and 3 abnormal) are printed on the card. The cards were handed out to the caregivers after their child's birth by the attending pediatrician or midwife. The card and the baby's stool color are checked at 4 weeks of age.

Home-based screening program in British Columbia in Canada was performed on 87,583 patients between 2014 and 2016 [10]. During the period of the program, six patients were identified as BA. Five in six were received this program; however, only three received KP within 60 days. The other two patients were identified as acholic stools by their families, but their general practitioners did not give further tests until late referral.

In general, early KP is considered as one of the factors of good prognosis of BA. In a Canadian cohort study, the native liver survival of the patients who received KP before 30 days of age had better through 10 years of observation [11]. In a French cohort study, KP within 30 days of age brought higher 5-year native liver survival [12]. Thus, earlier KP has been advocated to be performed around 30 days of age. Stool color card screening resulted in early detection of BA and fast KP, but could not find any BA patients before 30 days of life. The stool color card is a simple and inexpensive screening method. In areas where BA has not been screened, the introduction of the stool color card has been reported for its effectiveness of early diagnosis of BA and early KP and improved survival in native livers. However, aiming to detect BA at an earlier stage to improve prognosis, only the pale stool as a result of advanced bile duct obstruction might be somewhat difficult to achieve.

## 13.2 Serum Direct or Conjugated Bilirubin

Several studies have been performed for screening tests for BA using serum direct or conjugated bilirubin. Measurement of increasing direct or conjugated bilirubin is a most logical way for detecting BA by considering its basic pathology of intra and extrahepatic bile ducts, which are gradually obstructing after birth. In 2003, Powell et al. measured conjugated bilirubin in neonates younger than 28 days of life in the United Kingdom [13]. A total of 30,079 neonates were tested, and 23,415 samples (84.7%) could be analyzed. The remainders were inappropriate samples because of hemolysis (8.6%) and insufficient volume. Eleven patients were diagnosed with liver disease, and two of them had BA. A sensitivity, a specificity, and a positive predictive value of this test were 100%, 99.59%, and 10.3%, respectively. They concluded that serum conjugated bilirubin concentration might be a reliable marker for neonatal liver disease but not very accurate for detecting BA.

Harpavat et al. reported that 34 BA patients had elevated serum direct or conjugated bilirubin within the first 96 hours of age in 2011 [14]. In 2016, Hapavat et al. initiated a prospective study using two-step screening with direct or conjugated bilirubin [15]. They screened a total of 11,636 newborns at 4 Houston hospitals. One hundred and twenty-one infants were considered positive by screening in test 1 within less than 60 hours of life. The measurement of direct or conjugated bilirubin was repeated in test 2 at 2 to 3 weeks of age, and 11 infants continued to have positive test results. The 2 infants were diagnosed with BA and had positive results in both tests. Thus, sensitivity, specificity, and positive predictive value were 100%, 99.9%, and 18.2%, respectively. They expanded their evaluation of the two-step BA screening strategy and investigated 124,385 newborns at 14 south Texas hospitals in 2020 [16]. There were 1354 infants with positive screening results in test 1 within 60 hours of age. After test 2, 119 infants continued to have positive results. 7 out of 119 infants were finally diagnosed on BA. This test had a sensitivity of 100%, a specificity of 99.9%, and a positive predictive value of 5.9%.

Serum direct or conjugated bilirubin measurements are widely available and inexpensive. This measurement requires to draw blood because the concentration of serum direct or conjugated bilirubin, which has photosensitivity, is not measured with a dried blood spot. Serum direct or conjugated bilirubin screening appears to result in a feasible strategy for earlier detection and treatment of BA within 30 days of age.

## 13.3 Serum Bile Acid Measurement

Serum bile acid (SBA) has also been elevated with BA and cholestatic disease in neonates. SBA is more stable material and be able to be measured using the dried blood samples collected in the Guthrie test. Mushtaq et al. reported the possibility of SBA for BA screening [17]. They compared among cholestatic hepatobiliary disease patients (61 BA, 52 Idiopathic neonatal hepatitis, 17 Alagille syndrome, 15 $\alpha$

antitrypsin deficiency, 32 other diseases) and 708 normal newborns. The level of SB in BA was surely elevated. However, the sensitivity and specificity were 78.7% and 96.3%, respectively. In 2012, Zhou et al. investigated SBA in 8 BA patients, 17 neonatal jaundice, and 292 normal infants at 3–4 days of age [18]. Elevation of SBS in BA infants at 3–4 days of age might suggest the early occurrence of the bile duct obstruction around birth. Both the sensitivity and specificity were lower than expected 79.1% and 62.5%, respectively. Samples of SBA are easier to obtain and deliver than that of direct bilirubin. SBA screening has potential for screening of BA, but so far is not acceptable for BA screening with inadequate specificity.

## 13.4 Urinary Sulfated Bile Acid

Bile is synthesized in liver cells and discharged into the bile duct. In case of bile obstruction, as seen in BA or other cholestatic hepatobiliary diseases, water-soluble sulfated bile acid synthesized from bile reflux into the serum and then secreted in the urine as urinary sulfated bile acid (USBA). Comparing to the blood tests, USBA has less invasion of sampling and the advantage of safe handling of the samples [19]. Urine samples were collected in small plastic bottles by the caregivers at 14–30 days of age and kept frozen at −4 degree Celsius until USBA assay. Method of measurement was performed by the automated analyze with the direct enzymatic assay. USBA value was corrected with urine creatinine in consideration of immaturity of renal function. This test is commercially available at a cost of US$5. Subsequently, Obatake et al. measured both serum and urine bile acid levels at various times in BA patients and showed that they were correlated [20]. BA and cholestatic hepatobiliary diseases screening with USBA launched in Okinawa and Nagasaki Prefecture in Japan and continues to the present. In Nagasaki Prefecture, a total of 54,840 infants were screened with USBA between 2010 and 2018. This number represents about 60% of the number of births in the region. Elevated USBA levels were found in 1187 infants (2.16%) in the initial examination, and subsequent blood tests indicated that cholestatic liver disease was suspected in 56 infants. During the period, nine cases of BA have been diagnosed, and seven of them received USBA examination. Unfortunately, one out of seven patients was determined to be normal on the first USBA test. Later, blood test suspected BA because of prolonged jaundice, and the patients underwent KP at 111 days of age. This case was tested at 11 days of age, earlier than the protocol for USBA examination, suggesting that early neonatal USBA testing might be less likely to produce abnormal results than serum direct bilirubin testing. According to the 2018 JBAR report, preoperative USBA measurement was performed in 27 BA patients, and two of them were false-negative with normal values. Although the timing of the USBA tests in those two cases is not clear, the occurrence of false-negatives is major problem for screening, so the timing of the USBA tests needs to be discussed in the future.

## 13.5 Modified Color Card Screening

At present, the stool color card is the most widely used screening and seems to be superior in terms of economy and repeatability, but the problem is that it is a subjective judgment. In the mosaic stool mixed with light and a dark portion or the odd color stool not matched to the stool color card, sometimes it is difficult to classified to normal or abnormal stool. Bakshi et al. verified the reliability of pale stool identification among pediatric professionals [21]. They prepared three colors (five normal, three indeterminate, and four acholic stool) which were photographed by the digital camera with computer calibration for ambient light. The pediatric professionals included 36 pediatric doctors and 45 pediatric nurses in three different hospitals. Suspected BA stools were correctly identified in 62.8% (doctors; 62.7%, nurses; 62.9%) and failed to recognize in 37.2%. The results showed that even experienced professionals could not recognize stool color associated with BA. Two years' study in Canada, the color card was revised from 6 colors (3 normal and 3 abnormal) to 9 colors (3 normal and 6 abnormal) before starting the second year because of missing a BA patient by stool photo failure. In the Initial stool color card, only the color was printed. Currently, widely used color cards have not only the color but also the shape of the stool and help with judgment.

In the 2018 JBAR, 58 out of 152 BA patients (38%) at before 1 month old, 53 out of 151 patients (35%) at 1 month old, and 17 out of 131 patients (12.8%) after 1 month old declared to be having normal stool color before BA diagnosis. These stool colors judged to be normal were belong to the lightest normal stool color. The difference in color between the lightest normal stool color and the darkest abnormal stool color is subtle, and it is a true challenge for any professionals. However, there would still be a significant number of BA patients in the lightest normal stool color group. Between 2015 and 2016, we recruited caregivers to interview their infants' stool colors at the 1-month regular health checkup. A total of 2028 interviews were divided into two groups by age at examination. The mean ages at the examination for stool color were 14 ± 2 and 31 ± 4 days of age, respectively. The proportion of infants with the lightest normal stool color were 62.8% and 52.6%, respectively. Stool color seems to be darker with growth, although half of the caregivers recognized their infants' stool color belongs to the lightest normal group at 1 month of age. Nobody rules out the possibility that this lightest normal group includes patients with BA.

Recently, several researchers have attempted to objectively judge the stool color through a camera and computer programs. Franciscovich et al. first reported PoopMD as a mobile application for the identification of infant acholic stools [22]. PoopMD is based on color hexes that were captured from the Taiwan stool card and account for variations in hue and brightness.

Hoshino et al. announced the stool color evaluation system named Baby Poop in 2017 [23]. This program was integrated with pattern recognition and machine learning process utilizing the class-featuring information compression (CLAFIC) method. Baby Poop installed modified artificial intelligence (AI) technology. Judgment result displayed as not only "normal" or "caution / high probability of acholic stool" but also "indeterminate" for unrelated colors to images of the training data. Baba Poop was launched in 2016 as a free iPhone application for individual use. In 2019, a Clinical study has been started using the basic program of Baby Poop at 1-month health check in Kochi prefecture in Japan. AI technology is widely recognized for its evolution through deep learning and is advancing in all industrial fields. The field of medical care has been no exception, and AI has already been for disease diagnosis in practical use. If AI's high ability to distinguish the characteristics of substances can be applied to the screening field, it might replace the current stool color card screening diagnosed by the human eye. Even though developing an AI program is expensive, once the program is created, AI screening has the advantage of not having to pay for annual printing as color card and low maintenance costs. Moreover, since the stool color of newborns and infants changes daily depending on their stool property and the condition of their digestive system, it is risk to make a judgment of stool color at a temporary point. Digital technology might facilitate daily observation and diagnosis, because nowadays, most of the young mothers carry mobile phones in their pouch—even if they do not carry the maternity booklet with stool color cards.

## 13.6 Limits of Screening for BA and Future Prospects

As recounted above, so far, there are no perfect BA screening methods. Each screening tried to efficiently find out BA patients among the patients with cholestasis. Since there are no accurate BA assays currently, every screening strategy has produced a lot of false-positive cases and several false-negative cases as a result. Therefore, it is a matter of course for the occurrence of false-positive by current BA screenings. BA screening means the screening for the patients who have cholestatic diseases, including BA. The important point is how the BA patients are picked up among the patients with cholestasis. Repeated tests should be required to eliminate false positives, which cause a burden on caregivers and an increase in cost. As noted in the previous literature [24, 25], the stool color card strategy is cost-effective when comparing to no screening at all. It is necessary to further investigate to determine the cost-effectiveness among different screening modalities rather than comparing no screening to a single modality. Also, it is worth mentioning that when calculating costs associated with screening, not only direct but also indirect costs should be all taken into account.

Each screening has its advantages and disadvantages. Serum direct bilirubin assay has a potential for early detection of BA. However, several blood draws are needed to narrow down the patients with cholestasis. Stool color card screening is inexpensive and easily repeated; however, it is not good for temporary examination and seems more suitable for gradual clinical changes. Most reported screenings attempted to analyze their feasibility, potentiality, and economic efficiency by only one method in which they have been involved in. Even preoperative differential diagnosis of BA requires many examinations such as blood test, ultrasonography, CT, and scintigraphy, i.e., Taking advantage of respective screening characteristics, "Hybrid screening" might bring earlier diagnosis, earlier KP, and reduction of screening cost. Screening is one of the factors that have decreased the ages at diagnosis and KP in BA and contributed the improvement of prognosis. The screening will continue to be needed for early diagnosis of BA, and we expect collaborations between researchers and clinicians to lead a development of further effective screening methods.

## References


1. The Japanese Biliary Atresia Society and Department of Biliary Atresia Nationwide Registry. Summary of Japanese biliary atresia registry from 1989 to 2018. J Jpn Soc Pediatr Surg. 2018;2019(56):219–25.
2. WHO_PHP_34.pdf-WHO_PHP_34.pdf [internet]. Available from: http://whqlibdoc.who.int/php/WHO_PHP_34.pdf.
3. Matsui A, Dodoriki M. Screening for biliary atresia. Lancet. 1995;345:1181.
4. Gu YH, Yokoyama K, Kizuta K, et al. Stool color card screening for early detection of biliary atresia and long-term native liver survival: a 19-year cohort study in Japan. J Pediatr. 2015;166:897.e1–902.e1.
5. Matsui A. Screening for biliary atresia. Pediatr Surg Int. 2017;33:1305–13.
6. Hsiao CH, Chang MH, Chen HL, et al. Universal screening or biliary atresia using an infant stool color card in Taiwan. Hetatol. 2008;47:1233–40.
7. Lin JS, Chen SSC, Lu CL, et al. Reduction of the ages at diagnosis and operation of biliary atresia in Taiwan: 15-year population-based cohort study. World J Gastroenterol. 2015;21:13080–6.
8. Ramonet M. Stool color cards for screening for biliary atresia BA single topic conference. Bethesda, MD: National Institutes of Health. 2006: Sep; 12–13.

9. Wildhaber BE. Screening for biliary atresia: Swiss stool color card. Hepatology. 2011;54:367–8. https://doi.org/10.1002/hep.24346
10. Woolfson JP, Schreiber RA, Butler AE, et al. Province-wide biliary atresia home screening program in British Columbia: evaluation of first 2 years. J Pediatr Gastroenterol Nutr. 2018;66:845–9.
11. Schreiber RA, Barker CC, Roberts EA, et al. Canadian pediatric hepatology research group. Biliary atresia: the Canadian experience. J Pediatr. 2007;151:659–665, 665.el.
12. Serinet MO, Wildhaber BE, Broue P, et al. Impact of age at Kasai operation on its results in late childhood and adolescence: a rational basis for biliary atresia screening. Pediatrics. 2009;123:1280–6.
13. Powell JE, Keffler S, Kelly DA, et al. Population screening for neonatal liver disease. J Med Screen. 2003;10:112–6.
14. Hapavat S, Finegold MJ, Karpen SJ. Patients with biliary atresia have elevated direct/conjugated bilirubin levels shortly after birth. Pediatrics. 2011: 128; e1428–e1433. https://doi.org/10.1542/peds.2011–1869.
15. Hapavat S, Garcia-Prats JA, Shneider BL. Newborn bilirubin screening for biliary atresia. N Engl J Med. 2016;375:605–6.
16. Hapavat S, Garcia-Prats JA, Anaya C, et al. Diagnostic yield of newborn screening for biliary atresia using direct or conjugated bilirubin measurements. JAMA. 2020;323:1141–50.
17. Mushtaq I, Logan S, Morris M, et al. Screening for newborn infants for cholestatic hepatobiliary disease with tandem mass spectrometry. BMJ. 1999;319:471–7.
18. Zhou K, Lin N, Xiao Y, et al. Elevated bile acids in newborns with biliary atresia (BA). PLoS One. 2012;7:e49270. https://doi.org/10.1371/journal.pone.0049270
19. Muraji T, Harada T, Miki T, et al. Urinary sulfated bile acid concentrations in infants with biliary atresia and Brest-feeding jaundice. Pediatr Int. 2003;45:281–3.
20. Obatake M, Muraji T, Satoh S, et al. Urinary sulfated bile acids: a new simple urine test for cholestatis in infants and children. J Pediatr Surg. 2002;37:1707–8.
21. Bakshi B, Sutcliffe A, Akindolie M, et al. How reliably can paediatric professionals identify pale stool from cholestatic newborns? Arch Dis Child Fetal Neonatal Ed. 2012;97:F385–7.
22. Franciscovich A, Vaidya D, Doyle J, et al. PoopMD, a mobile health application, accurately identifies infant acholic stools. PLoS One. 2015;10:e0132270.
23. Hoshino E, Hayashi K, Suzuki M, et al. An iPhone application using a novel stool color detection algorithm for biliary atresia screening. Pediatr Surg Int. 2017;33:1115–21.
24. Mogul D, Zhou M, Intihar P, et al. Cost-effective analysis of screening for biliary atresia with the stool color card. J Pediatr Gastroenterol Nutr. 2015;60:91–8.
25. Schreiber RA, Masucci L, KZaczorowski J, et al. Home-based screening for biliary atresia using infant stool colour cards: a large-scale prospective cohort study and cost-effectiveness analysis. J Med Screen. 2014;21:126–32.

# Biliary Atresia: Signs and Symptoms, Prenatal Diagnosis

# 14

Jun Fujishiro

**Abstract**

Common clinical signs and symptoms suggestive of biliary atresia include jaundice, acholic stool, dark urine, and hepatomegaly. While acholic, pale, or clay-colored stools are well-known signs of biliary atresia, normal-colored stools do not exclude this diagnosis. Infants with biliary atresia may present with coagulopathy despite receiving oral vitamin K, owing to lack of absorption leading to its deficiency. About 5% of infants with biliary atresia are diagnosed or suspected prenatally. Biliary cystic lesions detected on prenatal ultrasonography can suggest biliary atresia and other biliary malformations, including choledochal cysts. Small, non-enlarging cysts may suggest biliary atresia rather than choledochal cysts. Some studies suggest that non-visualization of the fetal gallbladder may indicate biliary atresia; however, this association remains controversial. When biliary atresia is suspected, either postnatally by the above-mentioned signs and symptoms or prenatally by biliary cystic malformations or non-visualization of the fetal gallbladder, prompt investigation and subsequent treatment is necessary.

**Keywords**

Jaundice · Acholic stool · Hepatomegaly · Biliary cystic malformation · Non-visualization of the fetal gallbladder

## 14.1 Signs and Symptoms

The typical signs and symptoms of biliary atresia are jaundice, clay-colored or acholic stool, dark urine, and hepatomegaly in an otherwise healthy neonate (Table 14.1). The perinatal period is unremarkable in most patients.

J. Fujishiro (✉)
Department of Pediatric Surgery, Graduate School of Medicine, The University of Tokyo, Tokyo, Japan
e-mail: FUJISHIROJ-PSU@h.u-tokyo.ac.jp

**Table 14.1** Clinical sign and symptoms in biliary atresia

| | |
|---|---|
| Jaundice | Presenting sign |
| Acholic stools | Variable color (white, pale, clay, beige) |
| | Normal color stool DOES NOT exclude biliary atresia. |
| Dark urine | Due to the excretion of water-soluble bilirubin conjugates |
| Hepatomegaly | Common finding at presentation |
| Splenomegaly | Late sign suggestive of cirrhosis |
| Coagulopathy | Caused by vitamin K deficiency |
| | Occurs in infants with oral vitamin K supplementation. |

Prolongation of physiological neonatal jaundice can be the presentation in some cases, although jaundice occasionally appears 2 or 3 weeks after birth in infants with biliary atresia. According to the Japanese Biliary Atresia Registry, neonatal jaundice, normal-colored meconium, and yellow stools in the perinatal period are recognized in 71%, 75%, and 72% patients with biliary atresia, respectively [1]. More than half the patients passed normal meconium and yellowish stools just after birth. While clay-colored or acholic stool is a well-known finding of biliary atresia, it can also occur in patients with neonatal cholestasis from other causes. Direct observation of urine color, and more importantly, stool color, is important for assessing the jaundiced infant, as acholic stool and dark urine often indicate the presence of cholestasis and conjugated hyperbilirubinemia [2]. Dark urine is caused by the excretion of water-soluble bilirubin conjugates [3]. Urine might stain the nappy and coat the stool, leading to misidentification of the stool color. Various colors of stool, from white, clay-colored, beige, and even yellow, are observed in infants with biliary atresia on admission [3]. In infants younger than 1 month of age, approximately 1 month old, and more than 1 month old, 52, 56, and 82% of patients, respectively, passed apparently pale stools [1]. In addition, a study showed that 83% of infants with biliary atresia had a pale stool on admission [4]. Thus, the yellow- or normal-colored stool does not exclude the possibility of biliary atresia.


M. Nio (ed.), *Introduction to Biliary Atresia*, https://doi.org/10.1007/978-981-16-2160-4_14

The liver gradually increases in size and becomes firm in infants with biliary atresia, reflecting the duration of cholestasis. Most of these infants (94%–100%) have hepatomegaly on admission [4, 5]. Splenomegaly appears after the newborn period [2] and is a sign of portal hypertension [3]. Cholestasis, fat malabsorption, and deficiency of fat-soluble vitamins (vitamins A, D, E, and K) also occur in these infants. Coagulopathy, and most importantly intracranial bleeding, is occasionally encountered in patients with biliary atresia who have received oral vitamin K or no vitamin K supplementation. Due to poor absorption of long-chain fats and the catabolic state, failure to thrive becomes apparent later in the clinical course. Excessive feeding is a characteristic clinical sign of failure to thrive [3]. If not treated, biliary atresia is fatal within 2 to 3 years of life [6].

Several studies have evaluated the effectiveness of clinical signs and symptoms for differentiating biliary atresia from other causes of neonatal cholestasis. Some studies have suggested that hepatomegaly and a hard liver indicate biliary atresia [7, 8], but other studies showed that hepatomegaly was equally common in infants with biliary atresia and those with other causes of neonatal cholestasis [4, 5, 9]. The presence of acholic stool was reported to be more common in patients with biliary atresia [4, 5]. As none of these clinical signs and symptoms are specific, infants with these clinical features need further examination to diagnose biliary atresia.

## 14.2 Prenatal Diagnosis

While biliary atresia is known to develop during the perinatal period and affects only neonates and infants, prenatal diagnosis or suspicion of biliary atresia is relatively rare. From the Japanese Biliary Atresia Registry, 107 out of 2145 infants with biliary atresia (5.0%) were diagnosed prenatally [10]. A study also demonstrated that 5% of cases of biliary atresia were diagnosed prenatally [11]. Many prenatal diagnoses of biliary atresia are made by prenatal detection of biliary cystic malformations, which suggest diseases of the biliary tract, including biliary atresia and choledochal cysts (congenital biliary dilatation). Recently, there have been a few studies that suggest the possibility of prenatal diagnosis or suspicion of biliary atresia by non-visualization of the fetal gallbladder.

## 14.3 Biliary Cystic Malformation

Prenatal diagnosis or suspicion of biliary atresia by the detection of biliary cystic malformation has been reported since the 1980s. In the first case reported by Greenholz *et al.* [12], a cystic structure was detected by fetal ultrasonography at 32 weeks of gestation, and portoenterostomy was performed 76 hours after birth. Tsuchida *et al.* reported a case of prenatal diagnosis of cystic biliary atresia [13]. The cystic structure was identified at approximately 19 weeks of gestation, and repeat ultrasonography at 34 weeks of gestation confirmed that the cyst was located at the hepatic hilum and was communicating with the liver. Since these reports, there have been several case reports and case series on prenatal diagnosis of biliary atresia by detection of biliary cystic structures.

Two types of biliary atresia, type Ic (atresia of the distal common bile duct with cystic dilatation of the proximal part) and type IIId (atresia of the bile duct at the porta hepatis with cystic dilation of the common bile duct) according to the classification of the Japanese Biliary Atresia Society [14], were identified in those with the prenatal diagnosis of biliary cystic malformation [15–18]. Several case reports have suggested a possible change from type Ic to type IIId biliary atresia in cases with prenatally detected biliary cystic malformation [19, 20].

Differential diagnosis of prenatal cystic lesions in the upper abdomen includes cystic biliary malformations such as biliary atresia and choledochal cyst, duodenal atresia, duodenal duplication, and ovarian cysts [15]. With the recent advances in prenatal ultrasonography, prenatal detection of biliary cystic malformation and its distinction from other conditions (including duodenal atresia, ovarian cyst, and cystic lymphatic malformation) is possible during routine prenatal screening. However, the prenatal distinction between biliary atresia and choledochal cysts remains difficult and unreliable in fetuses with biliary cystic malformation. The size of the cyst and its change were reported to be useful for this distinction [16]. The cyst size was smaller in biliary atresia than in choledochal cysts [18]. The size remained unchanged or decreased in biliary atresia, while it increased in choledochal cysts [17]. The disappearance of prenatal biliary cysts in an infant with biliary atresia has been reported in the literature [19]. A study suggested that all patients with biliary cystic malformations smaller than 21 mm were diagnosed with biliary atresia [18]. However, there are several studies with conflicting results: a study showed a prenatal increase in cyst size in biliary atresia [16]. Another study demonstrated no difference in the size of prenatal cysts between biliary atresia and choledochal cysts [17]. Other characteristics that suggested biliary atresia were anechoic cysts, small cysts in the hepatic hilum, and an undetected or atrophic gallbladder [17, 21]. An atrophic gallbladder detected after birth can be an important parameter for differentiating biliary atresia from choledochal cysts [17].

There are several studies on the outcome of biliary atresia with prenatal detection of biliary cystic malformation. Many studies have shown good outcomes in these cases after the

Kasai operation [13, 16, 17, 22]. However, a case series reported that four out of five patients with biliary atresia diagnosed by prenatal or perinatal detection of biliary cystic malformation resulted in liver transplantation [18]. This discrepancy is presumably due to differences in the types of biliary atresia. While the majority of patients with a good prognosis were type Ic, all five patients in the study with poor outcomes [18] were type IIId.

An algorithm for the management of prenatally diagnosed cystic biliary malformations was advocated [15]. The algorithm emphasized the postnatal confirmation of the biliary origin of cysts and the assessment of biliary obstruction. The postnatal investigation is important for fetuses with prenatally detected biliary cystic malformations.

## 14.4 Non-Visualization of the Fetal Gallbladder

The fetal gallbladder can be observed at 14–16 weeks of gestation by transvaginal ultrasonography [23] and between 24 and 32 weeks of gestation by transabdominal ultrasonography [24]. Non-visualization of the fetal gallbladder is rare and occurs in 0.1–0.15% of pregnancies [23, 25]. When the fetal gallbladder is not seen during the second trimester, the differential diagnoses include isolated gallbladder agenesis, which is a benign condition with an incidence of 1/6300 [26], as well as severe diseases like biliary atresia and cystic fibrosis [11, 23, 27, 28].

Generally, the outcome of fetuses with non-visualization of the gallbladder as an isolated finding is good. In a large study, the gallbladder was not visualized in 34 fetuses among 29,749 pregnancies [23]. However, the gallbladder is visualized in the third trimester or postnatally in most cases. The gallbladder was later found in 13 and was not found in 5 out of 20 fetuses with non-visualization of the gallbladder as an isolated finding. The outcome of all 18 fetuses was good. In contrast, only 1 of 14 fetuses with non-visualization of the gall bladder associated with structural malformation was healthy. The other 13 included 5 cases of chromosomal abnormalities and 2 cases of cystic fibrosis.

The association between biliary atresia and non-visualization of the fetal gallbladder remains controversial. In a study that reviewed 5 case series, including 168 cases with non-visualization of the fetal gallbladder, none were associated with biliary atresia [29]. In another previous report, 5.8% of cases of isolated non-visualization of the fetal gallbladder and 17.6% of cases of non-isolated non-visualization of the fetal gallbladder were associated with biliary atresia [28]. Another study estimated a 3% probability of biliary atresia when non-visualization of the fetal gallbladder was confirmed on repeat sonograms [30]. This discrepancy can be explained by the fact that both non-visualization of the fetal gallbladder and biliary atresia are rare. Conversely, non-visualization of the gallbladder by prenatal ultrasound was relatively common in infants with biliary atresia. In a retrospective study that reviewed 25 cases of biliary atresia with good prenatal ultrasound images, 24% of cases had non-visualization of the fetal gallbladder [30].

When the gallbladder is not visualized in fetuses, it is difficult to prenatally distinguish between biliary atresia and other conditions (both severe diseases and benign conditions), especially in cases without other structural anomalies. Some studies suggest that amniotic fluid levels of digestive enzymes, namely gamma-glutamyl transpeptidase (GGTP), before 22 weeks of gestation, is useful for differentiation. GGTP is present in the amniotic fluid from 13–14 weeks of gestation, rises to a plateau at 17–18 weeks, and gradually decreases from 22–24 weeks due to the maturation of the anal sphincter muscle [28]. Abnormal levels of amniotic fluid enzymes have been used for the prenatal diagnosis of digestive tract anomalies, such as cystic fibrosis, intestinal obstruction, and biliary atresia [27, 28, 31]. The low level of GGTP in the amniotic fluid before 22 weeks of gestation was reported to suggest biliary atresia or cystic fibrosis [28, 32, 33]. The sensitivity and specificity of digestive enzymes in the amniotic fluid before 22 weeks were 90% and 80% for diagnosing biliary atresia or cystic fibrosis in fetuses with non-visualization of the gallbladder [28]. After 22 weeks of gestation, digestive enzyme activities in the amniotic fluid are physiologically low, making it difficult to detect abnormally low levels. Several small case series suggested that high fetal blood GGTP levels after 22 weeks of gestation were associated with biliary atresia [31, 34]. However, a definitive prenatal diagnosis of biliary atresia is not necessary, and prompt postnatal examination is essential for early diagnosis and subsequent treatment. Therefore, amniocentesis or fetal blood sampling is too invasive for the prenatal diagnosis of biliary atresia.

## 14.5 Conclusion

Many infants with biliary atresia are first suspected of having this condition by clinical signs and symptoms, and a small number of infants are suspected prenatally by fetal ultrasonography. As early Kasai portoenterostomy improves the outcome [35], infants suspected to have biliary atresia need prompt investigation for diagnosis. Health care providers for neonates and fetuses should have a thorough knowledge of clinical signs/symptoms and prenatal findings for early referral to pediatric gastroenterologists and pediatric surgeons.

## References


1. Nio M. Japanese biliary atresia registry. Pediatr Surg Int. 2017;33(12):1319–25.
2. Fawaz R, et al. Guideline for the evaluation of Cholestatic jaundice in infants: joint recommendations of the north American Society for Pediatric Gastroenterology, hepatology, and nutrition and the European Society for Pediatric Gastroenterology, hepatology, and nutrition. J Pediatr Gastroenterol Nutr. 2017;64(1):154–68.
3. Hartley JL, Davenport M, Kelly DA. Biliary atresia. Lancet. 2009;374(9702):1704–13.
4. Lee WS, Chai PF. Clinical features differentiating biliary atresia from other causes of neonatal cholestasis. Ann Acad Med Singap. 2010;39(8):648–54.
5. El-Guindi MA, et al. Design and validation of a diagnostic score for biliary atresia. J Hepatol. 2014;61(1):116–23.
6. Karrer FM, et al. Biliary atresia registry, 1976 to 1989. J Pediatr Surg. 1990;25(10):1076–80. discussion 1081
7. Humphrey TM, Stringer MD. Biliary atresia: US diagnosis. Radiology. 2007;244(3):845–51.
8. Sun S, et al. Analysis of clinical parameters that contribute to the misdiagnosis of biliary atresia. J Pediatr Surg. 2013;48(7):1490–4.
9. Robie DK, Overfelt SR, Xie L. Differentiating biliary atresia from other causes of cholestatic jaundice. Am Surg. 2014;80(9):827–31.
10. National Registration, Japanese Biliary Atresia Society [cited 2020 June, 30]; Available from: https://jbas.net/en/national-registration/.
11. Davenport M, Hadzic N. Prenatal diagnosis of liver and biliary tract disease. Semin Neonatol. 2003;8(5):347–55.
12. Greenholz SK, et al. Biliary atresia in the newborn. J Pediatr Surg. 1986;21(12):1147–8.
13. Tsuchida Y, et al. Antenatal diagnosis of biliary atresia (type I cyst) at 19 weeks' gestation: differential diagnosis and etiologic implications. J Pediatr Surg. 1995;30(5):697–9.
14. Kasai M, et al. A proposal of new classification of biliary atresia. J Jpn Soc Pediatr Surg. 1976;12(2):327–31.
15. Redkar R, Davenport M, Howard ER. Antenatal diagnosis of congenital anomalies of the biliary tract. J Pediatr Surg. 1998;33(5):700–4.
16. Saito T, et al. The perinatal transition of the hepatobiliary cyst size provides information about the condition of bile flow in biliary cystic malformation cases. J Pediatr Surg. 2006;41(8):1397–402.
17. Tanaka H, et al. Postnatal management of prenatally diagnosed biliary cystic malformation. J Pediatr Surg. 2015;50(4):507–10.
18. Tanaka N, et al. Diagnosis and management of biliary cystic malformations in neonates. J Pediatr Surg. 2010;45(11):2119–23.
19. Fujishiro J, et al. Disappearing cyst of the hepatic hilum in uncorrectable biliary atresia. Pediatr Surg Int. 2005;21(2):116–8.
20. Masumoto K, et al. A case of cystic biliary atresia with an antenatally detected cyst: the possibility of changing from a correctable type with a cystic lesion (I cyst) to an uncorrectable one (IIId). Pediatr Surg Int. 2011;27(1):99–102.
21. Casaccia G, et al. Cystic anomalies of biliary tree in the fetus: is it possible to make a more specific prenatal diagnosis? J Pediatr Surg. 2002;37(8):1191–4.
22. Davenport M. Biliary atresia: clinical aspects. Semin Pediatr Surg. 2012;21(3):175–84.
23. Blazer S, Zimmer EZ, Bronshtein M. Nonvisualization of the fetal gallbladder in early pregnancy: comparison with clinical outcome. Radiology. 2002;224(2):379–82.
24. Hertzberg BS, et al. Nonvisualization of the fetal gallbladder: frequency and prognostic importance. Radiology. 1996;199(3):679–82.
25. Bronshtein M, et al. Prenatal diagnosis of gall bladder anomalies—report of 17 cases. Prenat Diagn. 1993;13(9):851–61.
26. Bennion RS, Thompson JE Jr, Tompkins RK. Agenesis of the gallbladder without extrahepatic biliary atresia. Arch Surg. 1988;123(10):1257–60.
27. Ochshorn Y, et al. Clinical evaluation of isolated nonvisualized fetal gallbladder. Prenat Diagn. 2007;27(8):699–703.
28. Dreux S, et al. Relationship of non-visualization of the fetal gallbladder and amniotic fluid digestive enzymes analysis to outcome. Prenat Diagn. 2012;32(5):423–6.
29. Shen O, et al. Absent gallbladder on fetal ultrasound: prenatal findings and postnatal outcome. Ultrasound Obstet Gynecol. 2011;37(6):673–7.
30. Shen O, et al. Prenatal diagnosis of biliary atresia: a case series. Early Hum Dev. 2017;111:16–9.
31. Muller F, et al. Role of fetal blood sampling in cases of nonvisualization of fetal gallbladder. Ultrasound Obstet Gynecol. 2015;46(6):743–4.
32. Bardin R, et al. Nonvisualization of the fetal gallbladder: can levels of gamma-Glutamyl Transpeptidase in amniotic fluid predict fetal prognosis? Fetal Diagn Ther. 2016;39(1):50–5.
33. Boughanim M, et al. Nonvisualization of the fetal gallbladder by second-trimester ultrasound scan: strategy of clinical management based on four examples. Prenat Diagn. 2008;28(1):46–8.
34. Ruiz A, et al. Prenatal nonvisualization of the gallbladder: a diagnostic and prognostic dilemma. Fetal Diagn Ther. 2017;42(2):150–2.
35. Serinet MO, et al. Impact of age at Kasai operation on its results in late childhood and adolescence: a rational basis for biliary atresia screening. Pediatrics. 2009;123(5):1280–6.

# Intracranial Hemorrhage in Biliary Atresia

15

Akiko Yokoi

**Abstract**

Significant numbers of infants diagnosed with biliary atresia (BA) initially present with intracranial hemorrhage associated with vitamin K deficiency. Preventing and treating intracranial hemorrhage, which may lead to death or severe neurological sequelae in survivors, are important issues in the management of BA. Prophylactic vitamin K administration regimens are still insufficient to prevent intracranial hemorrhage in BA. The treatment of coagulopathy with intravenous vitamin K and fresh frozen plasma administration is effective within 24 hours. Urgent surgical intervention for intracranial hemorrhage including craniotomy followed by Kasai portoenterostomy may contribute to improving native liver survival. Early detection through nationwide screening of BA may confer advantages in preventing intracranial hemorrhage, as well as improving native liver survival; however, currently, no screening programs show an impact on intracranial hemorrhage in the management of BA.

**Keywords**

Intracranial hemorrhage · Vitamin K deficiency bleeding
Biliary atresia

A. Yokoi (✉)
Department of Pediatric Surgery, Kobe Children's Hospital, Kobe, Japan
e-mail: yokoi_kch@hp.pref.hyogo.jp

Intracranial hemorrhage is associated with malabsorption of fat-soluble vitamin K due to insufficient bile flow in BA.

## 15.1 Vitamin K deficiency bleeding

Vitamin K deficiency bleeding (VKDB) is classified as early (<24 hours after birth), classic (within days 2–7), and late (between 2 weeks and 6 months) [1]. Late VKDB is further classified as idiopathic without risk factors of vitamin K deficiency other than breastfeeding and secondary VKDB with risk factors such as malabsorption due to cholestasis. More than 80% of patients with late VKDB present with intracranial hemorrhage with a mortality rate of 20–50%.

## 15.2 Incidence of intracranial hemorrhage in BA

The incidence of intracranial hemorrhage in biliary atresia (BA) has been reported to vary according to the vitamin K prophylactic regimen and incidences of BA among countries. Hasselt et al. reported that 43% of patients with BA presented with intracranial hemorrhage with 25 mg of daily oral vitamin K administration in Denmark, which was reduced to 0% with 1 mg of weekly oral administration [2]. Takahashi et al. reported that intracranial hemorrhage occurs in 11.1% of patients with BA. We reported a rate of 22% in our series (Table 15.1) [3]. Based on the Japanese BA registry, the incidence of intracranial hemorrhage was 4.3% between 1989 and 2009.

## 15.3 Presentation of intracranial hemorrhage in BA

Intracranial hemorrhage associated with BA occurs as late VKDB, which occurs later than 2 weeks after birth. In the literature, the earliest ages at diagnosis in various series have


M. Nio (ed.), *Introduction to Biliary Atresia*, https://doi.org/10.1007/978-981-16-2160-4_15

**Table 15.1** Characteristics of patients in the periods before and after SCC implementation

| | Before SCC (2005–2011) | After SCC (2012–2018) | p |
|---|---|---|---|
| N=41 | 27 | 14 | |
| Gender (female) | 16 | 10 | 0.51 |
| Gestation week [weeks median (range)] | 39 (36–41) | 40 (37–41) | 0.26 |
| Birth weight [g median (range)] | 2864 (2105–3764) | 3084 (2560–3685) | 0.05 |
| Age at admission [days median (range)] | 64 (8–102) | 62 (0–86) | 0.47 |
| Preoperative laboratory data [median (range)] | | | |
| Total bilirubin (mg/dL) | 8.8 (6.0–19.8) | 9.2 (6.4–14.9) | 0.76 |
| Direct bilirubin (mg/dL) | 6.0 (3.4–12.9) | 5.4 (3.1–10.2) | 0.12 |
| AST (IU/L) | 155 (43–380) | 146 (37–275) | 0.50 |
| ALT (IU/L) | 101 (17–263) | 91.5 (16–289) | 0.80 |
| γ-GTP (IU/L) | 551 (120–2283) | 675 (74–1600) | 0.33 |
| Prolonged PT | 10/27 (37.0%) | 7/14 (50.0%) | 0.51 |
| VKDB | 8/27 (29.6%) | 5/14 (35.7%) | 0.73 |
| Intracranial hemorrhage | 6/27 (22.2%) | 3/14 (21.4%) | 1.00 |
| Age at surgery [days median (range)] | 70 (22–111) | 69.5 (25–97) | 0.88 |
| Liver transplantation | 15/27 (56.1%) | 8/14 (57.1%) | 1.00 |

SCC=stool color card, AST=aspartate aminotransferase, ALT=alanine aminotransferase, GTP, glutamyl transpeptidase, PT=prothrombin time, VKDB=vitamin K deficiency bleeding

been reported as 17 days [4], 35 days [5], 3 weeks [6], and 47 days [7].

The clinical symptoms in previously healthy infants include jaundice, poor sucking, poor activity, vomiting (non-bilious emesis), and seizures or other neurological findings such as anisocoria at the onset of intracranial hemorrhage.

In the initial laboratory tests, coagulopathy with direct hyperbilirubinemia is evident. The prothrombin time and activated partial thrombin time are significantly prolonged in infants with intracranial hemorrhage compared to those in infants without intracranial hemorrhage [7].

The location and distribution of intracranial bleeding vary [4–6, 8, 9]. Most cases present with subdural and subarachnoid hemorrhage, while intraparenchymal and intraventricular hemorrhage are noted as well. Bilateral involvement has also been reported.

## 15.4 Treatment of intracranial hemorrhage in BA

Coagulopathy should be corrected with prompt intravenous or intramuscular administration of vitamin K, which is normalized within 24 hours in patients with VKDB. Fresh frozen plasma is also effective to improve coagulopathy when considering further surgical intervention.

**Table 15.2** Comparison between patients with and without VKDB

| | VKDB (+) | VKDB (-) | p |
|---|---|---|---|
| N=41 | 13 | 28 | |
| Intracranial hemorrhage | 9 | | |
| Age at admission [days median (range)] | 66 (43–86) | 52 (0–86) | 0.03 |
| Preoperative laboratory data [median (range)] | | | |
| Total bilirubin (mg/dL) | 8.7 (7.2–19.8) | 9.0 (6.0–12.7) | 0.61 |
| Direct bilirubin (mg/dL) | 6.0 (4.0–12.9) | 6.0 (3.1–11.2) | 0.33 |
| Prolonged PT | 13 (100%) | 4 (14.3%) | <0.01 |
| Age at surgery [days median (range)] | 74 (59–97) | 59.5 (22–111) | 0.01 |
| Liver transplantation | 9 (69.2%) | 14 (50.0%) | 0.3 |

AST=aspartate aminotransferase, ALT=alanine aminotransferase, GTP, glutamyl transpeptidase, PT=prothrombin time, VKDB=vitamin K deficiency bleeding

Akiyama et al. described 8 of 15 patients presented intracranial hemorrhage underwent surgical evacuation of intracranial hematoma when a midline shift was identified on head computed tomography, while another 7 patients were treated conservatively without surgical intervention [4]. Takahashi et al. reported only 3 of 7 patients presented intracranial hemorrhage underwent craniotomy [7].

As patients become clinically stable after neurosurgical intervention, Kasai portoenterostomy should be planned without delays.

## 15.5 Consequence of intracranial hemorrhage in BA

Mortality is mainly due to liver failure, and the native liver survival rate is not significantly different in patients who had intracranial hemorrhage compared to that in patients who didn't have an eisode of intracranial hemorrhage (Table 15.2) [3]. However, 15% to 70% of patients who experienced intracranial hemorrhage developed neurological sequelae including mental retardation, epilepsy, hemiparesis, and cerebral palsy.

## 15.6 Prophylactic management of intracranial hemorrhage

Prophylactic vitamin K administration is essential to prevent VKDB in breastfed infants. Oral administration is feasible and widely accepted; however, it is difficult to prevent secondary VKDB with malabsorption in infants with cholestatic disease [10]. A comparison between patients who diagnosed with BA in the Netherlands and Denmark revealed that the Dutch regimen of increasing the daily oral dose to 150 mg from 25 mg fails to prevent VKDB, while the Danish regimen comprising a single dose of 2 mg administered intramuscularly at birth is effective in reducing VKDB. The National Institute for Clinical Excellence (NICE) in the United Kingdom recommends vitamin K prophylaxis as follows:

- All parents should be offered vitamin K prophylaxis for their babies to prevent the rare but serious and sometimes fatal disorder of VKDB.
- Vitamin K should be administered as a single dose of 1 mg intramuscularly, as this is the most clinically and cost-effective method of administration.
- If parents decline intramuscular vitamin K for their baby, oral vitamin K should be offered as a second-line option. Parents should be advised that oral vitamin K must be administered according to the manufacturer's instructions for clinical efficacy and will require multiple doses (NICE Clinical Guideline 37 2006).

The American Academy of Pediatrics recommendations on vitamin K are as follows:

- Vitamin K should be administered to all newborn infants as a single, intramuscular dose of 0.5 to 1 mg.
- Additional research should be conducted on the efficacy, safety, and bioavailability of oral vitamin K to prevent late VKDB.
- Healthcare professionals should promote awareness among families of the risks of late VKDB associated with inadequate vitamin K prophylaxis from current oral dosage regimens, particularly for newborns who are breastfed.

Despite those recommendations, refusal of intramuscular prophylactics has been highlighted due to parents' concerns about potential adverse effects and pain to the infant [9]. Thus, none of the regimens of vitamin K prophylactic administration are currently sufficient to prevent late VKDB.

## 15.7 Early detection of BA

BA is a progressive disease, and its early detection followed by Kasai portoenterostomy has been shown to improve outcomes. Nationwide screening of BA using stool color cards has been conducted in some countries such as Taiwan [11] and Japan [12] where the incidence of BA is high. In the United States, where the incidence of BA is much lower than that in Asia, screening using serum bilirubin or stool color cards has been advocated [13]. A mobile phone application for screening of stool color has been reported; however, no data have been shown regarding the efficacy for early detection of BA. Those screening for early detection of BA may contribute to not only improving outcomes but to reducing the incidence of intracranial hemorrhage. However, in our series, we did not observe improvements in the incidence of intracranial hemorrhage after implementation of the nationwide stool color card screening in Japan (Table 15.1) [3]. Further studies and improvements in screening programs are warranted to improve outcomes and prevent intracranial hemorrhage.

## 15.8 Summary

Intracranial hemorrhage, which is potentially life-threatening and may cause neurological sequelae, occurs in a significant number of patients. Oral vitamin K prophylactic regimens are insufficient to prevent intracranial hemorrhage as late VKDB because of fat-soluble vitamin K malabsorption with limited bile flow. Intramuscular vitamin K regimens may be effective; however, parents' compliance is an issue. Screening programs for the early detection of BA may have a potential impact on preventing intracranial hemorrhage, as well as improving native liver survival; however, to date, no data are available regarding the prevention of intracranial hemorrhage.

Intracranial hemorrhage should be treated as follows:

- Coagulopathy should be corrected with intravenous vitamin K injections with fresh frozen plasma immediately.
- Neurosurgeons should be consulted to evaluate the need for emergent evacuation of intracranial hematoma.
- Kasai portoenterostomy should be planned as soon as the patients become stable, which is feasible and may contribute to improving native liver survival.
- Long-term neurological sequelae should be evaluated.

## References

1. Araki S, Shirahata A. Vitamin K Deficiency Bleeding in Infancy. Nutrients. 2020;12(3):1. https://doi.org/10.3390/nu12030780.
2. van Hasselt PM, de Koning TJ, Kvist N, de Vries E, Lundin CR, Berger R, et al. Prevention of vitamin K deficiency bleeding in breastfed infants: lessons from the Dutch and Danish biliary atresia registries. Pediatrics. 2008;121(4):e857–63. https://doi.org/10.1542/peds.2007-1788.
3. Yokoi A, Isono K. Stool color card screening for early detection of biliary atresia. J Jpn Soc Pediatr Surg. 2019;55(5):945–50.
4. Akiyama H, Okamura Y, Nagashima T, Yokoi A, Muraji T, Uetani Y. Intracranial hemorrhage and vitamin K deficiency associated with biliary atresia: summary of 15 cases and review of the literature. Pediatr Neurosurg. 2006;42(6):362–7. https://doi.org/10.1159/000095566.
5. Miyasaka M, Nosaka S, Sakai H, Tsutsumi Y, Kitamura M, Miyazaki O, et al. Vitamin K deficiency bleeding with intracranial hemorrhage: focus on secondary form. Emerg Radiol. 2007;14(5):323–9. https://doi.org/10.1007/s10140-007-0632-y.

6. Per H, Arslan D, Gumus H, Coskun A, Kumandas S. Intracranial hemorrhages and late hemorrhagic disease associated cholestatic liver disease. Neurol Sci. 2013;34(1):51–6. https://doi.org/10.1007/s10072-012-0965-5.
7. Takahashi Y, Matsuura T, Yoshimaru K, Yanagi Y, Hayashida M, Taguchi T. Comparison of biliary atresia with and without intracranial hemorrhage. J Pediatr Surg. 2018;53(11):2245–9. https://doi.org/10.1016/j.jpedsurg.2018.04.031.
8. Alatas FS, Hayashida M, Matsuura T, Saeki I, Yanagi Y, Taguchi T. Intracranial hemorrhage associated with vitamin K-deficiency bleeding in patients with biliary atresia: focus on long-term outcomes. J Pediatr Gastroenterol Nutr. 2012;54(4):552–7. https://doi.org/10.1097/MPG.0b013e3182421878.
9. Bruton L, Hoffmann JA. Intracranial Hemorrhage in a Previously Healthy Infant. Clinical Pediatric Emergency Medicine. 2020;100763
10. Mihatsch WA, Braegger C, Bronsky J, Campoy C, Domellof M, Fewtrell M, et al. Prevention of Vitamin K Deficiency Bleeding in Newborn Infants: A Position Paper by the ESPGHAN Committee on Nutrition. J Pediatr Gastroenterol Nutr. 2016;63(1):123–9. https://doi.org/10.1097/MPG.0000000000001232.
11. Lin JS, Chen SC, Lu CL, Lee HC, Yeung CY, Chan WT. Reduction of the ages at diagnosis and operation of biliary atresia in Taiwan: A 15-year population-based cohort study. World J Gastroenterol. 2015;21(46):13080–6. https://doi.org/10.3748/wjg.v21.i46.13080.
12. Gu YH, Yokoyama K, Mizuta K, Tsuchioka T, Kudo T, Sasaki H, et al. Stool color card screening for early detection of biliary atresia and long-term native liver survival: a 19-year cohort study in Japan. J Pediatr. 2015;166(4):897–902. e1. https://doi.org/10.1016/j.jpeds.2014.12.063.
13. Goodhue C, Fenlon M, Wang KS. Newborn screening for biliary atresia in the United States. Pediatr Surg Int. 2017;33(12):1315–8. https://doi.org/10.1007/s00383-017-4159-3.

# Pathology of Biliary Atresia

# 16

Masayoshi Kage, Kennichi Tanikawa, and Hironori Kusano

## 16.1 Introduction

Biliary atresia (BA) displays characteristic pathological findings of the liver and choledochus in the hepatic hilum [1–4]. We will discuss them and compare them with the liver histological features in other two major diseases, namely Alagille syndrome (AGS) [5–7] and progressive familial intrahepatic cholestasis type 2 (PFIC2) [8, 9] that we need to distinguish from BA. Next, we will review the association between pathological changes of BA and the prognosis.

### 16.1.1 Histological Findings in BA

#### 16.1.1.1 Liver Histology

Characteristic histological indings in the liver in BA are fibrosis of biliary type, bile duct changes, and cholestasis. We explain each finding.

**Fibrosis**

Fibrosis first occurs in portal tract, and the portal tract gradually presents fibrous expansion. This fibrous expansion leads to the formation of portal to portal fibrous bridging. As fibrous expansion proceeds, the hepatic lobular architecture becomes distorted, leading to the development of biliary cirrhosis. Furthermore, patients with BA may develop hepatocellular carcinoma [1].

Fibrosis of BA is classified into four stages based on the degree of its progression to cirrhosis. Figure 16.1 shows a schematic diagram of the stage of hepatic fibrosis in BA proposed by Batts KP et al. [10]. Briefly, Stage 1: Mild portal fibrous expansion. Stage 2: Moderate portal fibrous expansion. Stage 3: Bridging fibrosis with distorted lobular architecture but no regenerative nodules. Stage 4: Biliary cirrhosis, consisting of nodules ad fibrous septa. The representative histology of each stage is shown in Fig. 16.2.

Figure 16.3 shows an autopsy case of BA in which the evolutional process to liver cirrhosis could be histologically observed.

It is known that in biliary atresia, liver fibrosis progresses rapidly, leading to cirrhosis. However, it is also known that the degree of fibrosis is not always related to the age at biopsy. Figure 16.4 shows the histology of liver biopsy at Kasai procedure, taken from two BA patients at the same age of 70-day-old. In the cases shown in Fig. 16.4a, liver fibrosis (Stage 1) is mild for patients with BA of this age, while advanced fibrosis (Stage 3) is the case in Fig. 16.4b.

**Bile Duct Changes**

We will discuss the main pathological findings of the proliferation of bile ductules and ductal plate malformation (DPM).

Significant proliferation of bile ductules occurs in the portal tracts and at the interface. The proliferated ductules contain irregularly dilated lumen. Bile plugs are often seen within the lumen of these ductules (Fig. 16.5). DPM appears as an irregular string of bead-like bile duct structures located slightly inside the interface of the portal area [1, 3, 4] (Figs. 16.6 and 16.7-a, b). Small capillaries are found in the center of these bile duct structures. DPM is usually observed together with the proliferation of ductules at the interface of the portal tracts.

DPM reportedly occurs in 20–40% of BA cases [1]. However, DPM is not specific to BA and also occurs in Caroli disease, congenital hepatic fibrosis, and other pediatric liver diseases [1, 2]. DPM can be recognized by immunohistochemistry (Fig. 16.7-b).

As regards the mechanism of DPM formation, in the pediatric period, the intrahepatic bile ducts form after the

M. Kage (✉)
Department of Medical Engineering, Junshin Gakuen University, Fukuoka, Japan
e-mail: masakage@med.kurume-u.ac.jp

K. Tanikawa · H. Kusano
Department of Pathology, Kurume University, Fukuoka, Japan


M. Nio (ed.), *Introduction to Biliary Atresia*, https://doi.org/10.1007/978-981-16-2160-4_16

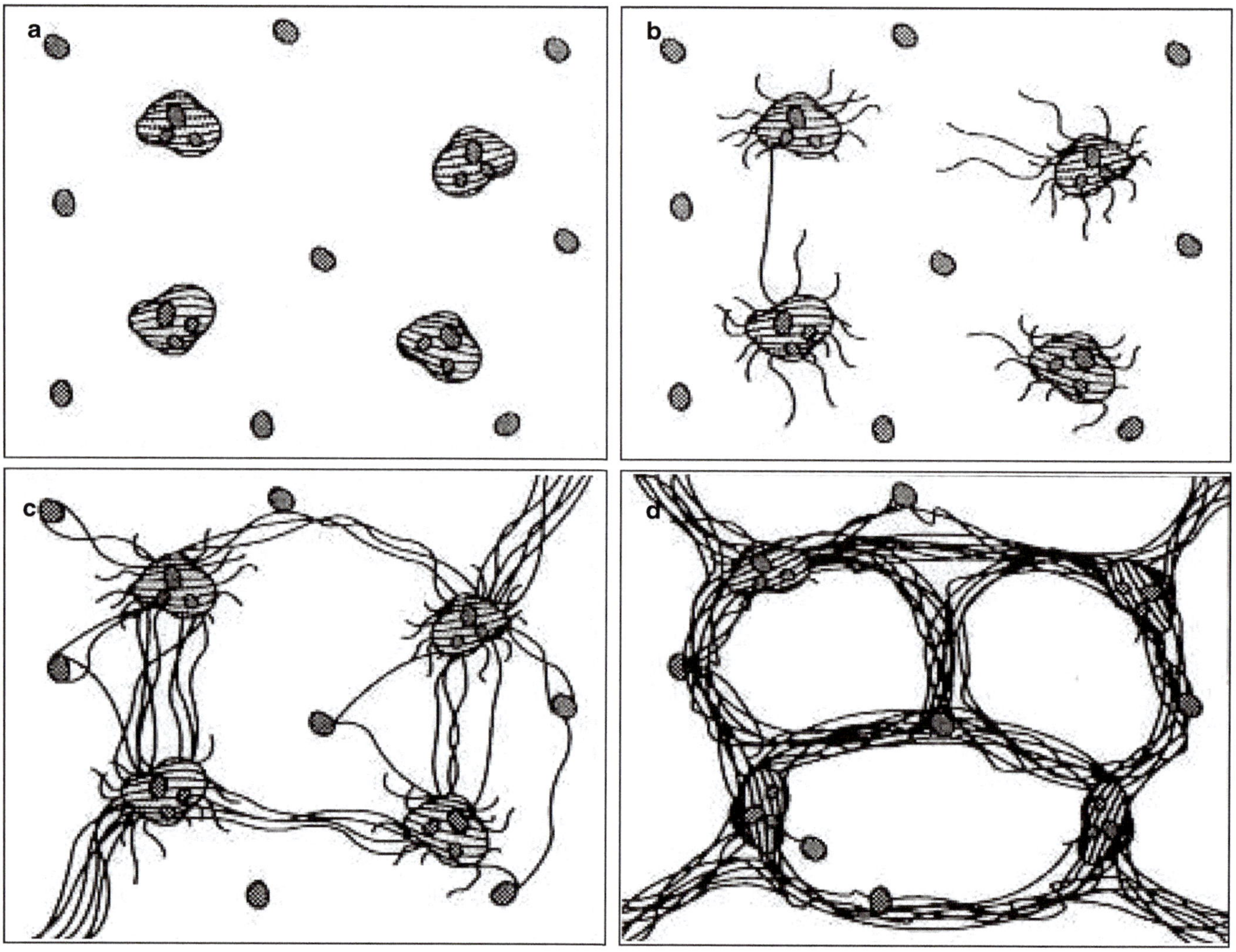


**Fig. 16.1** Schematic diagram of the stage of hepatic fibrosis in BA. **a**: Stage1; mild portal fibrosis, **b**: Stage 2; moderate portal fibrous expansion, Stage 3; advanced fibrosis with bridging fibrosis, Stage 4; biliary cirrhosis with the regenerative nodule. Reprinted from BATT (Ref. 10)

formation of the ductal plate. The formation of the ductal plate begins in the proximity of the hepatic hilum and gradually expands and gradually expands into the peripheral portal tract of the liver to form the intrahepatic bile ducts. DPM is regarded as a malformation of the ductal plate, which plays an important role in the development of the intrahepatic bile ducts.

In the evolutional process to cirrhosis in BA, damage to the interlobular bile ducts has usually increased and leads to bile duct loss. Some cases of BA are associated with paucity of interlobular bile ducts [11], particularly in the cirrhotic stage (Figs. 16.2-d and 16.3-c), and this is considered an exacerbation factor for BA. In other words, BA is included in vanishing bile duct syndrome. However, histological evaluation of the interlobular bile ducts can be difficult in BA cases which show ductular proliferation in the portal tracts. It can be difficult to distinguish between the proliferated ductules and normal interlobular bile ducts.

#### Cholestasis

Significant cholestasis is observed in both the hepatic lobules and intra-biliary system in BA. This feature is especially prominent in the central area. The hepatocytes with intracytoplasmic cholestasis swell and may display an acinar arrangement, with bile plugs in the acinus (Fig. 16.8), as well as in the bile duct lumen (Fig. 16.5). Further, hepatocytes may sometimes undergo giant cell transformation with multinuclei, having several to several tens of nuclei per cell (Fig. 16.9). The causes of giant cell transformation of the hepatocytes are unknown, but may be related to the fusion of hepatocytes or excessive nuclear division during regeneration of a hepatocyte. Giant cell transformation is a common finding in BA, but not specific. It is a common finding in infants with various diseases that develop cholestasis.

We have discussed the three most common and characteristic pathological features of the liver in BA. In addition to

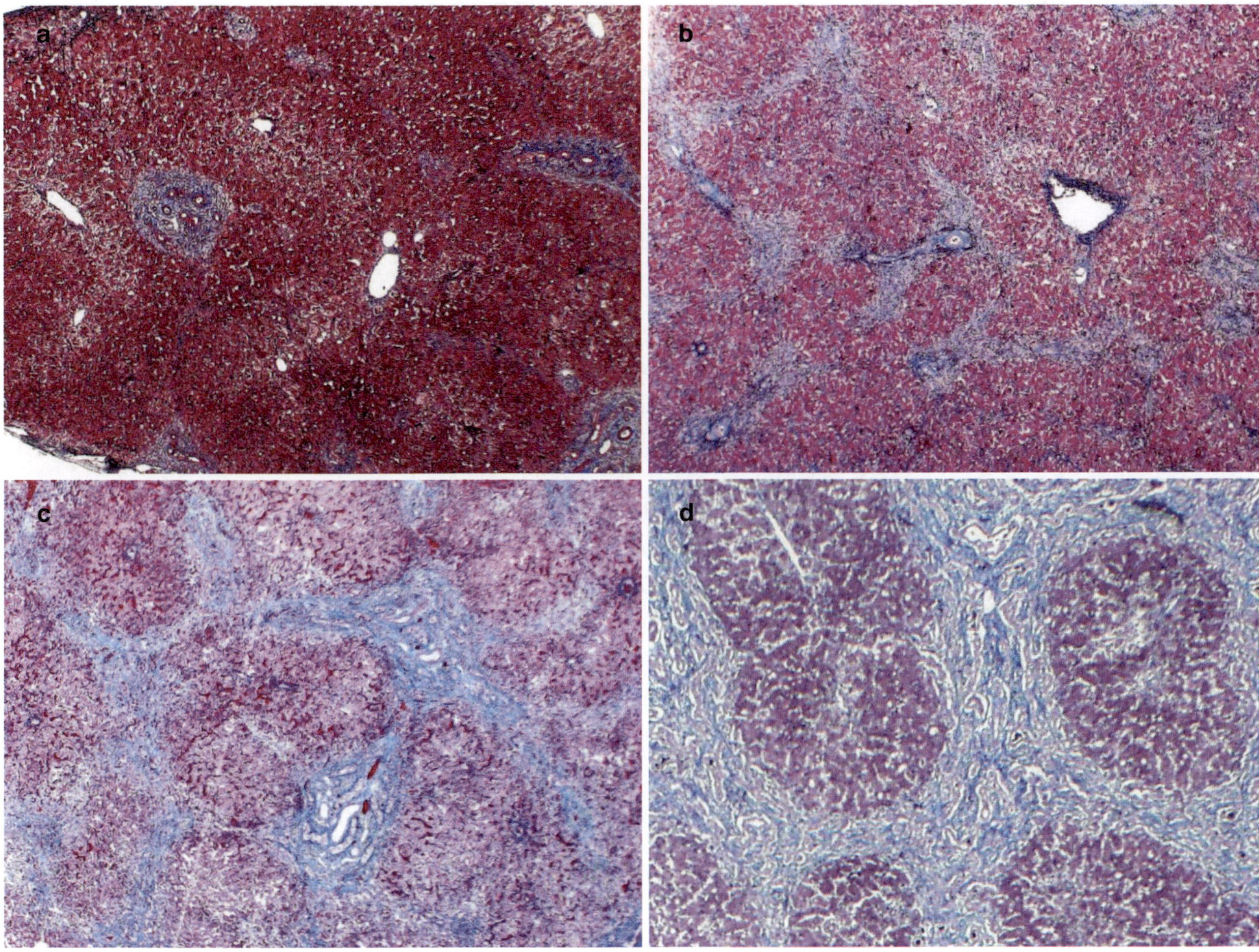


Fig. 16.2 Histological images of each stage of hepatic fibrosis in BA. **a**: Stage 1, **b**: Stage 2, Stage 3, Stage 4. (**a**, **b**, **c**: Wedge biopsy at Kasai procedure, d: Liver at autopsy, Masson trichrome stain)

these features, BA shows a variety of other hepatic findings. We will briefly explain them below.

### Extramedullary Hematopoiesis (EMH)

EMH is often observed in sinusoids in BA and the other diseases in cholestasis. The name reflects the fact that hematopoiesis occurs in the liver in the neo-natal period. EMH is a small focus, consisting of mixed myeloid and erythroid cells (Fig. 16.10), while focal necrosis is a small group of lytic necrosis of hepatocytes with infiltrate of lymphocytes and macrophages. EMH can at first glance be easily confused with focal necrosis, so care must be taken to distinguish the two findings.

### Necrosis and Apoptosis, and Inflammation

Cases of BA with giant cell changes in hepatocytes are often referred to as giant cell hepatitis. However, even if it is called hepatitis, it is histologically different from hepatitis caused by the hepatitis virus. Hepatocyte death, such as apoptosis, focal necrosis, and bridging necrosis, is usually found in acute or chronic viral hepatitis B or C. On the other hand, in BA, we seldom observe severe necroinflammation such as bridging necrosis or massive hepatic necrosis. However, apoptosis of hepatic cells is sometimes seen in BA (Fig. 16.11).

### Changes in the Portal Tracts Other than the Bile Ducts

Various degrees of lymphocytic infiltration are found in the portal tracts in BA. Mild eosinophilic infiltration may be sometimes found along with lymphocytic infiltration. Moreover, the hepatic arteries usually become thick, and the portal vein branches become narrowed in the portal tracts [12, 13].

### Differential Diagnosis

There are several diseases that need to be distinguished from BA when making a differential diagnosis. Of particular

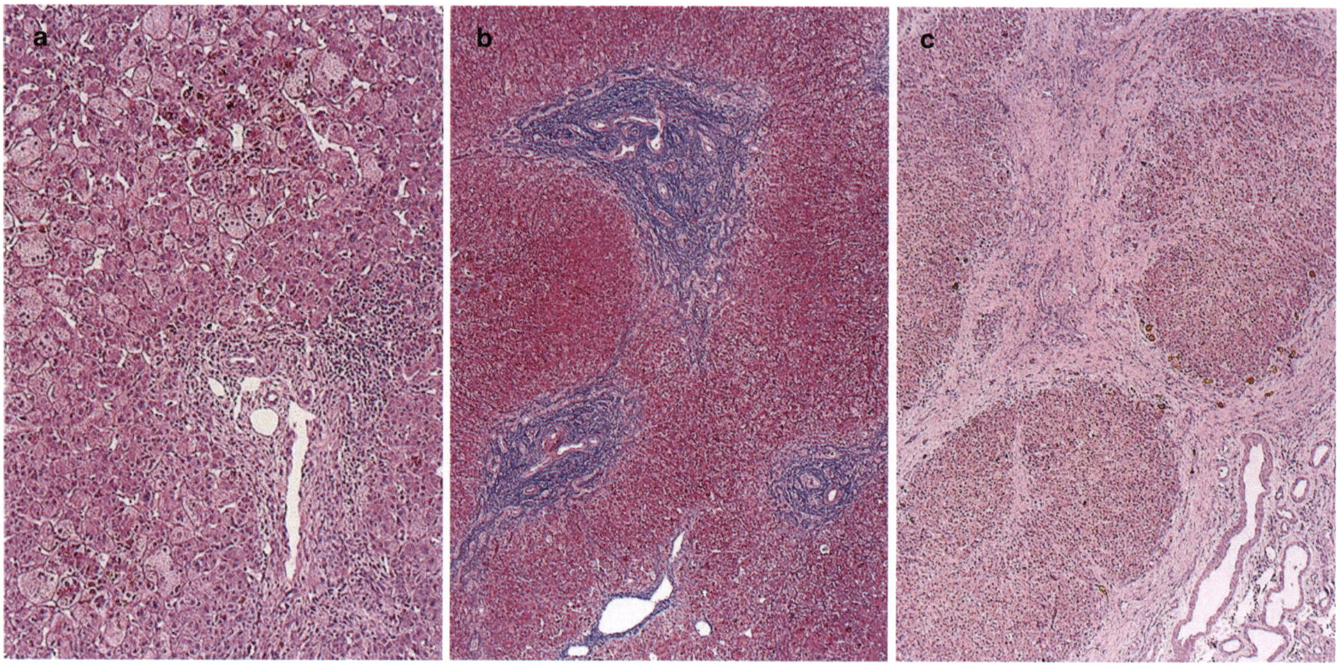


**Fig. 16.3** Histologically followed autopsy case of a girl with BA. She underwent the Kasai procedure at the age of 2 months under the diagnosis of BA (**a**). However, due to poor bile outflow, reoperation was performed at the age of 7 months (**b**), but cholestasis worsened. She died of multiple organ failure at the age of 1 year-7 months (**c**). **a**. Two months old. Mild portal fibrosis (Stage 1). **b**. Seven months old. Moderate fibrous expansion of the portal tracts (Stage 2). **c**. One year and 10 months old. Liver cirrhosis of biliary cirrhosis (Stage 4). Thick fibrous septa have no interlobular bile duct, suggesting vanishing bile duct syndrome. **a**, **c**: H.E. stain, **b**: Azan stain

importance are AGS [6, 7, 14] and PFIC2 [8, 9]. Next, we will discuss how to histologically distinguish BA from these two diseases.

## AGS

AGS is an autosomal dominant disorder and is caused by mutations in the human *Jagged 1*, which encodes a ligand for Notch 1 [15]. AGS primarily affects various organs, including the liver, heart and vascular system, eyes, face, and skeleton. The major clinical features are chronic cholestasis, peripheral pulmonary stenosis, butterfly vertebrae, ocular abnormalities (posterior embryotoxon), and characteristic facial features [7]. AGS has traditionally been diagnosed based on the paucity of the interlobular bile ducts on liver biopsy (Fig. 16.12) and the characteristic clinical findings.

The important histological findings to distinguish BA from AGS are the bile duct changes and fibrosis I portal tract. First, regarding the bile duct changes in AGS, the most important finding is paucity of the interlobular bile ducts. The paucity is determined by the ratio of the number of interlobular ducts (P) to that of interlobular bile ducts (B) (P/B) in the portal tract. When this ratio is 0.2 or less, there is considered to be a paucity of interlobular bile ducts. However, there are some cases of AGS in which such a paucity is not observed. In AGS, even when interlobular bile ducts are present, morphological abnormalities of the interlobular bile duct such as irregular lumen and decreased and disarrayed biliary epithelial cells may present (Fig. 16.13). Some cases of BA may present with the paucity of the bile duct, but in such cases, ductular proliferation and fibrosis in the portal tract are usually observed. Next, regarding fibrosis in the portal tract, it is absent or minor in AGS, while portal fibrous expansion is pronounced in BA even in the early stage. DPM is not usually found in AGS. These findings are differential points to distinguish two diseases.

Some BA patients who experience poor results after the Kasai procedure may actually be suffering from AGS. When the liver biopsy from such cases is reviewed, it is found that pathologically some of them should be diagnosed as AGS. These cases are usually diagnosed as BA based on findings of biliary obstruction in the hilum at the surgery. It has been reported that approximately 10% of AGS cases are complicated by extrahepatic biliary obstruction. It is not difficult to differentiate pathologically between AGS and BA. If AGS is pathologically suspected, a pathologist recommends the genetic testing for AGS. It is important to always keep in mind the possibility of AGS when making a pathological diagnosis of BA.

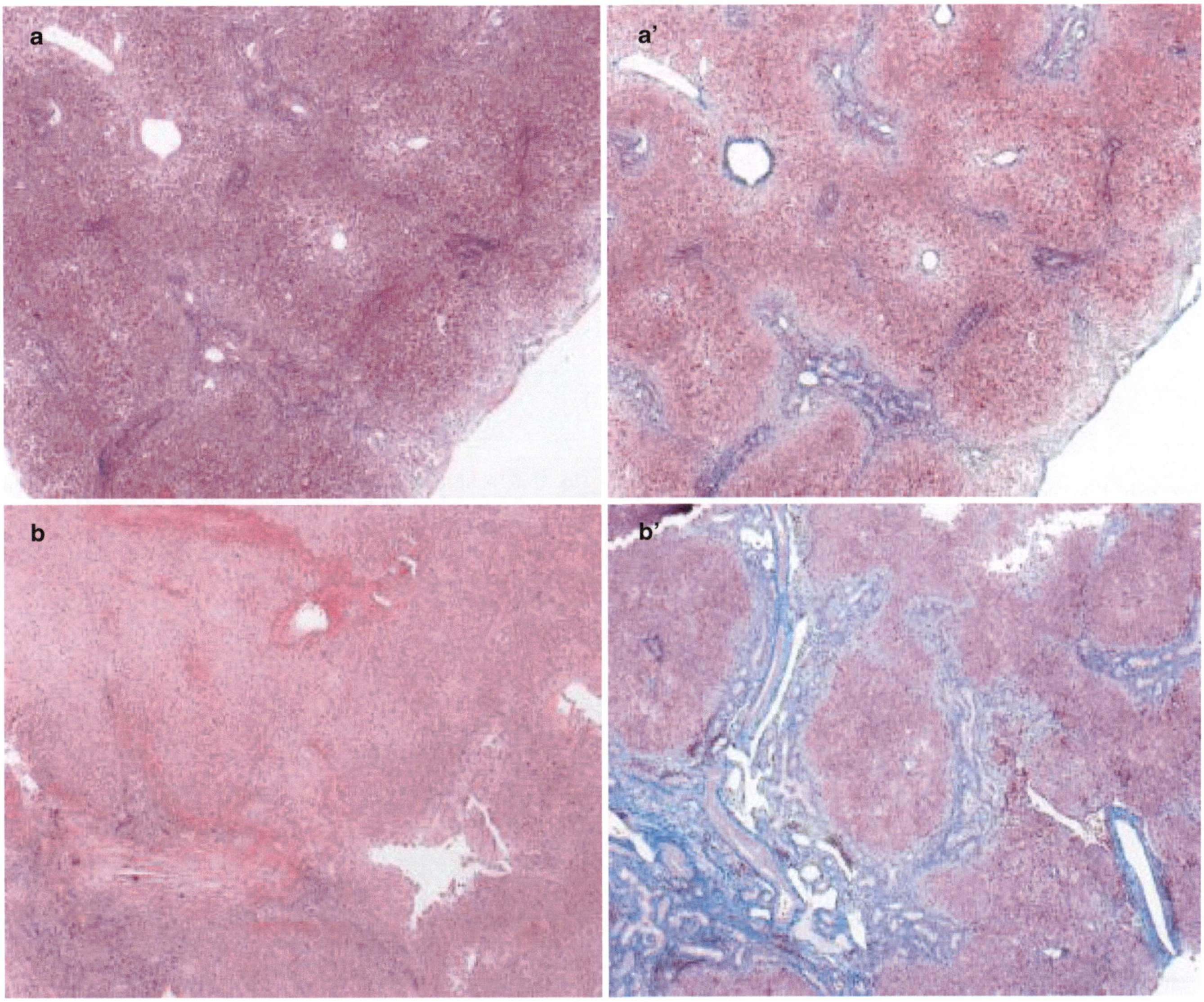


**Fig. 16.4** The pathological feature of liver biopsy of two BA patients at the same age of 70-day-old at Kasai procedure. 7-**a**: Mild fibrosis (Stage 1), 7-**b**: Advanced fibrosis (Stage 3). **a'** and **b'**: Masson trichrome stain

**PFIC2**

PFIC2 is a rare autosomal-recessive disorder of childhood caused by defects in the transporter of hepatocyte, namely bile salt export pump (BSEP) [8]. BSEP is present at the bile canaliculi of hepatocytes. PFIC2 usually causes progressive liver disease leading to cirrhosis.

PFIC2 is histologically similar to BA in that they both can appear with cholestasis, giant cell transformation, and fibrosis of the portal tracts (Fig. 16.14). One of the features that distinguishes BA from PFIC2 is the highly pronounced ductular proliferation accompanied by bile plug. On the other hand, necroinflammation is usually more prominent in PFIC2 than BA. Both diseases can develop biliary cirrhosis. In such cases in the cirrhotic stage, it is very difficult to distinguish between the two diseases. For a differential diagnosis, immunohistochemistry will be useful, because PFIC2 lacks the expression of BSEP (Fig. 16.15), whereas it is highly overexpressed in BA. When the clinical and histopathological findings suggest PFIC2, genetic testing for PFIC2 will be needed to confirm the diagnosis.

#### 16.1.1.2 Histology of the Obstruction of Bile Ducts at the Hepatic Hilum

One of the characteristics of BA is progressive inflammatory destruction and subsequent loss of the extrahepatic bile ducts and granulation tissue formation [1, 4] (Fig. 16.16), followed

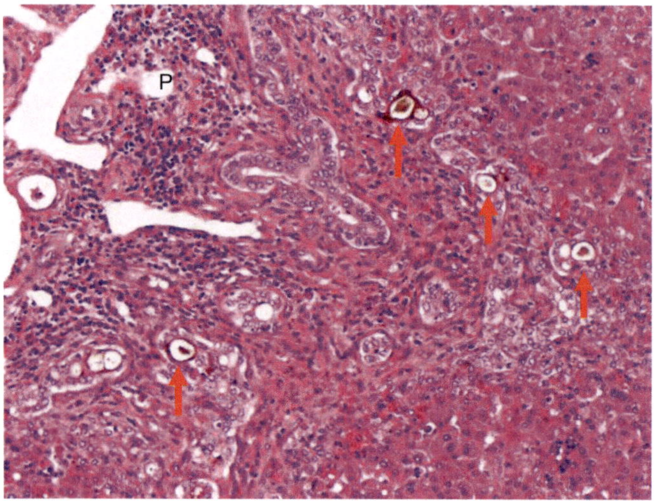


**Fig. 16.5** Bile ductular proliferation with bile plugs. The proliferated ductules contain bile plugs within the lumen (arrows)

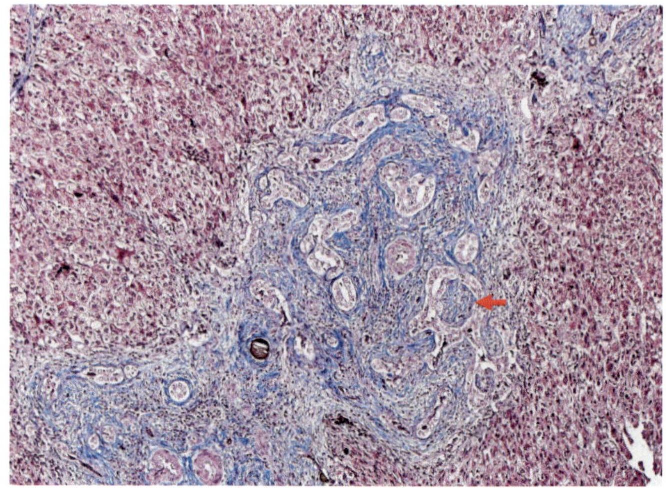

**Fig. 16.6** A histological finding of DPM at the medium-sized portal tract in BA with Masson trichrome stain. DPM is characterized by an irregular string of bead-like bile duct structures in the portal area. Small vessels in the center of these bile duct structures is found (arrow). DPM is clearly demonstrated by Masson trichrome stain

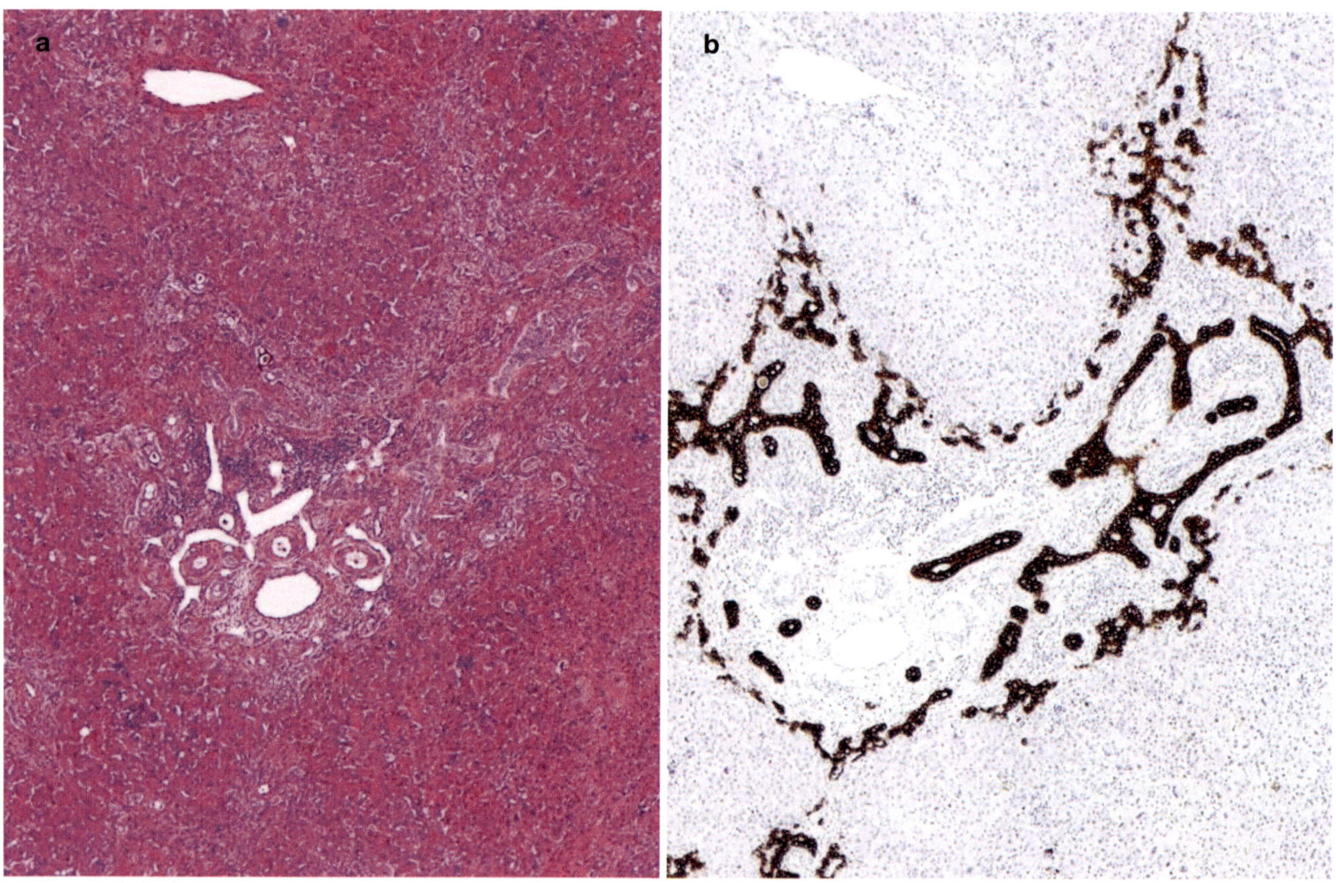


**Fig. 16.7** A histological finding of DPM at the periphery of the portal tract. **a**: Abnormal ductular structures in the portal tract. **b**. DPM can be clearly observed by immunohistochemistry using CK7

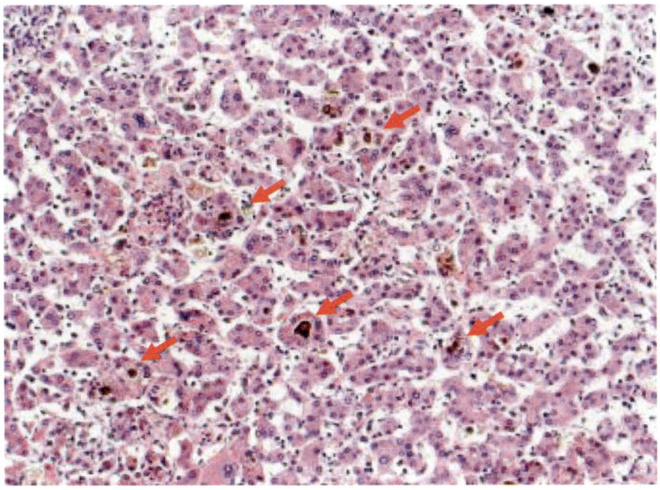

**Fig. 16.8** Cholestasis in the hepatic lobules in BA. Bile plugs are found in the center of the acinar arrangement of the hepatocytes (*arrows*)

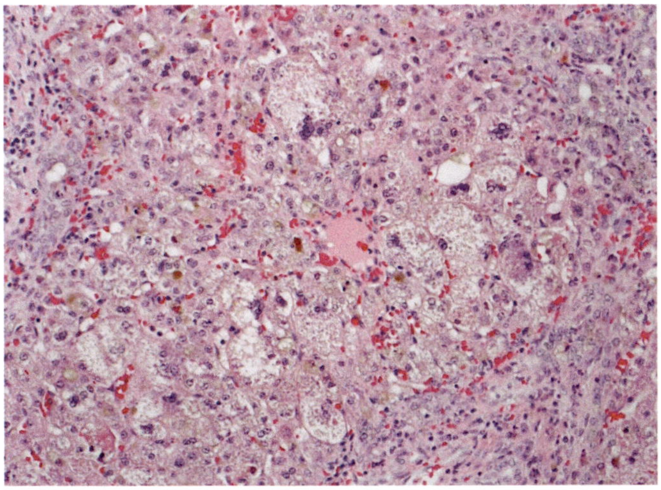

**Fig. 16.9** Giant cell transformation with multinuclear change of hepatocyte in BA

by fibrotic scarring. During this process, the bile ducts become obstructed. This progression matches the clinical findings in BA, namely changing from normal stool to acholic stool after birth.

Histologically the fibrotic connective tissue at the hepatic hilum has no normal bile ducts and may instead have bile duct-like structures measuring several tens to several hundred microns in diameter (microscopic bile ducts) (Fig. 16.17).

### 16.1.2 Usefulness of Liver Biopsy in BA

We will now discuss the usefulness of pre-operative percutaneous biopsy and biopsy at Kasai procedure in BA.

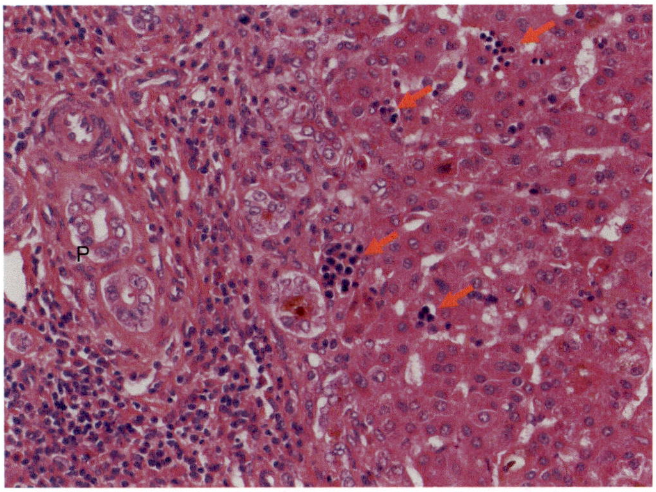


**Fig. 16.10** EMH of liver in BA. Scattered foci of EMH consist of the mixed myeloid and erythroid cell (*arrows*)

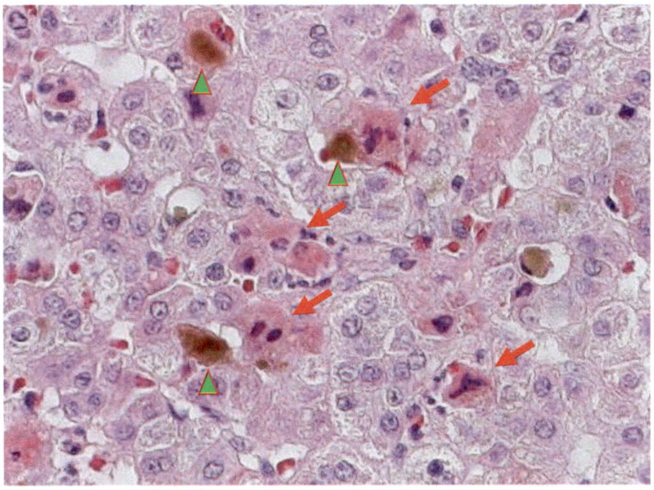

**Fig. 16.11** Apoptosis of hepatocytes in BA. Apoptotic hepatocytes of giant cell transformation (*arrows*)

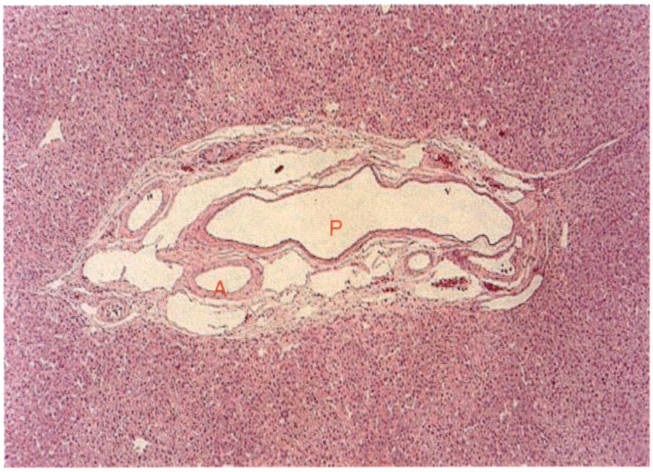


**Fig. 16.12** A histological finding of the liver in AGS. **a**: A case with AGS shows hepatic artery (**a**) and portal vein (p) but lacks interlobular bile duct in the portal tract without fibrosis

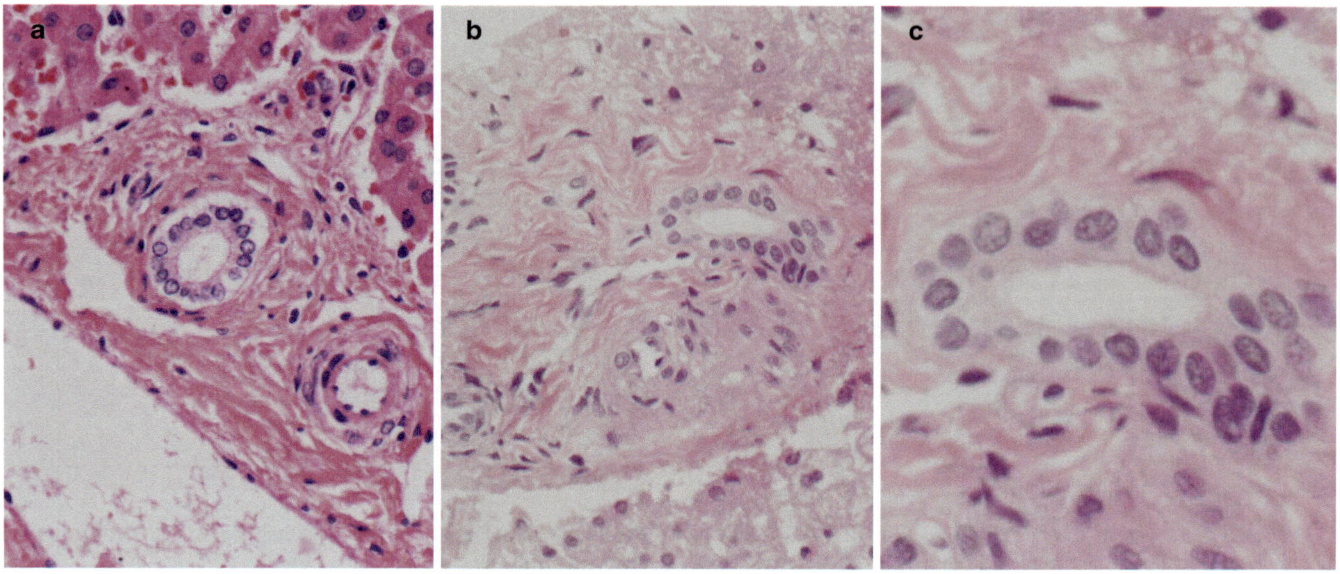


**Fig. 16.13** An interlobular bile duct of the liver in AGS. The interlobular bile duct shows an irregular luminal configuration and disarray of bile duct epithelial cells. **a**: normal control, **b**: interlobular bile duct in AGS, **c**: magnified "**b**"

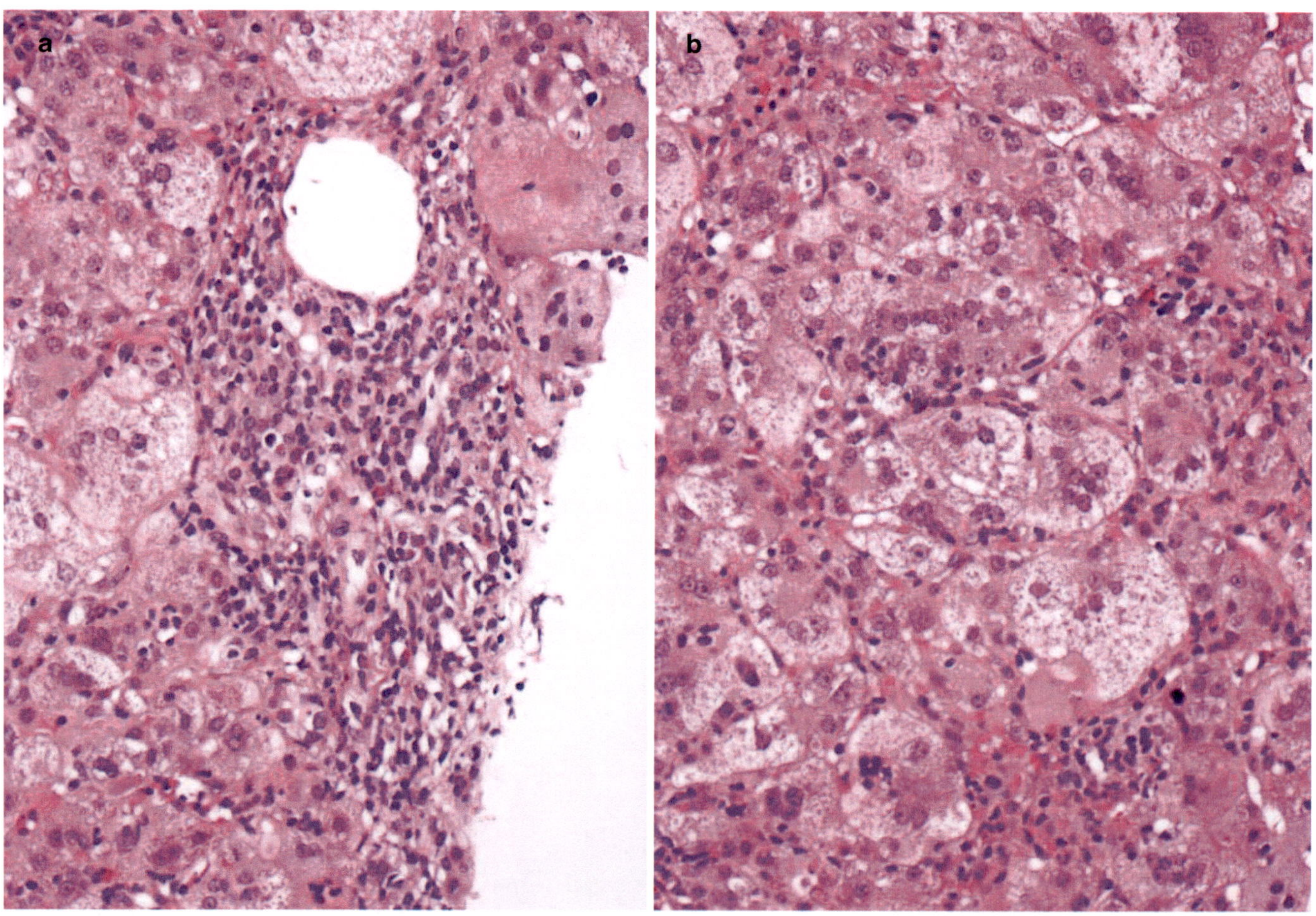


**Fig. 16.14** A histological finding of PFIC2. **a**: Mild fibrous expansion of the portal tract and hepatocytes arranged in a cobblestone pattern. **b**: Hepatic cords are disarranged. Hepatocytes show an acinar arrangement (*arrow*)

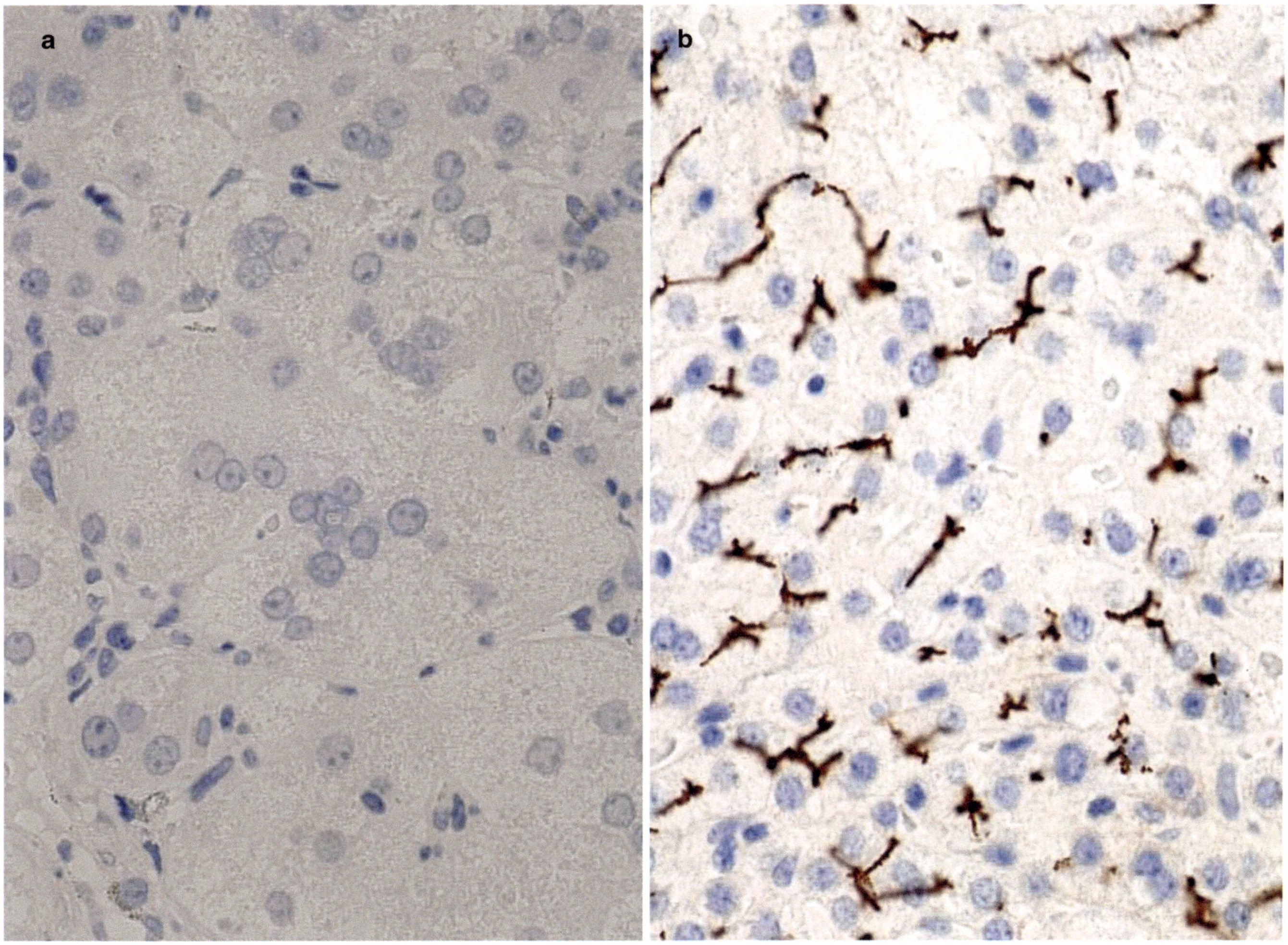


**Fig. 16.15** Immunohistochemistry for BSEP in PFIC 2. Immunohistochemistry clearly demonstrates BSEP expression at the bile canaliculi in normal control (**a**), but no expression in PFIC 2 (**b**)

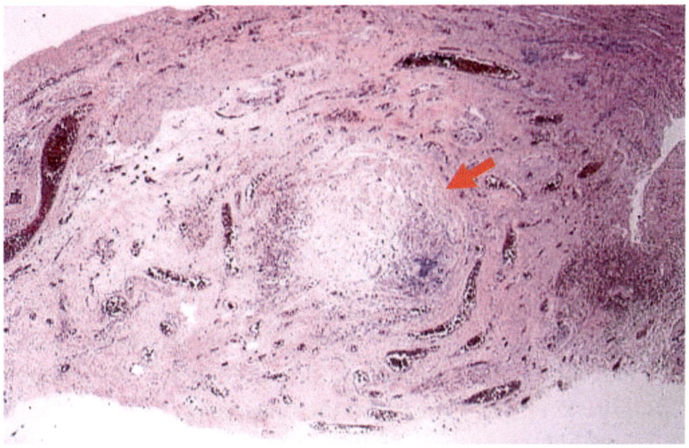

**Fig. 16.16** A histological finding of BA at the hepatic hilum taken at Kasai procedure. A progressively obstructed choledoch duct by inflammatory granulation (*arrow*)

#### 16.1.2.1 Pre-Operative Percutaneous Biopsy

Pre-operative liver biopsy is useful in diagnosing BA, and the specificity and sensitivity is high [16, 17]. However, the indications for liver biopsy need to be considered carefully, because the biopsies performed in the neonatal period to early infancy have a high risk of complications.

#### 16.1.2.2 Biopsy at Kasai Procedure

Biopsy at Kasai procedure is performed not only for the pathological diagnosis of BA, but also for accurate assessment for the current state of the disease, especially the degree of fibrosis. Furthermore, there are reports that histological findings from a biopsy at the Kasai procedure can help predict the prognosis. This will be discussed below.

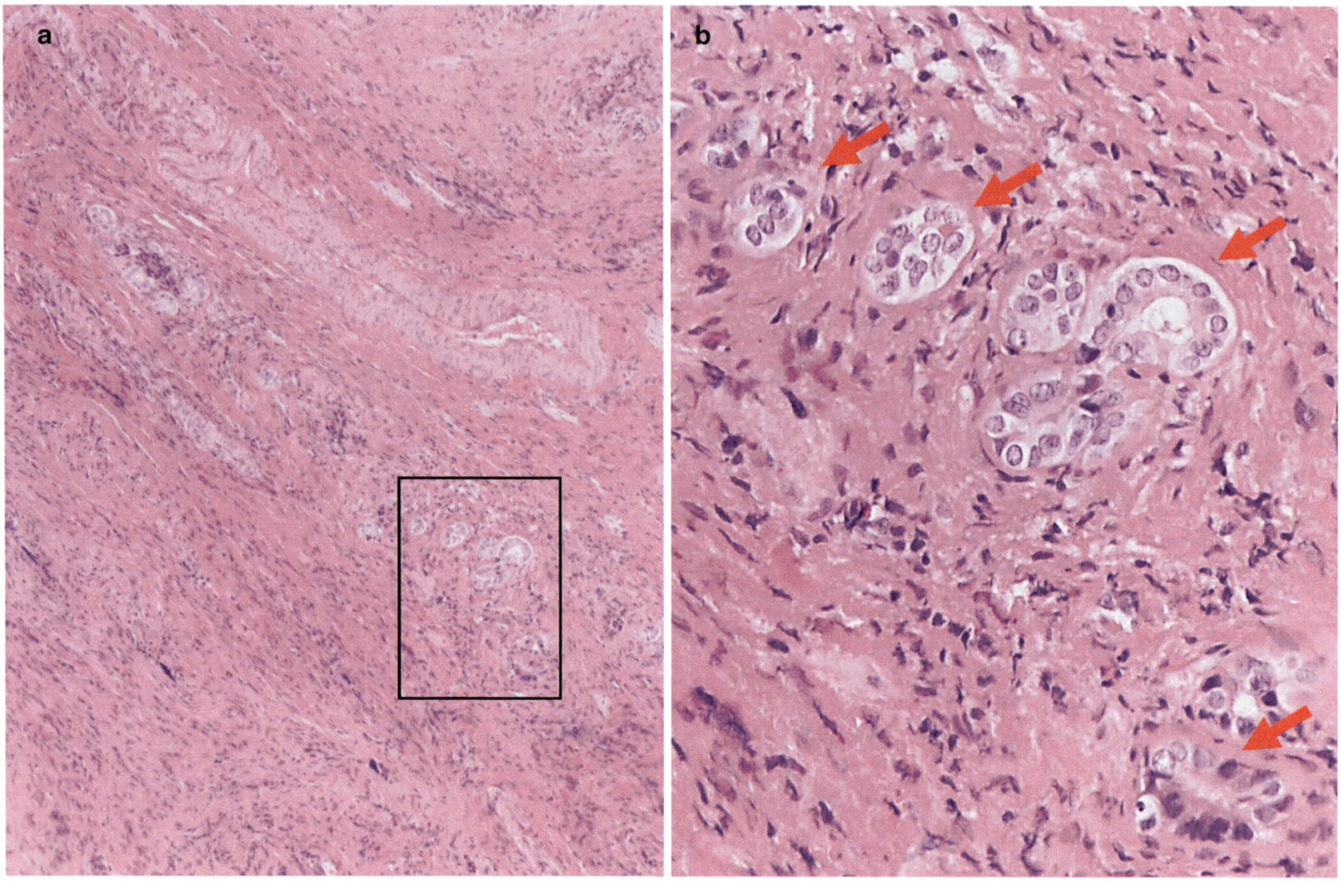


**Fig. 16.17** A histological finding of string-like fibrous cord at the hepatic hilum in BA. **a**: The scarred fibrous connective tissue has no choledoch duct, instead of micro bile ducts. **b**: A magnified view of the rectangle shows the micro bile duct (*arrow*)

### 16.1.3 Hepatopathological Findings and Prognosis

To date, many studies have examined the relationship between prognosis and histopathological findings in the liver and portal tracts at the time of the Kasai procedure. A variety of reports have been published, and they tend to show a certain degree of correlation between pathological findings in liver biopsy taken at the Kasai procedure and prognosis. We will describe the important histological findings, namely fibrosis, and DPM of the liver and changes of the hepatic hilum tissue, in BA that are reported to be related to the prognosis.

*Fibrosis*: Several studies have evaluated the relationship between the degree of hepatic fibrosis at the Kasai procedure and prognosis. It has been reported that severe hepatic fibrosis is associated with increased mortality [3].

*DPM*: It has been reported that the prognosis of BA complicated with DPM tends to be poorer than that without [3, 18]. On the other hand, the long-term prognosis has been reported to be favorable in cases without DPM and with the low degree of fibrosis and ductular proliferation [19]. It is also reported that biopsy at the Kasai procedure can help determine a treatment strategy. For example, the administration of high-dose steroids has been recommended in cases where the Kasai biopsy shows DPM and high levels of serum total bilirubin [20]. However, at present, there are very few reports recommending a specific treatment regimen based on histopathological findings from a liver biopsy.

*Hepatic Hilum Tissue*: The relationship between histopathological findings in the connective tissues of the hepatic hilum and the outcome after Kasai surgery has been studied [3]. The morphometrical study on the proliferated bile duct lumen in the connective tissue revealed favorable prognosis in cases where the number and diameter of bile duct lumen are large [21]. With regard to the prognostic significance of the morphology of these increased bile ducts, the results of a meta-analysis of five reports suggested that the larger the diameter of the microtubules, the better the long-term. It has also been reported that the smaller the diameter of the bile ducts at the hilum and the milder the inflammation, the lower the rate of survival.

## 16.2 Conclusion

We have discussed the findings in the liver and hepatic hilum tissue in BA. Biopsy is very important for the pathological diagnosis of BA, and is also useful in evaluating disease conditions. Going forward, it is desirable that the method of treating BA should be determined on the basis of liver histology.

## References


1. Robert EV, Portman BC. Developmental anomalies and liver disease in childhood. MacSween's pathology of the liver. In: Burt AD, Portman BC, Ferrell LD, editors. . Edinburgh: Churchill Livingstone Elsevier; 2012. p. 101–56.
2. Landing BH. Considerations of the pathogenesis of neonatal hepatitis, biliary atresia and choledochal cyst-the concept of infantile obstructive cholangiopathy. Prog Pediat Surg. 1974;6:113–39.
3. Russo P, Magee JC, Boitnott J, et al. Design and validation of the biliary atresia research consortium histologic assessment system for cholestasis in infancy. Clin Gastroenterol Hepatol. 2011;9: 357–62.
4. Roy P, Chatterjee U, Ganguli M, et al. A histopathological study of liver and biliary remnants with clinical outcome in cases of extrahepatic biliary atresia. Indian J Pathol Microbiol. 2010;53:101–5.
5. Desmet VJ. Congenital diseases of intrahepatic bile ducts: variations on the theme "ductal plate malformation". Hepatology. 1992;16:1069–83.
6. Dedic T, Jirsa M, Keil R, et al. Alagille syndrome mimicking biliary atresia in early infancy. PLoS One. 2015;10(11):e0143939.
7. Turnpenny PD, Ellard S. Alagille syndrome: pathogenesis, diagnosis and management. Eur J Hum Genet. 2012;20:251–7.
8. Davit-Spraul A, Fabre M, Branchereau S, et al. *ATP8B1* and *ABCB11* analysis in 62 children with normal gamma-glutamyl transferase progressive familial intrahepatic cholestasis (PFIC): phenotypic differences between PFIC1 and PFIC2 and natural history. Hepatology. 2010;51:1645–55.
9. Knisely AS, Strautnieks SS, Meier Y, et al. Hepatocellular carcinoma in ten children under five years of age with bile salt export pump deficiency. Hepatology. 2006;44:478–86.
10. Batts KP. J Ludwig. An update on terminology and reporting. Am J Surg Pathol. 1995;19:1409–17.
11. Nietgen GW, Vacanti JP, Perez-Atayde AR. Intrahepatic bile duct loss in biliary atresia despite portoenterostomy: a consequence of ongoing obstruction? Gastroenterology. 1992;102:2126–33.
12. Ho CM, Shioda K, Shirasaki K, et al. The pathogenesis of biliary atresia: a morphological study of the hepatobiliary system and the hepatic artery. J Pediatr Gastroenterol Nutr. 1993;16:53–60.
13. dos Santos JL, da Silveria TR, da Silva VD, et al. Medial thickening of hepatic artery branches in biliary atresia. A morphometric study. J Pediatr Surg. 2005;40:637–42.
14. Kaye AJ, Rand EB, Munoz PS, Spinner NB, Flake AW, Kamath BM. Effect of Kasai procedure on hepatic outcome in Alagille syndrome. J Pediatr Gastroenterol Nutr. 2010;51:319–21.
15. Oda T, Elkahloun AG, Pike BL, et al. Mutations in the human jagged 1 gene are responsible for the Allagile syndrome. Nat Genet. 1997;16:235–42.
16. Zerbini MC, Gallucci SD, Maezono R, et al. Liver biopsy in neonatal cholestasis: a review on statistical grounds. Mod Pathol. 1997;10:793–9.
17. Sira MM, El-Guindi MA, Saber MA, et al. Differential hepatic expression of CD56 can discriminate biliary atresia from other neonatal cholestatic disorders. Eur J Gastroenterol Hepatol. 2012;24:1227–33.
18. Vukovic J, Grizelj R, Bojanic K, et al. Ductal plate malformation in patients with biliary atresia. Eur J Pediatr. 2012;171:1799–804.
19. Sookpotarom P, Vejchapipat P, Chittmittrapap S, et al. Short-term results of Kasai operation for biliary atresia: experience from one institution. Asian J Surg. 2006;29:188–92.
20. Arii R, Koga H, Arakawa A, et al. How valuable is ductal plate malformation as a predictor of clinical course in postoperative biliary atresia patients? Pediatr Su rg Int. 2011;27:275–7.
21. Mirza Q, Kvist N, Petersen BL. Histologic features of the portal plate in extrahepatic biliary atresia and their impact on prognosis—a Danish study. J Pediatr Surg. 2009;44:1344–8.

# Biomarkers of Biliary Atresia

# 17

Tatsuki Mizuochi and Ken-ichiro Konishi

**Abstract**

Since the definitive diagnosis of biliary atresia (BA) currently depends on surgical cholangiography, identification of noninvasive biomarkers for BA is urgently needed to simplify the diagnostic algorithm and ideally avoid an operative procedure. Recently, serum matrix metalloproteinase-7 (MMP-7) has shown promise in diagnosing BA, achieving a more favorable area under the receiver operating characteristic curves than other noninvasive biomarkers of BA, with better sensitivity and specificity. Serum γ-glutamyl transpeptidase (GGT), also used for the diagnosis of BA, is considered insufficient as a single marker, especially considering the effects of an infant's age on normal values. Bile acid concentrations in serum, urine, stool, and duodenal fluid, serum micro RNAs (miR) such as miR-140-3p, miR-200b/429, miR-4429, and miR-4689, and serum concentrations of cytokines such as macrophage inflammatory protein-3α and interleukin-33 also have been suggested as diagnostic markers of BA. At present, we believe that a combination of biomarkers such as serum MMP-7 with GGT offers better accuracy for diagnosis of BA than any single biomarker in current use.

**Keywords**

Noninvasive diagnostic marker · Serum matrix metalloproteinase-7 · Serum γ-glutamyl transpeptidase

T. Mizuochi (✉)
Department of Pediatrics and Child Health, Kurume University School of Medicine, Kurume, Japan
e-mail: mizuochi_tatsuki@kurume-u.ac.jp

K.-i. Konishi
Department of Pediatrics and Child Health, Kurume University School of Medicine, Kurume, Japan

Department of Pediatric Surgery, Graduate School of Medicine, The University of Tokyo, Tokyo, Japan

## 17.1 Introduction

Biliary atresia (BA) is the most common cause of neonatal cholestasis, accounting for 40% to 50% of liver transplants in children [1]. Idiopathic neonatal hepatitis, neonatal intrahepatic cholestasis caused by citrin deficiency, and Alagille syndrome are among other causes of neonatal cholestasis that can confound the diagnosis of BA, despite some differences in disease characteristics. As the only definitive diagnostic procedure in BA is operative cholangiography [2], the use of noninvasive biomarkers for the diagnosis of BA is hoped to simplify the diagnostic process and provide an alternative to surgical procedures.

Characteristics sought in biomarkers for BA are noninvasiveness, repeatability of measurement over the course of illness, sensitivity to changes in disease status, ease of clinical use, and specificity for BA. Preferring more noninvasive markers, we did not consider liver biopsy in this review, focusing instead on serum, urine, duodenal fluid, and stool samples. A list of potential diagnostic biomarkers for BA is given in Table 17.1. Details of these options, such as diagnostic accuracies, are outlined in Table 17.2.

## 17.2 MMP-7

As a marker for BA, serum matrix metalloproteinase-7 (MMP-7) has shown better values for areas under receiver operating characteristic curves (AUC) than other biomarkers (Table 17.2) [3–6]. Previous studies have considered MMP-7 as a diagnostic or prognostic marker for various cancers, including cholangiocarcinoma, pancreatic carcinoma, and gastric cancer, as well as for lung and liver fibrosis [22–26]. Studying a North American population, Lertudomphonwanit et al. reported higher serum MMP-7 concentrations in infants with BA than in infants with other cholestatic diseases. The AUC was 0.970, with sensitivity and specificity of 97.0% and 91.0%, respectively [3]. In a Chinese population, Yang et al. reported an AUC of 0.990, with the sensitivity of 98.7%


M. Nio (ed.), *Introduction to Biliary Atresia*, https://doi.org/10.1007/978-981-16-2160-4_17

and specificity of 95.0% [4], while Wu et al. reported an AUC of 0.960, the sensitivity of 97.3%, and specificity of 83.2% in a Taiwanese population [5]. Most recently, Jiang et al. reported an AUC of 0.983 with sensitivity and specificity of 95.2% and 93.1% in another Chinese population [6]. Although cutoff values and patient cohorts differed among these studies, all demonstrated that MMP-7 showed higher AUC, sensitivity, and specificity than other noninvasive markers for BA.

The close relationship between MMP-7 and BA suggests that MMP-7 could be involved in the pathogenesis of BA. In paraffin-embedded sections of the human liver, gallbladder, and extrahepatic bile ducts, Lertudomphonwanit et al. [3] demonstrated minimal or no immunostaining for MMP-7 in parenchymal or nonparenchymal cells of normal liver. In contrast, this protein was detected in the cytoplasm of epithelial cells lining normal gallbladder, extrahepatic bile ducts, and surrounding peribiliary glands. In most liver biopsy samples from BA patients, however, MMP-7 also was evident in epithelial cells lining intrahepatic bile ducts—a difference that suggests that the increased serum MMP-7 in BA might reflect a response to tissue injury.

Previous reports have demonstrated that serum MMP-7 concentrations correlated positively with those of γ-glutamyl transpeptidase (GGT), while in combination, the two markers slightly improved diagnostic accuracy but without statistical significance difference compared with MMP-7 alone [3–6]. Yang et al. found that using both MMP-7 and GGT in a composite model did not substantially improve AUC, sensitivity, or specificity [4]. However, when Lertudomphonwanit et al. [3] used MMP-7 and GGT together, they attained an AUC of 0.98, considering their data to be preliminary evi-

**Table 17.1** Biomarkers for diagnosis of BA

| Sample | Biomarker |
|---|---|
| Serum | MMP-7 |
| | GGT |
| | Bile acids (TCA, GCDCA, and TCDCA) |
| | Micro RNAs (miR-140-3p, miR-200b/429, miR-4429 and miR-4689) |
| | Cytokines (MIP3a and IL-33) |
| | Hyaluronic acid |
| Urine | Bile acids (sulfated bile acid) |
| | Metabolomics profiles (N-acetyl-d-mannosamine and alpha-aminoadipic acid) |
| Duodenal fluid | Bile acids (total bile acid concentration) |
| Stool | Bile acids (total bile acid concentration and secondary bile acid concentration) |

BA, biliary atresia; MMP-7, matrix metalloproteinase-7; GGT, γ-glutamyl transpeptidase; TCA, tauro-cholic acid; GCDCA, glycol-chenodeoxycholic acid; TCDCA, tauro-chenodeoxycholic acid; miR, microRNA; MIP3a, macrophage inflammatory protein-3 alpha; IL-33, interleukin-33

**Table 17.2** Characteristics of biomarkers for diagnosis of BA

| Sample | Biomarker | Author, Year [reference] | Total subjects | Subjects with BA | Sensitivity, % | Specificity, % | AUC |
|---|---|---|---|---|---|---|---|
| Serum | MMP-7 | Lertudomphonwanit, 2017 [3] | 245 | 175 | 97.0 | 91.0 | 0.970 |
| | | Yang, 2018 [4] | 207 | 75 | 98.7 | 95.0 | 0.990 |
| | | Wu, 2019 [5] | 100 | 36 | 97.3 | 83.2 | 0.960 |
| | | Jiang, 2019 [6] | 288 | 187 | 95.2 | 93.1 | 0.983 |
| | GGT | Chen,2016 [7] | 1469 | 1338 | NA | NA | 0.843 |
| | | Dillman, 2019 [8] | 41 | 13 | 100.0 | 77.8 | 0.850 |
| | TCA | Zhou, 2012 [9] | 317 | 8 | 79.1 | 62.5 | 0.820 |
| | TCDCA/CDCA ratio | Zhou, 2015 [10] | 96 | 53 | 88.7 | 83.9 | 0.923 |
| | GCDCA | Golden, 2018 [11] | 50 | 16 | 100.0 | 83.3 | 0.875 |
| | GCDCA/CDCA ratio | Zhao, 2020 [12] | 103 | 34 | 85.3 | 81.3 | 0.870 |
| | miR-200b/429 cluster | Zahm, 2012 [13] | 48 | 24 | 70.8 | 91.7 | 0.806 |
| | miR-140-3p | Peng, 2016 [14] | 146 | 44 | 66.7 | 79.1 | 0.750 |
| | miR-4429 | Dong, 2016 [15] | 75 | 45 | 83.3 | 80.0 | 0.789 |
| | miR-4689 | Dong, 2016 [15] | 75 | 45 | 66.7 | 80.0 | 0.722 |
| | MIP3a | Chen, 2019 [16] | 76 | 31 | 86.7 | 83.3 | 0.881 |
| | IL-33 | Behairy, 2020 [17] | 90 | 30 | 96.7 | 95.0 | 0.995 |
| | Hyaluronic acid | Ukarapoklu, 2007 [18] | 25 | 10 | 70.0 | 77.8 | NA |
| Urine | Sulfated bile acid | Muraji, 2003 [19] | 676 | 16 | 100.0 | NA | NA |
| | N-acetyl-d-mannosamine | Li, 2018 [20] | 101 | 25 | NA | NA | 0.910 |
| | Alpha-aminoadipic acid | Li, 2018 [20] | 101 | 25 | NA | NA | 0.950 |
| Duodenal fluid | Total bile acids concentration | Fukuoka, 2018 [21] | 37 | 16 | 100.0 | 76.2 | 0.993 |

BA, biliary atresia; AUC, area under the receiver operating characteristic curve value; MMP-7, matrix metalloproteinase-7; GGT, γ-glutamyl transpeptidase; TCA, tauro-cholic acid; GCDCA, glycol-chenodeoxycholic acid; TCDCA, tauro-chenodeoxycholic acid; CDCA, chenodeoxycholic acid; miR, microRNA; MIP3a, macrophage inflammatory protein-3 Alpha; IL-33, interleukin-33; NA, not available dence favoring the combination. We believe that combining MMP-7 with other biomarkers such as GGT could improve diagnosis in BA.

MMP-7 was found to correlate with age in BA patients [4–6], which could reflect earlier development of liver fibrosis in BA than in other cholestatic diseases of infancy. However, previous results concerning fibrosis and the ages of children have varied. One study reported a positive correlation in older children using Metavir fibrosis staging, while another study in infants using Scheuer fibrosis staging found no correlation in infants between age at the time of diagnosis and severity of fibrosis [3, 27]. Positive correlations between MMP-7 and fibrosis suggest that the tissue remodeling activity of MMP-7 may promote liver fibrosis [5, 28]. Further study is needed to clarify whether serum MMP-7 can be considered a reliable biomarker for liver fibrosis in BA.

## 17.3 GGT

Serum GGT has been used in the diagnosis of BA [7, 8, 29, 30]. Cheng et al. reported that GGT showed a favorable AUC of 0.869 with sensitivity and specificity of 82.8% and 81.6% in infants 61 to 90 days old, but a poorer AUC of 0.712 (sensitivity, 76.6%; specificity, 62.5%) in infants older than 121 days [7]. GGT exceeding 300 U/L or increasing by 6 U/L or more daily has been used to differentiate BA from neonatal hepatitis, with sensitivity and specificity of 85% and 88%; several authors consider GGT concentrations exceeding 300 U/L to be useful in identifying patients with BA [30, 31].

Cabrera-Abreu et al. [29] have emphasized that infants have a higher reference range for GGT at birth, gradually declining to reach the adult range after 7 months of age. Specifically, GGT in healthy infants is highest in those less than 1 month old (47.4 ± 21.2 IU/L), reduced at 1 to 3 months (26.8 ± 23.1 IU/L), and lowest at 5 to 7 months. Despite a significant correlation between GGT and age, few studies have considered the age when evaluating the diagnostic value of GGT in suspected BA [31]. Mario et al. suggested that the reliability of GGT was lower among infants 4 to 8 weeks old, with considerable overlap of serum GGT in patients with BA and other patients with neonatal hepatitis [30]. Although GGT is helpful in the diagnosis of BA, it is insufficient as a single marker, largely because of the age dependence of the reference range.

## 17.4 Bile Acids

Synthesized in the liver from cholesterol, bile acids serve as important regulatory molecules. Given that hepatocytes secrete primary bile acids and maintain a stable systemic bile acid pool, dysregulated bile acid synthesis and metabolism often point to hepatobiliary disease [32], so serum bile acid analyses can be highly useful liver function tests for screening or differential diagnosis [33], such as in BA [34], intrahepatic cholestasis of pregnancy [35], and bile acid synthetic defects [36].

Serum bile acid analysis recently has been investigated as a rapid, noninvasive, and inexpensive additional diagnostic tool for differentiating BA from other cholestatic diseases [9–11]. Zhou et al. reported that measurement of tauro-cholic acid in dried blood spots from newborns could be used in early screening for BA, with an AUC of 0.820, sensitivity of 79.1%, and specificity of 62.5% [9]. Golden et al. found higher serum glyco-chenodeoxycholic acid concentrations in BA than in other cholestatic disease (AUC, 0.875; sensitivity, 100%; and specificity, 83.3%) [11]. Another investigator reported elevated glyco-chenodeoxycholic acid concentrations in sera from infants with BA, while another study concluded that serum tauro-chenodeoxycholic acid was elevated in BA [10, 12]. Cholic acid and chenodeoxycholic acid are primary bile acids synthesized in human pericentral hepatocytes and are thought to perform a hepatoprotective function. These bile acids may be useful in the diagnosis of BA, but uncertainty about conjugation pathway abnormalities that might occur in BA may create confusion.

Fukuoka et al. reported that total bile acid concentrations in duodenal fluid aspirated through an inserted tube could rule BA in or out with high accuracy (AUC, 0.993; sensitivity, 100%; and specificity, 76.2%) [21]. Although fluid collection can be performed safely and rapidly, it is not completely noninvasive.

Nguyen et al. studied noninvasively obtained specimens, specifically stool samples. They reported that total bile acid content was reduced in stools from children with the cholestatic disease compared to healthy controls, with samples from BA patients having much lower content than others from patients with parenteral nutrition-associated cholestasis or healthy controls [37]. Lack of intestinal bacterial interaction with conjugated bile acids in BA could account for reduced content of unconjugated and secondary bile acids.

## 17.5 Micro RNAs

Micro RNAs (miR) are short, noncoding RNAs that regulate target genes via transcript degradation or translational repression. Recent studies have identified stable miR populations in cell-free plasma and serum preparations. Profiling of circulating miR can detect altered expression or release from injured and diseased tissues and sometimes can distinguish among similar disorders [13, 38–40]. Previously reported candidate biomarkers for diagnosis of BA include miR-

140-3p [14], miR-200b/429 [13], miR-4429, and miR-4689 [15], but these show lower sensitivity and specificity than more conventional biomarkers and have not undergone prospective validation. Including retrospective validation in a larger, independent sample set, Zahm et al. [13] confirmed a serum miR cluster, miR-200b/429, to be significantly increased in BA, using serum samples from the Childhood Liver Disease Research and Education Network's prospective longitudinal study of cholestasis in infancy. The results suggested that miR-200b/429 may have diagnostic promise (AUC, 0.806; sensitivity, 70.8%; and specificity, 91.7%). Elevated circulating miR-200b/429 might represent an indication for accelerating the diagnostic workup of an infant with jaundice, or it might prove useful as a population-based screening test. Peng et al. [14] reported a study characterizing circulating miR in patients with BA using a next-generation sequencing platform, identifying a distinct plasma profile of 15 miR that may be involved in the onset and progression of BA has been identified. Those authors found that decreased plasma miR-140-3p could distinguish BA from other neonatal cholestatic disorders. Dong et al. [15] identified 13 differentially expressed miR using Agilent miR microarray expression profiling. Moreover, eight differentially expressed miR were selected for validation analysis by qRT-PCR using independent serum samples from infants with BA versus. Other cholestatic diseases, and four miR, including miR-150-3p, miR-4429, miR-4689, and miR-92a-3p, were differentially expressed. The AUC for miR-4429 was 0.789, with sensitivity of 83.3% and specificity of 80.0%; for miR-4689, the AUC was 0.722 with sensitivity of 66.7% and specificity of 80.0%. These results suggest that miR-4429 and miR-4689 might serve as diagnostic biomarkers of BA. Further investigation in a large cohort is needed to confirm these previously reported findings, establish reliable diagnostic thresholds for BA, and compare or combine miR with other markers as a diagnostic strategy.

## 17.6 Cytokines

Ongoing inflammation in BA leads to progressive scarring of the liver with severe fibrosis resulting in cirrhosis. These events are likely to result from the release of proinflammatory cytokines by immune cells in the portal tracts surrounding bile ducts [41]. Since induction and maintenance of systemic and local inflammatory responses are believed to play a pivotal role in pathogenesis, inflammatory responses have been evaluated as markers of BA. Chen et al. reported that serum assays for macrophage inflammatory protein-3α, a Th17-associated cytokine, could significantly increase the accuracy of BA diagnosis (AUC, 0.881; sensitivity, 86.7%; and specificity, 83.3%) [16]. Behairy et al. reported that interleukin-33, an important factor in the pathogenesis of liver damage during acute and chronic hepatitis, may have diagnostic value in infants with BA (AUC, 0.995; sensitivity, 96.7%; and specificity, 95.0%) [17].

## 17.7 Others

Ukarapol et al. reported that serum hyaluronic acid, a marker for liver dysfunction and liver fibrosis, was significantly more elevated in BA than in neonatal hepatitis (sensitivity and specificity, 70.0% and 77.8%). Hyaluronic acid is a hepatically produced, high molecular weight glycosaminoglycan in the extracellular matrix that is degraded in liver sinusoids [18].

Muraji et al. reported a statistically significant difference in urinary sulfated bile acid concentrations between infants with BA and those with other etiologies for cholestasis [19].

Li et al. reported that urinary N-acetyl-d-mannosamine and α-aminoadipic acid were highly accurate at distinguishing BA from neonatal hepatitis using urinary metabolomic profiles. AUCs of urinary N-acetyl-d-mannosamine and alpha-aminoadipic acid were 0.910 and 0.950, respectively, suggesting that they might serve as biomarkers in differentiating BA from neonatal hepatitis [20].

## 17.8 Conclusion

At present, we believe that a combination of serum MMP-7 and serum GGT concentrations represents the best option for prompt noninvasive diagnosis of BA, provided that allowance is made for the age-related elevation and decline of normal serum GGT values early in life. Ongoing assessment of roles for bile acid analysis, miR, cytokines, and other candidate markers remains important.

## References

1. Sundaram SS, Mack CL, Feldman AG, Sokol RJ. Biliary atresia: indications and timing of liver transplantation and optimization of pretransplant care. Liver Transpl. 2017;23(1):96–109. https://doi.org/10.1002/lt.24640.
2. Hartley JL, Davenport M, Kelly DA. Biliary atresia. Lancet. 2009;374(9702):1704–13. https://doi.org/10.1016/s0140-6736(09)60946-6.
3. Lertudomphonwanit C, Mourya R, Fei L, Zhang Y, Gutta S, Yang L, et al. Large-scale proteomics identifies MMP-7 as a sentinel of epithelial injury and of biliary atresia. Sci Transl Med. 2017;9(417) https://doi.org/10.1126/scitranslmed.aan8462.
4. Yang L, Zhou Y, Xu PP, Mourya R, Lei HY, Cao GQ, et al. Diagnostic accuracy of serum matrix Metalloproteinase-7 for biliary atresia. Hepatology. 2018;68(6):2069–77. https://doi.org/10.1002/hep.30234.
5. Wu JF, Jeng YM, Chen HL, Ni YH, Hsu HY, Chang MH. Quantification of serum matrix Metallopeptide 7 levels may

assist in the diagnosis and predict the outcome for patients with biliary atresia. J Pediatr. 2019;208:30–7.e1. https://doi.org/10.1016/j.jpeds.2018.12.006.
6. Jiang J, Wang J, Shen Z, Lu X, Chen G, Huang Y, et al. Serum MMP-7 in the diagnosis of biliary atresia. Pediatrics. 2019;144(5) https://doi.org/10.1542/peds.2019-0902.
7. Chen X, Dong R, Shen Z, Yan W, Zheng S. Value of gamma-Glutamyl Transpeptidase for diagnosis of biliary atresia by correlation with age. J Pediatr Gastroenterol Nutr. 2016;63(3):370–3. https://doi.org/10.1097/mpg.0000000000001168.
8. Dillman JR, DiPaola FW, Smith SJ, Barth RA, Asai A, Lam S, et al. Prospective assessment of ultrasound shear wave Elastography for discriminating biliary atresia from other causes of neonatal cholestasis. J Pediatr. 2019;212:60–5.e3. https://doi.org/10.1016/j.jpeds.2019.05.048.
9. Zhou K, Lin N, Xiao Y, Wang Y, Wen J, Zou GM, et al. Elevated bile acids in newborns with biliary atresia (BA). PLoS One. 2012;7(11):e49270. https://doi.org/10.1371/journal.pone.0049270.
10. Zhou K, Wang J, Xie G, Zhou Y, Yan W, Pan W, et al. Distinct plasma bile acid profiles of biliary atresia and neonatal hepatitis syndrome. J Proteome Res. 2015;14(11):4844–50. https://doi.org/10.1021/acs.jproteome.5b00676.
11. Golden J, Zagory JA, Fenlon M, Goodhue CJ, Xiao Y, Fu X, et al. Liquid chromatography-mass spectroscopy in the diagnosis of biliary atresia in children with hyperbilirubinemia. J Surg Res. 2018;228:228–37. https://doi.org/10.1016/j.jss.2018.03.021.
12. Zhao D, Zhou K, Chen Y, Xie W, Zhang Y. Development and validation of bile acid profile-based scoring system for identification of biliary atresia: a prospective study. BMC Pediatr. 2020;20(1):255. https://doi.org/10.1186/s12887-020-02169-8.
13. Zahm AM, Hand NJ, Boateng LA, Friedman JR. Circulating microRNA is a biomarker of biliary atresia. J Pediatr Gastroenterol Nutr. 2012;55(4):366–9. https://doi.org/10.1097/MPG.0b013e318264e648.
14. Peng X, Yang L, Liu H, Pang S, Chen Y, Fu J, et al. Identification of circulating MicroRNAs in biliary atresia by next-generation sequencing. J Pediatr Gastroenterol Nutr. 2016;63(5):518–23. https://doi.org/10.1097/mpg.0000000000001194.
15. Dong R, Shen Z, Zheng C, Chen G, Zheng S. Serum microRNA microarray analysis identifies miR-4429 and miR-4689 are potential diagnostic biomarkers for biliary atresia. Sci Rep. 2016;6:21084. https://doi.org/10.1038/srep21084.
16. Chen P, Zhong Z, Jiang H, Chen H, Lyu J, Zhou L. Th17-associated cytokines multiplex testing indicates the potential of macrophage inflammatory protein-3 alpha in the diagnosis of biliary atresia. Cytokine. 2019;116:21–6. https://doi.org/10.1016/j.cyto.2019.01.002.
17. Behairy OG, Elsadek AE, Behiry EG, Elhenawy IA, Shalan NH, Sayied KR. Clinical value of serum Interleukin-33 biomarker in infants with neonatal cholestasis. J Pediatr Gastroenterol Nutr. 2020;70(3):344–9. https://doi.org/10.1097/mpg.0000000000002565.
18. Ukarapol N, Wongsawasdi L, Ong-Chai S, Riddhiputra P, Kongtawelert P. Hyaluronic acid: additional biochemical marker in the diagnosis of biliary atresia. Pediatr Int. 2007;49(5):608–11. https://doi.org/10.1111/j.1442-200X.2007.02423.x.
19. Muraji T, Harada T, Miki K, Moriuchi T, Obatake M, Tsugawa C. Urinary sulfated bile acid concentrations in infants with biliary atresia and breast-feeding jaundice. Pediatr Int. 2003;45(3):281–3. https://doi.org/10.1046/j.1442-200x.2003.01710.x.
20. Li WW, Yang Y, Dai QG, Lin LL, Xie T, He LL, et al. Non-invasive urinary metabolomic profiles discriminate biliary atresia from infantile hepatitis syndrome. Metabolomics. 2018;14(7):90. https://doi.org/10.1007/s11306-018-1387-z.
21. Fukuoka T, Bessho K, Tachibana M, Satomura Y, Konishi A, Yasuda K, et al. Total bile acid concentration in duodenal fluid is a useful preoperative screening marker to rule out biliary atresia. J Pediatr Gastroenterol Nutr. 2018;67(3):383–7. https://doi.org/10.1097/mpg.0000000000002037.
22. Leelawat K, Narong S, Wannaprasert J, Ratanashu-ek T. Prospective study of MMP7 serum levels in the diagnosis of cholangiocarcinoma. World J Gastroenterol. 2010;16(37):4697–703. https://doi.org/10.3748/wjg.v16.i37.4697.
23. Kuhlmann KF, van Till JW, Boermeester MA, de Reuver PR, Tzvetanova ID, Offerhaus GJ, et al. Evaluation of matrix metalloproteinase 7 in plasma and pancreatic juice as a biomarker for pancreatic cancer. Cancer Epidemiol Biomark Prev. 2007;16(5):886–91. https://doi.org/10.1158/1055-9965.Epi-06-0779.
24. Morais A, Beltrão M, Sokhatska O, Costa D, Melo N, Mota P, et al. Serum metalloproteinases 1 and 7 in the diagnosis of idiopathic pulmonary fibrosis and other interstitial pneumonias. Respir Med. 2015;109(8):1063–8. https://doi.org/10.1016/j.rmed.2015.06.003.
25. Hung TM, Chang SC, Yu WH, Wang YW, Huang C, Lu SC, et al. A novel nonsynonymous variant of matrix metalloproteinase-7 confers risk of liver cirrhosis. Hepatology. 2009;50(4):1184–93. https://doi.org/10.1002/hep.23137.
26. Irvine KM, Wockner LF, Hoffmann I, Horsfall LU, Fagan KJ, Bijin V, et al. Multiplex serum protein analysis identifies novel biomarkers of advanced fibrosis in patients with chronic liver disease with the potential to improve diagnostic accuracy of established biomarkers. PLoS One. 2016;11(11):e0167001. https://doi.org/10.1371/journal.pone.0167001.
27. Kerola A, Lampela H, Lohi J, Heikkilä P, Mutanen A, Hagström J, et al. Increased MMP-7 expression in biliary epithelium and serum underpins native liver fibrosis after successful portoenterostomy in biliary atresia. J Pathol Clin Res. 2016;2(3):187–98. https://doi.org/10.1002/cjp2.50.
28. Harpavat S. MMP-7: the next best serum biomarker for biliary atresia? J Pediatr. 2019;208:8–9. https://doi.org/10.1016/j.jpeds.2019.01.026.
29. Cabrera-Abreu JC, Green A. Gamma-glutamyltransferase: value of its measurement in paediatrics. Ann Clin Biochem. 2002;39(Pt 1):22–5. https://doi.org/10.1258/0004563021901685.
30. Rendón-Macías ME, Villasís-Keever MA, Castañeda-Muciño G, Sandoval-Mex AM. Improvement in accuracy of gamma-glutamyl transferase for differential diagnosis of biliary atresia by correlation with age. Turk J Pediatr. 2008;50(3):253–9.
31. Liu CS, Chin TW, Wei CF. Value of gamma-glutamyl transpeptidase for early diagnosis of biliary atresia. Zhonghua Yi Xue Za Zhi (Taipei). 1998;61(12):716–20.
32. Song P, Zhang Y, Klaassen CD. Dose-response of five bile acids on serum and liver bile acid concentrations and hepatotoxicity in mice. Toxicol Sci. 2011;123(2):359–67. https://doi.org/10.1093/toxsci/kfr177.
33. Kawasaki H, Yamanishi Y, Miyake M, Mura T, Ikawa S. Age- and sex-related profiles of serum primary and total bile acids in infants, children and adults. Tohoku J Exp Med. 1986;150(3):353–7. https://doi.org/10.1620/tjem.150.353.
34. Suzuki M, Muraji T, Obatake M, Nio M, Ito K, Suzuki K, et al. Urinary sulfated bile acid analysis for the early detection of biliary atresia in infants. Pediatr Int. 2011;53(4):497–500. https://doi.org/10.1111/j.1442-200X.2010.03268.x.
35. Tribe RM, Dann AT, Kenyon AP, Seed P, Shennan AH, Mallet A. Longitudinal profiles of 15 serum bile acids in patients with intrahepatic cholestasis of pregnancy. Am J Gastroenterol. 2010;105(3):585–95. https://doi.org/10.1038/ajg.2009.633.
36. Haas D, Gan-Schreier H, Langhans CD, Rohrer T, Engelmann G, Heverin M, et al. Differential diagnosis in patients with suspected bile acid synthesis defects. World J Gastroenterol. 2012;18(10):1067–76. https://doi.org/10.3748/wjg.v18.i10.1067.
37. Nguyen M, Dossa A, Zagory J, Golden J, Roberts A, Fu X, et al. Liquid chromatography-mass spectroscopy as a tool in the

rapid diagnosis of biliary atresia: a pilot study. J Pediatr Surg. 2016;51(6):923–6. https://doi.org/10.1016/j.jpedsurg.2016.02.053.
38. Lawrie CH, Gal S, Dunlop HM, Pushkaran B, Liggins AP, Pulford K, et al. Detection of elevated levels of tumour-associated microRNAs in serum of patients with diffuse large B-cell lymphoma. Br J Haematol. 2008;141(5):672–5. https://doi.org/10.1111/j.1365-2141.2008.07077.x.
39. Mitchell PS, Parkin RK, Kroh EM, Fritz BR, Wyman SK, Pogosova-Agadjanyan EL, et al. Circulating microRNAs as stable blood-based markers for cancer detection. Proc Natl Acad Sci U S A. 2008;105(30):10513–8. https://doi.org/10.1073/pnas.0804549105.
40. Chen X, Ba Y, Ma L, Cai X, Yin Y, Wang K, et al. Characterization of microRNAs in serum: a novel class of biomarkers for diagnosis of cancer and other diseases. Cell Res. 2008;18(10):997–1006. https://doi.org/10.1038/cr.2008.282.
41. Bessho K, Bezerra JA. Biliary atresia: will blocking inflammation tame the disease? Annu Rev Med. 2011;62:171–85. https://doi.org/10.1146/annurev-med-042909-093734.

# Differential Diagnosis of Biliary Atresia

# 18

Daiki Abukawa

**Abstract**

Biliary atresia is the most common causative disease of neonatal cholestasis. Causes of neonatal cholestasis that should be distinguished from biliary atresia include various diseases, such as congenital biliary dilatation, genetic diseases, metabolic disorders, infections, and idiopathic neonatal hepatitis. In cases with neonatal cholestasis, biliary atresia is considered first, and diagnosis and treatment are performed as quickly as possible. If biliary atresia is suspected or cannot be excluded, intraoperative cholangiogram should be performed earlier. If biliary atresia is negative, various tests for differential diagnosis of intrahepatic cholestasis are performed.

## 18.1 Introduction

Neonatal cholestasis is defined biochemically as prolonged elevation of serum conjugated bilirubin levels beyond the first 14 days of life [1]. It is classified as either extrahepatic biliary obstruction or intrahepatic cholestasis, depending on the site of injury.

Biliary atresia is the most common causative disease of neonatal cholestasis [2]. Infants with suspected biliary atresia should be evaluated as quickly as possible, as the success of surgical interventions (hepatoportoenterostomy, Kasai's procedure) declines with increasing age at surgery.

D. Abukawa (✉)
Department of General Pediatrics, Gastroenterology and Hepatology, Miyagi Children's Hospital, Sendai, Miyagi, Japan
e-mail: dabukawa@miyagi-children.or.jp

## 18.2 Causes of Neonatal Cholestasis

Diseases that should be differentiated from biliary atresia are diverse and can be classified into the categories shown in Table 18.1.

Cholestatic jaundice affects approximately 1 in every 2500 term infants [2]. The most common causes of cholestatic jaundice in the first months of life include biliary atresia (25%–40%) and an array of individually uncommon genetic disorders (25%) [2], such as Alagille syndrome and progressive familial intrahepatic cholestasis (PFIC). Many cases in which the cause cannot be identified are classified as "idiopathic" neonatal hepatitis (INH) (Table 18.2) [3]. Cholestasis in premature infants often results from complete parenteral nutrition or sepsis.

Figure 18.1 shows a conceptual approach to the group of diseases presenting as neonatal cholestasis [1]. Biliary atresia and congenital biliary dilatation (choledochal cyst) are typical diseases that cause extrahepatic biliary obstruction. The mechanisms of intrahepatic cholestasis include intrahepatic bile duct injury (hypoplasia/paucity) and hepatocellular injury. On the other hand, diseases that cause hepatocellular injury include metabolic diseases (such as citrin deficiency), infectious diseases (such as cytomegalovirus infection), and genetic diseases (such as PFIC). Exclusion of all of these diseases leads to a diagnosis of INH.

Here we present an outline of diseases that must be differentiated from biliary atresia.

### 18.2.1 Extrahepatic Biliary Obstruction

#### 18.2.1.1 Congenital Biliary Dilatation (Choledochal Cyst)

Congenital biliary dilatation is a congenital dysplasia in which the extrahepatic and intrahepatic bile ducts, including the common bile duct, dilate locally to form a cyst or spindle shape and is complicated by pancreaticobiliary maljunction (PBM) [4]. The mechanism of PBM is predominantly


M. Nio (ed.), *Introduction to Biliary Atresia*, https://doi.org/10.1007/978-981-16-2160-4_18

**Table 18.1** Causes of neonatal cholestasis

| |
|---|
| Extrahepatic biliary obstruction |
| Biliary atresia |
| Congenital biliary dilatation (Choledochal cyst) |
| Inspissated bile/plug syndrome |
| Cholelithiasis or biliary sludge |
| Tumors/masses |
| Neonatal sclerosing cholangitis |
| Spontaneous perforation of the bile ducts |
| Infections |
| Viral |
| Adenovirus, cytomegalovirus, echovirus, enterovirus, herpes simplex virus, HIV, parvovirus B19, rubella |
| Bacterial |
| Urinary tract infection, sepsis, syphilis |
| Protozoal |
| Toxoplasma |
| Genetic disorders |
| Alagille syndrome |
| Alpha-1 antitrypsin deficiency |
| ARC syndrome (arthrogryposis-renal dysfunction-cholestasis) |
| Cystic fibrosis |
| Progressive familial intrahepatic cholestasis (types 1 to 5) |
| NISCH syndrome (neonatal ichthyosis sclerosing cholangitis) |
| Neonatal Dubin–Johnson syndrome |
| Inborn errors of metabolism |
| Disorders of carbohydrate metabolism |
| Galactosemia |
| Fructosemia |
| Glycogen storage disease type IV |
| Disorders of amino acid metabolism |
| Tyrosinemia type 1 |
| Citrin deficiency |
| Disorders of lipid metabolism |
| Wolman's disease (acidic lipase deficiency) |
| Niemann–Pick's disease type C |
| Gaucher's disease type II |
| Inborn errors of bile acid metabolism |
| Bile acid synthesis defect (type 1 to 6) |
| Cerebrotendinous xanthomatosis |
| Amidation defects |
| Zellweger spectrum disorders |
| Smith–Lemli–Opitz syndrome |
| Mitochondrial disorders |
| Congenital disorders of glycosylation |
| Phosphomannomutase 2 deficiency |
| Phosphoglucomutase 1 deficiency |
| Mannosephosphate isomerase deficiency |
| Alloimmune conditions |
| Neonatal hemochromatosis (gestational alloimmune liver disease) |
| Toxic conditions |
| Intestinal failure-related liver disease |
| Drugs |
| Miscellaneous |
| "Idiopathic" neonatal hepatitis |
| Nonsyndromic paucity of the interlobular bile ducts |
| Shock/hypoperfusion |
| Intestinal obstruction |
| Hypothyroidism |
| Hypopituitarism |

**Table 18.2** Etiologies of conjugated hyperbilirubinemia in infancy by disease category

| | Total number | % of total |
|---|---|---|
| Idiopathic neonatal hepatitis | 440 | 26.00 |
| Extrahepatic biliary atresia | 438 | 25.89 |
| Infection | 194 | 11.47 |
| TPN-associated cholestasis | 109 | 6.44 |
| Metabolic disease | 74 | 4.37 |
| Alpha-1 antitrypsin deficiency | 70 | 4.14 |
| Perinatal hypoxia/ischemia | 62 | 3.66 |
| Interlobular bile duct paucity | 42 | 2.48 |
| Choledochal cyst | 36 | 2.13 |
| Hypopituitarism/hypothyroidism | 33 | 1.95 |
| Hemolysis | 24 | 1.42 |
| Inspissated bile syndrome | 23 | 1.36 |
| Progressive familial intrahepatic cholestasis (PFIC) | 17 | 1.00 |
| Alagille syndrome | 16 | 0.95 |
| Cystic fibrosis | 15 | 0.9 |
| Other | 99 | 5.85 |
| Total | 1692 | 100.00 |

Ref. [3] Gottesman LE, et al.: BMC Pediatrics 2015; 15: 192–199

thought to be dysplasia of the ventral pancreas that occurs by approximately 4 weeks of fetal life.

Congenital biliary dilatation is more common in Asia than in Europe and the United States and affects approximately 1 in 1000 live births in Japan [5]. The male-to-female ratio is approximately 1:3 and is common among young women.

The main symptoms include abdominal pain, vomiting, jaundice, and fever. Most affected infants have cystic dilation and develop obstructive jaundice, occasionally with perforation of the dilation and complications of biliary peritonitis.

Abdominal ultrasonography is useful for screening for congenital biliary dilatation, and dilation of the common bile duct and intrahepatic bile duct is the trigger for diagnosis. Abdominal computed tomography (CT) and magnetic resonance imaging are used to evaluate the morphology of the extrahepatic and intrahepatic biliary system, PBM, and protein plug/bile duct stones, whereas magnetic resonance cholangiopancreatography is used to examine pancreatic lesions. Finally, intraoperative cholangiography is performed to confirm the presence or absence of PBM.

Choledochal cyst must be distinguished from biliary atresia type I cyst. In infants with the choledochal cyst, the intrahepatic bile ducts are normal or dilated rather than sclerosed. Ultrasonographic findings suggestive of choledochal cyst rather than biliary atresia include larger cyst size, dilated intrahepatic bile duct, and a normal-appearing gallbladder [6].

Surgery using hepatic jejunal Roux-Y anastomosis removes the dilated extrahepatic bile duct and reconstructs the biliary tract. Cholangiocarcinoma can occur at a high rate from the dilated bile duct if it remains; therefore, all dilated

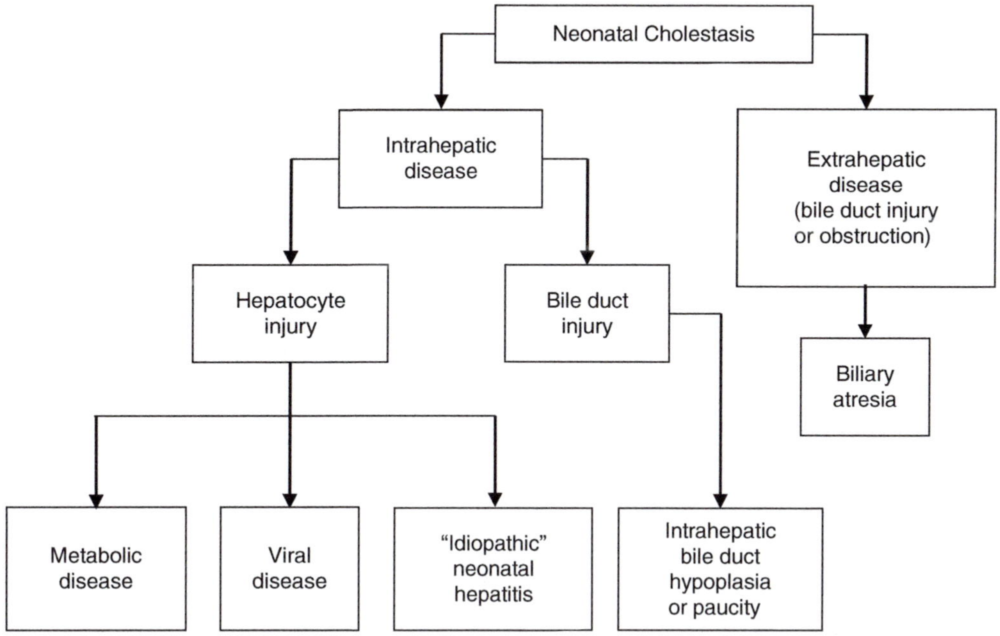


**Fig. 18.1** A conceptual approach to the group of diseases presenting as neonatal cholestasis. (Ref. [1] Hassan HHA, Balistreri WF: Neonatal cholestasis. In Nelson Textbook of Pediatrics, 20th ed., 2015; 2092–2100)

extrahepatic bile ducts are resected. The long-term prognosis of this disease is generally good; however, cholangitis, intrahepatic stones, pancreatitis, and pancreatolithiasis may occur.

### 18.2.2 Infections

Bacterial, protozoan, and viral infections can cause cholestasis. The rate of cholestasis due to infection varies significantly between studies and is likely population-dependent [3]. Commonly acquired pathogens include cytomegalovirus, toxoplasmosis, rubella, herpes, and syphilis. Infrequent causes include echovirus, adenovirus, and parvovirus B19. Bacterial infections with Gram-positive and Gram-negative bacteria, such as urinary tract infections, are also associated with neonatal cholestasis. Bacterial infections also contribute to cholestasis in infants who receive parenteral nutrition [7].

### 18.2.3 Genetic Disorders

#### 18.2.3.1 Alagille Syndrome

In Alagille syndrome, mutations in either the *JAG1* gene (chromosome 20p12) or the *NOTCH2* gene, which encodes the receptor for Jagged1, lead to abnormal development and differentiation via the Notch signaling pathway. More than 90% of patients have mutations in the *JAG1* gene [8]. Although Alagille syndrome shows autosomal dominant inheritance and is often observed in families, sporadic cases are also frequent.

Alagille syndrome is classically defined as intrahepatic bile duct hypoplasia as well as at least three of the five following major symptoms: cholestasis, dysmorphic facies (broad nasal bridge, triangular facies, and deep-set eyes), cardiovascular abnormalities (e.g., peripheral pulmonary stenosis), vertebral bone abnormalities (butterfly vertebrae), and ophthalmic abnormalities (e.g., posterior embryotoxon). Renal disorders and brain and systemic vascular malformations may also be present.

Cholestasis mostly develops in early infancy and presents as jaundice and acholic stool. While the prognosis is good in cases in which cholestasis decreases or disappears with age, 30%–50% of cases with liver symptoms in infancy eventually require liver transplantation [9]. Cases with complex cardiac malformations have a poor prognosis. Hepatoportoenterostomy (Kasai's procedure) is not beneficial and is not recommended [10]. A longitudinal follow-up study of a cohort of pediatric patients with Alagille syndrome showed the survival rate without transplantation was 24% at age 18 years. Approximately 40% of patients with the native liver that survived until age 20 years had portal hypertension [11].

#### 18.2.3.2 Alpha-1 Antitrypsin (ATT) Deficiency

AAT deficiency is an autosomal recessive disorder. Its prevalence varies considerably between countries and affects 1 in 2000–5000 Caucasians in Europe and the United States, but it is extremely rare in Japan, in which approximately 20 cases have been reported [12]. Diagnosis is based on low serum AAT levels and identification of the *SERPINA1* genotype.

In vivo, AAT deficiency leads to cholestatic liver disease in children and early-onset emphysema in adults. Cholestasis begins within the first few months of life, and approximately 65% of cases develop severe liver disease [13, 14]. Liver transplantation improves the prognosis of infants with severe liver disease. Prognosis for life is good if liver damage is not severe in childhood.

#### 18.2.3.3 Cystic Fibrosis (CF)

CF is an autosomal recessive genetic disorder caused by a mutation in the cystic fibrosis transmembrane conductance regulator (*CFTR*) gene localized on chromosome 7q31. The frequency varies depending on ethnicity. CF occurs in approximately 1:3200 Caucasians in the United States [15]; however, it is rare in Japan, where it affects approximately 1 in 1.87 million live births [16].

Classic symptoms of CF include abdominal distension (≥50%) or meconium ileus (approximately 15%) immediately after birth, heavy and frequent steatorrhea due to exocrine pancreatic insufficiency, poor weight gain, and respiratory tract infections that occur in approximately 50% of cases within the first year of life.

Neonatal cholestasis is a rare symptom of CF and occurs in <5% of CF patients [17]. In affected infants, jaundice and hepatomegaly recover slowly. Infants with CF develop meconium ileus or steatorrhea and are more likely to fail to thrive.

#### 18.2.3.4 PFIC

PFIC develops in infancy and presents as severe chronic intrahepatic cholestasis with a progressive and fatal course. Its basic pathology is thought to be abnormalities in the bile excretion mechanism in hepatocytes, especially impaired transport of bile acid from hepatocytes to the bile canaliculus.

PFIC shows an autosomal recessive inheritance and is classified into several different subtypes based on its genetic etiology [18].

The most common type of PFIC that appears in infancy is PFIC2, which is caused by a mutation in the *ABCB11* gene [19]. Affected infants tend to have a rapid and severe course with marked elevations of serum bile acids and refractory pruritus, occasionally with coagulopathy due to poor vitamin K absorption. Serum gamma-glutamyl transpeptidase (γ-GTP) levels tend to be normal despite severe cholestasis.

PFIC1 (*ATP8B1* gene mutation) [18], also known as Byler's disease, and PFIC4 (*TJP2* gene mutation) [20] can appear at any time during infancy and tend to be associated with severe cholestasis. Like PFIC2, γ-GTP levels are normal.

PFIC3 (*ABCB4* gene mutation) [21] is distinguished from other types of PFIC by high levels of γ-GTP.

Several new genes, such as PFIC5 (*NR1H4* gene mutation), have been identified as causing the PFIC phenotype [22].

Clinical symptoms include progressive jaundice, hepatosplenomegaly, marked pruritus, thickened skin, clubbed finger, failure to thrive, and deficiency of fat-soluble vitamins. All types show a poor prognosis, progress to biliary cirrhosis, and most patients die due to liver failure by age 20 years. PFIC2 progresses faster than PFIC1 and progresses to cirrhosis and liver failure at an early stage.

There is no medical cure for PFIC, and drug therapy is used to reduce jaundice and pruritus. High-dose administration of fat-soluble vitamins is essential. Surgery, such as partial extrabiliary diversion and liver transplantation, is required. However, after liver transplantation, PFIC1 presents with various complications, such as chronic diarrhea, pancreatitis, and fatty degeneration of the graft, and the post-transplant prognosis of PFIC1 is not always favorable.

#### 18.2.3.5 Neonatal Dubin–Johnson Syndrome (DJS)

DJS is an autosomal recessive disorder resulting from mutations in the ATP-binding cassette subfamily C member 2 (*ABCC2*)/multidrug resistance-associated protein 2 (*MRP2*) gene that causes either an absent or deficient expression of this transporter protein [23]. The MRP2 transporter is located in the canalicular membrane of hepatocytes as well as in apical membranes of other polarized cells such as enterocytes and renal tubular cells.

DJS rarely is diagnosed in the neonatal period; when DJS uncommonly presents with severe cholestasis at that age, the term "neonatal DJS" is used [24]. All ten patients with neonatal DJS reported in Japan exhibited cholestasis, evident as prolonged jaundice with or without acholic stools and elevated serum direct bilirubin as well as γ-GTP or total bile acid levels [25]. Furthermore, only 38% (3 of 8) patients who underwent liver biopsy exhibited grossly black liver or melanin-like pigment deposits in hepatocytes, which are characteristic findings in adults with DJS [25]. Neonatal DJS is recognized as one of the diseases that need to be differentiated from biliary atresia.

### 18.2.4 Inborn Errors of Metabolism

#### 18.2.4.1 Galactosemia

Galactosemia is caused by a congenital abnormality of galactose-metabolizing enzyme, which is typified by galactose-1-phosphate uridyltransferase (GALT) deficiency. The frequency of occurrence in Japan is approximately 1 in 900,000 births [26].

In GALT deficiency, increased hepatotoxicity due to elevated galactose-1-phosphate levels leads to symptoms such as discomfort, anorexia, diarrhea, vomiting, poor weight gain, and difficulty in stopping bleeding after blood collection are observed at an early stage in newborns. Galactosemia causes hypoglycemia, renal tubular disorders, cataracts, and liver disorders (e.g., jaundice, hepatosplenomegaly, elevated liver enzymes), as well as coagulopathies and hemolytic anemia. Since high galactose levels promote the growth of

*Escherichia coli*, infectious diseases such as sepsis and meningitis are likely to occur. Galactosemia is fatal if lactose is not removed from the diet [27].

#### 18.2.4.2 Tyrosinemia

Hereditary tyrosinemia type 1 is caused by fumarylacetoacetate hydrolase deficiency and leads to progressive liver disease, renal tubular acidosis, and neuropathy in infancy. The frequency is estimated to be 1 in 100,000–120,000 worldwide but is thought to be lower in Japan [28].

Cholestasis and coagulopathy present in early infancy and are often disproportionate to the apparent degree of liver disease. Patients exhibit increased urinary excretion of succinylacetone and markedly elevated serum tyrosine levels.

#### 18.2.4.3 Citrin Deficiency

Citrin deficiency is an inborn error of metabolism due to an abnormality in the *SLC25A13* gene and leads to neonatal intrahepatic cholestasis due to citrin deficiency (NICCD). Citrin is a transport protein localized in the inner mitochondrial membrane, and loss of citrine function leads to impaired urea and protein synthesis, aerobic glycolysis, gluconeogenesis, and energy metabolism, which result in various symptoms [29].

Citrin deficiency is common in East and Southeast Asia, and there are a few reports from Europe and the United States. The frequency of carriers in Japan is 1/65 births, and the theoretical prevalence is 1/17,000 births [30].

Approximately 40% of NICCDs identified during newborn mass screening show high levels of galactose, methionine, and phenylalanine, while others present with jaundice and pale yellow or acholic stools [31]. Laboratory findings include hyperbileacidemia, coagulopathy, hypoproteinemia, hypoglycemia, and transient elevation of multiple amino acids, such as citrulline, threonine, methionine, and tyrosine. Liver histology shows extensive fatty liver with large and small lipid droplets and cholestasis.

In most patients with NICCD, symptoms usually disappear within the first year of life. After an apparently healthy period (adaptation/compensation period) from infancy to adulthood, approximately 20% of patients will go on to develop adult-onset type II citrullinemia [29].

Formulas containing medium-chain triglycerides, lactose-free formulas, fat-soluble vitamins, and ursodeoxycholic acid are used to treat NICCD. Patients should aim to eat low-carbohydrate, high-protein, and high-fat foods; avoid excessive sugar and alcohol intake. Intravenous hyperalimentation and Glyceol®, a formulation of concentrated glycerin and fructose given to patients with intracranial hypertension, is contraindicated [32].

#### 18.2.4.4 Other Metabolic Liver Disorders

Inborn errors of bile acid metabolism [33], disorders of lipid metabolism, such as Wolman's disease (acidic lipase deficiency), Niemann–Pick's disease type C, and Gaucher's disease type II, as well as various mitochondrial disorders [34] may be accompanied by neonatal cholestasis.

### 18.2.5 Alloimmune Conditions

#### 18.2.5.1 Neonatal Hemochromatosis

Neonatal hemochromatosis is a gestational alloimmune liver disease (GALD) that is unrelated to hereditary hemochromatosis. GALD is caused by transplacental passage of reactive maternal immunoglobulins and is characterized by liver failure and hepatic and extrahepatic iron accumulation (hemosiderosis) during the neonatal period [35]. Newborns show signs of severe liver failure, such as coagulopathy, ascites, and hypoalbuminemia. Liver transplantation is necessary for infants who do not respond to exchange transfusion and treatment with high-dose intravenous immunoglobulin [36].

### 18.2.6 Toxic Conditions

#### 18.2.6.1 Intestinal Failure-Related Liver Disease (IFALD)

IFALD is defined as liver disease resulting from medical and surgical management for bowel failure, such as short bowel syndrome [37]. Parenteral nutrition plays an important role in the etiology of the disease. IFALD is especially common in premature infants with short bowel syndrome.

### 18.2.7 INH

INH was once considered to be a typical disease that needed to be differentiated from biliary atresia. However, the causative genes of metabolic and hereditary diseases have been identified as a result of advances in genetic analysis, and the number of cases with definitive diagnosis has increased [38]. Therefore, the frequency and significance of INH in neonatal cholestasis are decreasing [2].

Cases with perinatal abnormalities, such as premature and/or low-birth-weight infants [39], and neonatal asphyxia [40], often present with intrahepatic cholestasis; however, most are transient and have a good prognosis. Such cases have recently been termed transient neonatal cholestasis [41], which refers to a group of diseases that are almost identical to conventional INH. Parenteral nutrition is an important factor causing transient neonatal cholestasis, and being small for gestational age (SGA) and neonatal surgery are additional risk factors [39].

Most patients develop overt jaundice, acholic or pale yellow stools, and dark yellow urine within the first 2 months of life, although the stool color often fluctuates. Poor weight gain, hepatomegaly and splenomegaly are often observed. Laboratory findings usually show elevation of direct bilirubin, aspartate transaminase (AST), alanine aminotransferase (ALT), and total bile acids.

Liver histology often reveals giant cell hepatitis (appearance of multinucleated giant cells) with cholestasis, but this is not a specific finding. Expanded portal tracts with marked fibrosis and bile duct proliferation, which are characteristic features of biliary atresia, are usually absent.

The prognosis for neonatal hepatitis is generally good, with jaundice disappearing within 6 months of age and liver function normalizing within 12 months. Treatment predominantly comprises nutritional management and fat-soluble vitamin supplementation. The Combined used of ursodeoxycholic acid and other drugs for cholestasis is used for patients with prolonged jaundice or severe liver cholestasis.

## 18.3 Approach to Differential Diagnosis of Biliary Atresia

### 18.3.1 Diagnosis/Treatment Flowchart

In cases with suspected neonatal cholestasis, biliary atresia is considered first, and diagnosis and treatment are promptly performed as follows (Fig. 18.2):

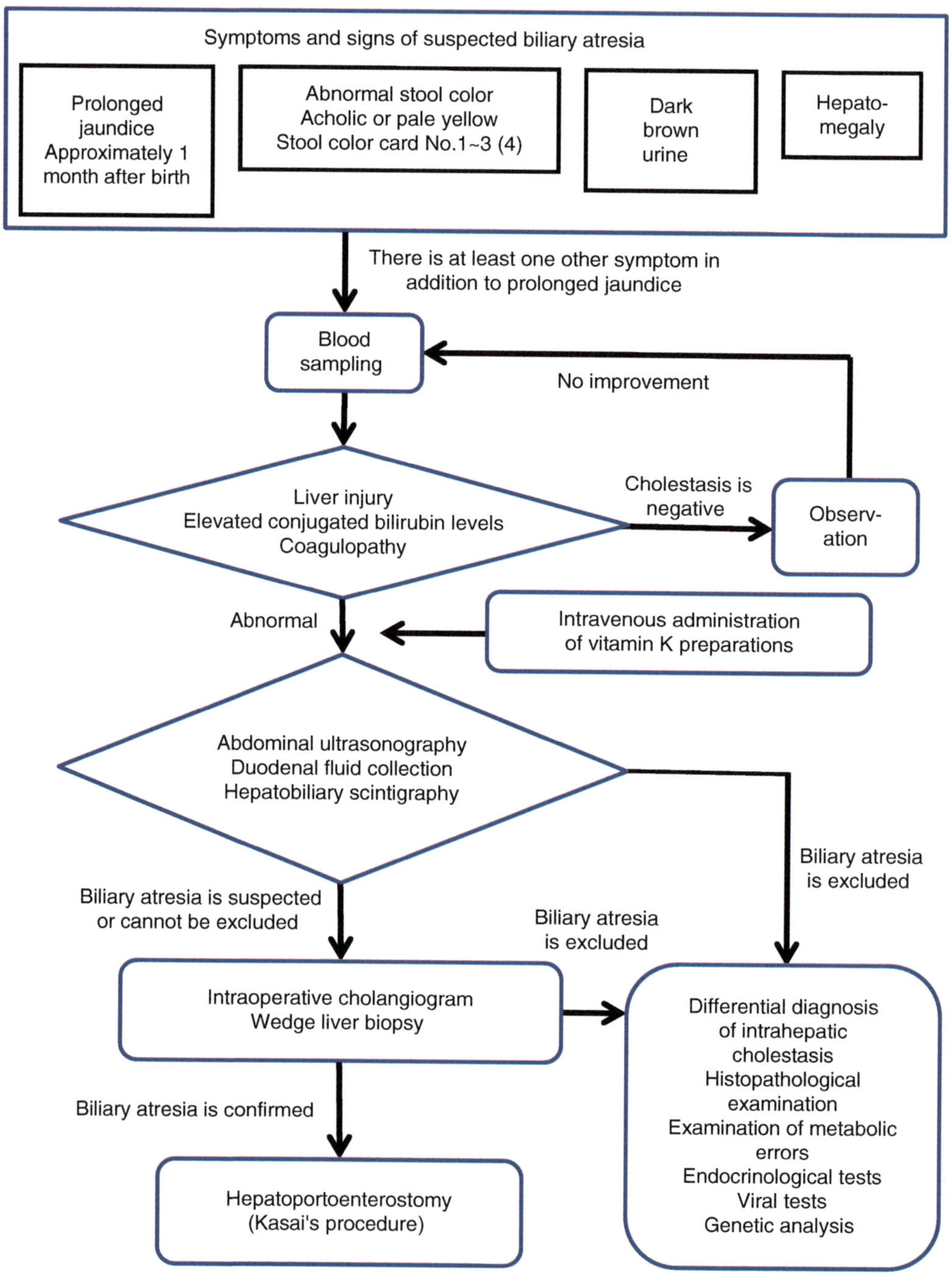


**Fig. 18.2** Diagnosis and treatment flowchart for biliary atresia and neonatal cholestasis

- If acholic stools or persistent jaundice are present in the early stages of neonates to infants, check for dark brown urine and hepatomegaly and perform a blood sampling test including conjugated bilirubin.
- If cholestatic liver injury is observed, abdominal ultrasonography, duodenal fluid collection, hepatobiliary scintigraphy, and other examinations should be performed immediately as a differential diagnosis of biliary atresia.
- For cases with coagulopathy, check for intracranial hemorrhage by head CT scan and ensure intravenous administration of vitamin K preparations.
- If biliary atresia is suspected or cannot be excluded, intraoperative cholangiogram should be performed earlier. Hepatoportoenterostomy (Kasai's procedure) is then performed if the diagnosis is confirmed.
- If biliary atresia is negative, various tests for differential diagnosis of intrahepatic cholestasis are performed.

### 18.3.2 Symptoms/Physical Findings

The main symptoms of biliary atresia include jaundice, acholic to pale yellow stool, dark brown urine, hepatomegaly, and bleeding tendency due to vitamin K deficiency.

Abnormal stool color is an important indicator for biliary atresia diagnosis, but in many cases the yellow stool color after birth gradually fades to pale yellow (beige). The Japanese Biliary Atresia Registry revealed that stool color at admission was gray in 61.1%, pale yellow in 28.8%, and yellow in 5.0% of cases [42], and it was noted that some patients presented with yellowish stools. Screening using a stool color card was shown to increase the number of early diagnoses and improve the autologous liver survival rate; therefore, it is desirable to screen for biliary atresia using the stool color card in the Maternal and Child Health Handbook [43]. It is also recommended that healthcare providers directly examine patients' stools [2].

Of all cases of biliary atresia in Japan, 4.7% are first diagnosed with the disorder due to intracranial hemorrhage resulting from vitamin K deficiency [42]. Such cases are common at about 2 months of age. Early diagnosis of biliary atresia is extremely important since the mortality and neurological sequelae rates increase due to complications of intracranial hemorrhage.

Although the general condition is often initially good, symptoms of chronic liver diseases, such as increased jaundice, poor weight gain, hepatosplenomegaly, dilatation of abdominal wall vein, ascites, and abdominal distension, gradually become prominent after 3–4 months of age. Other fat-soluble vitamin deficiencies (vitamin D-deficient rickets, neurological complications due to vitamin E deficiency) should also be noted.

### 18.3.3 Laboratory Analyses

If hepatomegaly, stool color abnormality, or dark brown urine is observed in addition to prolonged jaundice, it is strongly recommended to perform a blood test that includes conjugated bilirubin. Close examination for differentiation of biliary atresia should also be performed if cholestasis is suspected.

Cholestasis is easily overlooked as there are many cases of unconjugated bilirubin, such as physiological jaundice (up to 2–3 weeks after birth) and breast milk jaundice (up to 2–3 months after birth), in the early stages in newborns and infants. Even if persistent jaundice is found during a one-month medical examination, it is not easy to perform blood sampling in all cases. However, if a one-month medical examination fails to detect biliary atresia, the diagnosis may be made after the second month of life, and the risk of intracranial hemorrhage increases. If prolonged jaundice is found during a one-month medical examination, it should not be diagnosed as breast-fed jaundice just because the patient is breastfed. Blood sampling should be actively performed if cholestasis is suspected based on symptoms and findings.

If serum total bilirubin levels are $<5$ mg/dL and conjugated bilirubin levels are $\geq 1.0$ mg/dL, serum conjugated bilirubin levels are judged to be obstructive jaundice [2]. If total bilirubin levels are $\geq 5$ mg/dL and conjugated bilirubin accounts for $\geq 20\%$ of total bilirubin, it is judged to be obstructive jaundice [2]. In addition, high serum levels of AST, ALT, γ-GTP, alkaline phosphatase, and total bile acid are often observed.

High serum γ-GTP levels are useful as an adjunct diagnosis of biliary atresia. If there is obstructive jaundice in addition to high serum γ-GTP levels, congenital biliary dilatation, citrin deficiency, and Alagille syndrome should be considered in addition to biliary atresia. Conversely, INH, PFIC, and inborn errors of bile acid metabolism should be considered if serum γ-GTP levels are low or normal.

It is strongly recommended to perform a blood coagulation test and administer vitamin K preparations intravenously in children with cholestasis suspected of having biliary atresia.

### 18.3.4 Further Differential Diagnosis

Abdominal ultrasonography, duodenal fluid collection, hepatobiliary scintigraphy, and other examinations should be performed immediately as a further differential diagnosis if biliary atresia is suspected or cannot be excluded. In patients with coagulopathy, it is important to check for intracranial hemorrhage using head CT scan and administer a vitamin K preparation intravenously.

Evaluation via intraoperative cholangiogram and histological examination of the duct remnant are considered the gold standard to diagnose biliary atresia [2]. Intraoperative cholangiogram should be performed earlier if there is a possibility of biliary atresia based on the above examinations. Hepatoportoenterostomy (Kasai's procedure) should then be performed if the diagnosis is confirmed. Wedge liver biopsy is usually performed simultaneously.

The usefulness of these modalities is explained in detail in the next chapter.

On the other hand, if biliary atresia is excluded, histopathological examination, examination of metabolic errors, endocrinological tests, viral tests, and genetic analysis should be considered for the differential diagnosis of intrahepatic cholestasis. Comprehensive genetic analysis using next-generation sequencing is useful for diagnosis when a genetic disease is suspected to be the cause of neonatal cholestasis [44–46]. It has become possible to comprehensively analyze the exon region of multiple genes responsible for genetic cholestasis, including Alagille syndrome and PFIC, and make a definitive diagnosis.

## References


1. Hassan HHA, Balistreri WF. Neonatal cholestasis. In: Kliegman R, Stanton BF, St Geme J, Nina Schor N, editors. Nelson textbook of pediatrics. 20th ed. Philadelphia: Elsevier; 2015. p. 2092–100.
2. Fawaz R, Baumann U, Ekong U, et al. Guideline for the evaluation of cholestatic jaundice in infants: joint recommendations of the North American Society for Pediatric Gastroenterology, Hepatology, and Nutrition and the European Society for Pediatric Gastroenterology, Hepatology, and Nutrition. J Pediatr Gastroenterol Nutr. 2017;64:154–68.
3. Gottesman LE, Del Vecchio MT, Aronoff SC. Etiologies of conjugated hyperbilirubinemia in infancy: a systematic review of 1692 subjects. BMC Pediatr. 2015;15:192–9.
4. Ragot E, Mabrut JY, Ouaïssi M, et al. Pancreaticobiliary maljunctions in European patients with bile duct cysts: results of the multicenter study of the French Surgical Association (AFC). World J Surg. 2017;41:538–45.
5. Singham J, Yoshida EM, Scudamore CH. Choledochal cysts: part 1 of 3: classification and pathogenesis. Can J Surg. 2009;52:434–40.
6. Kim WS, Kim IO, Yeon KM, et al. Choledochal cyst with or without biliary atresia in neonates and young infants: US differentiation. Radiology. 1998;209:465–9.
7. Sondheimer JM, Asturias E, Cadnapaphornchai M. Infection and cholestasis in neonates with intestinal resection and long-term parenteral nutrition. J Pediatr Gastroenterol Nutr. 1998;27:131–7.
8. Kamath BM, Baker A, Houwen R, et al. Systematic review: the epidemiology, natural history, and burden of Alagille syndrome. J Pediatr Gastroenterol Nutr. 2018;67:148–56.
9. Kamath BM, Spinner NB, Piccoli AD. Alagille syndrome. In: Suchy FJ, Sokol RJ, Balistreri WF, editors. Liver disease in children. 4th ed. Cambridge: Cambridge Univ. Press; 2014. p. 216–33.
10. Kaye AJ, Rand EB, Munoz PS, et al. Effect of Kasai procedure on hepatic outcome in Alagille syndrome. J Pediatr Gastroenterol Nutr. 2010;51:319–21.
11. Kamath BM, Ye W, Goodrich NP, et al. Outcomes of childhood cholestasis in Alagille syndrome: results of a multicenter observational study. Hepatol Commun. 2020:4(3).
12. Information Center for Specific Pediatric Chronic Diseases, Japan. Available from: https://www.shouman.jp/disease/details/08_15_139/. Accessed 4 Oct 2020.
13. Sveger T. Liver disease in alpha1-antitrypsin deficiency detected by screening of 200,000 infants. N Engl J Med. 1976;294:1316–21.
14. Mostafavi B, Piitulainen E, Tanash HA. Survival in the Swedish cohort with alpha-1-antitrypsin deficiency, up to the age of 43–45 years. Int J Chron Obstruct Pulmon Dis. 2019;14:525–30.
15. Hamosh A, FitzSimmons SC, Macek M Jr, et al. Comparison of the clinical manifestations of cystic fibrosis in black and white patients. J Pediatr. 1998;132:255–9.
16. Information Center for Specific Pediatric Chronic Diseases, Japan. Available from: https://www.shouman.jp/disease/details03_06_008/. Accessed 4 Oct 2020.
17. Sokol RJ, Durie PR. Recommendations for management of liver and biliary tract disease in cystic fibrosis. Cystic Fibrosis Foundation hepatobiliary disease consensus group. J Pediatr Gastroenterol Nutr. 1999;28(Suppl. 1):S1.
18. Srivastava A. Progressive familial intrahepatic cholestasis. J Clin Exp Hepatol. 2014;4:25–36.
19. Knisely AS, Strautnieks SS, Meier Y, et al. Hepatocellular carcinoma in ten children under five years of age with bile salt export pump deficiency. Hepatology. 2006;44:478–86.
20. Sambrotta M, Strautnieks S, Papouli E, et al. Mutations in *TJP2* cause progressive cholestatic liver disease. Nat Genet. 2014;46:326–8.
21. Degiorgio D, Colombo C, Seia M, et al. Molecular characterization and structural implications of 25 new *ABCB4* mutations in progressive familial intrahepatic cholestasis type 3 (PFIC3). Eur J Hum Genet. 2007;15:1230–8.
22. Gomez-Ospina N, Potter CJ, Xiao R, et al. Mutations in the nuclear bile acid receptor FXR cause progressive familial intrahepatic cholestasis. Nat Commun. 2016;7:10713.
23. Erlinger S, Arias IM, Dhumeaux D. Inherited disorders of bilirubin transport and conjugation: new insights into molecular mechanisms and consequences. Gastroenterology. 2014;146:1625–38.
24. Lee JH, Chen HL, Chen HL, et al. Neonatal Dubin- Johnson syndrome: long-term follow-up and MRP2 mutations study. Pediatr Res. 2006;59:584–9.
25. Towaga T, Mizuochi T, Sugiura T, et al. Clinical, pathologic, and genetic features of neonatal Dubin-Johnson syndrome: a multicenter study in Japan. J Pediatr. 2018;196:161–7.
26. Information Center for Specific Pediatric Chronic Diseases, Japan. Available from: https://www.shouman.jp/disease/details/08_05_060/. Accessed 4 Oct 2020.
27. Holton JB, et al. Galactosemia. In: Scriber CR, et al., editors. The metabolic &molecular bases of inherited disease. New York: McGraw-Hill; 2001. p. 1807–20.
28. Information Center for Specific Pediatric Chronic Diseases, Japan. Available from: https://www.shouman.jp/disease/details/08_01_002/. Accessed 4 Oct 2020.
29. Saheki T, Kobayashi K. Mitochondrial aspartate glutamate carrier (citrin) deficiency as the cause of adult-onset type II citrullinemia (CTLN2) and idiopathic neonatal hepatitis (NICCD). J Hum Genet. 2002;47:333–41.
30. Tabata A, Sheng JS, Ushikai M, et al. Identification of 13 novel mutations including a retrotransposal insertion in *SLC25A13* gene and frequency of 30 mutations found in patients with citrin deficiency. J Hum Genet. 2008;53:534–45.
31. Ohura T, Kobayashi K, Tazawa Y, et al. Clinical pictures of 75 patients with neonatal intrahepatic cholestasis caused by citrin deficiency (NICCD). J Inherit Metab Dis. 2007;30:139–44.

32. Saheki T, Inoue K, Tushima A, et al. Citrin deficiency and current treatment concepts. Mol Genet Metab. 2010;100(Suppl. 1):S59–64.
33. Heubi JE, Setchell KD, Bove KE. Inborn errors of bile acid metabolism. Semin Liver Dis. 2007;27:282–94.
34. Molleston JP, Sokol RJ, Karnsakul W, et al. Evaluation of the child with suspected mitochondrial liver disease. J Pediatr Gastroenterol Nutr. 2013;57:269–76.
35. Whitington PF. Gestational alloimmune liver disease and neonatal hemochromatosis. Semin Liver Dis. 2012;32:325.
36. Fischer HS, Staufner C, Sallmon H, et al. Early exchange transfusion to treat neonates with gestational alloimmune liver disease: an 11-year cohort study. J Pediatr Gastroenterol Nutr. 2020;70:444.
37. Lacaille F, Gupte G, Colomb V, et al. Intestinal failure-associated liver disease: a position paper of the ESPGHAN working Group of Intestinal Failure and Intestinal Transplantation. J Pediatr Gastroenterol Nutr. 2015;60:272–83.
38. Balistreri WF, Bezerra JA. Whatever happened to "neonatal hepatitis"? Clin Liver Dis. 2006;10:27–53.
39. Champion V, Carbajal R, Lozar J, et al. Risk factors for developing transient neonatal cholestasis. J Pediatr Gastroenterol Nutr. 2012;55:592–8.
40. Herzog D, Chessex P, Martin S, et al. Transient cholestasis in newborn infants with perinatal asphyxia. Can J Gastroenterol. 2003;17:179–82.
41. Jacquemin E, Lykavieris P, Chaoui N, et al. Transient neonatal cholestasis: origin and outcome. J Pediatr. 1998;133:563–7.
42. Japanese Biliary Atresia Registry. Available from: https://jbas.net/data-en/initial/total_number.pdf. Accessed 4 Oct 2020.
43. Gu YH, Yokoyama K, Mizuta K, et al. Stool color card screening for early detection of biliary atresia and long-term native liver survival: a 19-year cohort study in Japan. J Pediatr. 2015;166:897–902.
44. Togawa T, Sugiura T, Ito K, et al. Molecular genetic dissection and neonatal/infantile intrahepatic cholestasis using targeted next-generation sequencing. J Pediatr. 2016;171:171–7.
45. Nicastro E, Di Giorgio A, Marchetti D, et al. Diagnostic yield of an algorithm for neonatal and infantile cholestasis integrating next generation sequencing. J Pediatr. 2019;211:54–62.
46. Moreira-Silva H, Maio I, Bandeira A, et al. Metabolic liver diseases presenting with neonatal cholestasis: at the crossroad between old and new paradigms. Eur J Pediatr. 2019;178:515–23.

# Diagnostic Modalities for Biliary Atresia

# 19

Miyuki Kohno

**Abstract**

Early diagnosis of biliary atresia (BA) is necessary because the timing of surgery affects the prognosis. The diagnostic imaging techniques for BA include invasive and noninvasive methods. The noninvasive methods include ultrasonography (US), duodenal tube test, hepatobiliary scintigraphy, magnetic resonance cholangiopancreatography, and endoscopic retrograde cholangiopancreatography; whereas the invasive methods include cholangiography, exploratory laparoscopy, and preoperative liver biopsy. As no method has 100% diagnostic accuracy, the limitations of each must be considered. The US is the most basic of the noninvasive method and has high diagnostic accuracy. Parameters including triangular cord sign, gallbladder abnormalities, and hepatic subcapsular flow can be evaluated. The invasive tests have high diagnostic accuracy but have the disadvantage of delaying radical surgery for BA. Accordingly, the Japanese guidelines suggest that preoperative liver biopsy should not be performed.

**Keywords**

Biliary atresia · Diagnostic methods · Ultrasonography
Duodenal tube test · Hepatobiliary scintigraphy
Magnetic resonance cholangiopancreatography
Laparoscopy · Cholangiography · Percutaneous liver biopsy

## 19.1 Introduction

Biliary atresia (BA) is a serious disease that results in biliary cirrhosis unless bile drainage is performed by Kasai portoenterostomy. Early diagnosis is necessary because the timing of surgery affects the prognosis.

If BA is suspected by stool color or jaundice screening, blood biochemistry tests, and diagnostic modalities are performed. However, it is important to note that no modality has 100% diagnostic accuracy. If the diagnostic judgment remains difficult after imaging examinations have been performed and there is a strong suspicion of biliary atresia, definitive diagnosis by trial laparotomy and direct cholangiography is required.

This chapter describes the diagnostic imaging examinations suitable for BA, including noninvasive and invasive methods.

## 19.2 Diagnostic Modalities for Biliary Atresia

### 19.2.1 Plain Radiographs of the Chest/abdomen

Plain radiographs are important for assessing hepatosplenomegaly and also in screening for biliary atresia splenic malformation (BASM) syndrome, which occurs in ~10% of cases of BA and is associated with polysplenia [1]. If BASM syndrome is suspected, ultrasonography, CT, and MRI can reveal internal abnormalities and the positional relationships associated with BA. As the concomitant rate of congenital heart diseases is high, ultrasonography (US) should be performed to assess the hemodynamics.

M. Kohno (✉)
Department of Pediatric Surgery, Kanazawa Medical University, Ishikawa, Japan
e-mail: miyuki@kanazawa-med.ac.jp


M. Nio (ed.), *Introduction to Biliary Atresia*, https://doi.org/10.1007/978-981-16-2160-4_19

## 19.2.2 Ultrasonography

US is a simple, noninvasive, and highly diagnostic imaging modality that is first performed when BA is suspected. In many cases, US avoids unnecessary invasive procedures. The quality of the US examination is operator dependent.

Abdominal US includes examination of the liver, gallbladder, extrahepatic bile duct, and spleen, and evaluation for the presence of situs inversus, polysplenia/asplenia, and other congenital anomalies associated with BASM syndrome [1, 2].

Although it is not always easy to visualize the extrahepatic bile duct in normal infants, technical advances in US have improved its visibility, and BA can be ruled out if the extrahepatic bile duct can be observed from the hilar region to the papilla of Vater. Inability to identify the common bile duct (CBD) is an important finding; however, the CBD may be visible on US in patients with type IIIa BA.

Type I BA occurs in ~10% of cases of BA and is characterized by occlusion of the CBD with a patent hepatic bile duct. In type I cysts, the extrahepatic bile duct is expanded in cystic form, which must be differentiated from choledochal cysts (Fig. 19.1). Although it may be difficult to distinguish cysts in the hilum of the liver from biliary dilatation in US, it is reported that BA should be suspected in the case that cyst size decreases before and after birth and the gallbladder atrophies after birth [3].

The US parameters for suspected BA include presence of a ventral high-intensity band in the hepatic bifurcation (termed triangular cord, TC), nonidentification of the GB, GB length, abnormal GB morphology, loss of GB contractibility, enlarged hepatic artery diameter, nonvisualization of the CBD, and the presence of hepatic subcapsular flow (HSF). The difficulty in identifying the CBD in healthy infants even with a high-resolution probe may explain why absence of the CBD is not more widely used for diagnosis.

A high-frequency probe is used for these assessments, and the infant must have fasted for 4 hours prior.

#### 19.2.2.1 Triangular Cord Sign (Fig. 19.2)

The presence of an echogenicity on the ventral side of the portal bifurcation is termed triangular cord (TC) sign. Histologically, TC is due to residual fibrous obstructive tissue in the hilum of the liver. The cutoff value in terms of TC thickness is reported to vary from 2 to 4 mm or more [4, 5].

In a meta-analysis of 20 studies from 1990 to 2015, Zhou et al. [4] reported that the TC sign had the summary sensitivity of 74% and summary specificity of 97% for the diagnosis of BA. In a meta-analysis of 17 studies from 1996 to 2015, Yoon et al. [5] reported the summary sensitivity of 85% and summary specificity of 97% for the diagnosis of BA. In mild cases of BA, TC sign might not be detected on US at an early stage, but become more apparent as the disease develops. Zhou et al [6] suggested that thickness >2 mm should be considered a positive finding.

#### 19.2.2.2 Gallbladder Abnormalities (Fig. 19.3)

Gallbladder abnormalities (GBAs) include absence of a gallbladder, small gallbladder size, abnormal shape and wall of the gallbladder, and no contraction of the gallbladder. In terms of gallbladder shape, discontinuous or absent mucosal lining, indistinct wall, and irregular outer margin are regarded as abnormal [7]. No contraction of the gallbladder describes a gallbladder that does not contract after feeding. The CBD can be confirmed by US in CBD type IIIa of the lower bile duct classification. US may also be useful for gallbladder visualization and observation of gallbladder contraction.

Regarding diagnostic performance for detection of gallbladder abnormalities, Zhou et al [4] reported that in 19 studies, US yielded the summary sensitivity of 85% and summary specificity of 92%; and in 10 studies, the summary sensitivity for absent gallbladder was 28%, and specificity of 99%. In their meta-analysis, Yoon et al [5] reported that diagnostic

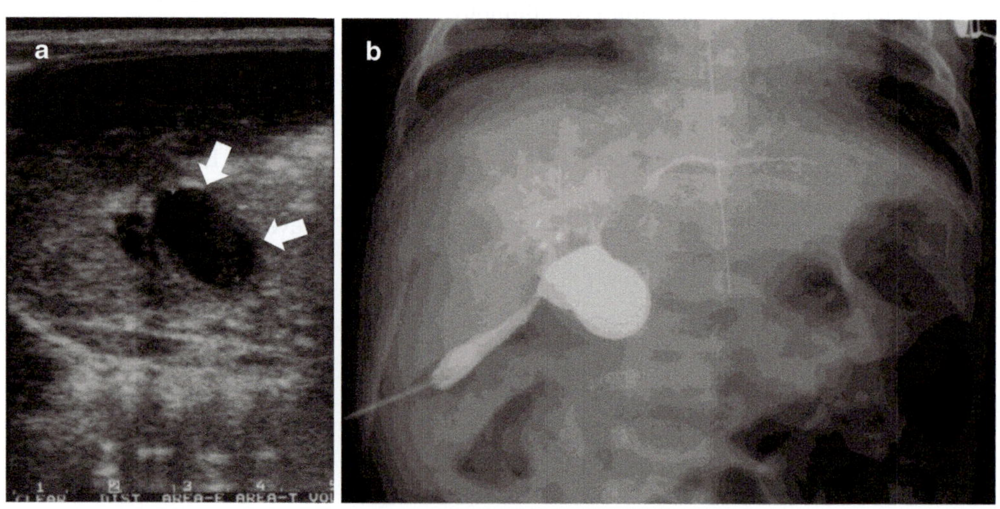


**Fig. 19.1** A 6-week-old girl with type 1 cystic BA. Ultrasound shows a cystic lesion (white arrows) at the porta hepatis (A). Intraoperative cholangiography depicts the intrahepatic bile duct, but the CBD is occluded and outflow of contrast medium into the duodenum is not observed (B)

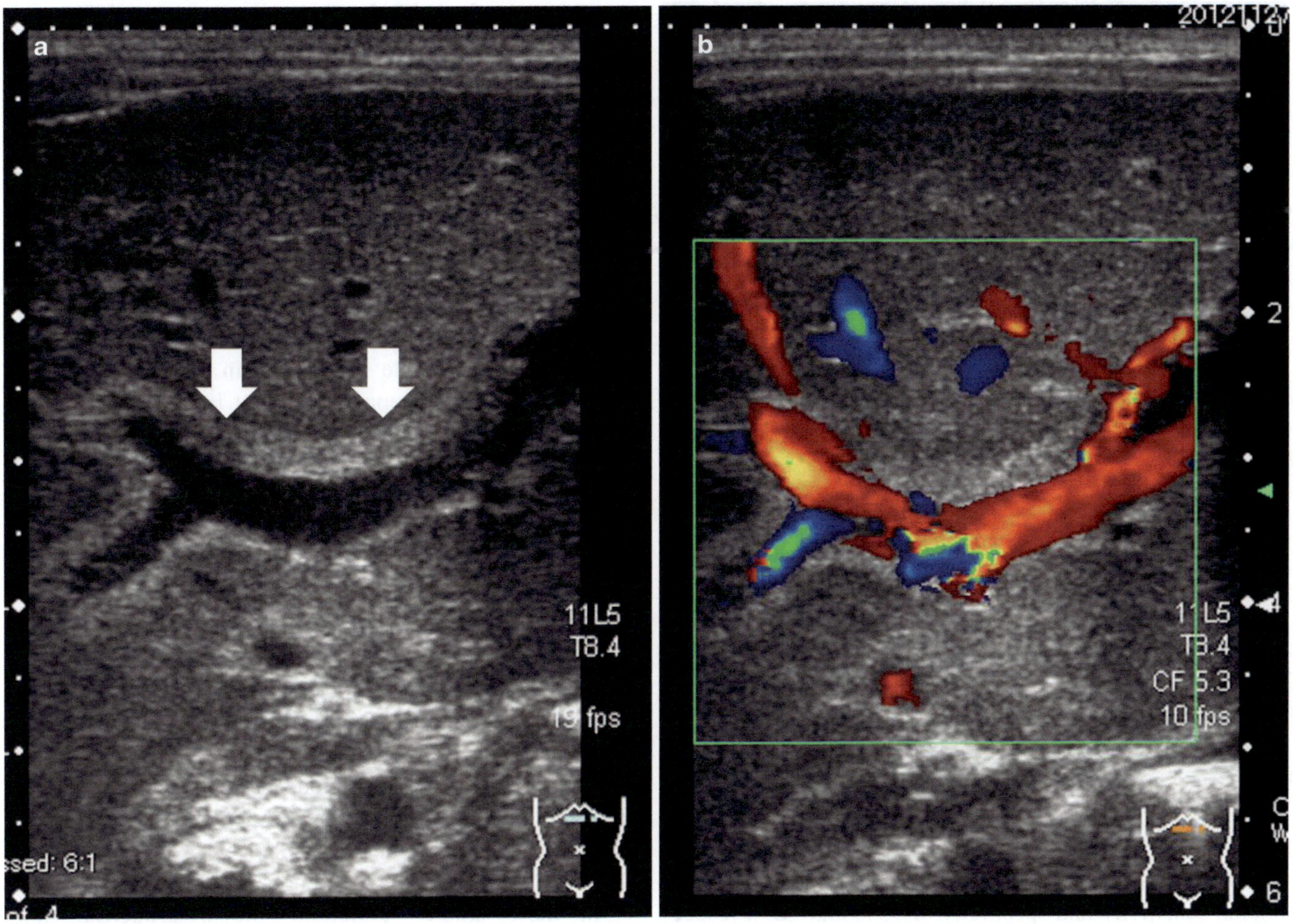


**Fig. 19.2** A 3-week-old girl with BA (III-b1-ν). Ultrasonography shows the TC sign (white arrows) on the ventral side of the portal vein bifurcation (A). Color Doppler clearly shows blood flow in the portal vein and distinguishes the vessel from the TC sign (B)

performance of the most common cutoff sizes for GB length (<1.5 cm or <1.9 cm) in 8 studies had the sensitivity of 50%–100% and specificity of 68%–99%. Regarding the diagnostic performance for characterizing GBA in 4 studies, the sensitivity was 85%–96% and specificity was 82%–95%. In two studies of loss of contractility, the sensitivity was 93% and 94% and specificity was 53% and 70%. In two studies regarding nonvisualization of the CBD, the sensitivity was 86% and 93%, and specificity was 92% in each.

The criteria for determining GBAs vary between studies, which might help explain discrepancies in diagnostic accuracy among them. A more objective gallbladder classification system that unifies all of these criteria would improve the diagnostic accuracy [4].

#### 19.2.2.3 Enlarged Hepatic Artery Diameter

US color Doppler study revealed a larger diameter of the hepatic artery (HAD) in patients with BA compared with that in patients with other causes of cholestasis and in control subjects. Enlargement of the hepatic artery may be a compensatory change to improve the blood supply to the biliary tree [8]. The cutoff value varies depending on the criteria used for HAD expansion, and is reported as >1.5 mm [9] and as >1.9 mm [6].

In a meta-analysis, Yoon et al [5] found that in four studies, enlarged HAD showed the sensitivity of 72%–100% and specificity of 70%–89% for BA.

#### 19.2.2.4 Hepatic Subcapsular Flow

Hepatic arterial flow over the surface of the liver on color Doppler US imaging, termed hepatic subcapsular flow (HSF), has been described in patients with BA by Lee et al [10]. HSF occurs as a result of hyperplastic and hypertrophic changes in branches of the hepatic artery and has been observed at the stage of disease when bridging fibrosis leads to features of overt biliary cirrhosis [11].

Recent studies have confirmed that HSF could be used as a clinical marker with high capacity for discriminating BA. A meta-analysis of nine studies performed between 2009 and 2017 by Sun et al [12] reported the values for

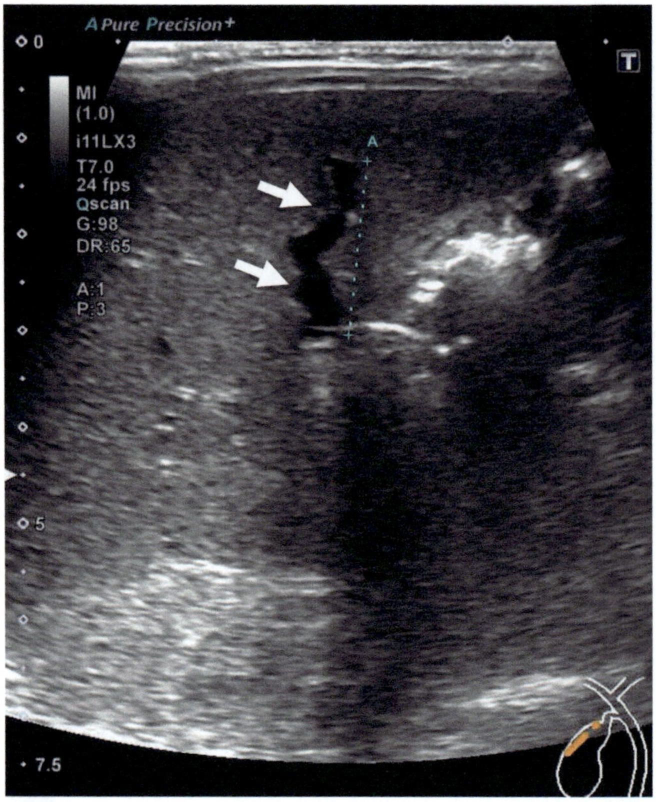


**Fig. 19.3** A 5-week-old boy with BA (III-b1-ν). Irregularity of the gallbladder wall is seen on longitudinal US

pooled sensitivity and specificity of 95% and 92%, respectively, of HSF for the diagnosis of BA.

#### 19.2.2.5 Shear Wave Elastography

Shear wave elastography (SWE) is a relatively recent technique for quantifying liver stiffness as a measure of liver fibrosis. SWE has been shown to be useful in the detection of BA, especially in the absence of TC sign and abnormal gallbladder [13]. SWE can be used to establish the presence of fibrosis and to assess its progression over time. SWE is calculated as shear wave speed (m/s) or as Young's modulus (kPa).

Regarding the diagnostic performance of SWE for BA, Wang et al [14] reported the sensitivity of 97.4% and specificity of 100% for a cutoff value of 8.68 kPa; Zhou et al [15] reported the sensitivity of 81.4% and specificity of 66.7% for a cutoff value of 10.2 kPa; and Duan et al [16] reported the sensitivity of 84.3% and specificity of 89.7% for a cutoff value of 12.35 kPa. Dillman et al [17] reported that diagnostic performance was better for 2-D than for point US SWE technique. Using a cutoff value of >1.84 m/s, 2D US SWE had the sensitivity of 92.3% and specificity of 78.6%.

The use of SWE combined with grayscale US findings might enable substantial expedition in the workup for suspected BA.

### 19.2.3 Duodenal Tube Test

The duodenal tube test (DTT) evaluates the presence or absence of excretion of bile into the duodenum based on the composition of collected duodenal juice. Bile flowing from the papilla of Vater is collected by catheter in the third part of the duodenum (placed transnasally under fluoroscopy and fixed in position) and duodenal juice is collected.

The collected liquid is tested for pH, total bilirubin, direct bilirubin, total bile acid, and amylase. The pH and amylase values indicate whether the sample has been collected from the correct site. If bile is detected in the duodenal juice, patency of the extrahepatic bile duct is proven and BA is excluded. Note that magnesium sulfate administration causes the gallbladder to contract and promote biliary excretion. If bile excretion can be confirmed by the color of the juice or from the test results, the test can be completed in about 1 hour. Otherwise, collection can continue for up to 24 hours.

Larrosa-Haro et al, Meisheri et al, and Meisheri et al [18–20] in which the outcome of DTT was assessed by the color of duodenal juice reported the high sensitivity (97%–100%) and relatively low specificity (60%–93.7%).

Fukuoka et al and Yoshii et al [21, 22] researched quantitative and objective parameters from previous subjective evaluations of the color of duodenal juice, and reported that the ratio of total bile acid in the duodenal fluid (dTBA)/serum (S) gamma-glutamyltransferase (GGT) was the best discriminator between BA and non-BA.

In these studies evaluating the dTBA/sGGT ratio, Fukuoka et al. [21] reported the sensitivity and specificity of 100% with a cutoff value of 0.076 μmol/U, while Yoshii et al. [22] reported the sensitivity of 98.0% and specificity of 100% with a cutoff value of 0.014 μmol/U.

DTT may be the most valuable and noninvasive diagnostic method for detecting BA in patients with cholestasis.

### 19.2.4 Hepatobiliary Scintigraphy

Hepatobiliary scintigraphy (HS) plays an important role in the diagnosis of neonatal cholestasis as it can rule out BA. The procedure is noninvasive and seldom requires sedation. Confirmation of excretion of radionuclide from the liver into the digestive tract (Fig. 19.4) indicates patency of the biliary system and rules out BA.

In Western countries, $^{99m}$Tc-IDA derivatives (iminodiacetic acid) are generally used as the radionuclide, whereas $^{99m}$Tc-PMT ($^{99m}$Tc-N-pyrudoxy-5-methyltryptophan) is most commonly used in Japan. Intravenously injected $^{99m}$Tc-PMT has rapid blood clearance, fast hepatobiliary transit, low urinary excretion, and no intestinal reabsorption. $^{99m}$Tc-PMT and $^{99m}$Tc-IDA derivatives have very similar pharmacokinetics [23, 24], and $^{99m}$Tc-PMT

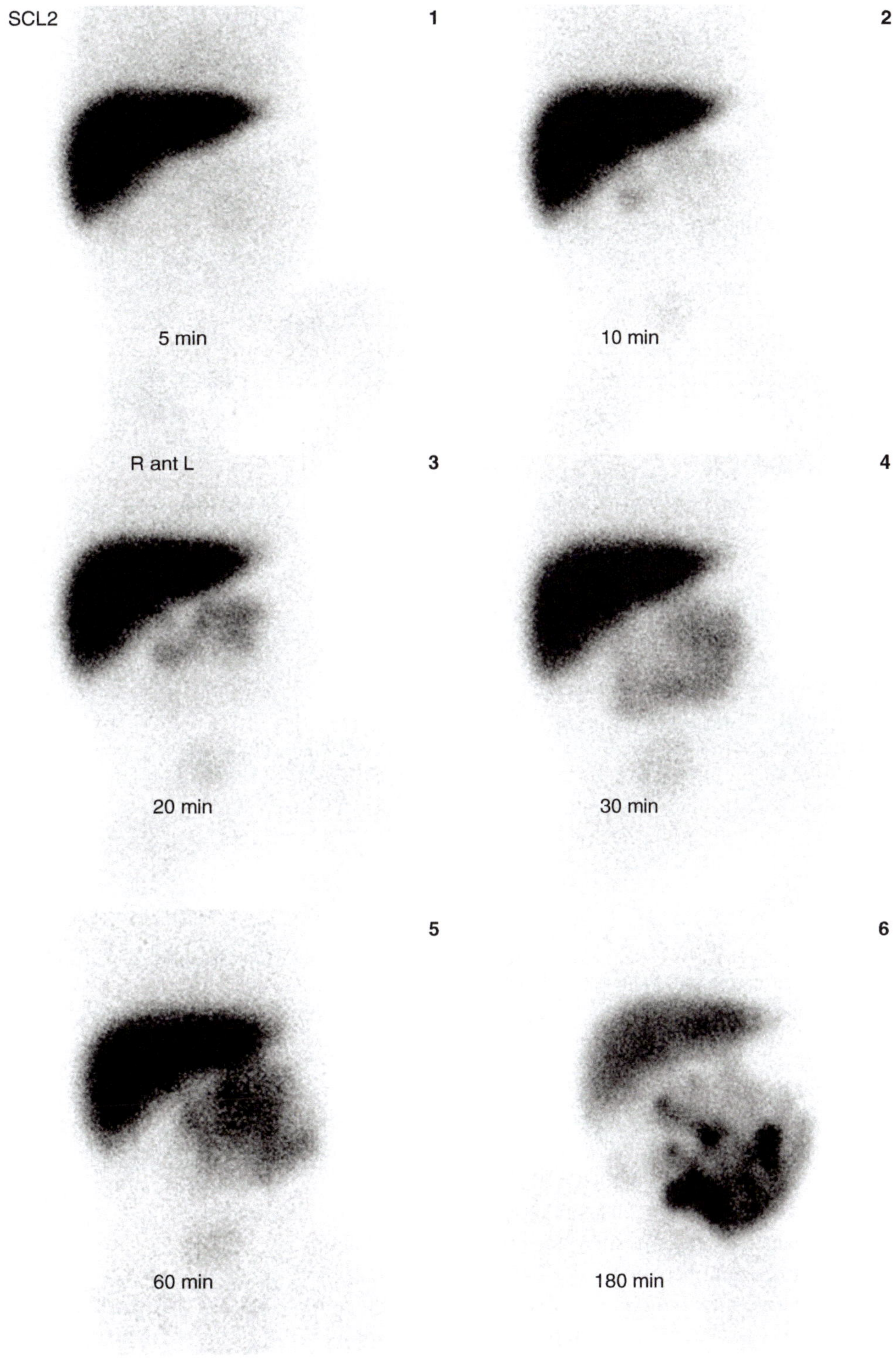


**Fig. 19.4** A 4-week-old infant who was true-negative for BA. The extrahepatic ducts were visualized at 10 min after injection, and duodenal excretion was visualized at 20 min after injection on $^{99m}$ Tc-PMT scintigraphy

has the additional advantage of being much more resistant to high bilirubin levels (close to 20 mg/dL) compared with $^{99m}$Tc-IDA derivatives [23] However, intestinal excretion may not be seen if the total bilirubin level is >6 mg/dL. BA is more likely if excretion into the intestinal tract is not observed (Fig. 19.5); however, delayed excretion or a false negative result due to neonatal hepatitis can make it difficult to distinguish between BA and neonatal hepatitis.

In a meta-analysis of 81 studies between 1981 and 2011, Kianifar et al [25] reported an overall sensitivity of 98.7% (range, 98.1%–99.2%) and specificity of 70.4% (range, 68.5%–72.2%) of HS for the diagnosis of BA. In a meta-analysis in 18 studies between 1985 and 2016, Wang et al

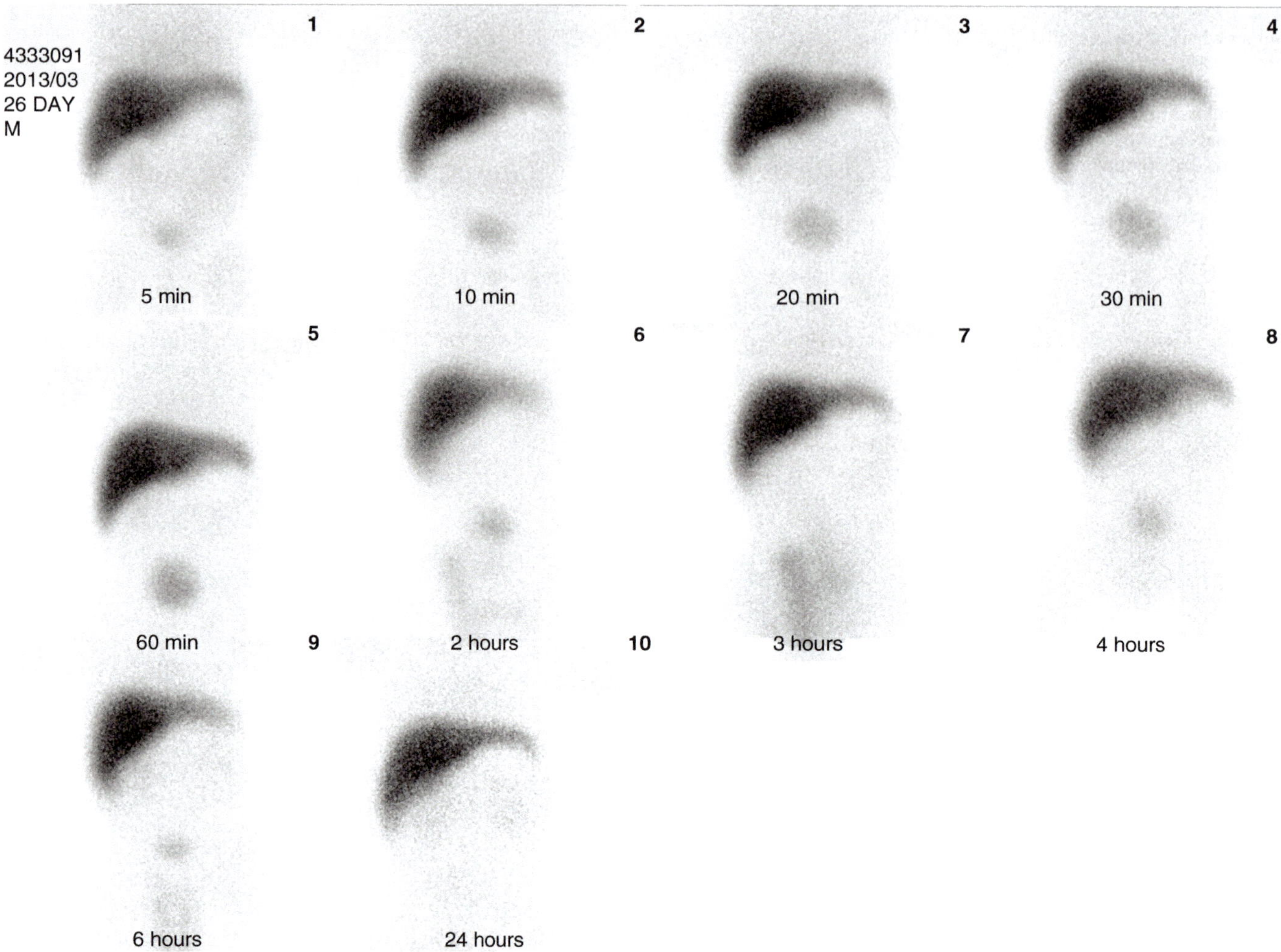


**Fig. 19.5** True-positive BA in a 3-week-old infant. $^{99m}$Tc-PMT trace shows normal uptake in the liver at 5 minutes after injection, but no intestinal excretion was visualized at 24 hours

[26] reported the pooled sensitivity of 96% (range, 94%–97%) and pooled specificity of 73% (70%–76%) of HS for the diagnosis of BA. Two $^{99m}$Tc-PMT scintigraphy studies [22, 24] performed in Japan both showed the sensitivity of 100%, but specificity was 82.4% and 53.3%, respectively.

Hepatobiliary scintigraphy suffers from low specificity, which means that false-positive results are a major shortcoming in neonatal hepatitis [24]. Tsuda et al [24] reported that HS in combination with serum γ-GTP level monitoring could reduce the number of false positives. Phenobarbital is sometimes given prior to HS to increase the specificity of HS [27]. However, another study reported no improvement with phenobarbital [28]. Because the use of phenobarbital is time consuming, it is less suitable for patients in whom an early diagnosis is required.

In terms of temporal resolution, Guan et al and Zhou et al [29, 30] reported that 6-hour HS has the same diagnostic effect as traditional 24-hour HS.

### 19.2.5 Computed Tomography

Computed tomography (CT) and contrast-enhanced CT are not reported as effective for diagnosing BA, but can be performed to evaluate anatomical abnormalities such as BASM syndrome.

### 19.2.6 Magnetic Resonance Cholangiopancreatography

Magnetic resonance cholangiopancreatography (MRCP) is a noninvasive technique for visualizing the biliary system, including the intrahepatic bile duct, extrahepatic bile duct, and primary branches of the gallbladder. If a normal biliary system is confirmed by visualization of the biliary system, BA can be ruled out. In MRI of infants and children, useful information cannot be obtained without deep sedation, which has its own risks, and informed consent from the caregiver is required. Liu et al evaluated the diagnostic value of 3-dimensional MRCP for BA in a large cohort of cholestatic infants and neonates, and they reported the specificity of 36% and sensitivity of 99% [31].

Wang et al [26] reported the sensitivity of 96% and specificity of 58% for MRI diagnosis of BA in a meta-analysis of 5 studies conducted between 2002 and 2014. Although previous studies reported that MRI had low specificity for the diagnosis of BA, more recent studies have reported improvements in sensitivity and specificity. Kim et al [32] specified three MRI features (visibility of CBD, abnormality of GB, and triangular cord thickness >5.1 mm) as good discriminators for the diagnosis of BA, and an MRI-based decision tree using these findings showed the sensitivity of 97.3%, specificity of 94.8%, and accuracy of 96.2%.

Lin et al [33] postulated that the presence of an enlarged T2-hyperintense structure at the porta hepatis might be an alternative quantitative MRI measurement for diagnosis of BA, particularly when the US or other image findings are inconclusive. The optimum cutoff value of the enlarged T2-hyperintense structure for diagnosing BA was 3.1 mm, for sensitivity of 98% and specificity of 98%.

When US or other imaging findings are inconclusive, MRI may be an alternative useful quantitative measure for the diagnosis of BA.

### 19.2.7 Endoscopic Retrograde Cholangiopancreatography

Endoscopic retrograde cholangiopancreatography (ERCP) has become safer, with less complications even in infants, due to the reduced size of endoscopes and development of instruments. However, as it requires high technical expertise under general anesthesia and carries a substantial risk of complications, ERCP should be undertaken only at a center experienced in performing this procedure in infants [34], and only if a proper diagnosis cannot be made by less invasive examinations [34]. If ERCP is chosen, a surgical intervention must be prepared in time.

Shanmugam et al [35] reported the high sensitivity (100%) and specificity (87.5%) of ERCP in differentiating BA from other forms of neonatal jaundice. They reported that clinical complications can be effectively avoided, and a low rate of technical failure (6%). Keil et al [36] reported the sensitivity of 86% and specificity of 94% of ERCP for the diagnosis of BA. Cannulation of the papilla failed in 9 of 104 patients (7.7%). Negm et al [37] reported that ERCP was successful in 224 of 251 patients (89.2%) and failed in 10.8%, with no procedure-related complications. Sensitivity of ERCP for diagnosing BA was 100% and specificity was 78.5%.

### 19.2.8 Percutaneous Cholecystocholangiography/diagnostic Laparoscopy and Laparoscopic Cholangiography

#### 19.2.8.1 Percutaneous Cholecystocholangiography (PTCC)

PTCC can exclude BA in patients with suspected BA but in whom the US findings are negative or equivocal and gallbladder length is >1.5 cm on US.

PTCC is an invasive procedure that requires moderate sedation or general anesthesia, but is less invasive for infants compared with laparoscopic cholangiography. It may be a safe and effective tool for early exclusion of BA in infants in whom BA is clinically suspected but the US findings are equivocal. PTCC could prevent unnecessary laparoscopic cholangiography [38].

Jensen et al [39] reported the sensitivity of 100% and specificity of 86% of PTTC for the diagnosis of BA. PTCC was not attempted in 7/53 patients (13%) because hepatic US performed at the time of PTCC failed to identify a GB. Complications occurred in 4/46 (8.7%) who underwent PTCC. No failures and no complications are reported in the studies of Nwomeh et al [40] and Lee et al [41].

PTCC can reduce the need for more invasive diagnostic procedures such as exploratory laparotomy. However, strict selection criteria must be used to prevent failure of this procedure, including US identification of gallbladder size.

#### 19.2.8.2 Diagnostic Laparoscopy and Laparoscopic Cholangiography

Laparoscopic cholangiography is reported to be as invasive as PTCC, and can avoid unnecessary laparotomy [42]. The gallbladder hitch technique (which corresponds to atrophic gallbladder) has been reported and its success rate is increasing [43, 44]. The usefulness of diagnostic laparoscopy has been reported previously [45–48]. It can be used to diagnose BA and enables radical surgery to be performed quickly. Compared with needle biopsy, laparoscopic assessment has the advantage of a thorough assessment of the entire liver, gallbladder, CBD, and hepatic hilum, using magnified inspection. Zhou et al [48] reported the value of hepatic subcapsular spider-like telangiectasia sign observed by laparoscopy in diagnosing BA, with an accuracy of 100% and specificity of 97.8%.

### 19.2.9 Preoperative Percutaneous Liver Biopsy

Preoperative percutaneous liver biopsy is generally performed for the differential diagnosis of BA if the diagnosis is inconclusive by other tests, including percutaneous cholangiography. Although it is reported to have the highest correct diagnosis rate among all tests, it is invasive and the frequency of complications is 6.9%–18% [49, 50]. The complications include bleeding, pain, peritoneum, hemothorax, pneumothorax, and pleural effusion. In addition, the collected biopsy material may be inadequate, and the interval needed to repeat a biopsy may have an adverse effect on bile drainage [51]. The pathological diagnosis of BA is problematic due to histological changes over time, the overlapping of histological features in the many diseases that cause cholestasis in infants, and the lengthy time to complete the pathological evaluation (2–3 days).

A meta-analysis of 22 studies (n = 1231) by Lee et al [52] conducted between 1967 and 2014 showed the pooled sensitivity of 91.2% and pooled specificity of 93.0%.

Russo et al [53] reported the sensitivity of 88.4% and specificity of 92.7% for the diagnosis of BA in 227 needle biopsies. The meta-analysis of 11 studies (n = 646) by Wang et al [26] between 1985 and 2016 reported the pooled sensitivity of 98% and specificity of 93%. The Japanese Guidelines for the Medical Treatment of Biliary Atresia [54] recommend that pre-operative liver biopsy should not be performed because it delays radical surgery and interferes with early treatment.

## References


1. Davenport M, Tizzard S, Underhill J, et al. The biliary atresia splenic malformation: A 28-year single-center retrospective review. J Pediatr. 2006;149:393–400.
2. Nizery L, Chardot C, Sissaoui S, et al. Biliary atresia: Clinical advances and perspectives. Clin Res Hepatol Gastroenterol. 2016;40:281–7.
3. Tanaka H, Sasaki H, Wada M, et al. Postnatal management of prenatally diagnosed biliary cystic malformation. J Pediatr Surg. 2015;50:507–10.
4. Zhou L, Shan Q, Tian W, et al. Ultrasound for the diagnosis of biliary atresia: A meta-analysis. AJR. 2016;206:W73–82.
5. Yoon HM, Suh CH, Kim JR, et al. Diagnostic performance of sonographic features in patients with biliary atresia: A systematic review and meta-analysis. J Ultrasound Med. 2017;36:2027–38.
6. Zhou L-Y, Wang W, Shan Q-Y, et al. Optimizing the US diagnosis of biliary atresia with a modified triangular cord thickness and gallbladder classification. Radiology. 2015;277:181–91.
7. Kim S-S, Kim M-J, Lee M-J, et al. Ultrasonographic findings of type IIIa biliary atresia. Ultrasonography. 2014;33:267–74.
8. El-Guindi MA-S, Sira MM, Konsowa HA-S, et al. Value of hepatic subcapsular flow by color Doppler ultrasonography in the diagnosis of biliary atresia. J Gastroenterol Hepatol. 2013;28:867–72.
9. Kim WS, Cheon JE, Youn BJ, et al. Hepatic arterial diameter measured with US: adjunct for US diagnosis of biliary atresia. Radiology. 2007;245:49–55.
10. Lee MS, Kim M-J, Lee MJ, et al. Biliary atresia: Color Doppler US findings in neonates and infants. Radiology. 2009;252:282–9.
11. dos Santos JL, da Silveira TR, da Silva VD, et al. Medial thickening of hepatic artery branches in biliary atresia. A morphometric study. J Pediatr Surg. 2005;40:637–42.
12. Sun C, Wu B, Pan J, et al. Hepatic subcapsular flow as a significant diagnostic marker for biliary atresia: A meta-analysis. Dis Markers. 2020;5262565 https://doi.org/10.1155/2020/5262565.
13. Leschied JR, Dillman JR, Bilhartz J, et al. Shear wave elastography helps differentiate biliary atresia from other neonatal/infantile liver diseases. Pediatr Radiol. 2015;45:366–75.
14. Wang X, Qian L, Jia L, et al. Utility of shear wave elastography for differentiating biliary atresia from infantile hepatitis syndrome. J Ultrasound Med. 2016;35:1475–9.
15. Zhou L-Y, Jiang H, Shan Q-Y, et al. Liver stiffness measurements with supersonic shear wave elastography in the diagnosis of biliary atresia: a comparative study with grey-scale US. Eur Radiol. 2017;27:3474–84.
16. Duan X, Peng Y, Liu W, et al. Does supersonic shear wave elastography help differentiate biliary atresia from other causes of cholestatic hepatitis in infants less than 90 days old? Compared with Grey-Scale US. BioMed Res Int. 2019;2019:9036362. https://doi.org/10.1155/2019/9036362.
17. Dillman JR, DiPaola F, Smith SJ, et al. Prospective assessment of ultrasound shear wave elastography for discriminating biliary atresia from other causes of neonatal cholestasis. J Pediatr. 2019;212:60–5.
18. Larrosa-Haro A, Caro-López AM, Coello-Ramírez P, et al. Duodenal tube test in the diagnosis of biliary atresia. J Pediatr Gastroenterol Nutr. 2001;32:311–5.
19. Meisheri IV, Kasat LS, Kumar A, et al. Duodenal intubation and test for bile – a reliable method to rule out biliary atresia. Pediatr Surg Int. 2002;18:392–5.
20. Boskovic A, Kitic I, Prokic D, et al. Predictive value of hepatic ultrasound, liver biopsy, and duodenal tube test in the diagnosis of extrahepatic biliary atresia in Serbian infants. Turk J Gastroenterol. 2014;25:170–4.
21. Fukuoka T, Bessho K, Tachibana M, et al. Total bile acid concentration in duodenal fluid is a useful preoperative screening marker to rule out biliary atresia. J Pediatr Gastroenterol Nutr. 2018;67:383–7.
22. Yoshii D, Inomata Y, Yamamoto H, et al. The duodenal tube test is more specific than hepatobiliary scintigraphy for identifying bile excretion in the differential diagnosis of biliary atresia. Surg Today. 2020;20 https://doi.org/10.1007/s00595-020-02010-w.
23. Kato-Azuma M. Tc-99m(Sn)-N-Pyridoxylaminates: A new series of hepatobiliary imaging agents. J Nucl Med. 1982;23:517–27.
24. Tsuda N, Shiraishi S, Sakamoto F, et al. Tc-99m PMT scintigraphy in the diagnosis of pediatric biliary atresia. Jap J Radiol. 2019;37:841–9.
25. Kianifar HR, Tehranian S, Shojaci P, et al. Accuracy of hepatobiliary scintigraphy for differentiation of neonatal hepatitis from biliary atresia: systematic review and meta-analysis of the literature. Pediatr Radiol. 2013;43:905–19.
26. Wang L, Yang Y, Chen Y, et al. Early differential diagnosis methods of biliary atresia: a meta-analysis. Pediatr Surg Int. 2018;34:363–80.
27. Kwatra N, Shalaby-Rana E, Narayanan S, et al. Phenobarbital-enhanced hepatobiliary scintigraphy in the diagnosis of biliary atresia: two decades of experience at a tertiary center. Pediatr Radiol. 2013;43:1365–75.
28. Malik D, Khan SH, Ali SW, et al. Comparison of phenobarbitone and ursodeoxycholic acid in drug-augmented hepatobiliary scintigraphy for excluding the diagnosis of obstructive cholestasis in neonatal cholestasis syndrome. Nucl Med Commun. 2015;36:827–32.
29. Guan YX, Chen Q, Wan SH, et al. Effect of different time phases of radionuclide hepatobiliary scintigraphy on the differential diagnosis of congenital biliary atresia. Genet Mol Res. 2015;14:3862–8.
30. Zhou H, Li J, Wei H, et al. A novel timesaving and semiquantitative method for radionuclide hepatobiliary scintigraphy for suspected biliary atresia. Ann Palliat Med. 2020;9:63–9.

31. Liu B, Cai J, Xu Y, et al. Three-dimensional magnetic resonance cholangiopancreatography for the diagnosis of biliary atresia in infants and neonates. PLoS One. 2014;9(2):e88268. doi:10.1371
32. Kim YH, Kim M, Shin HJ, et al. MRI-based decision tree model for diagnosis of biliary atresia. Europ Radiol. 2018;28:3422–31.
33. Lin DC, Wu KY, Sun FJ, et al. A quantitative image analysis using MRI for diagnosis of biliary atresia. Clin Imaging. 2019;53:186–90.
34. Moyer V, Freese DK, Whitington PF, et al. Guideline for the evaluation of cholestatic jaundice in infants: recommendations of the North American Society for Pediatric Gastroenterology, Hepatology and Nutrition. J Pediatr Gastroenterol Nutr. 2004;39:115–28.
35. Shanmugam NP, Harrison PM, Devlin J, et al. Selective use of endoscopic retrograde cholangiopancreatography in the diagnosis of biliary atresia in infants younger than 100 days. J Pediatr Gastroenterol Nutr. 2009;49:435–41.
36. Keil R, Snajdauf J, Rygl M, et al. Diagnostic efficacy of ERCP in cholestatic infants and neonates – a retrospective study on a large series. Endoscopy. 2010;42:121–6.
37. Negm AA, Petersen C, Markowski A, et al. The role of endoscopic retrograde cholangiopancreatography in the diagnosis of biliary atresia: 14 years' experience. Eur J Pediatr Surg. 2018;28:261–7.
38. Zhou L, Chen S, Chen H, et al. Percutaneous US-guided cholecystocholangiography with microbubbles for assessment of infants with US findings equivocal for biliary atresia and gallbladder longer than 1.5 cm: A pilot study. Radiology. 2018;286:1033–9.
39. Jensen MK, Biank VF, Moe DC, et al. HIDA, percutaneous transhepatic cholecysto-cholangiography and liver biopsy in infants with persistent jaundice: can a combination of PTCC and liver biopsy reduce unnecessary laparotomy? Pediatr Radiol. 2012;42:32–9.
40. Nwomeh BC, Caniano DA, Hogan M. Definitive exclusion of biliary atresia in infants with cholestatic jaundice: the role of percutaneous cholecysto-cholangiography. Pediatr Surg Int. 2007;23:845–9.
41. Lee SY, Kim GC, Choe B, et al. Efficacy of US-guided percutaneous cholecystocholangiography for the early exclusion and type determination of biliary atresia. Radiology. 2011;261:916–22.
42. Huang L, Wang W, Liu G, et al. Laparoscopic cholecystocholangiography for diagnosis of prolonged jaundice in infants, experience of 144 cases. Pediatr Surg Int. 2010;26:711–5.
43. Houben CH, Wong HY, Mou WC, et al. Hitching the gallbladder in laparoscopic-assisted cholecystocholangiography: a simple technique. Pediatr Surg Int. 2013;29:953–5.
44. Kishore R, Kisku SMC, Thomas RJ, et al. Laparoscopic cholangiogram in biliary atresia: a refinement in the gallbladder hitch technique. Pediatr Surg Int. 2018;34:395–8.
45. Senyüz OF, Yeşildağ E, Emir H, et al. Diagnostic laparoscopy in prolonged jaundice. J Pediatr Surg. 2001;36:463–5.
46. Alkan M, Tutus K, Fakıoglu E, et al. Laparoscopy-assisted percutaneous cholangiography in biliary atresia diagnosis: Comparison with open technique. Gastroenterol Res Pract. 2016;2016:5637072.
47. Okazaki T, Ochi T, Nakamura H, et al. Needle liver biopsy has potential for delaying Kasai portoenterostomy and is obsolete for diagnosing biliary atresia in the laparoscopic era. J Pediatr Surg. 2019;54:2570–3.
48. Zhou Y, Jiang M, Tang S-T, et al. Laparoscopic finding of a hepatic subcapsular spider-like telangiectasis sign in biliary atresia. World J Gastroenterol. 2017;23:7119–28.
49. Azzam RK, Alonso EM, Emerick KM, et al. Safety of percutaneous liver biopsy in infants less than three months old. J Pediatr Gastroenterol Nutr. 2005;41:639–43.
50. Chaudhry Z, Forget S, Nguyen V-H, et al. The role of liver biopsy in investigation of cholestatic liver disease in infancy. Journal of the Canadian Association of Gastroenterology. 2019;2:51–6.
51. Lemoine C, Melin-Aldana H, Brandt K, et al. The evolution of early liver biopsy findings in babies with jaundice may delay the diagnosis and treatment of biliary atresia. J Pediatr Surg. 2020;55:866–72.
52. Lee JYJ, Sullivan K, El Demellawy D, et al. The value of preoperative liver biopsy in the diagnosis of extrahepatic biliary atresia: A systematic review and meta-analysis. J Pediatr Surg. 2016;51:753–61.
53. Russo P, Magee JC, Anders RA, et al. Key histopathological features of liver biopsies that distinguish biliary atresia from other causes of infantile cholestasis and their correlation with outcome: a multicenter study. Am J Surg Pathol. 2016;40:1601–15.
54. Guidelines for the Medical Treatment of Biliary Atresia. Japanese Biliary Atresia Society. 2018. Herusu Shuppan, Co. Inc. pp. 40-58 (in Japanese)

# 20 Preoperative Management and Direct Cholangiography

Yasushi Fuchimoto

**Abstract**

Biliary atresia is the absence of bile excretion, which is important for fat absorption. For this reason, a fat-soluble vitamin deficiency is often found at the time of diagnosis. Among the fat-soluble vitamins, vitamin K is a particular problem at the time of surgery. Since vitamin K is closely related to blood coagulation, it is important to supplement the patient with sufficient vitamin K preoperatively to stop the bleeding tendency during radical surgery. Fresh frozen plasma (FFP) is also necessary to prevent the tendency to bleed intraoperatively.

Ultrasonography, hepatobiliary scintigraphy, and duodenal fluid testing are often used to diagnose biliary atresia. If biliary atresia is suspected on these evaluations, the final diagnosis must be made by means of exploratory laparotomy and intraoperative cholangiography. Intraoperative cholangiography is usually performed by cannulation into the gallbladder. Intraoperative cholangiography is not only useful for the definitive diagnosis of biliary atresia, but also plays an important role in the classification of the disease and is useful in predicting the prognosis and determining postoperative treatment. However, there are cases in which the gallbladder is so highly atrophic that cholangiography is not possible.

**Keywords**

Fat-soluble vitamin · Vitamin K · Coagulability
Intraoperative cholangiogram · Intrahepatic bile ducts
Extrahepatic bile ducts

Y. Fuchimoto (✉)
Department of Pediatric Surgery, IUHW School of Medicine, Narita, Japan
e-mail: yfuchimoto@iuhw.ac.jp

## 20.1 Preoperative Management

In biliary atresia, fat-soluble vitamins are often poorly absorbed due to bile stasis; therefore, vitamin A, D, E, and K supplementation should be considered. Particularly, Vitamin K is important to improve the coagulation function and should be administered intravenously (vitamin K2 supplementation, 2 mg/dose iv intravenously for 2 days before surgery).

As preoperative bowel preparation, the patient should not eat for 24 hours before the operation, and an enema should be administered the night before the operation and the morning of the operation. Antibiotics should be administered prior to the operation. Two units of MAP and two units of FFP should be kept ready for transfusion.

## 20.2 Direct Cholangiography

In cases of suspected biliary atresia, blood investigations and imaging studies are performed. Ultrasonography, hepatobiliary scintigraphy, and duodenal fluid examination are usually performed. Recently, ERCP and PTC for evaluating biliary ducts have been suggested [1, 2, 3, 4, 5]; however, these procedures are often difficult to perform because of their technical and invasive nature. If the gallbladder is of normal size, the laparoscopic procedure might be minimally invasive [6].

The differential diagnosis of biliary atresia includes infantile hepatitis and bile duct paucity. Recent advances in fetal ultrasonography have led to an increasing number of cases in which it is difficult to differentiate biliary atresia [7, 8] from congenital bile duct dilatation for cysts of the biliary system in the neonatal period. Early and accurate diagnosis is necessary because the treatment of the two diseases is quite different.

Cholangiography helps to evaluate the patency of the intrahepatic bile ducts and the bile ducts on the duodenal side and reveals the presence or absence of extrahepatic bile duct obstruction [9]. To confirm the diagnosis, lapa-


M. Nio (ed.), *Introduction to Biliary Atresia*, https://doi.org/10.1007/978-981-16-2160-4_20

rotomy and intraoperative cholangiography should be performed, and if a cholestatic obstruction is present, Kasai surgery (hilar jejunal anastomosis) should be performed as soon as possible.

Cholangiography is also an essential test to determine the type of disease as it has been reported that cholangiography findings are useful in predicting the prognosis. Nio et al. reported a significantly higher rate of transplant-free survival and overall survival with types I and I cysts compared to types II and III [10]. Furthermore, Karrer et al. reported that cholangiographic findings strongly influenced survival. Proximal duct patency (correctable) was found to have the best prognosis, followed by patent distal ducts, while totally obliterated extrahepatic ducts had the worst prognosis (5-year survival rates of 62%, 38%, and 72%, respectively) [11].

The method of intraoperative cholangiography is shown. The abdomen was opened, an incision was made in the gallbladder, a 4 Fr polyvinyl chloride tube was inserted, and a 4–0 suture was placed around the insertion site with the help of a drawstring suture. If the gallbladder is atrophic and the catheter cannot be inserted easily, a 22- or 24-G indwelling venous needle tube is inserted. The contrast was injected with Urografin 60% (Bayer). Care must be taken to avoid the contamination of the catheter with air.

Biliary atresia is classified into two main types: no bile ducts in the liver (type II or III) (Fig. 20.1) or bile ducts in the liver (type I or Icyst) (Fig. 20.2) by contract images from the gallbladder. Nio et al. stated that intrahepatic bile duct structures (type I or I cysts) were further classified as cloudy, tree, or mixed types (Fig. 20.3), with survival rates of 50%, 100%, and 97%, respectively, without transplantation [10]. The cloudy type, in which the preexisting dendritic structure is lost, is considered as the typical intrahepatic bile duct finding in biliary atresia. However, there are more than a few cases in which the existing intrahepatic bile ducts connected to the hepatic ducts are partially preserved. Therefore, a certain percentage of tree-type cases with extensive preexisting intrahepatic bile ducts might involve congenital biliary dilatation rather than biliary atresia. Type II is a rare main type, but in some cases, the intrahepatic bile ducts on contrast image from the common hepatic duct show a tree-type

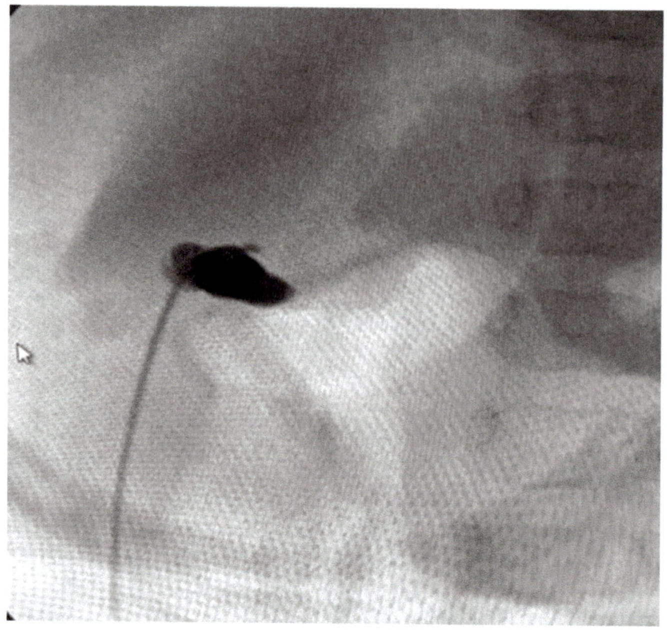

Fig. 20.1 Intrahepatic bile ducts are not visualized by contract images from the gallbladder (type II or III)

(Fig. 20.4). The intrahepatic bile ducts in biliary atresia may show a variety of images, as shown by contrast image findings of type I cyst intrahepatic bile ducts (Figs. 20.2a, 20.2b, and 20.2c).

Among the cases in which the hilar bile ducts are grossly combined in a woven mass, there is a type I or I cyst in which the intrahepatic bile ducts appear on cholangiography. In these cases, the diagnosis was type III based on the gross findings alone. Therefore, cholangiography, regardless of the gross findings, is essential for an accurate diagnosis [12, 13].

A high incidence of abnormalities in pancreatic and bile duct maljunction is found as a secondary finding in the lower bile duct classification of patent common bile duct as subtype "a" (Fig. 20.5). Furthermore, the lower bile duct classification subtype "d" shows a cystic structure that does not communicate with the intrahepatic bile ducts. Therefore, cystography can be used to determine whether the patient has a type III-d or type II common bile duct by performing a cystogram if the cyst is found in the extrahepatic bile ducts (Fig. 20.6).

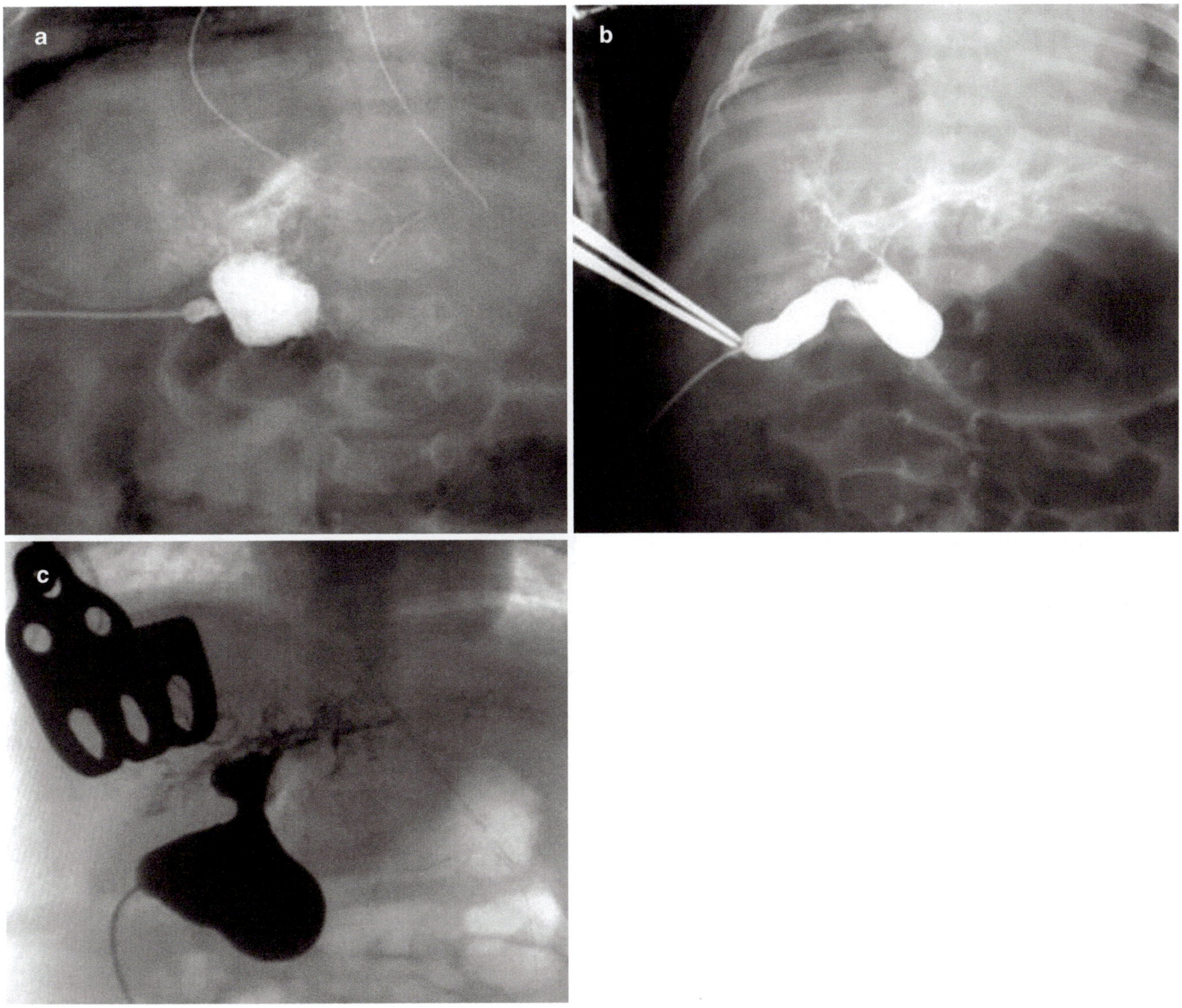



**Fig. 20.2** (**a**, **b**, **c**) Intrahepatic bile ducts of type I cyst by contract images from the gallbladder, show a variety of images, although they are extremely small

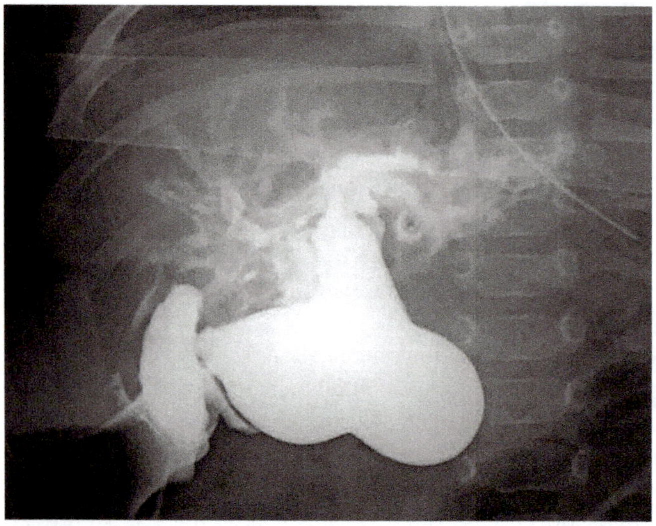

Fig. 20.3 Intrahepatic bile duct finding in I cyst mixed type

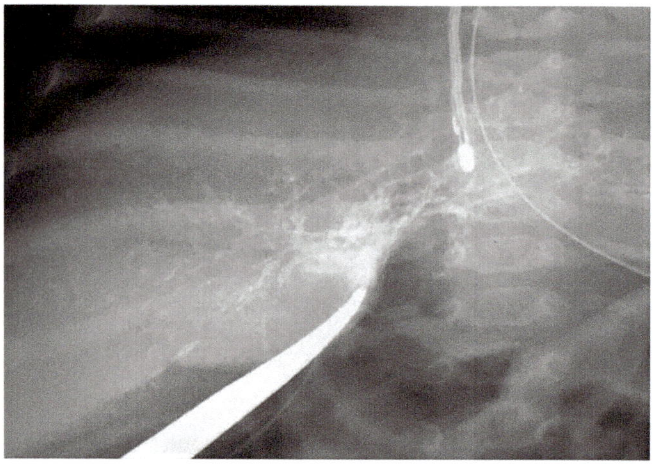

Fig. 20.4 Intrahepatic bile duct finding in Type II tree-type

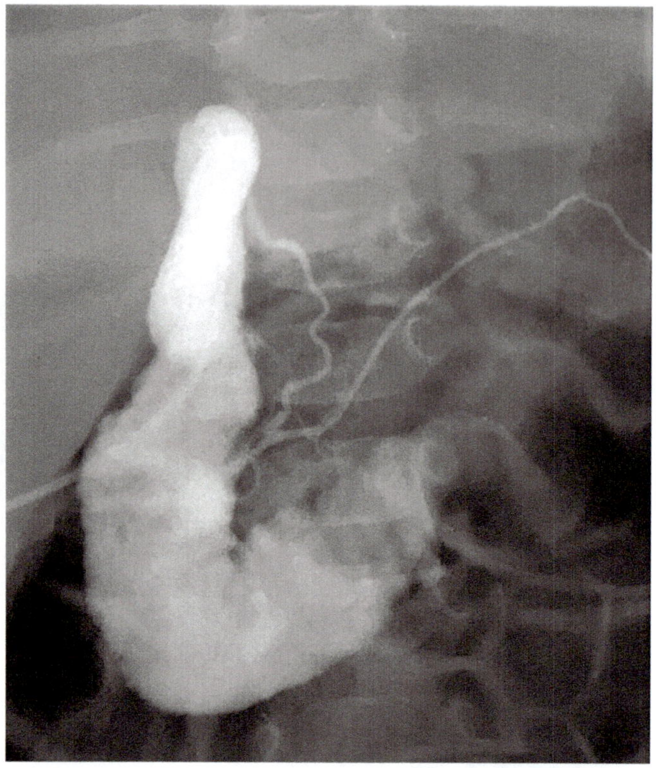

Fig. 20.5 The subtype "a" indicates patency of the distal common bile duct. In this case, it is accompanied by pancreatic and bile duct maljunction

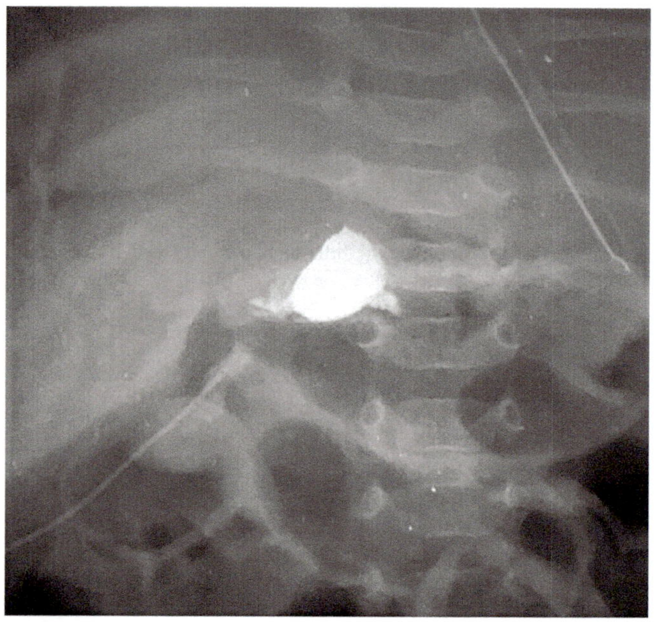

Fig. 20.6 The figure shows a cyst in the extrahepatic bile duct, which is classified as type III , subtype "d", because it does not communicate with the intrahepatic bile duct and the distal common bile duct is unclear

## References


1. Howard ER, Nunnerley HB. Percutaneous cholangiography in prolonged jaundice of childhood. J R Soc Med. 1979;72(7):495–502.
2. Shanmugam NP, Harrison PM, Devlin J, Peddu P, Knisely AS, Davenport M, et al. Selective use of endoscopic retrograde cholangiopancreatography in the diagnosis of biliary atresia in infants younger than 100 days. J Pediatr Gastroenterol Nutr. 2009;49(4):435–41.
3. Liu B, Cai J, Xu Y, Peng X, Zheng H, Huang K, et al. Three-dimensional magnetic resonance cholangiopancreatography for the diagnosis of biliary atresia in infants and neonates. PLoS One. 2014;9(2):e88268.
4. Parra D, Fecteau A, Daneman A. Findings in percutaneous cholangiography in two cases of type III cystic biliary atresia (with ultrasound correlation). BJR Case Rep. 2016;2(2):20150377.
5. Saito T, Terui K, Mitsunaga T, Nakata M, Kuriyama Y, Higashimoto Y, et al. Role of pediatric endoscopic retrograde cholangiopancreatography in an era stressing less-invasive imaging modalities. J Pediatr Gastroenterol Nutr. 2014;59(2):204–9.
6. Alkan M, Tutus K, Fakioglu E, Ozden O, Hatipoglu Z, Iskit SH, et al. Laparoscopy-assisted percutaneous cholangiography in biliary atresia diagnosis: comparison with open technique. Gastroenterol Res Pract. 2016;2016:5637072.
7. Davenport M, Hadzic N. Prenatal diagnosis of liver and biliary tract disease. Semin Neonatol. 2003;8(5):347–55.
8. Okada T, Sasaki F, Ueki S, Hirokata G, Okuyama K, Cho K, et al. Postnatal management for prenatally diagnosed choledochal cysts. J Pediatr Surg. 2004;39(7):1055–8.
9. Hays DM, Woolley MM, Snyder WH Jr, Reed GGJ, Landing BH. Diagnosis of biliary atresia: relative accuracy of percutaneous liver biopsy, open liver biopsy, and operative cholangiography. J Pediatr. 1967;71(4):598–607.
10. Nio M, Sano N, Ishii T, Sasaki H, Hayashi Y, Ohi R. Long-term outcome in type I biliary atresia. J Pediatr Surg. 2006;41(12):1973–5.
11. Karrer FM, Lilly JR, Stewart BA, Hall RJ. Biliary atresia registry, 1976 to 1989. J Pediatr Surg 1990;25(10):1076–1080; discussion 81.
12. Hasegawa T, Sasaki T, Kimura T, Sawai T, Nose K, Kamata S, et al. Prenatal ultrasonographic appearance of type IIId (uncorrectable type with cystic dilatation) biliary atresia. Pediatr Surg Int. 2002;18(5–6):425–8.
13. Masumoto K, Kai H, Oka Y, Otake R, Yoshizato T, Miyamoto S, et al. A case of cystic biliary atresia with an antenatally detected cyst: the possibility of changing from a correctable type with a cystic lesion (I cyst) to an uncorrectable one (IIId). Pediatr Surg Int. 2011;27(1):99–102.

# Operative Procedures: Open Kasai Procedure

21

Masaki Nio, Hideyuki Sasaki, Ryuji Okubo, Masatoshi Hashimoto, and Yudai Nakajima

**Abstract**

In biliary atresia, the extrahepatic biliary tract is completely obstructed, showing various morphologic patterns of obstruction on a case-by-case basis. Hepaticoenterostomy is performed when the hepatic duct is sufficiently open for anastomosis with the intestinal tract (correctable type) in types I and II. However, such a disease type is rare, and Kasai portoenterostomy is performed in most cases. In this procedure, the extrahepatic biliary remnant containing obstructed bile ducts is transected at the appropriate level and removed. Then, the intestine is anastomosed to the liver tissue at the hepatic hilum covering the resected area of the removed remnant. We present our current techniques for open Kasai portoenterostomy.

**Keywords**

Biliary atresia · Kasai portoenterostomy · Operative techniques

## 21.1 Introduction

The non-correctable type of biliary atresia is a lethal disease for which surgical treatment is impossible. In 1957, Morio Kasai performed Roux-en-Y hepatic portoenterostomy as the first intentional corrective surgery for biliary atresia, namely, Kasai portoenterostomy, at Tohoku University Hospital on a babyboy with non-correctable biliary atresia [1]. The patient survived with his native liver for a very long time [2]. In the 70 years since that surgery, in addition to improvements in the outcomes of Kasai portoenterostomy, liver transplantation has also improved the surgical results of biliary atresia. Researchers recently reported that the role of liver transplantation exceeded that of Kasai portoenterostomy in the treatment of this disease [3]. However, the choice of candidates for primary liver transplantation is not always easy [4]; moreover, maintaining a good quality of life with the native liver is a great advantage for Kasai portoenterostomy. Therefore, Kasai portoenterostomy is still the first-line treatment modality for biliary atresia. One of the many efforts made by pediatric surgeons has been to improve surgical techniques in biliary atresia. In Tohoku University Hospital, various modifications of surgical procedures have been carried out by Kasai and his successors [5]. Based on this background, in this chapter, we introduce our techniques for Kasai portoenterostomy, which we currently consider to be the standard procedure in our hospital.

## 21.2 Concept of Kasai Portoenterostomy

A previous concept in biliary atresia held that the extrahepatic bile duct was primarily obstructed due to severe inflammation of unknown etiology that, if untreated, would subsequently lead to intrahepatic cholestasis and, ultimately, biliary liver cirrhosis.

Although the etiology remains unknown, the disease process has gradually been revealed. Current evidence indicates that the whole hepatobiliary system involving the liver tissue and intra- and extrahepatic biliary tree is affected by severe inflammatory insult in biliary atresia. Due to the damage of the hepatobiliary system, in addition to the destruction of the intra- and extrahepatic biliary tree, bile formation is reduced. Importantly, the changes in the hepatic parenchyma and intrahepatic bile ducts are reversible due to their regenerative nature, although obstructive changes in the damaged extrahepatic bile ducts are irreversible.

M. Nio (✉) · M. Hashimoto · Y. Nakajima
Department of Pediatric Surgery, Tohoku University Graduate School of Medicine, Sendai, Japan
e-mail: mnio@ped-surg.med.tohoku.ac.jp; hashimoto@ped-surg.med.tohoku.ac.jp; nakajima@ped-surg.med.tohoku.ac.jp

H. Sasaki · R. Okubo
Department of Pediatric Surgery, Tohoku University Graduate School of Medicine, Sendai, Japan

Secretariat of The Japanese Biliary Atresia Society, Sendai, Japan
e-mail: h-sasaki@ped-surg.med.tohoku.ac.jp; okubo@ped-surg.med.tohoku.ac.jp


M. Nio (ed.), *Introduction to Biliary Atresia*, https://doi.org/10.1007/978-981-16-2160-4_21

The intrahepatic biliary system is damaged to various degrees, with some cases showing a paucity of intralobular bile ducts in the neonatal period [6]. However, the intrahepatic biliary system is subsequently reestablished, forming a network-shaped structure of proliferative bile ducts [7]. The fine network of the intrahepatic bile ducts continues to the hepatic hilum, while the biliary drainage route is obstructed by the fibrotic extrahepatic biliary remnant present before Kasai portoenterostomy. Therefore, when the fibrous remnant, including the ends of the biliary network, is surgically removed, and hepatic portoenterostomy is performed, the bile coming from the liver tissue to the opening of the bile duct at the resected area through the biliary network collects in the anastomosed intestine [8]. This is the concept of Kasai portoenterostomy. Pediatric surgeons assist in the last step of the recovery process of this disease by making a drainage route between the hepatic hilum and intestine with appropriate techniques and timing as possible. Successful Kasai portoenterostomy allows the natural establishment of the mucosal anastomosis between the bile ducts and the intestine and, ultimately, completion of the biliary drainage route.

## 21.3 Kasai Portoenterostomy Techniques

### 21.3.1 Surgical Preparation

Before surgery, an enema is performed to empty the colon. The patient is placed in a supine position, general anesthesia is introduced, and a pillow is placed under the back to raise the surgical field of the hepatic hilum.

### 21.3.2 Confirmation of the Biliary Atresia Diagnosis and Dissection of the Extrahepatic Biliary Remnant

After confirming the diagnosis of biliary atresia by cholangiography through a small laparotomy just above the gallbladder, the wound is extended using a right subcostal (or upper abdominal transverse) incision. To gain exposure, some surgeons recommended liver mobilization by dividing the falciform and left triangular ligaments and to evert the liver outside of the abdominal cavity [9]. We do not employ this procedure as we feel that it is stressful for patients. A wedge-shaped liver biopsy specimen is obtained.

In type III cases, which show atresia at the porta hepatis and are the most common type of biliary atresia, Kasai portoenterostomy is performed. In type I (atresia of the common bile duct) and type II (atresia of the hepatic ducts), hepaticoenterostomy is performed when the hepatic duct is sufficiently open for anastomosis with the intestine. However, in some cases of types I and II, which are associated with narrowed hepatic ducts confirmed by cholangiography, redosurgery is required following hepaticoenterostomy due to insufficient postoperative bile drainage or recurrent jaundice [10]. We routinely employ Kasai portoenterostomy in such cases.

The procedure starts from the dissection of the gallbladder and cystic duct. The peritoneum of the hepatoduodenal ligament is incised and dissected, and the major vessels are identified. The cystic artery is ligated and divided, preserving the branches of the cystic artery to the right lobe of the liver as much as possible. In patients with advanced liver fibrosis, dilated lymphatic vessels occasionally run through the hepatoduodenal ligament. These lymphatic vessels are divided after coagulation or ligation because damage to these vessels may cause postoperative ascites. The left hepatic artery is then identified and taped. The right hepatic artery is then also taped. However, this artery runs behind the extrahepatic remnant in many cases and may be difficult to identify at this stage. In such cases, the fibrotic common bile duct is dissected and taped beforehand, paying attention to avoid damaging the portal vein located behind (Fig. 21.1). The fibrotic common bile duct is ligated and divided at the level of the upper margin of the duodenum. The extrahepatic biliary remnant is then dissected toward the hepatic hilum. The right hepatic artery and its branches are exposed without difficulty at this stage. When the liver parenchyma of S3 and S4 is fused to cover the round ligament of the liver, it is divided using electrocautery to open up the Rex recess and visualize the anatomy of the umbilical portion of the portal vein and the left hepatic artery. Dissection between the arterial branches and the remnant is further advanced toward the hepatic hilum. Then, the anterior surface of the portal vein is exposed, and the dissection between the portal vein and the remnant is advanced cranially and bilaterally. The right and left branches of the portal vein are not taped to avoid interfering with the portal flow during the surgery.

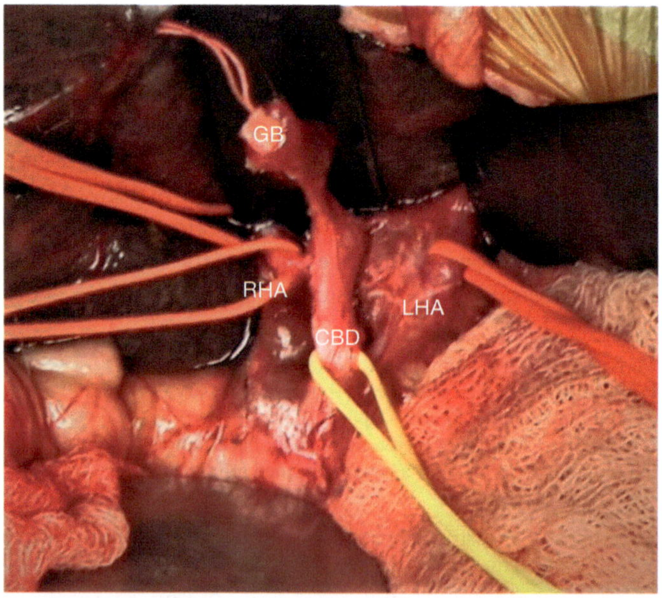

Fig. 21.1 Dissection of the hepatic artery and the fibrotic common bile duct. (CBD, common bile duct; GB, gallbladder; LHA, left hepatic artery; RHA, right hepatic artery)

Small branches of the portal vein to the caudate lobe of the liver through the remnant are carefully dissected, ligated, and divided (Fig. 21.2). Usually, 3–5 small portal branches are divided, and the caudate lobe is exposed.

### 21.3.3 Transection of the Fibrous Extrahepatic Bile Duct Remnant

Following dissection between the fibrous remnant and surrounding vessels, the remnant is then transected (Fig. 21.3). The remnant is totally removed within the range between the quadrate and the caudate lobes and between the right and left branches of the portal vein. At the central part of the remnant, small incisions are made using electrocautery along the borders between the remnant and the quadrate lobe and between the remnant and the caudate lobe. Then, the tips of a pair of right-angle forceps are placed between the remnant and the underlining liver capsule (Fig. 21.4), and the remnant is vertically divided between the tips of the forceps by electrocautery (Fig. 21.5). These techniques allow the thickness of the fibrous remnant to be evaluated during the transection of the remnant and allow total removal of the remnant without damaging the hepatic capsule. If the remnant remains after the vertical division and the liver capsule is not well exposed, the tips of the forceps are again placed beneath the remnant, and the remnant is further divided in the same way. In cases where the liver capsule is unintentionally injured during this maneuver, the transection of the remnant is started, confirming the liver capsule, paying attention not to further damage the liver capsule. The liver capsule is well exposed at the central part of the hepatic hilum between the

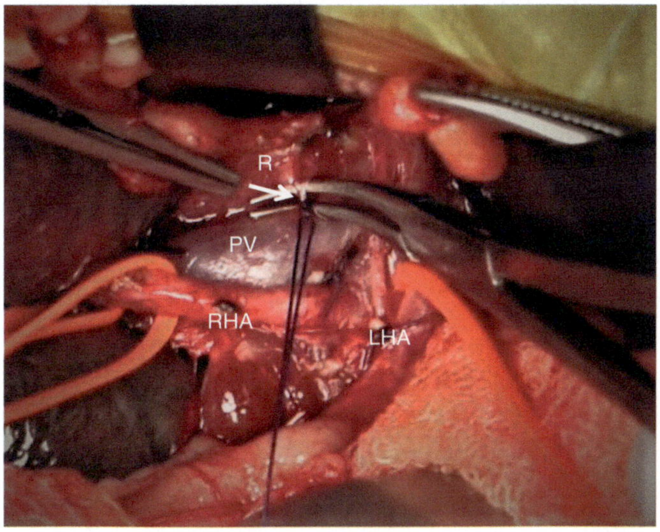


Fig. 21.2 Division of the branches of the portal vein. The venous branch (arrow) from the portal vein to the caudate lobe of the liver through the remnant. (LHA, left hepatic artery; PV, portal vein; R, remnant; RHA, right hepatic artery)

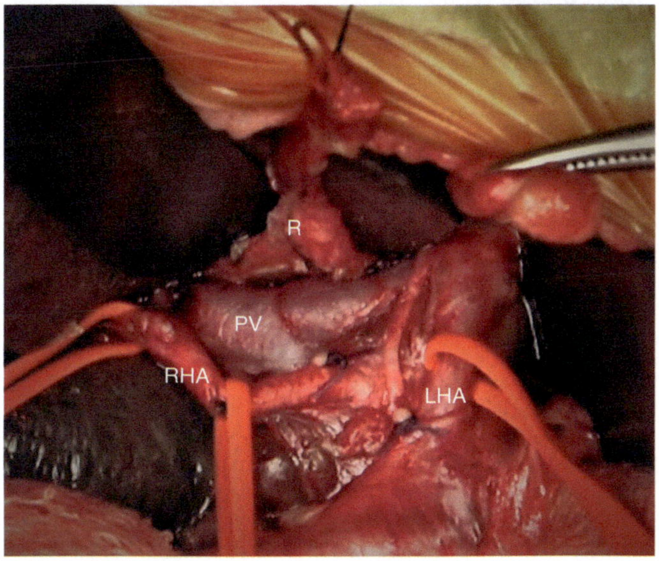


Fig. 21.3 Dissection of the extrahepatic biliary remnant. (LHA, left hepatic artery; R, remnant; RHA, right hepatic artery)

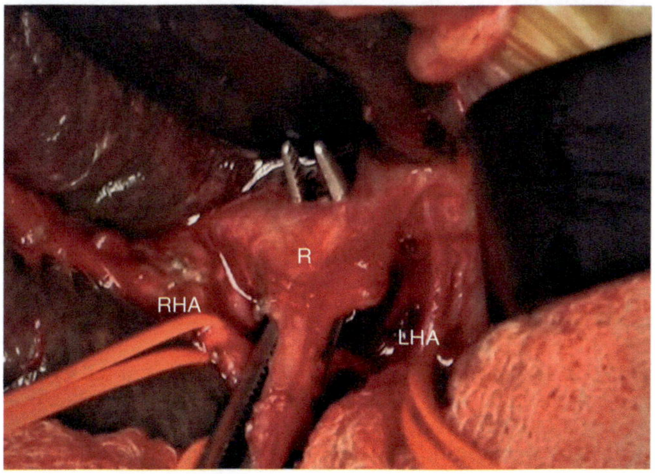


Fig. 21.4 Division of the remnant 1. Tips of a pair of right-angle forceps are placed between the remnant and the underlining liver capsule. (R, remnant)

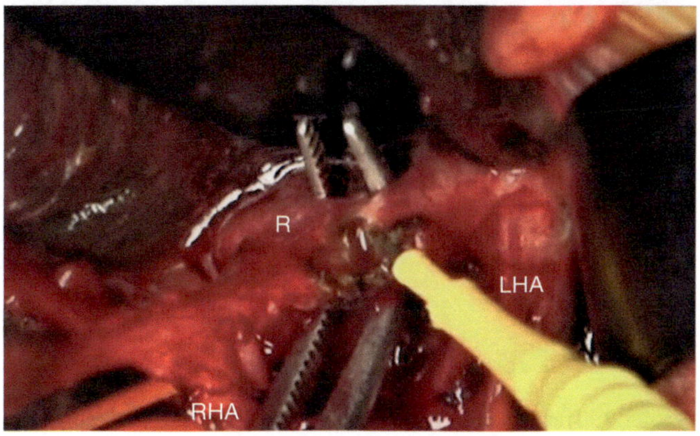


Fig. 21.5 Division of the remnant 2. The remnant (R) is vertically divided between the tips of the forceps using electrocautery. (LHA, left hepatic artery; R, remnant; RHA, right hepatic artery)

quadrate and caudate lobes. The right and left parts of the remnant are transected independently on the level of the liver capsule using scissors (Figs. 21.6, 21.7 and 21.8). No electric devices are applied at this point. Again, the transected surfaces of the remnant on both the right and left sides should be on the same plane as the surrounding liver capsule (Fig. 21.9). As the blood vessels are well separated from the remnant, only limited bleeding is encountered during and after the remnant transection. Oozing from the transected surfaces is usually controlled by irrigation with hot saline and gauze packing. The width of the transected area between the right and left portal branches is evaluated and usually ranges between 15 and 25 mm.

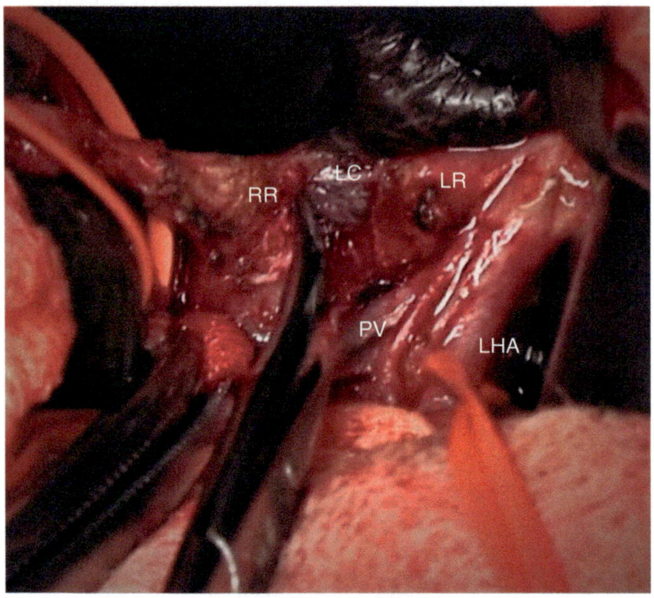


**Fig. 21.6** Transection of the remnant 1. The right part of the remnant is transected to the level of the liver capsule using scissors. (LC, liver capsule; LHA, left hepatic artery; LR, left part of the remnant; R, remnant; RHA, right hepatic artery; RR, right part of the remnant)

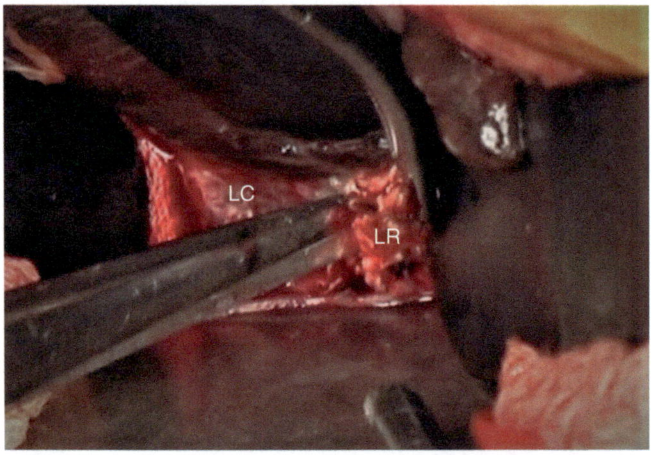


**Fig. 21.7** Transection of the remnant 2. The left part of the remnant is transected to the level of the liver capsule. (LC, liver capsule; LR, left part of the remnant)

### 21.3.4 Preparation of Roux-En-Y Limb and Creation of the Antireflux Spur Valve

While gauze packing the transected area, the Roux-en-Y limb is prepared. The second branches of the jejunal vessels are ligated and divided, and the jejunum is transected approximately 15–20 cm from the Treitz's ligament. The oral end of the jejunum is anastomosed to the side of the distal jejunum by interrupted sutures using 5-0 monofilament absorbable suture materials, preparing for 50 cm (or

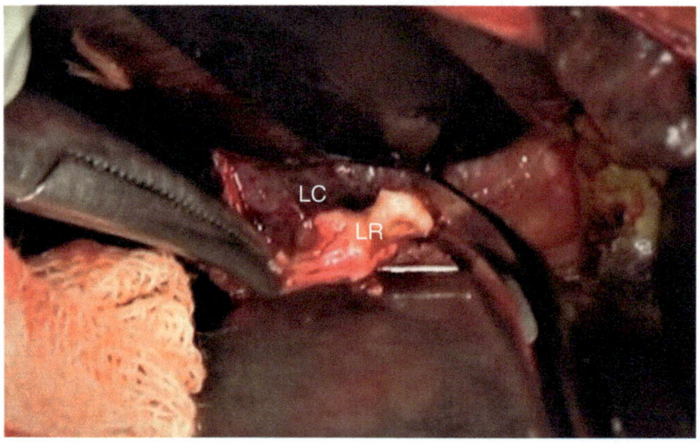


**Fig. 21.8** Transection of the remnant 3. The left part of the remnant is transected from the left side. (LC, liver capsule; LR, left part of the remnant)

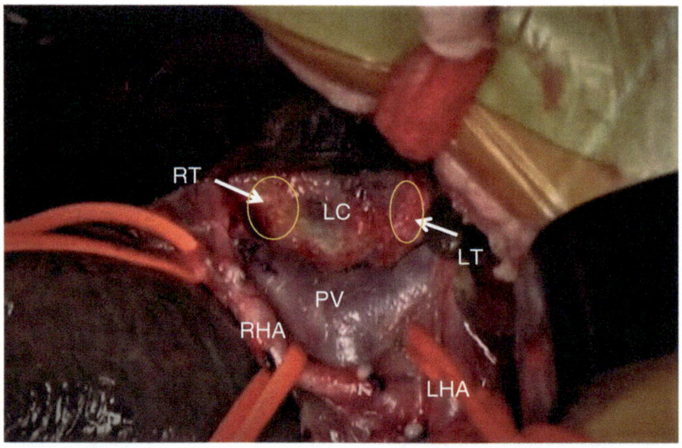


**Fig. 21.9** Transection of the remnant 4. The remnant is transected. The transected surfaces (yellow circles) of the right and left sides and the liver capsule, which is exposed between the transected surfaces, are at the same level. (LC, liver capsule; LHA, left hepatic artery; LR, left part of the remnant; LT, transected surface of the left side; R, remnant; RHA, right hepatic artery; RR, right part of the remnant; RT, transected surface of the right side)

10 cm/kg weight for patients weighing less than 5 kg) of the Roux-en-Y limb. An antireflux intestinal spur valve is then created [11]. The seromuscular layer of the Roux-en-Y limb opposed to the jejunum is hemi-circumferentially removed as far as 2 cm from the Rou-en-Y anastomosis (Figs. 21.10 and 21.11). The exposed submucosal layer of the Roux-en-Y limb is covered by the seromuscular layer of the confronting jejunal wall by interrupted sutures using 5-0 monofilament absorbable suture materials (Fig. 21.12). After valve function is confirmed, the space between the Roux-en-Y limb and jejunum is closed with several stitches. The end of the Roux-en-Y limb is raised to the hepatic hilum through the retrocolic approach. The Roux-en-Y limb is then fixed to the mesocolon by several stitches 15 cm from the end of the Roux-en-Y limb. After cannulating a catheter into the Roux-en-Y limb from the end, it is irrigated with a sufficient volume of warm saline. Kasai portoenterostomy is performed in end-to-end or end-to-back rather than end-to-side fashion to prevent long-term complications related to pouch formation following end-to-side anastomosis. The end of the Roux-en-Y limb is then trimmed and adjusted to the size of the transected area of the remnant.

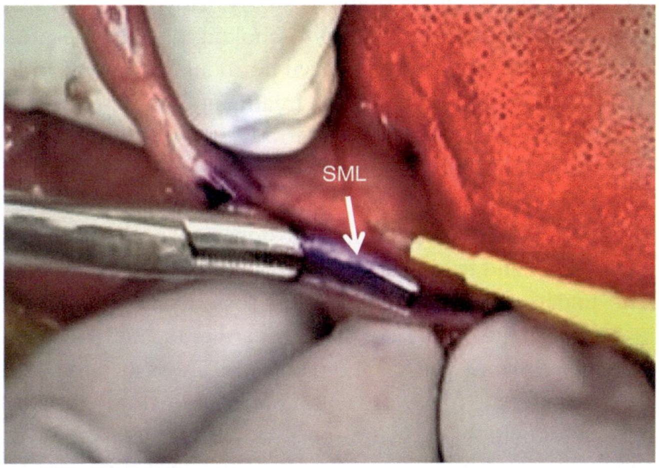


**Fig. 21.10** Creation of the spur valve 1. The seromuscular layer of the Roux-en-Y limb is dissected. (SML, seromuscular layer)

### 21.3.5 Hepatic-Portojejunostomy

Kasai portoenterostomy is performed by interrupted stitches using 5-0 monofilament absorbable suture materials. Before starting anastomosis, hemostasis from the resected surfaces is confirmed. A small amount of oozing is usually spontaneously controlled during the anastomosis of the posterior row. Stitches of the posterior row are placed between the posterior aspect of the transected area and the jejunum. Especially at both the right and left ends of the anastomosis, small and shallow stitches should be placed between the lateral side of the transected remnant and the jejunum. Attention should be paid not to place stitches on the transected surface and to avoid covering the transected surface by the anastomosed jejunum. In contrast, at the central part of the anastomosis of the posterior row, stitches are placed with sufficient bites between the caudate lobe and jejunum. A total of 8–10 stitches are placed on the posterior row, and the suture materials are then tied in order from the center to both the right and left sides (Fig. 21.13). Before starting the anastomosis of

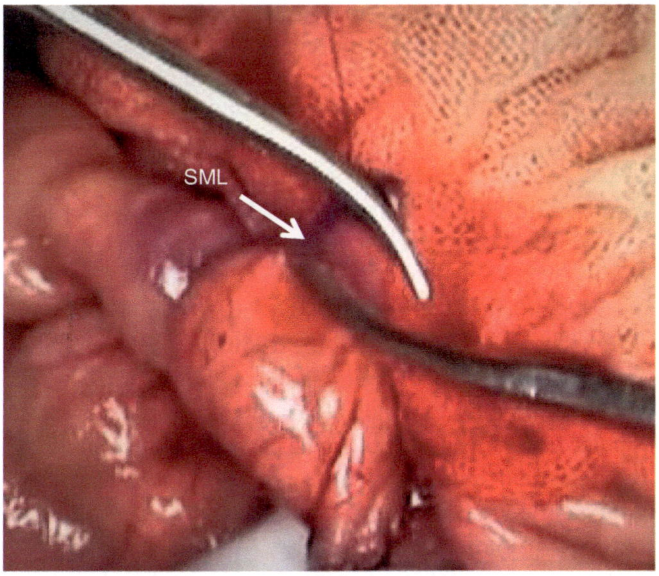


**Fig. 21.11** Creation of the spur valve 2. The seromuscular layer is hemi-circumferentially removed. (SML, seromuscular layer)

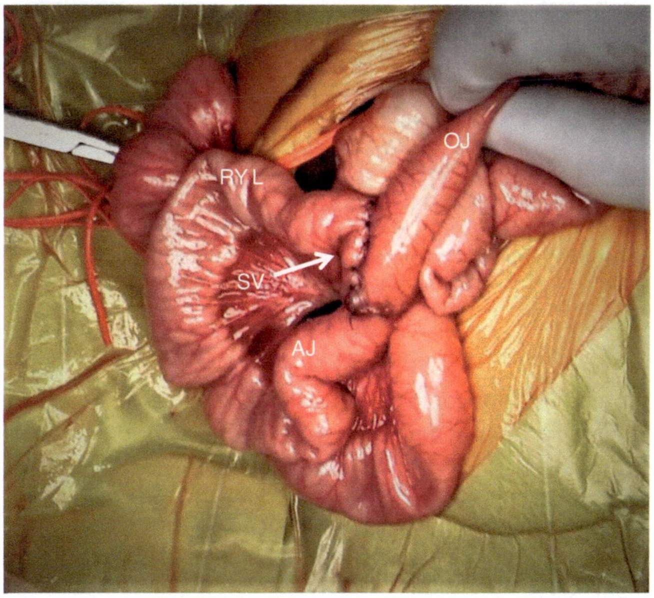


**Fig. 21.12** Creation of the spur valve 3. A spur valve is created. (AJ, anal jejunum; OJ, oral jejunum; RYL, Roux-en-Y limb, SV, spur valve)

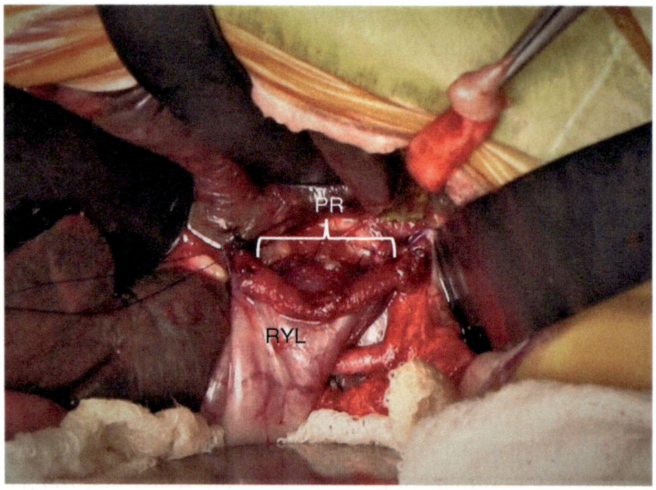


**Fig. 21.13** Anastomosis of the posterior row. The anastomosis of the posterior row is completed. (PR, posterior row; RYL, Roux-en-Y limb)

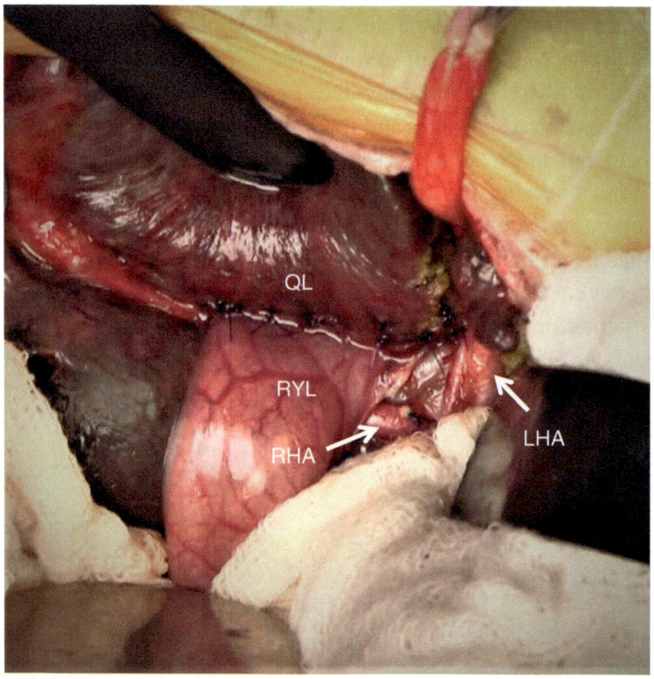


**Fig. 21.14** Anastomosis of the anterior row. Kasai portoenterostomy is completed. (LHA, left hepatic artery; QL, quadrate lobe of the liver; RHA, right hepatic artery; RYL, Roux-en-Y limb)

the anterior row, complete hemostasis at the hepatic hilum is confirmed. During the anastomosis of the anterior row, sufficient bites are used in the quadrate lobe. After all, stitches are placed between the quadrate lobe and the jejunum, the suture materials are tied in order (Fig. 21.14). A total of 20–25 stitches are generally placed in Kasai portoenterostomy. Additional stitches are placed if reinforcement of the anastomosis is required.

### 21.3.6 Drain Placement and Abdominal Closure

Intraperitoneal lavage is performed using a sufficient volume of warm saline. A closed drain is placed in the Winslow's Fossa, and the end of the drain is pulled through from the right lower abdominal wall. The liver and intestine of the operative field are covered with an anti-adhesive agent such as Seprafilm®, and the abdomen is closed layer by layer.

## 21.4 Revision of Kasai Portoenterostomy

Bile drainage is achieved in most patients with biliary atresia following Kasai portoenterostomy. However, in some cases, bile drainage stops due to cholangitis for other reasons. In these patients, redo Kasai portoenterostomy is indicated when anti-cholangitis treatment, choleretics, or corticosteroids are ineffective. However, the indications for liver transplantation should also be considered. We perform redo Kasai portoenterostomy to carefully assess patient condition, including the pattern of postoperative bile drainage, patient age, and the hepatic functional reserve [12]. Patients who undergo early Kasai portoenterostomy are increasing in number. According to data from the Japanese Biliary Atresia Registry (JBAR), neonatal cases are associated with the best outcome following Kasai portoenterostomy (https://jbas.net/en/national-registration/). However, the outcome of some patients who undergo Kasai portoenterostomy during the neonatal period is not good. The operative age might be too early for these patients, in whom the bile formation might still be reduced, or the network-shaped intrahepatic biliary reconstruction mentioned above might be undeveloped. Thus, an additional indication for Redo Kasai portoenterostomy may need to be considered for patients with unfavorable postoperative course following early neonatal surgery [6].

## 21.5 Technical Standardization of Kasai Portoenterostomy

Many modifications to the biliary reconstruction procedure have been proposed between the 1960s and 1990s, mainly aiming to prevent cholangitis. Among them, the Suruga II procedure, a total external biliary conduit procedure, was popular from the late 1980s to the early 1990s in Japan [13]. The intestinal antireflux valve procedure was also commonly employed [14, 15]. Ultimately, the original Kasai portoenterostomy with long (40–60 cm) Roux-en Y limb has become the most popular procedure. This trend of modifications in the 1990s was largely influenced by the wide-

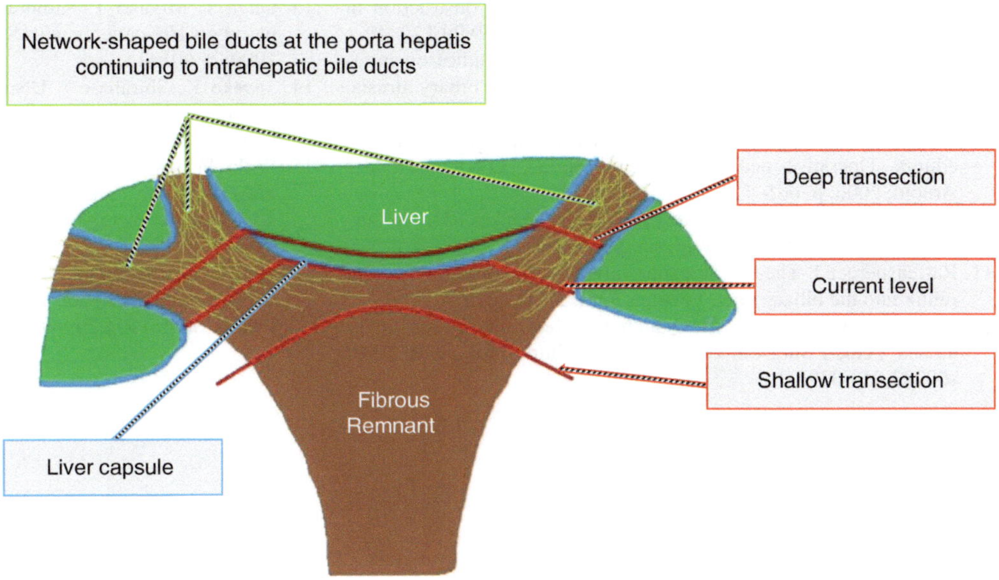


**Fig. 21.15** Image showing the level of transection. Currently, the remnant is transected at the level of the liver capsule (blue line, current level). If the transection level is too shallow, the network of bile ducts (light green fine network) connected to the intrahepatic bile ducts may not reach the transected surface (shallow transection). If the level is too deep, damage to the liver parenchyma may disturb continuous biliary drainage (deep transection)

spread of liver transplantation. More recently, the intestinal antireflux valve procedure has been revisited due to the lower incidence of cholangitis. According to JBAR data, the incidence of cholangitis was 10 points lower in the intestinal antireflux valve procedure than for the original Kasai procedure, while the jaundice clearance rate was equivalent between the two procedures. Thus, we continue to use the intestinal antireflux valve procedure. The two types of intestinal valves are the spur- [11] and intussuscepted-type [14] valves. We used both valves simultaneously in some cases in the 1990s in double-valve Kasai portoenterostomy. However, as the preventive effect of double valves was not superior to a single valve and late complications related to the intussuscepted-type valve were encountered, we currently use only the spur valve. Furthermore, we believe that the most important point of Kasai portoenterostomy is not the modification of biliary reconstruction, including valve formation, but rather the appropriate remnant transection and anastomosis procedures. While complete resection of the remnant is the basic procedure, wider and deeper dissection are associated with better outcomes to some extent [16]. However, we experienced worsened outcomes if the transection level was too deep [5]. Thus, we stress that the transection level should be maintained at the same level as the surrounding liver capsule (Fig. 21.15). The current procedure was developed based on the historical background of our department and JBAR data. While it remains unknown whether the current procedure is the ideal one, it is associated with comparable outcomes to the best ones in the history of our department. Therefore, we consider it our standardized procedure and employ essentially the same procedure for all patients with biliary atresia for the past 20 years. Following our current procedure, jaundice clearance (to a total bilirubin level of <2.0 mg/dL) and 10-year native liver survival were achieved in 80–90% and approximately 70–75% of patients, respectively [5]. However, maintaining jaundice clearance rates above 90% remains difficult. Further refinement of surgical techniques might be an important issue. However, universal employment of early surgery, hopefully during the neonatal period, as well as the appropriate indication for revision surgery, maybe essential for achieving better surgical outcomes of Kasai portoenterostomy. Most important is the elucidation of the etiology of biliary atresia, and new treatment strategies should be developed based on the pathophysiology.

**Conflicts of Interest** The authors declare no conflicts of interest associated with this manuscript.

## References


1. Kasai M, Suzuki S. A new operation for "noncorrectable" biliary atresia; hepatic portoenterostomy. (in Japanese) Shujutsu (Operation). 1959;13:733–9.
2. Kasai M, Ohi R, Chiba T, Hayashi Y. A patient with biliary atresia who died 28 years after hepatic portojejunostomy. J Pediatr Surg. 1988;23:430–1. https://doi.org/10.1016/s0022-3468(88)80441-x.
3. LeeVan E, Matsuoka L, Cao S, Groshen S, Alexopoulos S. Biliary-enteric drainage vs primary liver transplant as initial treatment for children with biliary atresia. JAMA Surg. 2019;154:26–32.
4. Uto K, Inomata Y, Sakamoto S, Hibi T, Sasaki H, Nio M. A multicenter study of primary liver transplantation for biliary atresia in Japan. Pediatr Surg Int. 2019;35:1223–9. https://doi.org/10.1007/s00383-019-04553-7. Epub 2019 Sep 18
5. Nio M, Wada M, Sasaki H, Kazama T, Tanaka H, Kudo H. Technical standardization of Kasai portoenterostomy for biliary atresia. J Pediatr Surg. 2016;51:2105–8. https://doi.org/10.1016/j.jpedsurg.2016.09.047.
6. Tanaka H, Sasaki H, Hashimoto M, Nio M. Re-do Kasai procedure in a preterm infant. J Pediatr Surg Case Rep. 2020; https://doi.org/10.1016/J.EPSC.2019.101220.

7. Ohi R, Kasai M, Takahashi T. Intrahepatic biliary obstruction in congenital bile duct atresia. Tohoku J Exp Med. 1969;99:129–49.
8. Chiba T, Kasai M, Sasano N. Histopathological studies on intrahepatic bile ducts in the vicinity of porta hepatis in biliary atresia. Tohoku J Exp Med. 1976;118:199–207.
9. Davenport M. Surgery for biliary atresia. In: Spitz L, Coran AG, editors. Operative pediatric surgery. 6th ed. London: Hodder Arnold; 2006. p. 661–72.
10. Lilly JR, Hall RJ, Vasquez-Estevez J, Karrer F, Shikes RH. The surgery of "correctable" biliary atresia. J Pediatr Surg. 1987;22:522–5.
11. Raffensperger J. The use of a spur valve in a roux loop to prevent reflux into the biliary tract. J Pediatr Surg. 2000;35:1014–5.
12. Nio M, Sasaki H, Tanaka H, Okamura A. Redo surgery for biliary atresia. Pediatr Surg Int. 2013;29:989–93. https://doi.org/10.1007/s00383-013-3396-3.
13. Ohya T, Miyano T, Kimura K. Indication for portoenterostomy based on 103 patients with Suruga II modification. J Pediatr Surg. 1990;25:801–4.
14. Tanaka K, Shirahase I, Utsunomiya H, Katayama T, Uemoto S, Asonuma K, et al. A valved hepatic portoduodenal intestinal conduit for biliary atresia. Ann Surg. 1991;213:230–5.
15. Saeki M, Nakano M, Hagane K, Shimizu K. Effectiveness of an intussusceptive antireflux valve to prevent ascending cholangitis after hepatic portojejunostomy in biliary atresia. J Pediatr Surg. 1991;26:800–3.
16. Toyosaka A, Okamoto E, Okasora T, Nose K, Tomimoto Y, Seki Y. Extensive dissection at the porta hepatis for biliary atresia. J Pediatr Surg. 1994;29:896–9.

# Operative Procedures: Laparoscopic Kasai Procedure

22

Hiroo Uchida, Chiyoe Shirota, and Takahisa Tainaka

**Abstract**

Recently, many reports have shown that the outcomes of Laparoscopic Kasai Portoenterostomy (Lap Kasai PE) are comparable to those of open Kasai portoenterostomy. We have established surgical procedures for Lap Kasai PE. We performed an umbilical Mercedes incision for multiple purposes. We prefer using the AirSeal® Intelligent Flow System as a pneumoperitoneum and a 3 mm bipolar cautery. Laparoscopic surgery is not very different from open surgery. The dissection of the porta hepatis is similar to that in laparotomy. The fibrous biliary remnants were not entirely resected.

Lap Kasai PE provides excellent visibility for the resection of the fibrous biliary remnants in the hilar plate, which can ensure good results. The results are expected to be equivalent to those of open surgery.

**Keywords**

Biliary atresia · Portoenterostomy · Laparoscopic operation · Fibrous biliary remnants · Hilar plate

Laparoscopic Kasai portoenterostomy (Lap Kasai PE) was introduced by Esteves in 2002 [1]. With rapid advances in minimally invasive surgery, the replacement of open Kasai portoenterostomy with Lap Kasai PE is currently being considered [2, 3]. Recently, many reports have shown that the outcomes of Lap Kasai PE are comparable to those of open Kasai portoenterostomy [4–6].

We perform laparoscopic surgery for almost all cases of biliary atresia. We have established surgical procedures for Lap Kasai PE. The advantage of laparoscopic surgery is that it is minimally invasive; this means it is less painful, causes smaller wounds, and enables a faster recovery than open surgery. Laparoscopic surgery is beneficial not only for the patients, but also for the surgeons. The surgeons can visualize the hepatic hilum in a magnified view. They can share the surgical field using one monitor. All surgical procedures can be recorded and verified later. The recorded operative procedures can be easily performed throughout the body. The operative procedure we used for our patient is described below.

## 22.1 Preoperative Preparation

A decrease in bile excretion into the intestinal bilirubin can lead to vitamin K malabsorption; therefore, intravenous vitamin K should be administered before surgery to maintain coagulation ability. No other special pretreatment is performed for laparoscopic surgery.

## 22.2 Surgical Procedure

### 22.2.1 Position and Port Insertion

The patient was positioned at the foot of the operating table in a supine frog position under general anesthesia. The surgeon stood at the patient's foot; an assistant with a camera was positioned at the patient's left, and another assistant at the patient's right. A multichannel port with two 5-mm ports was inserted from an umbilical Mercedes incision, which can provide a wide enough fascial opening with minimal esthetic impact (Fig. 22.1a). One was a camera port, and the other was an assistant port for suction or securing the field of view. We prefer using the AirSeal® Intelligent Flow System as a pneumoperitoneum to secure the working space and operative vision. This system ensures that the pneumoperitoneum pressure remains constant despite the opening and closing of the port and suction. Without this pneumoperitoneum device, it is difficult to deal with accidental bleeding.

H. Uchida (✉) · C. Shirota · T. Tainaka
Department of Pediatric Surgery, Nagoya University School of Medicine, Nagoya, Japan
e-mail: hiro2013@med.nagoya-u.ac.jp


M. Nio (ed.), *Introduction to Biliary Atresia*, https://doi.org/10.1007/978-981-16-2160-4_22

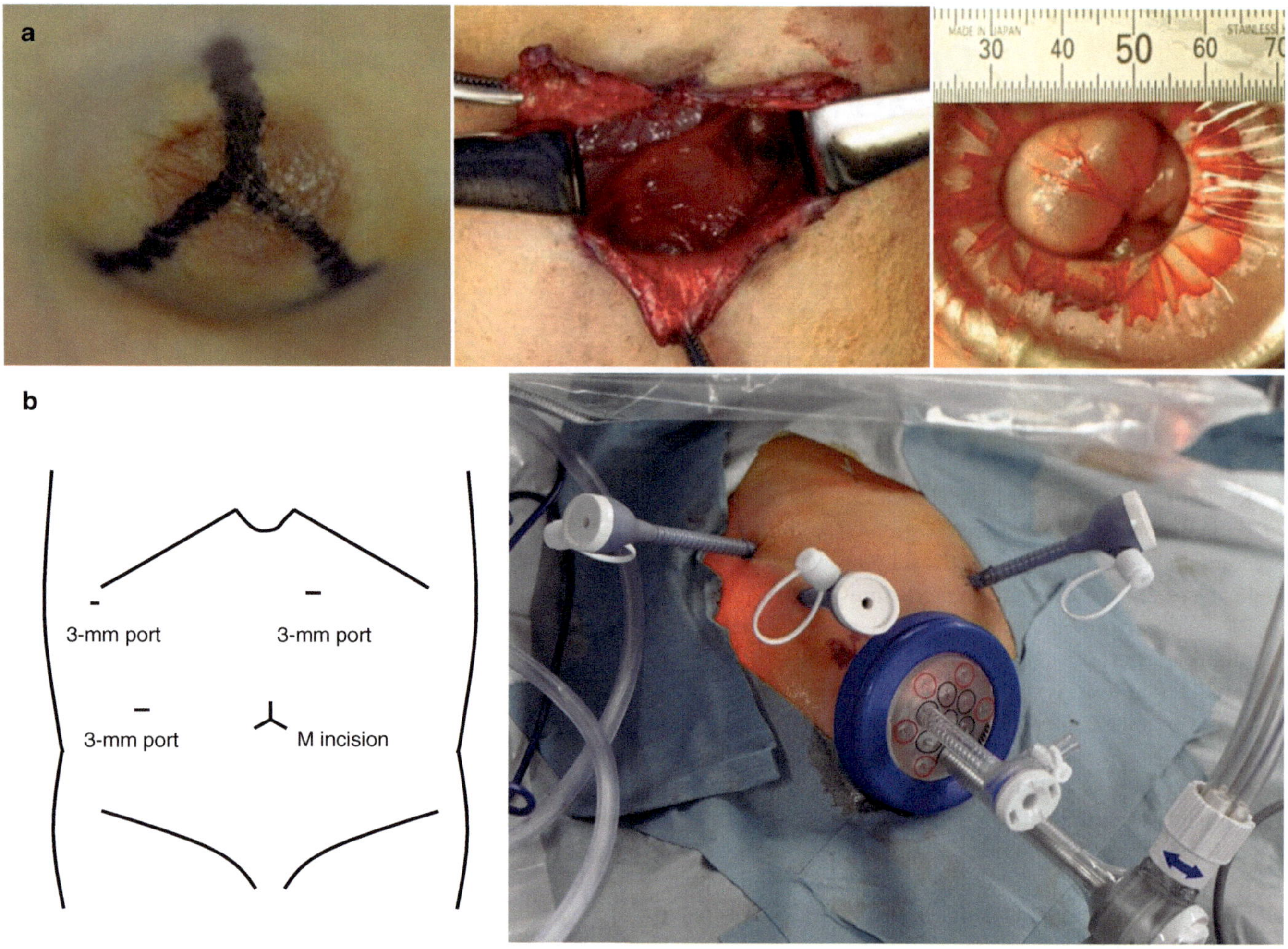


Fig. 22.1 Umbilical Mercedes Benz incision and Port alignment. (**a**) Umbilical Mercedes Benz incision. (**b**) Port alignment

Two 3-mm ports were inserted into the right abdomen and upper left abdomen as the working ports. The upper left abdominal port was inserted considerably into the upper abdomen, assuming a hilar jejunal anastomosis. The other port inserted into the upper right abdomen was the assistant port (Fig. 22.1b).

### 22.2.2 Cholangiography

A laparoscope was inserted, and the liver surface was observed. If the Makibishi sign (Fig. 22.2a) is visible, it is a strong indicator of biliary atresia. In order to make a definitive diagnosis of biliary atresia and a rapid intraoperative pathological diagnosis, a liver biopsy must first be performed, followed by cholangiography. The gallbladder was punctured using a 20-G needle, and a contrast study was performed (Fig. 22.2b). The findings confirmed the diagnosis of biliary atresia.

### 22.2.3 Securing the Surgical Field

The teres hepatis ligament of the liver was pulled up toward the epigastric region and the gallbladder was pulled to the upper right abdomen to view the hepatic hilum (Figs. 22.2c and 22.2d).

### 22.2.4 Identification of Common Bile Duct Cord-like Tissue and Approaching the Hilar Region

The operative procedure was performed using 3-mm forceps. The fibrous remnants of the common bile duct were identified on the cranial side of the duodenum near the surface of the hepatoduodenal ligament and dissected with ligation. This cord-like tissue is easily found in most cases (Fig. 22.3a). If the cord-like tissue is firmly lined up in the hilum of the liver, the cranial margin must be searched, but if the cord-like

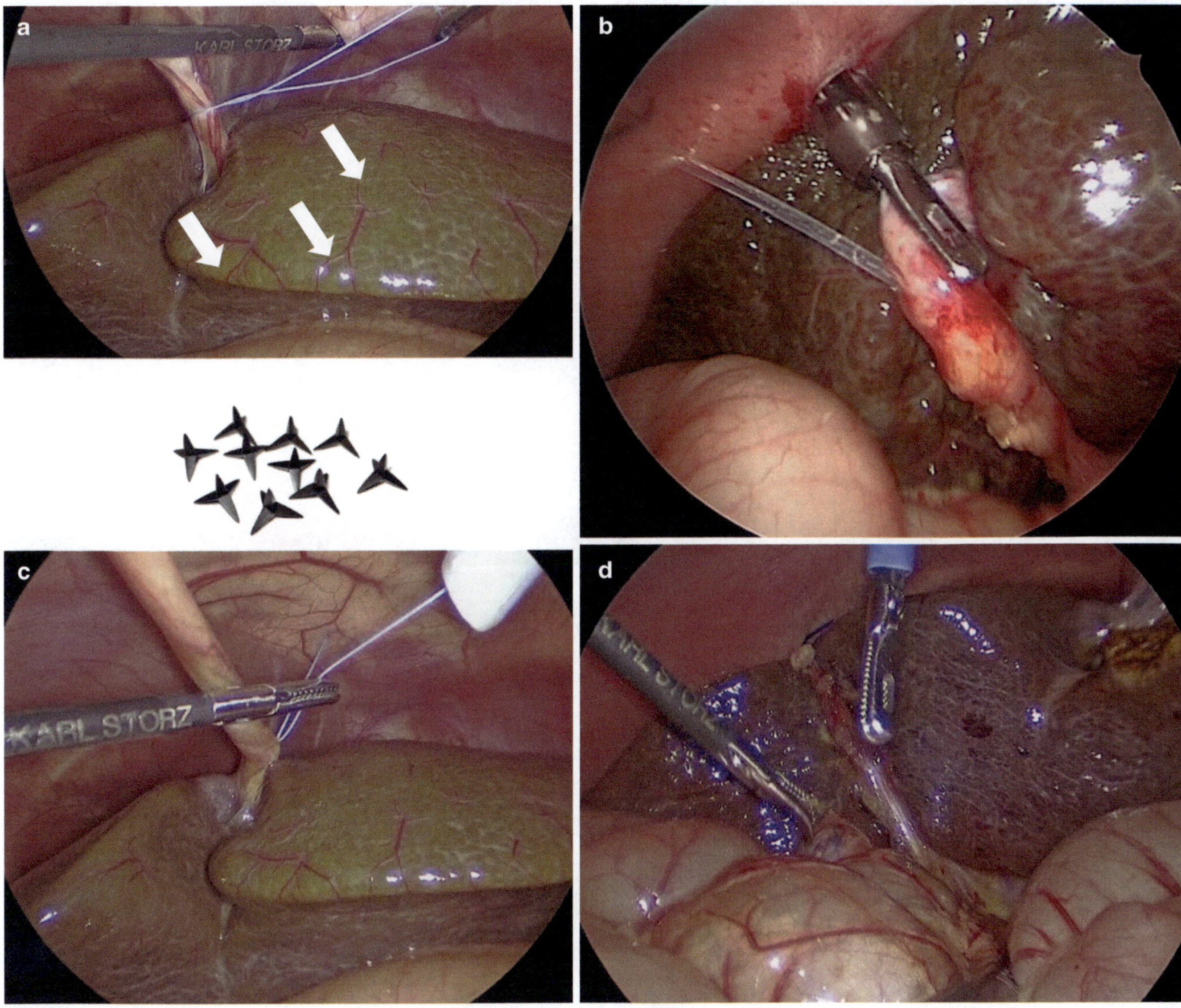


Fig. 22.2 Diagnosis of biliary atresia and elevation of the teres hepatis ligament and gallbladder for a fine view of porta hepatis. (**a**) Makibishi sign. (**b**) Liver biopsy and cholangiography. (**c**) Elevation of the teres hepatis ligament. (**d**) Elevation of gallbladder

tissue is considerably thin, this step is not necessary (Fig. 22.3b). The hepatic hilum was directly approached and detached. The cranial margin of the portal vein was found (Fig. 22.3c). If there are many fibrous remnants in the hepatic hilum, it takes some time to identify the portal vein (Fig. 22.3d).

### 22.2.5 Dissection of the Hepatic Hilum

After locating the cranial edge of the portal vein, the branches of the caudate lobe were cut off by bipolar cautery (Figs. 22.4a and 22.4b). The median branch of the hepatic artery was dissected since it crossed the hilum of the liver (Figs. 22.4c and 22.4d). First, the fibrous biliary remnants in the hepatic hilum were separated from the center of the porta hepatis toward the right porta hepatis (Fig. 22.5a). The fibrous biliary remnants were not entirely resected. A few remnants were preserved at the surface of the porta hepatis (Figs. 22.5b and 22.5c). The hepatic capsule must not be broken. The right porta hepatis extended to the point where the artery of the right anterior segment branch of the hepatic artery and portal vein entered the liver (Fig. 22.5d).

After the fibrous remnants in the right hepatic hilum were resected, the remaining fibrous remnants were separated from the center to the left porta hepatis (Fig. 22.6a). The depth of resection was the same on the right and left sides (Figs. 22.6b and 22.6c). Often, the fibrous remnants in the

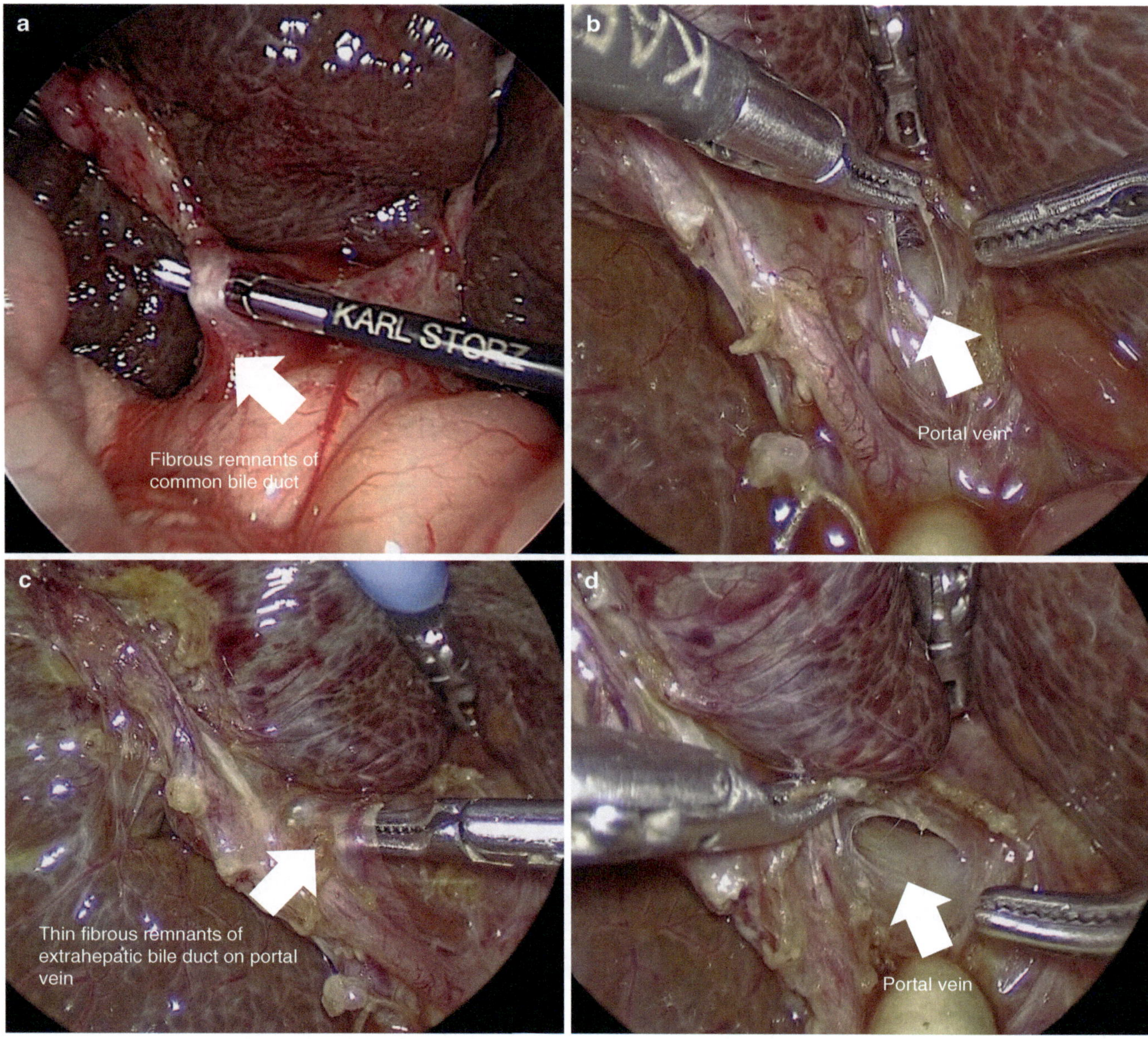


**Fig. 22.3** Identification of the fibrous biliary remnants and portal vein. (**a**) The fibrous remnants of the common bile duct. (**b**) The portal vein on the port hepatis. (**c**) The fibrous remnants of the common hepatic duct on portal vein. (**d**) The portal vein on the port hepatis

left are thinner than those on the right side. The left porta hepatis was dissected up to the point where the left branch of the portal vein entered the liver (Fig. 22.6d). Then, total resection of the fibrous remnants was performed at the porta hepatis (Fig. 22.6e).

### 22.2.6 Establishing the Roux-En-Y Limb with Exteriorization Via the Umbilical Mercedes Incision

We laparoscopically confirmed the presence of the ligament of Treitz and measured 15 cm of the jejunum. At 45 cm distal to the efferent cut end, the afferent limb was anastomosed. The roux limb was transferred in the retrocolic route, and an incision was made in the anterior wall. Then, the completed Roux-en-Y limb was returned to the abdominal cavity. After confirming that there were no twists in the intestinal tract, we closed the Petersen defect (Fig. 22.7a).

### 22.2.7 Portoenterostomy

Portoenterostomy was performed between the liver parenchyma and the roux limb using 5–0 monofilament sutures. The anastomosis was started in the 9 o'clock position. The first suture was made from the right edge of the fibrous remnants to the hepatic parenchyma (Fig. 22.7b). On the dorsal

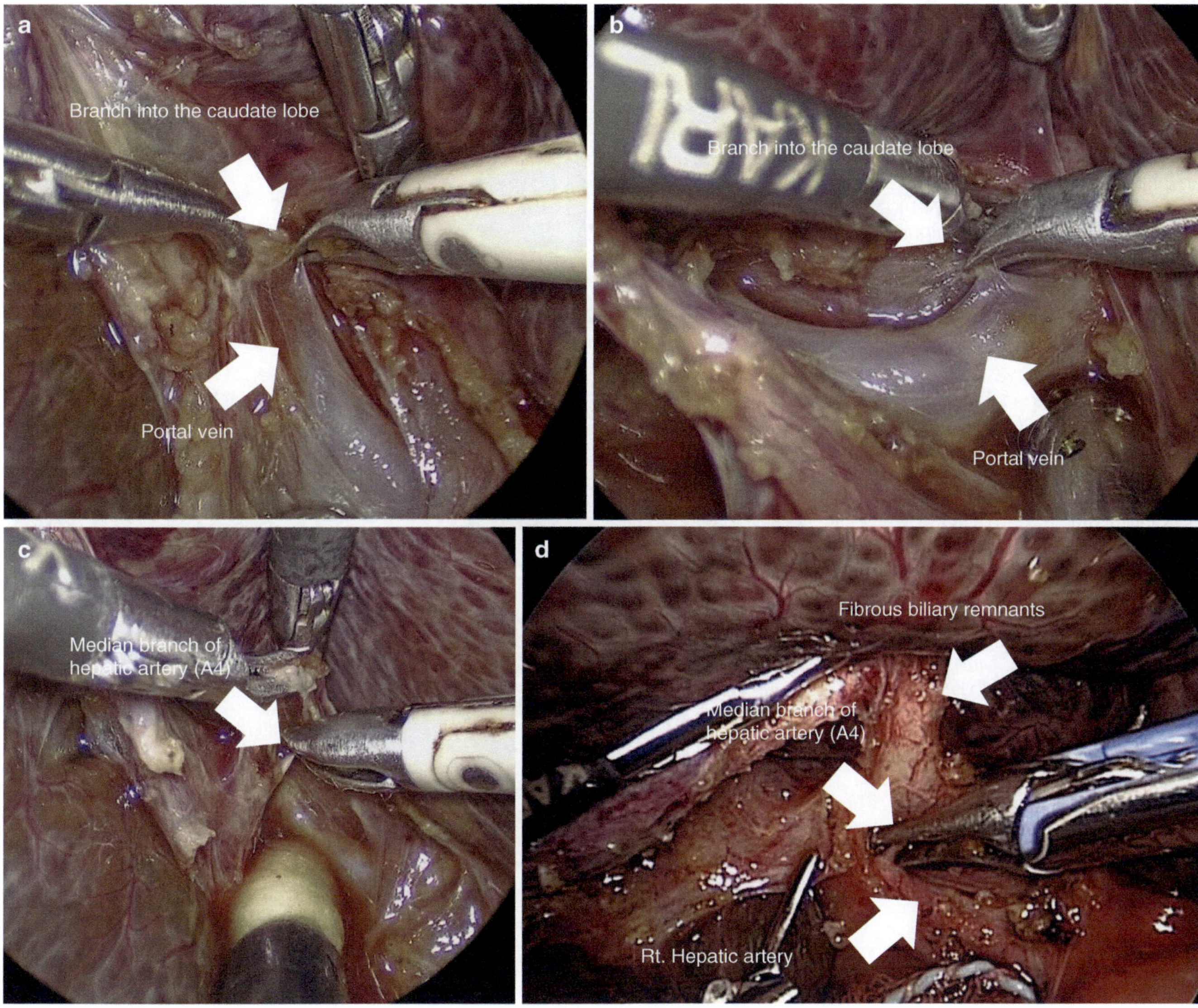


**Fig. 22.4** Preparation for resection of fibrous remnants at the hepatic hilum. (**a, b**) The branches of the portal vein are cut off by 3 mm bipolar cautery. (**c, d**) The median branch of the hepatic artery is dissected by 3 mm bipolar cautery

side, the hepatic parenchyma behind the portal vein was anastomosed to the jejunum (Figs. 22.7c and 22.7d). The fifth suture was made from the liver at 2 o'clock position in the hilum to the left edge of the dissection (Fig. 22.7e).

The anterior wall was sutured from the liver toward the boundary between the hilar dissection and hepatic parenchyma (Fig. 22.8a). Three or four stitches were made. The portoenterostomy was performed, covering all the transecting fibrous biliary remnants (Fig. 22.8b).

### 22.2.8 Drain Insertion and Abdominal Closure

After cleaning the abdominal cavity, the muscular layer at the port insertion site was sutured. A 10-Fr break drain was inserted into the dorsal site of the portoenterostomy from the port skin incision on the right abdomen since the muscular layer in the peritoneal insertion site was different from that in the port insertion site. By doing so, it is possible to prevent the omentum from escaping after the drain is removed. Finally, the portoenterostomy site was glazed with anti-adhesive agents (Fig. 22.8c). The operation was thus completed. Postoperative wounds, including the shape of the navel, showed good healing (Fig. 22.8d).

## 22.3 Postoperative Management

Postoperative management was the same as for laparotomy. Antibiotics were discontinued 48 hours after the operation, and oral drinking was started 3 days after the operation. Oral prednisolone was started 5 days after the operation. The dose was reduced every 5 days in the following sequence: 4, 2, 1, to 0.5 mg/kg. Ursodeoxycholic acid was administered intra-

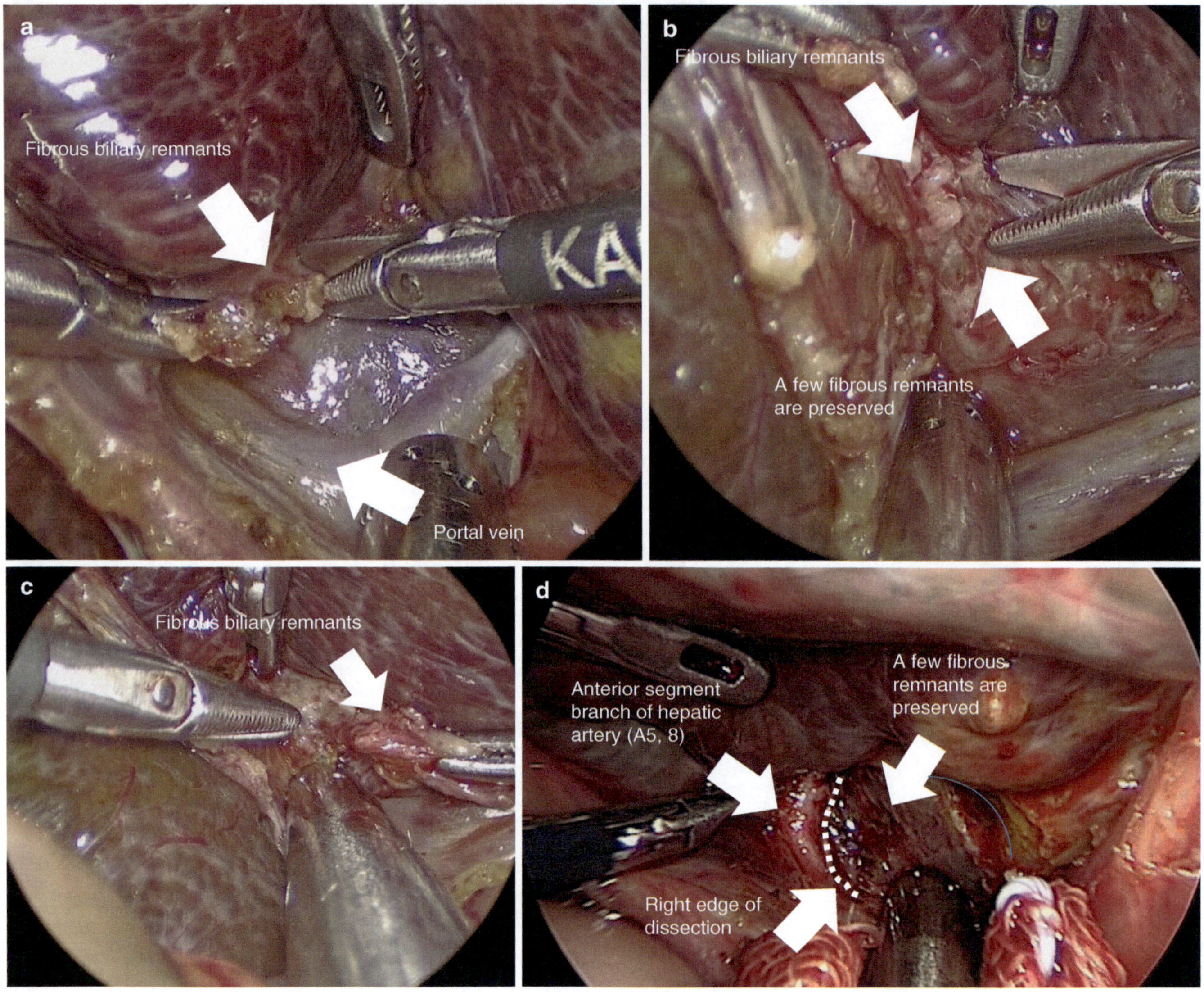


**Fig. 22.5** Dissection of fibrous remnants at right porta hepatis. The fibrous biliary remnants at the porta hepatis are not completely resected. (**a, b, c, d**) The fibrous biliary remnant cone is dissected from the center of the porta hepatis toward the right edge of the porta hepatis

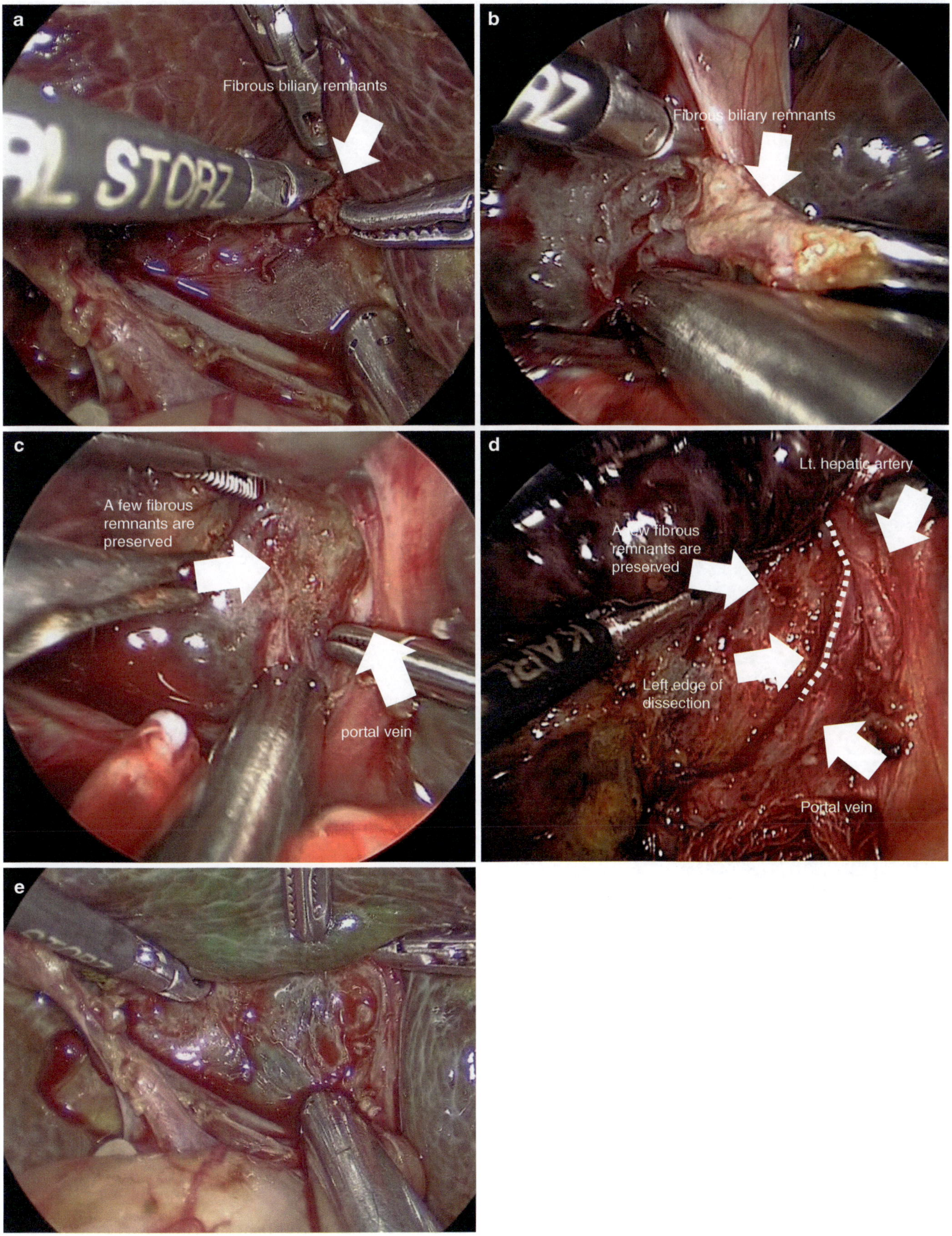


**Fig. 22.6** Resection of fibrous remnants at left porta hepatis. The fibrous biliary remnants at the porta hepatis are not completely resected. (**a, b, c, d**) The fibrous biliary remnant cone is dissected from the center of the porta hepatis toward the left edge of the porta hepatis. (**e**) Total resection of fibrous remnants at the porta hepatic

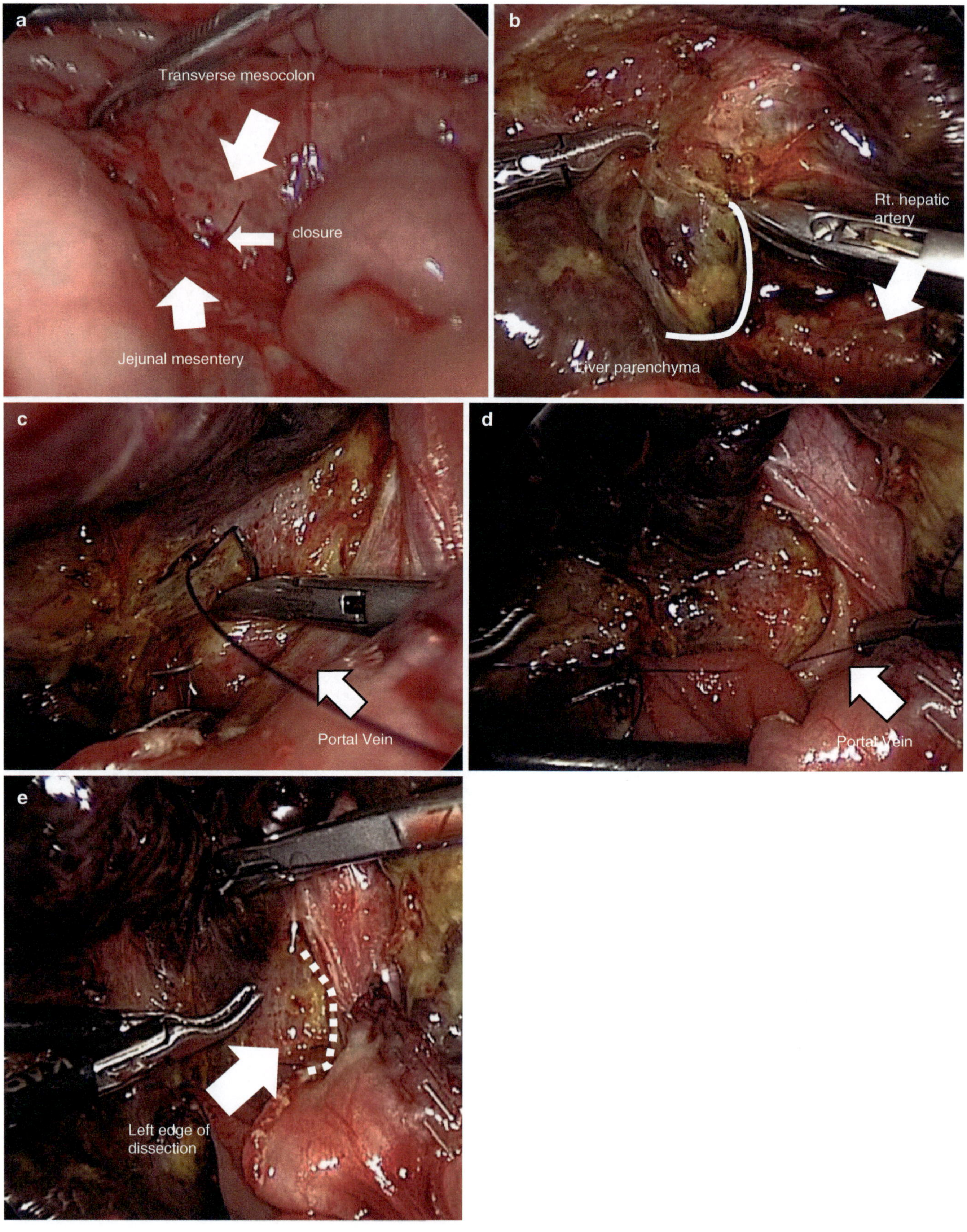


**Fig. 22.7** Portoenterostomy at the dorsal site of the porta hepatis. (**a**) Closure of Petersen's defect. (**b**) First stitch: liver parenchyma at the right side of the porta hepatis. (**c**) Third stitch: liver parenchyma at the dorsal site of portal vein. (**d**) Third stitch: from liver parenchyma at the dorsal site of portal vein to Roux limb. (**e**) Fifth stitch: from liver parenchyma to the left edge of the dissection

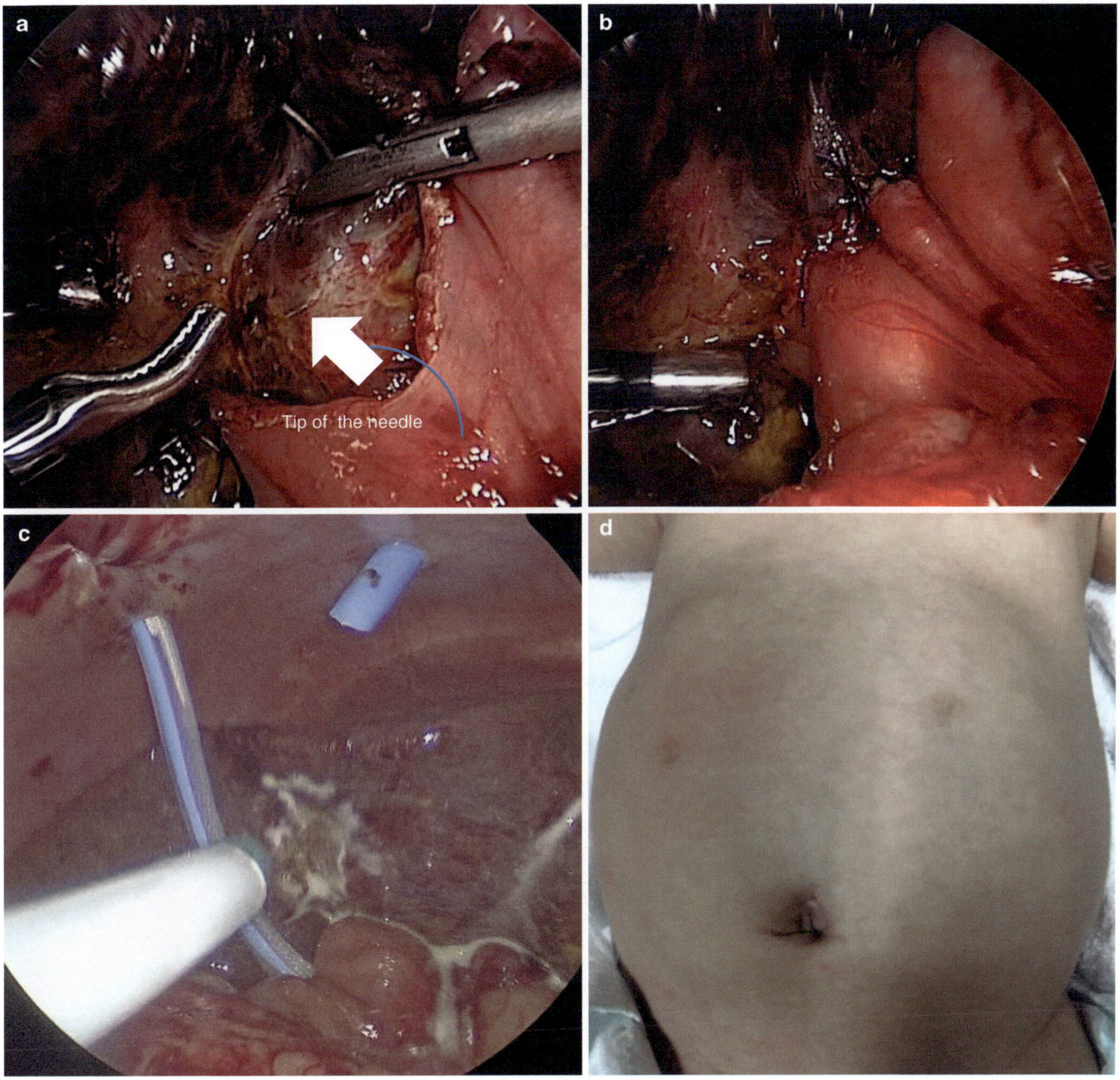


Fig. 22.8 Portoenterostomy at the abdominal site and postoperative wounds. (**a**) The anterior wall is sutured from the liver toward the boundary between the hilar dissection area and the liver parenchyma. (**b**) The portoenterostomy is covering all the transecting fibrous biliary remnants. (**c**) Glazing with anti-adhesive agents. (**d**) 2 months after the operation

venously from the day after surgery, and oral Urso was (20 mg/kg) was prescribed when oral administration was started.

Laparoscopic surgery is not very different from open surgery. The dissection of the porta hepatis is similar to that in laparotomy. The fibrous biliary remnants were not entirely resected. A few remnants were preserved at the surface of the porta hepatis to ensure the hepatic capsule is not broken. However, if bleeding from the portal vein occurs, it should be stopped with the AirSeal® system. When bleeding occurs, it is necessary to use various techniques under laparoscopy, including the Pringle maneuver.

Lap Kasai PE provides excellent visibility for the resection of the fibrous biliary remnants in the hilar plate, which can ensure good results. The results are expected to be equivalent to those of open surgery.

## References

1. Esteves E, et al. Laparoscopic Kasai portoenterostomy for biliary atresia. Pediatr Surg Int. 2002;18:737–40.
2. Lishuang M, et al. Laparoscopic portoenterostomy versus open portoenterostomy for the treatment of biliary atresia: a systematic review and meta-analysis of comparative studies. Pediatr Surg Int. 2015;31:261–9.
3. Hussain MH, et al. Outcomes of laparoscopic Kasai portoenterostomy for biliary atresia: a systematic review. J Pediatr Surg. 2017;52:264–7.
4. Murase N, et al. A new era of laparoscopic revision of Kasai Portoenterostomy for the treatment of biliary atresia. Biomed Res Int. 2015;2015:173014.
5. Nakamura H, et al. Comprehensive assessment of prognosis after laparoscopic portoenterostomy for biliary atresia. Pediatr Surg Int. 2016;32:109–12.
6. Shirota C, et al. Laparoscopic Kasai portoenterostomy is advantageous over open Kasai portoenterostomy in subsequent liver transplantation. Surg Endosc. 2020;34:3375–81.

# Reoperative Portoenterostomy in Biliary Atresia

# 23

Takeshi Saito

**Abstract**

As liver transplantation (LT) has become the treatment of choice for irreversible end-stage liver failure even among biliary atresia (BA) patients, the roles and indications for reoperative portoenterostomy have changed markedly over the last several decades. Accumulated data based on approximately 400 revisions from among over 3000 initial BA operations revealed a complete jaundice clearance rate following the second portoenterostomy of nearly 40%. It is true that a group of BA patients with a history of revision surgery can achieve long-term native liver survival (NLS) and biochemical status comparable to those without such a history, but no consensus has yet been reached regarding indications for revision. One possibly robust indication that has been suggested focuses on bile drainage transit after first portoenterostomy, particularly the decrease in total bilirubin over the first-month post-first Kasai operation. Given the shortage of donors for LT and that social and ethical issues related to living donor transplantation remain to be resolved, reoperative portoenterostomy has played a key role in selected BA cases by offering long-term NLS or delaying the need for LT.

**Keywords**

Revision · Indication · Timing · Native liver survival Prognosis · Bilirubin · Liver transplantation · Living donor liver transplantation

T. Saito (✉)
Department of Pediatric Surgery, Graduate School of Medicine, Chiba University, Chiba, Japan

Division of Pediatric Surgery, Chiba Children's Hospital, Chiba, Japan
e-mail: t.situ218@pref.chiba.lg.jp

## Abbreviations

AST: Aspartate aminotransferase
BA: Biliary atresia
DB: Direct bilirubin
γ-GTP: Gamma-glutamyl transpeptidase
JBAR: Japanese Biliary Atresia Registry
JCR: Jaundice clearance rate
LDLT: Living donor liver transplantation
LT: Liver transplantation
NLS: Native liver survival
NLSR: Native liver survival rate
TB: Total bilirubin

## 23.1 Introduction

Until several decades ago, liver transplantation (LT) was not widely available around the globe, and reoperative portoenterostomy was commonly performed to restore bile flow when postoperative scar tissue formation obstructed microducts draining bile into the porta hepatis [1]. Compared to some Western countries, the revision was particularly common in Japan [1], where the introduction of LT was markedly delayed [2], largely due to social and legal reasons. However, given the sufficiently improved outcomes with living donor LT (LDLT), the role of reoperation has changed dramatically, to the point where this intervention now plays a more minor role in the treatment algorithm for BA. According to the Japanese Biliary Atresia Registry (JBAR) [3], which had accumulated the largest number (over 3000) of new BA cases as of 2017, the reoperation rate was 8% for the 2008–2017 period, down from 21% for 1991–2000 (Fig. 23.1).

The negative effects of revision on LT have been an issue of focus, particularly for transplant surgeons [4, 5]. This has often made pediatric surgeons hesitant to explore chances for performing redo surgery. However, the donor shortages seen even in Western countries and the ethical ramifications of


M. Nio (ed.), *Introduction to Biliary Atresia*, https://doi.org/10.1007/978-981-16-2160-4_23

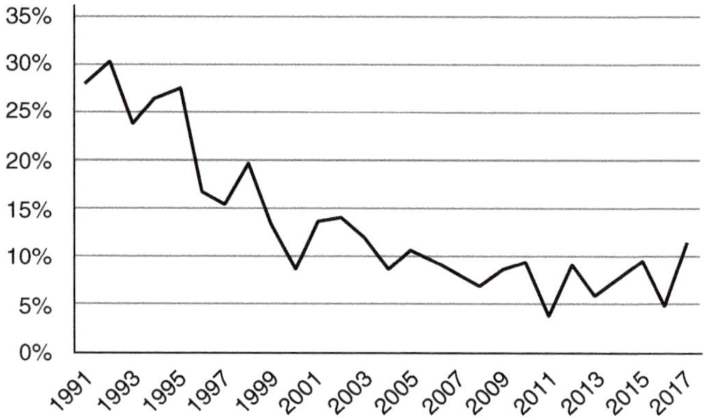


**Fig. 23.1** Transition of revision rate for BA surgery. Compared to the 1990s, the revision rate in the 2000s has fallen to nearly 10% of all initial BA portoenterostomies

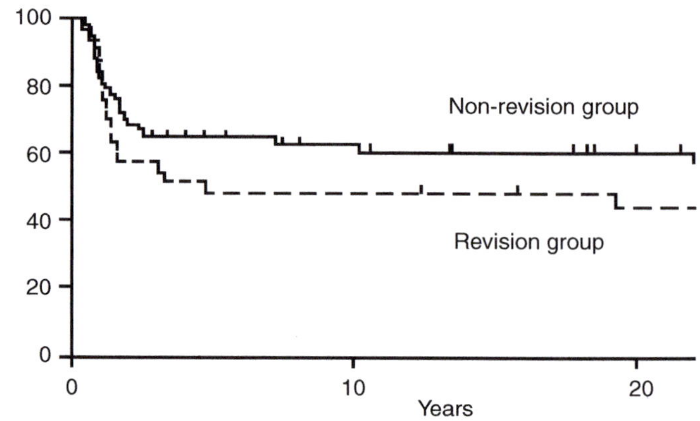


**Fig. 23.2** Kaplan-Meier curves for NLSR by revision status. Kaplan-Meier curves for NLS among post-portoenterostomy BA patients at our institution revealed overall 10- and 20-year NLSRs of 57% and 54%, with 49% and 45% for the revision group, and 63% and 61% for the non-revision group. NLS: native liver survival, NLSR: native liver survival rate

exposing healthy donors to hepatectomy for LDLT have meant that the possible roles of redo operations following failed initial portoenterostomy have not been completely eliminated.

This chapter reviews the significance of and indications for the second portoenterostomy based on relatively recently published articles, with judicious consideration of the effects on possible subsequent LT.

## 23.2 Significance of Reoperative Kasai Portoenterostomy

The JBAR demonstrated trustworthy short-term results of reoperation following failed Kasai with the largest accumulation of clinical data, collected from 3361 patients registered during the 1988–2017 period [3]. A total of 311 reoperations were performed during the 19 years from 1999 to 2017, with a subsequent jaundice clearance rate (JCR) of 40.2%, while 42.6% of those undergoing re-reoperations cleared jaundice [3]. Those rates are lower than the 60.8% JCR after the first Kasai operation [3], but undoubtedly prove that some cases undergoing redo surgery are able to accomplish native liver survival (NLS). Unfortunately, data on long-term results of revision are lacking from the JBAR registry.

Long-term native liver survival rates (NLSRs) after revision have varied between previous papers [6–9]. Our group demonstrated fairly good long-term NLSRs of 49% and 45% at 10 and 20 years post-revision (Fig. 23.2) [6], respectively, comparable to those described in two other reports [7, 8]. On the other hand, Nakamura et al. reported poorer outcomes of a 25% NLSR at 10 years and 16% at 20 years [9]. These discrepancies could be due to underlying differences across institutions and surgical services. In previous studies showing preferable results, a limited number of highly experienced surgeons followed clearly determined perioperative policies with regard to revision surgeries, resulting in excellent survival outcomes [6–8]. Conversely, in the study by Nakamura et al., some surgeons across the multiple centers involved might have performed revision surgeries without the benefit of a universal procedural policy, leading to greater disparities in outcomes [9]. These conflicting results on the long-term outcome seem insufficient to preclude revision for failed initial portoenterostomy.

Few papers have been published on not only long-term NLS, but also the biochemical status of these cases [6, 9]. Our group did not find any significant difference between 20-year-old BA native liver survivors with and without a history of revision in terms of admission rates for the treatment of postoperative cholangitis (46% vs. 40%) and/or portal hypertension (38% vs. 15%) at age 10–20 years, rates of patients not treated for cholangitis or portal hypertension at age 10–20 years (31% vs. 55%), or frequency of portopulmonary vascular abnormalities (8% vs. 10%) or hepatolithiasis (8% vs. 10%) [6]. In addition, concerning hepatobiliary function-associated laboratory indices at 20 years old, the investigated data did not show any significant differences except for AST and γ-GTP (Table 23.1) [6]. We conclude that the biochemical conditions of 20-year-old BA survivors are quite similar post-portoenterostomy, regardless of whether revision or only the initial surgery was performed. Rather, chances of achieving long-term NLS and/or delaying the timing of LT can be provided with the additional option of redo surgery for carefully selected cases.

## 23.3 Impact of Reoperative Portoenterostomy on Results of LT

Several reports, particularly those by transplant surgeons, have been critical of the performance of reoperative portoenterostomy surgery, citing greater blood loss and greater frequency of bowel perforation during transplant among BA

**Table 23.1** Comparison of laboratory data between 20-year-old BA native liver survivors with and without revision

| | With revision (n = 13) | Without revision (n = 20) | *p*-value |
|---|---|---|---|
| PLT (×10³/μL) | 152 ± 63 | 208 ± 94 | 0.11 |
| AST (U/L) | 80.5 ± 61.9 | 35.8 ± 24.9 | 0.02 |
| ALT (U/L) | 78.2 ± 66.4 | 38.0 ± 32.9 | 0.051 |
| TB (mg/dL) | 1.2 ± 0.90 | 0.8 ± 0.48 | 0.15 |
| γ-GTP (U/L) | 208.2 ± 231.8 | 110.5 ± 166.7 | 0.047 |
| Total protein (g/dL) | 7.0 ± 0.546 | 7.2 ± 0.343 | 0.38 |
| Cholinesterase (U/L) | 233.0 ± 69.1 | 252.8 ± 59.7 | 0.44 |
| TBA (μmol/l) | 52.0 ± 35.6 | 51.7 ± 84.7 | 0.13 |
| Abnormal laboratory data | 92% | 60% | 0.06 |

*ALT* alanine aminotransferase, *AST* aspartate aminotransferase, *BA* biliary atresia, *GTP* glutamyl transpeptidase, *PLT* platelets, *TB* total bilirubin, *TBA* total bile acids

recipients with revision than among those without [4, 5]. Another consistent finding, however, is that a history of single revision following portoenterostomy does not significantly increase mortality during LT compared to portoenterostomy alone without revision [4, 5]. A different group also showed comparable long-term post-LT survival between patients who had and had not undergone revision prior to LT, suggesting that second portoenterostomy might play an important role in delaying the need for LT [7].

## 23.4 Social and Ethical Issues Associated with LT

When discussing the significance of revision, social and ethical issues associated with the implementation of LT should also be taken into account. Donors represent a limited resource, even in Western countries where deceased-donor transplant is much more widely accepted. Delays in the performance of LT by additional revision for failed first Kasai might extend the time available to identify a suitable donor [7]. On the other hand, in countries where LDLT is the predominant procedure for LT (including Japan, where more than 95% of all LTs are LDLT [2]), the ethical ramifications of inflicting harm on healthy donors cannot be dismissed. A report from the Japanese Liver Transplantation Society with the highest integrity disclosed that 8.4% of living donors suffered complications of liver donation that exceeded grade II by Clavien score [10]. A previous report suggested that most LDLT donors return to baseline physical or mental quality of life within 6 months after transplantation [11], while the long-term effects have yet to be sufficiently investigated [12]. More importantly, the fundamental perspective is, as stated in the Declaration of Istanbul, that even in light of dramatically improved LT results, a positive outcome for a recipient does not justify inflicting harm on living donors [13].

## 23.5 Indications for Reoperative Kasai Portoenterostomy

Indications for redo surgery have changed in accordance with the advancement of LT, particularly LDLT, as well as its significance. Even though good (sufficient) post-portoenterostomy biliary drainage has been regarded as a prerequisite for revision [1, 7, 8, 14], differing definitions of "good (sufficient) biliary drainage" are in use. This confuses decision-making processes regarding reoperative portoenterostomy. Some authors have suggested that a total bilirubin (TB) value ≥2.0 mg/dL within a particular post-portoenterostomy interval [7, 14] is indicative of good biliary drainage, while others argue for a TB of 1.2 mg/dL [8]. Based on statistical analyses of 33 cases (35%) undergoing reoperation among the 95 cases of first Kasai for BA, comparing a variety of indices between those who did and did not accomplish 10-year NLS following redo procedures due to failed first portoenterostomy, we revealed the importance of the rate of change in TB up to 3–4 weeks post-portoenterostomy as an index of good postoperative biliary drainage [6]. Receiver operating characteristic curves for these parameters clearly demonstrated that the rate of change in TB over the first 4 weeks post-portoenterostomy offered the most accurate indicator of prognosis, with an area under the curve of 0.85 for a cut-off of −0.131 mg/dL/day (sensitivity, 0.79; specificity, 0.83) [6]. Applying this finding to a clinical scenario, BA cases in which TB levels fell at least 3.7 mg/dL during the first 4 weeks following the first portoenterostomy would qualify for revision [6].

Meanwhile, jaundice clearance prior to revision is preferable, but not an absolute prerequisite, based on the fact that some BA patients with persistent jaundice following first Kasai have successfully achieved long-term NLS without jaundice by undergoing redo operation [6, 8]. In addition, the clinical factors expected to affect prognosis after reoperative portoenterostomy such as age at first and second Kasai operations, lowest post-first portoenterostomy level (TB, direct bilirubin, and γ-GTP) prior to revision, and the interval between the first and second portoenterostomies proved to be less sensitive for predicting the outcome of revision [6].

## 23.6 Timing of Reoperation

The optimal timing of redo operation has varied in accordance with studies, and no consensus has yet been reached. Reoperations performed promptly [15], within 15 days [16] or 30 days [17] after cessation of bile drainage, and even beyond 90 days [18] or possibly within 1 year [19] following initial portoenterostomy have been suggested. However, the levels of evidence supporting each concept remain quite low.

## 23.7 Operative Procedure

Although the curettage, boring, and resection of fibrous tissue covering the porta hepatis have been suggested as suitable surgical procedures for revision [16], firm evidence in support of specific methods remains lacking. However, previous studies suggesting favorable outcomes of redo surgery advocated re-excision of scar tissue and further dissection of the hilar plate after the complete or partial takedown of the portoenterostomy, followed by re-anastomosis [6–8, 20].

## 23.8 Conclusion

Considering the reportedly favorable long-term outcomes in BA patients with a history of revision comparable to those without such history and the social and ethical issues related to LT, performing redo-Kasai just once for failed first portoenterostomy should be approved for carefully selected BA cases. One promising indication for revision is the rate of change in TB during the first-month post-portoenterostomy. Patients who show a decrease in TB of >3.7 mg/dL over the first-month post-portoenterostomy appear to represent suitable candidates for revision if good biliary drainage following first portoenterostomy cannot be maintained.

**Conflict of Interest** The authors report no conflicts of interest.

## References


1. Nio M, Sasaki H, Tanaka H, Okamura A. Redo surgery for biliary atresia. Pediatr Surg Int. 2013;29:989–93.
2. Umeshita K, Inomata Y, Furukawa H, Kasahara M, Kawasaki S, Kobayashi E, et al. Liver transplantation in Japan: registry by the Japanese liver transplantation society. Hepatol Res. 2016;46:1171–86.
3. Japanese Society for Biliary Atresia. Japanese biliary atresia registry 2017. J Jpn Soc Pediatr Sug. 2019;55:291–7.
4. Sugawara Y, Makuuchi M, Kaneko J, Ohkubo T, Mizuta K, Kawarasaki H. Impact of previous multiple portoenterostomies on living donor liver transplantation for biliary atresia. Hepato-Gastroenterology. 2004;51:192–4.
5. Urahashi T, Ihara Y, Sanada Y, Wakiya T, Yamada N, Okada N, et al. Effect of repeat Kasai hepatic portoenterostomy on pediatric live-donor liver graft for biliary atresia. Exp Clin Transplant. 2013;11:259–63.
6. Saito T, Terui K, Mitsunaga T, Nakata M, Komatsu S, Yoshida H. Significance and indications for reoperative portoenterostomy in biliary atresia in light of long-term outcome. J Hepatobiliary Pancreat Sci. 2018;25:275–80.
7. Bondoc AJ, Taylor JA, Alonso MH, Nathan JD, Wang Y, Balistreri WF, et al. The beneficial impact of revision of Kasai portoenterostomy for biliary atresia: an institutional study. Ann Surg. 2012;255:570–6.
8. Shirota C, Uchida H, Ono Y, Murase N, Tainaka T, Yokota K, et al. Long-term outcomes after revision of Kasai portoenterostomy for biliary atresia. J Hepatobiliary Pancreat Sci. 2016;23:715–20.
9. Nakamura H, Kawano T, Yoshizawa K, Nakajima H, Suda K, Koga H, et al. Long-term follow-up for anicteric survival with native liver after redo Kasai: a first report. J Pediatr Surg. 2016;51:2109–12.
10. Hashikura Y, Ichida T, Umeshita K, Kawasaki S, Mizokami M, Mochida S, et al. Donor complications associated with living donor liver transplantation in Japan. Transplantation. 2009;88:110–4.
11. Parikh ND, Ladner D, Abecassis M, Butt Z. Quality of life for donors after living donor liver transplantation: a review of the literature. Liver Transpl. 2010;16:1352–8.
12. Dew MA, Butt Z, Humar A, DiMartini AF. Long-term medical and psychosocial outcomes in living liver donors. Am J Transplant. 2017;17:880–92.
13. Participants in the International Summit on Transplant Tourism and Organ Trafficking Convened by the Transplantation Society and International Society of Nephrology in Istanbul, Turkey, April 30–May 2, 2008. The Declaration of Istanbul on organ trafficking and transplant tourism. Transplantation. 2008;86:1013–8.
14. Hasegawa T, Kimura T, Sasaki T, Okada A, Mushiake S. Indication for redo hepatic portoenterostomy for insufficient bile drainage in biliary atresia: re-evaluation in the era of liver transplantation. Pediatr Surg Int. 2003;19:256–9.
15. Lilly JR, Karrer FM, Hall RJ, Stellin GP, Vasquez-Estevez JJ, Greenholz SK, et al. The surgery of biliary atresia. Ann Surg. 1989;210:289–94. discussion 294–6
16. Saeki M, Nakano M, Kuroda T, Kaneshiro R, Torikai G, Sakamoto S. Analysis of re-hepatic portojejunostomy for biliary atresia. Jpn J Pediatr Surg. 1997;29:972–6.
17. Ohi R, Hanamatsu M, Mochizuki I, Ohkohchi N, Kasai M. Reoperation in patients with biliary atresia. J Pediatr Surg. 1985;20:256–9.
18. Ando H, Kaneko K, Ono Y, Tainaka T, Sumida W. Value of reoperation after Kasai portoenterostomy in the times of liver transplantation for biliary atresia. Jpn J Pediatr Surg. 2008;40:119–22.
19. Nishi T, Yamamoto H, Kashimura T. The results of long-term follow-up after reoperation for biliary atresia: analysis of the timing for reoperation. Jpn J Pediatr Surg. 1997;29:928–33.
20. Mendoza MM, Chiang JH, Lee SY, Kao CY, Chuang JH, Tiao MM, et al. Reappraise the effect of redo-Kasai for recurrent jaundice following Kasai operation for biliary atresia in the era of liver transplantation. Pediatr Surg Int. 2012;28:861–4.

# Operation Procedure: Living Donor Liver Transplantation for Biliary Atresia

24

Mureo Kasahara, Akinari Fukuda, and Seisuke Sakamoto

**Abstract**

Biliary atresia is the most common indication for liver transplantation in pediatric population. This chapter provide surgical technique and the comprehensive factors that might influence the outcomes of patients with biliaryt atresia who undergo living donor liver transplantation in the largest pediatric organ transplantation center in Japan. Surgical technique involves the donor surgery, the recipient vascular and biliary reconstructions including surgical tips. The donor body mass index, ABO incompatibility, graft type, recipient age, center experience and transplant era were found to be significant predictors of the overall graft survival. Adolescent age (12 to <18 years) was associated with a significantly worse long-term graft survival rate than younger or older ages. We conclude that living donor live rtransplantation for biliary atresia is a safe and effective treatment modality that does not compromise living donors. The optimum timing for living donor liver transplantation is crucial for a successful outcome, and early referral to transplantation center can improve the short-term outcomes of liver transplantation for biliary atresia. Further investigation of the major cause of death in liver transplanted recipients with biliary atresia in the long-term is essential, especially among adolescents.

**Keywords**

Living donor liver transplantation · Living donor
Liver transplantation · Pediatric liver transplantation
Biliary atresia · Portal vein reconstruction

M. Kasahara (✉) · A. Fukuda · S. Sakamoto
Organ Transplantation Center, National Center for Child Health and Development, Tokyo, Japan
e-mail: kasahara-m@ncchd.go.jp

## Abbreviations

BA: biliary atresia
BMI: body mass index
BW: body weight
DDLT: deceased donor liver transplantation
LDLT: living donor liver transplantation
GRWR: graft-recipient body weight ratio
LT: liver transplantation

## 24.1 Introduction

The Kasai operation has dramatically improved the outcomes in children with biliary atresia (BA); however, most patients with BA ultimately require liver transplantation (LT) even after a successful Kasai procedure [1, 2]. BA is still one of the most common indications for pediatric LT [3–7]. Untreated infants succumb to either liver cirrhosis or liver failure, or both within a year or two of birth [8]. Indications for LT in patients with post-Kasai BA include persistent hyperbilirubinemia, liver cirrhosis, liver failure, gastrointestinal bleeding due to portal hypertension, growth retardation, pruritus, progressive intrapulmonary shunting, hepatopulmonary syndrome, and repeated cholangitis, either alone or in combination [9]. Pediatric end-stage liver disease score over 10 points is one of the good makers for indication of LT in pediatric patient with BA. Several large studies from outstanding global institutions have reported the excellent long-term outcomes after pediatric LT for BA, given that the 5-year recipient survival rate ranges from 82% to 98% [10–14].

The first successful pediatric living donor liver transplantation (LDLT) operation was performed in 1989 by Strong RY from Australia for Japanese patients with BA, which brought a new light to the field of LT, particularly in Asia [15, 16]. This technical innovation was soon implemented for the treatment of pediatric patients with end-stage liver disease in Japan (1989), Hongkong (1993), Taiwan (1994),


M. Nio (ed.), *Introduction to Biliary Atresia*, https://doi.org/10.1007/978-981-16-2160-4_24

South Korea (1994), and mainland China (1995) due to the lack of deceased donor liver transplantation (DDLT) [17]. Asian pediatric LT physicians have made great innovations from the initial adult-pediatric LDLT to adult–adult LDLT, and from using a left lateral segment graft to left/right lobe, and even a monosegment graft for the small babies [18, 19]. Furthermore, donation by hepatitis B core antibody (HBcAb)-positive and ABO-incompatible donors can be safely performed with perioperative anti-HB virus treatment and desensitization of preformed antibodies [20–22].

The first LDLT operation in Japan was performed for a pediatric patient with BA in 1989. According to the Japanese Liver Transplantation Society registration, which is mandatory dataset of all LT cases in Japan, during the 28-year period from November 1989 to December 2017, LT has been performed in 8347 cases. Currently, 300 ~ 350 LDLTs and 100 DDLTs are performed each year. Overall, 3173 LDLTs were performed in children of <18 years of age over the same period, which accounts for 36.8% of all LDLT procedures [23]. In the United States, pediatric LT cases accounted for 7.3% of the total LT volume [24]. Of note, the proactive performance of pediatric LDLT in Japan has led to such enormous differences in comparison to most Western countries, including the United States and Europe.

In Japan, the annual number of LDLT cases has decreased since 2005. Donor death caused by adult-to-adult LDLT with an extended right lobe graft with nonalcoholic steatohepatitis donor was, for example, reported in May 2003 [25]. This was paralleled by an overall 50% increase in deceased liver donation since the revision of the organ transplant law in 2010. Maximal efforts have been made to reduce living donor morbidity/mortality and to increase the number of deceased donors in Japan. Indeed, during the same period, DDLT was indicated in 447 cases, 63 (14.1%) of which were pediatric cases [26].

Regarding the indication of pediatric LDLT in Japan, cholestatic liver diseases represented by BA account for 64.0% of cases, followed by metabolic liver disease in 9.0% (urea cycle disorders, 50%; organic acidemia, 19%; Wilson's disease, 10%; glycogen storage disease, 9%, etc.) and acute liver failure in 9.0%, with over all the patient survival of 80.1% in 25 years [26].

In this chapter, the standard operation procedure of LDLT in the National Center for Child Health and Development, Tokyo, Japan, was demonstrated in detail.

## 24.2 Living Donor Surgical Procedure

### 24.2.1 Graft Selection in Pediatric Living Donor Liver Transplantation

The potential living donors are strictly limited to three degree of the family members in Japan. The donors were evaluated using liver function tests, viral infection tests, and blood type, anatomical variations, and graft size were evaluated with computed tomography (CT) volumetry. Three dimensional evaluation of vascular and biliary anatomy can be achieved with CT and MRI. This method is easier and more precise than conventional CT. Graft selection was made according to the graft-recipient body weight ratio (GRWR), given that 4.0% ≥ GRWR ≥ 1.0% is the ideal graft size for successful outcomes in pediatric LDLT [27]. Namely, reduced left lateral segment graft was applied for the recipient's body weight (BW) ≤ 5.0 kg without portal hypertension such as neonatal acute liver failure and metabolic liver disease, left lateral segment of 5.0 kg < BW ≤ 25 kg, left lobe of 25 kg < BW ≤ 50 kg, and right lobe of BW < 50 kg are recommended as a graft selection in LDLT setting (Fig. 24.1). The plane of liver resection and graft type was determined before planned LDLT on the basis of a precise imaging study.

### 24.2.2 Skin Incision

A 10–12 cm midline incision is made in the upper abdomen while leaving the donor's xiphoid process intact (Fig. 24.1). Following careful laparotomy, the round ligament of the liver is tied up with 2-0 silks and incised. At this point, the ligating liver side is left uncut and held with a mosquito clamp so that it is available for the later extension of the operational area and the mobilization procedure during hepatectomy. Since the falciform ligament of the liver is fixed to the diaphragm in the recipient, care must be taken not to make it too short on the liver side. The surgeons hook one right and one left costal arch traction to extend the operational area (Fig. 24.2). The abdominal cavity is inspected to exclude any abnormal lesions.

### 24.2.3 Mobilization of the Liver

The liver surface is held with the surgeon's left hand towards the caudal side and the fibrotic tissue of the anterior surface of the left and middle hepatic veins is dissected to expose the

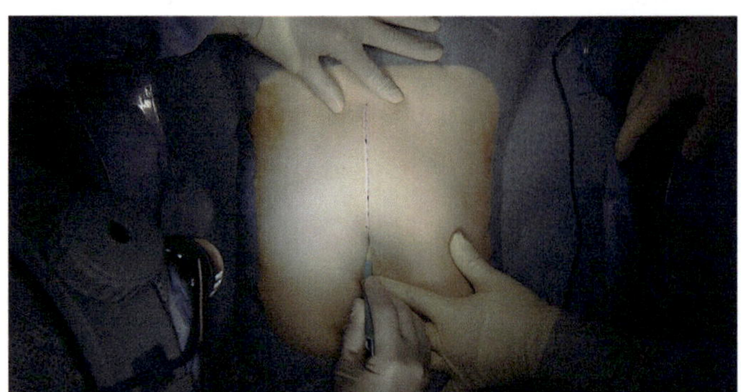

Fig. 24.1 A 10–12 cm midline incision is made in the upper abdomen was made in the donor

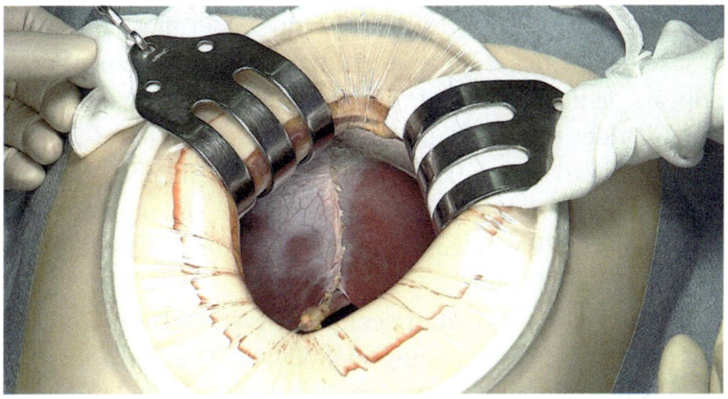

Fig. 24.2 Kent tractions are placed to extend the operation area

anterior surface. The lateral segment is lifted, and the towel is placed in front of the spleen for its protection. The triangular and hepatogastric ligaments were then dissected from the liver, and the hepatic veins were isolated. The left phrenic vein usually runs along the ligament where it is attached to the diaphragm, but in certain cases, it may also run inside the left triangular ligament before it enters the left hepatic vein. In these cases, the surgeon should double ligate the left phrenic vein and incise it so that later it will be easier to clump the left hepatic vein to secure enough cuff for reconstruction.

### 24.2.4 Isolation of Left Hepatic Artery

The lateral segment is then lifted up, and the lesser omentum is incised close to the liver. This must be carefully done as in 20% of the donor's accessory left hepatic artery emerges from the left gastric artery. If there is an accessory left hepatic artery, it should be preserved as long as possible and is usually dissected out to the bifurcation of the left gastric artery.

The serous membrane on the left ventral side of the hepatoduodenal ligament is detached at the level of the left hepatic duct, and the left hepatic artery is identified. The artery should be manipulated gently during the dissection (Fig. 24.3). Forceful stretching or pinching of the artery with forceps can easily cause intimal injury, dissection, and hematoma in the arterial wall. Subsequently, the left hepatic duct is identified. After dissecting the very loose connective tissues behind the left hepatic duct and left hepatic artery, the left portal vein can be isolated by dissecting several caudate branches. Given the left hepatic artery and left portal vein were isolated from Glisson's sheath, the sheath around the left bile duct was left undisturbed as much as possible to maintain the blood supply to the biliary system.

### 24.2.5 The Bile Duct Preparation

To begin with preparing the bile duct dissection, the hepatic hilar lesion is detached. After the left hepatic duct is identified, a small Sugita Clip is applied to the predetermined cut

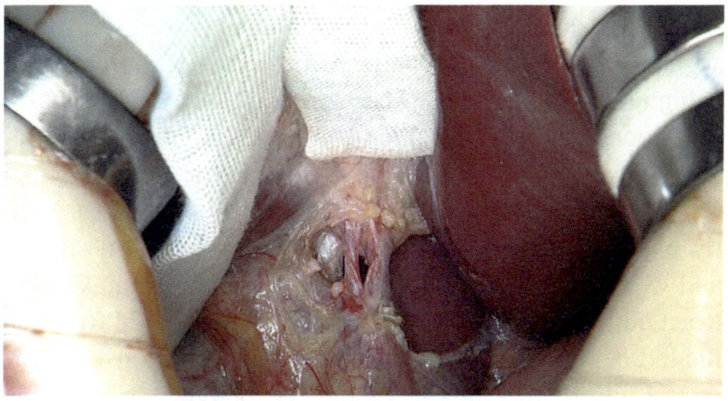

Fig. 24.3 The artery should be manipulated gently during the dissection. There are two left hepatic arteries arising from the proper hepatic artery

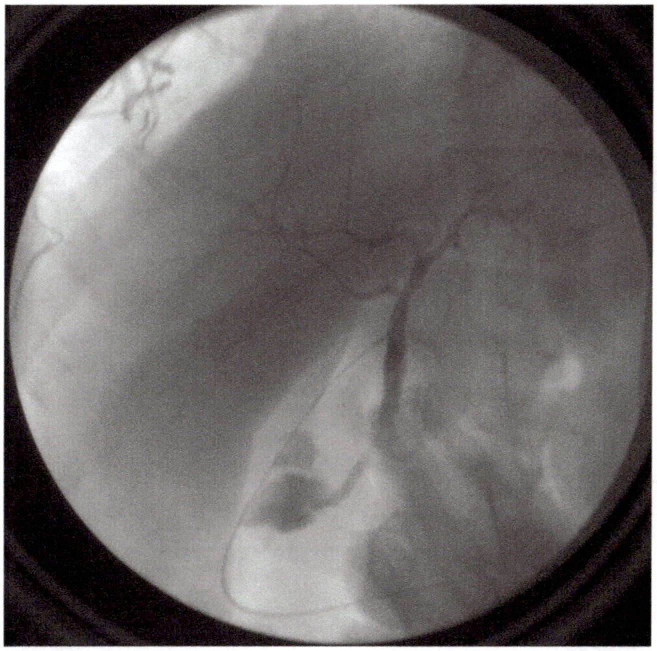

Fig. 24.4 Intraoperative cholangiogram shows posterior duct was drained into the left bile duct

line on the left bile duct. Cholecystectomy and intraoperative cholangiogram with C-arm were performed to confirm the exact biliary anatomy and cutting line of the left bile duct (Fig. 24.4). Once the cutting line on the hepatic duct is determined by consulting findings from cholangiography, 5-0 Prolene stitch was made as a landmark of the cutting line.

### 24.2.6 Parenchymal Dissection of the Liver

When the mobilization of the liver and the preparation of the vessels and bile duct is completed, a cutting line is marked on the liver surface with a cautery approximately 5 ~ 10 mm right side of the falciform ligament (Trans hilar approach). On both sides of the predetermined cutting line at the liver edge, 3-0 Prolene suture is attached as traction sutures to spread the opening. Liver biopsy is taken from the tip of segment 4. Then the hepatic parenchyma was transected using ultrasonic aspirator and bipolar electric cautery without blood vessel clumping and without the graft manipulation (Fig. 24.5). At the middle of the parenchymal transection, the left hepatic duct and the hilar plate was gently isolated at previously determined site with 3-0 silk tie and C-arm cholangiography is applied again to make sure exact cutting plane of the left hepatic duct (Fig. 24.6). Then the left hepatic duct was cut sharply at the previously determined site at the middle of the parenchymal transection (Fig. 24.7). The stump of the main bile duct is closed with 6-0 PDS suture, while the left hepatic duct is left open to allow drainage of bile (Fig. 24.8). Behind the left hepatic duct, a remnant hilar plate can be seen as a stiff fibrous tissue that can be suture ligated with 5-0 Prolene. In some cases, the orifice of hepatic ducts from segment 1 or 4 appears on the cutting side close to the left hepatic duct, segment 4 duct reconstruction is not necessary, and it can be simply closed with 6-0 Prolene. Once the left hepatic duct is cut, the left portal vein can be easily seen, and remnant segment 1 portal branch can be ligated to elongate the left portal vein.

For the parenchymal dissection, curved DeBakey forceps are used as a guide hanging manoeuver. The tip of the forceps is inserted between the caudate lobe and the left lateral segment from the head direction of the left portal vein. The forceps should be lifted slightly upwards and used as a guide in cutting the parenchyma. The parenchyma dissection is continued toward the root of the left hepatic vein. The tissue around the left hepatic vein (Laennec's capsule) is separated, and the confluence of the left and middle hepatic vein is exposed using CUSA and the cautery. Although the left hepatic vein is the only drainage vein in the left lateral segment graft, there are two veins as the graft includes the main branch and the individual superficial branched. In some cases, V2 and 3 are independently drain into inferior vena cava. These variations can easily be identified with preoperative 3D-CT scan, and venoplasty is made as bench surgery.

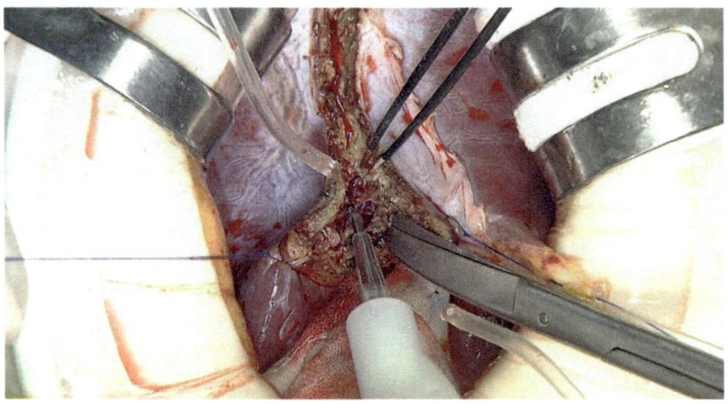

**Fig. 24.5** The hepatic parenchyma was transected using ultrasonic aspirator and bipolar electric cautery without blood vessel clumping and without the graft manipulation

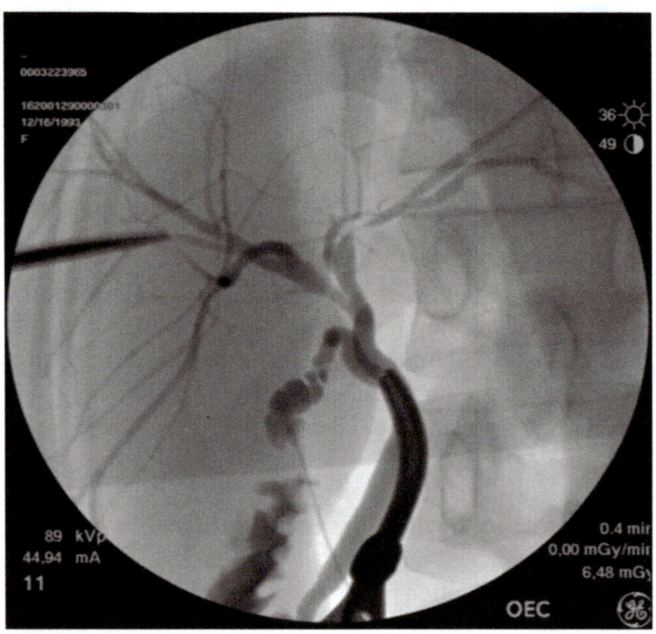


**Fig. 24.6** C-arm cholangiography is applied again to make sure the exact cutting plane of the left hepatic duct

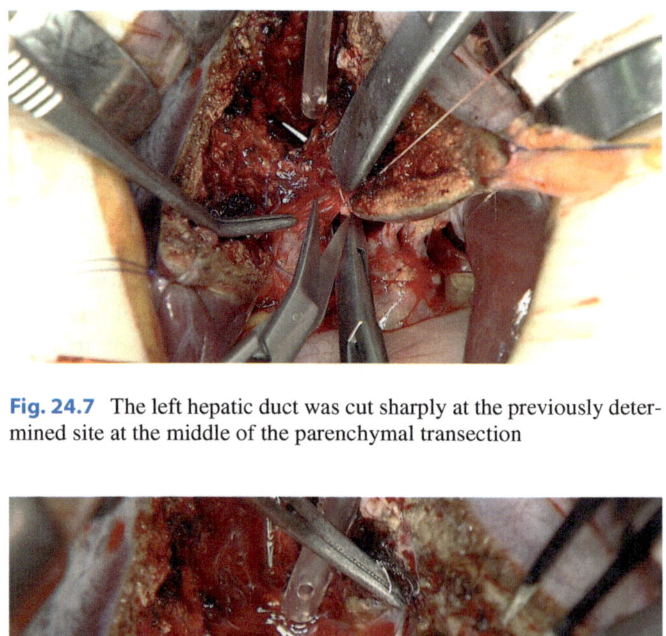

**Fig. 24.7** The left hepatic duct was cut sharply at the previously determined site at the middle of the parenchymal transection

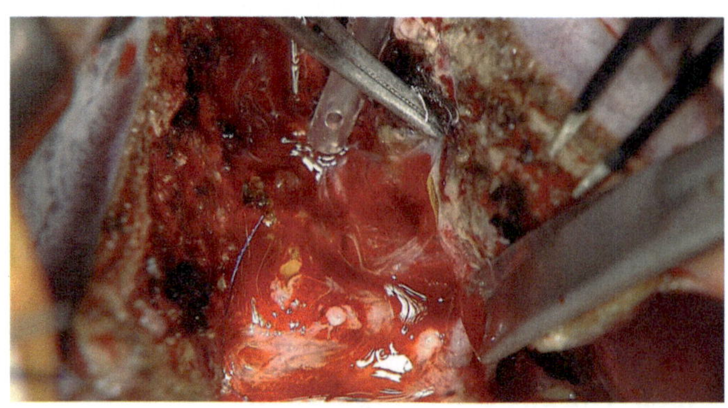

**Fig. 24.8** The stump of the main bile duct is closed with 6-0 PDS suture, while the left hepatic duct is left open to allow drainage of bile

At the end of the dissection, the donor is systematically administered 1000 units of intravenous heparin. After transection of the left hepatic artery, left portal vein, and left hepatic vein, the isolated graft was perfused ex situ through the left portal vein with 4 °C Histidine-tryptophan-ketoglutarate solution (800 ~ 1000 ml). The hepatic veins of the graft were measured and prepared on the back table for feasible venous anastomosis, and the graft was preserved until the recipient is ready for implantation (Fig. 24.9).

Before the closure of the donor abdomen, the surgeon should discuss with the recipient team whether the recipient requires a vein graft for vascular reconstruction. Especially in the BA patient with attenuated portal vein, the vascular graft is sometimes necessary for portal vein reconstruction as an interposition vein graft. We prefer to use the left ovarian vein in female donors and the inferior mesenteric vein in male donors.

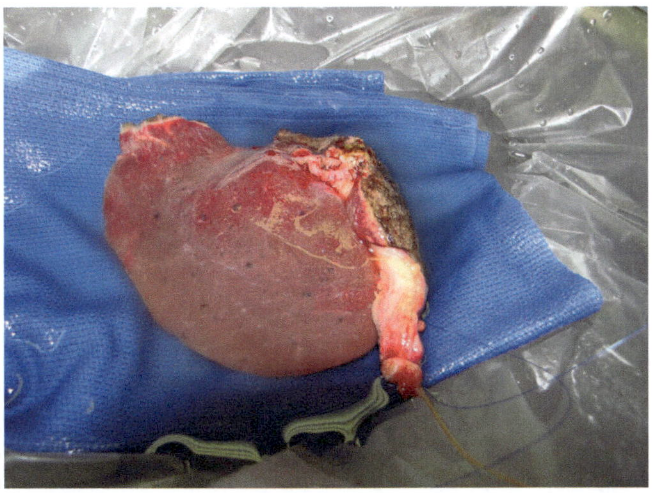

Fig. 24.9 The isolated graft was perfused ex situ through the left portal vein with 4 °C Histidine-tryptophan-ketoglutarate solution

## 24.3 Back Table Procedure

Sterilized crush ice should be prepared in advance, and histidine-tryptophan-ketoglutarate (HTK) solution should be stored at 4 °C in a refrigerator or on ice. As a washout and preservation solution, we use HTK solution because of the short preservation time in LDLT and the low viscosity and potassium concentration. The irrigation tube is cannulated ex situ through the left portal vein and flush with 1000 ml HTK solution. After the portal vein perfusion, the bile duct is washed with 5 ml HTK solution using a 24G cannula. At the same time, the anatomy of the graft hepatic duct and veins should be carefully reconfirmed on the back table. Once all the procedures are completed, the graft is weighed and stored at 4 °C in cold HTK solution until the recipient is ready for implantation.

If the V2 and V3 drain into the inferior vena cava separately, the wall of the veins are sutured together with 6-0 Prolene continuously (with or without patch), and the newly constructed hepatic vein is anastomosed with the recipient hepatic vein (Figs. 24.10 and 24.11).

### 24.3.1 Living Donor Recipient Operation for Biliary Atresia

The most important issue on transplanting the patient with BA is preoperative imaging study of the anatomy. The BA patients frequently show cardiac and vascular anomaly which should be paid attention prior to planned LDLT [28]

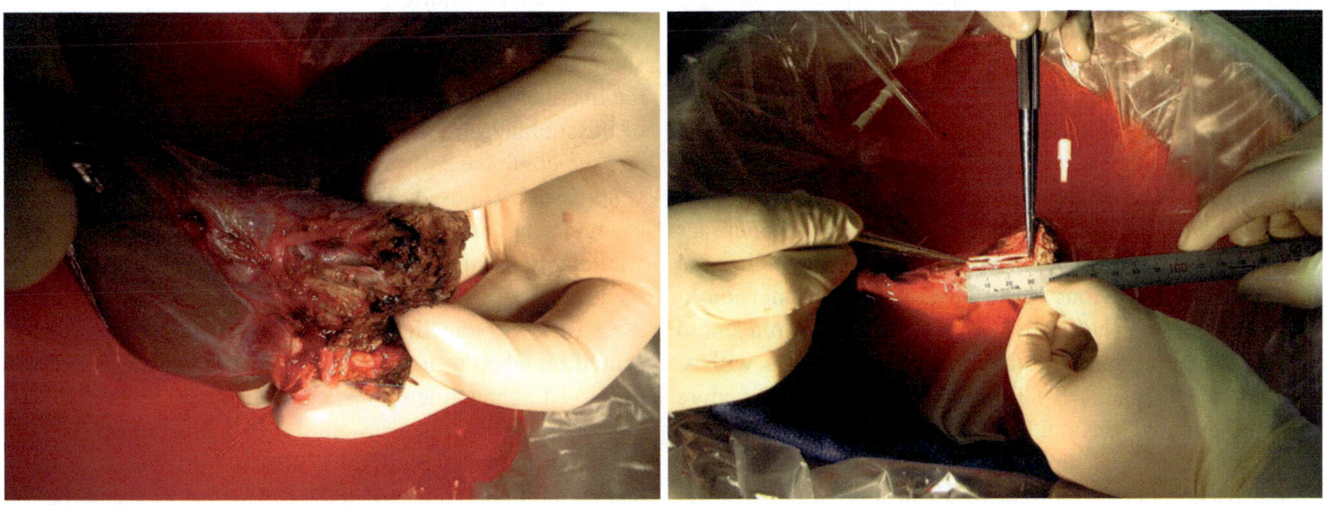

Fig. 24.10 If there are separate V2 and V3 opening, the wall of the veins are sutured together with 6-0 Prolene continuously, and the newly constructed hepatic vein is anastomosed with the recipient hepatic vein

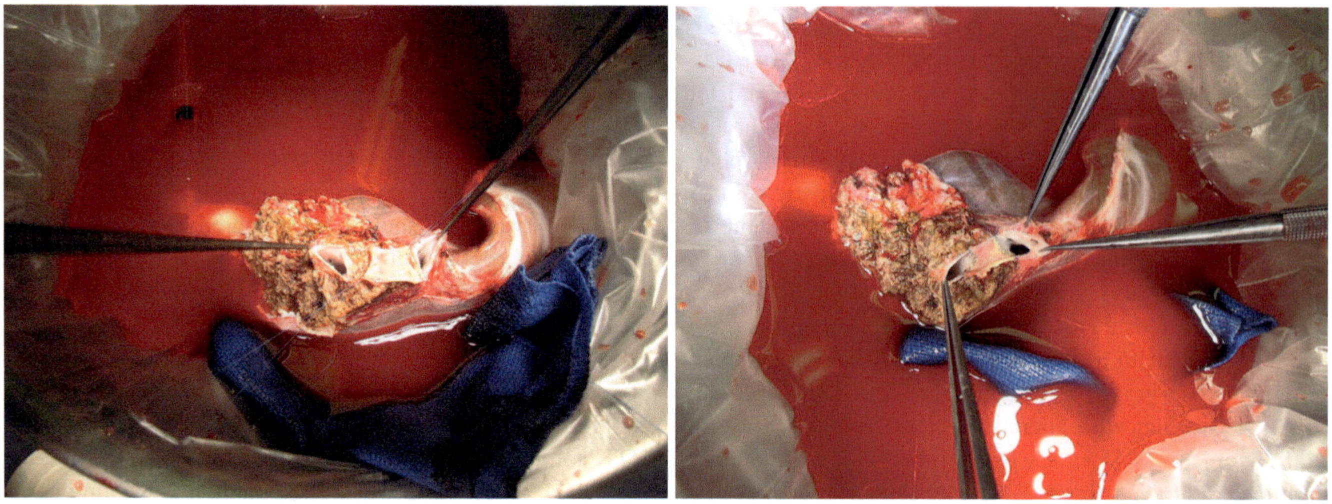

**Fig. 24.11** The wall of the V2 and V3 vein are sutured together with the graft's Falciform ligament interposition

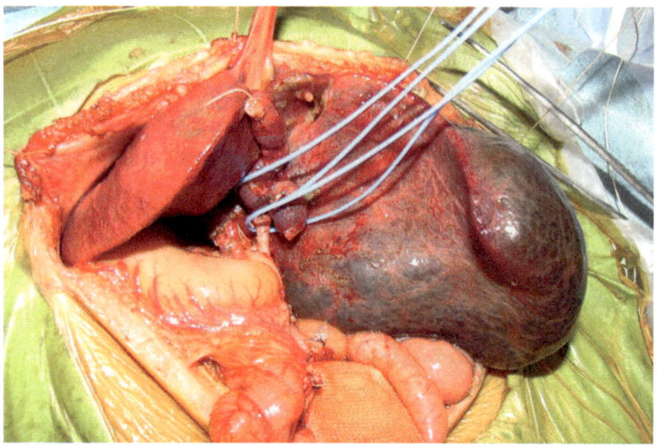

**Fig. 24.12** Biliary atresia with situs inversus

(Fig. 24.12). The patient with a repeated episode of cholangitis, re-do Kasai procedure, hepatic bilomas is strongly associated with attenuated portal vein, which sometimes cause postoperative portal vein complications and even mortality [29].

Skin incision might be another key for successful LT in the recipients with BA. Almost 100% of the patient with BA had Kasai procedure prior to LDLT in Japan. As children grew up, previous Kasai Operation goes up; it sometimes goes up almost on the chest wall. Make a low-down incision (not follow the previous Kasai Scar) with wide incision to get wide space for the relatively big graft for children and to prevent bowel congestion during the manipulation will be recommended (Fig. 24.13). Recently laparoscopic procedure has been initiated in Kasai procedure as a minimum invasive procedure. It has been reported that the recipient with laparoscopic Kasai operation might result in less vascular/bowel complications in subsequent transplantation surgery, as a consequence of less frequent bowel adhesion and hepatic hilus inflammation (Fig. 24.14). If Lap Kasai procedure could be done without compromising the micro bile ducts around the porta hepatis by an expert surgeon, it would be quite beneficial for the patient with BA [30].

### 24.3.2 Mobilization of the Liver

A bilateral subcostal incision combined with upper midline extension to the xiphoid is preferred for recipient total hepatectomy. If the recipient has multiple laparotomies, including Kasai operation and/or an episode of spontaneous bacterial peritonitis, an extraperitoneal approach can be initially taken to prevent bowel injuries. In the case of notable development of the collateral vessels from paraumbilical veins through the peritoneal fatty tissue to the xiphoid process, an extraperitoneal approach can be also employed to avoid collateral injuries.

The falciform ligament is dissected carefully from the suprahepatic vena cava using cautery as the ligament around the liver contains fine collateral vessels. The anterior surface of the suprahepatic inferior vena cava is carefully dissected, and the confluence of major hepatic veins and suprahepatic vena cava is exposed. The towel was placed under the left triangular ligament before it is divided with cautery to prevent any heat injury to the tissue under the left lateral segment. The left lateral segment is then retracted up-ward, and the gastric hepatic ligament is opened with cautery. Care should be taken to locate a replaced left hepatic artery and preserved as much length as possible, since it may be used for hepatic artery reconstruction. The ligamentum venosum (Arantius ligament) is divided near the inferior vena cava, and the peritoneum between the Spiegelius lobe and the left side of the inferior vena cava is incised up from the bottom of the Spiegelius lobe. There are dens adhesions of the stom-

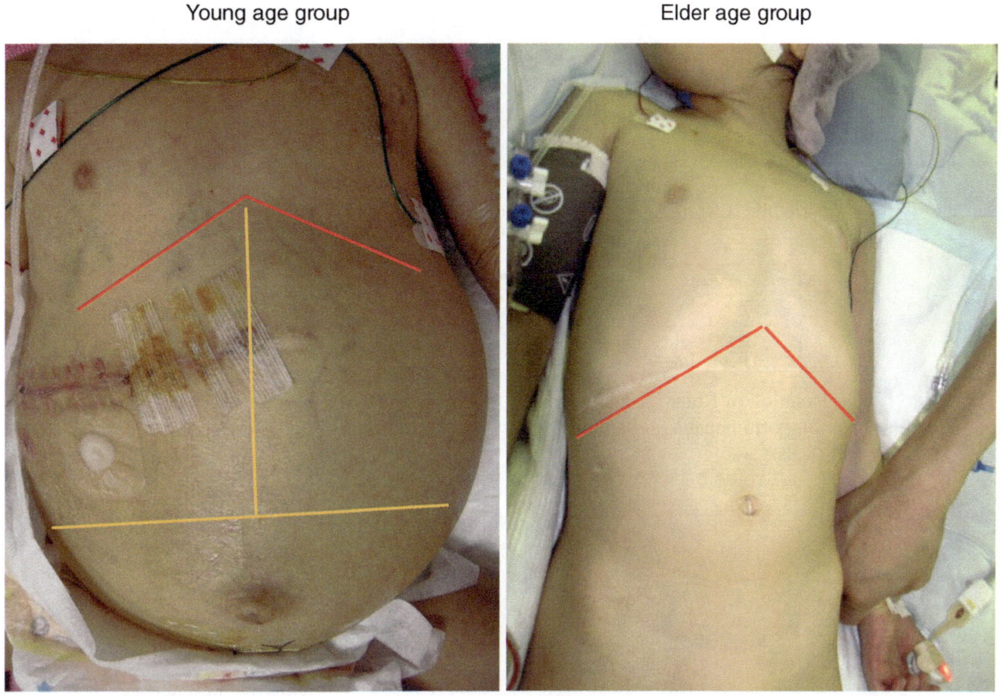


**Fig. 24.13** Previous Kasai Scar in the patient with biliary atresia according to the age group

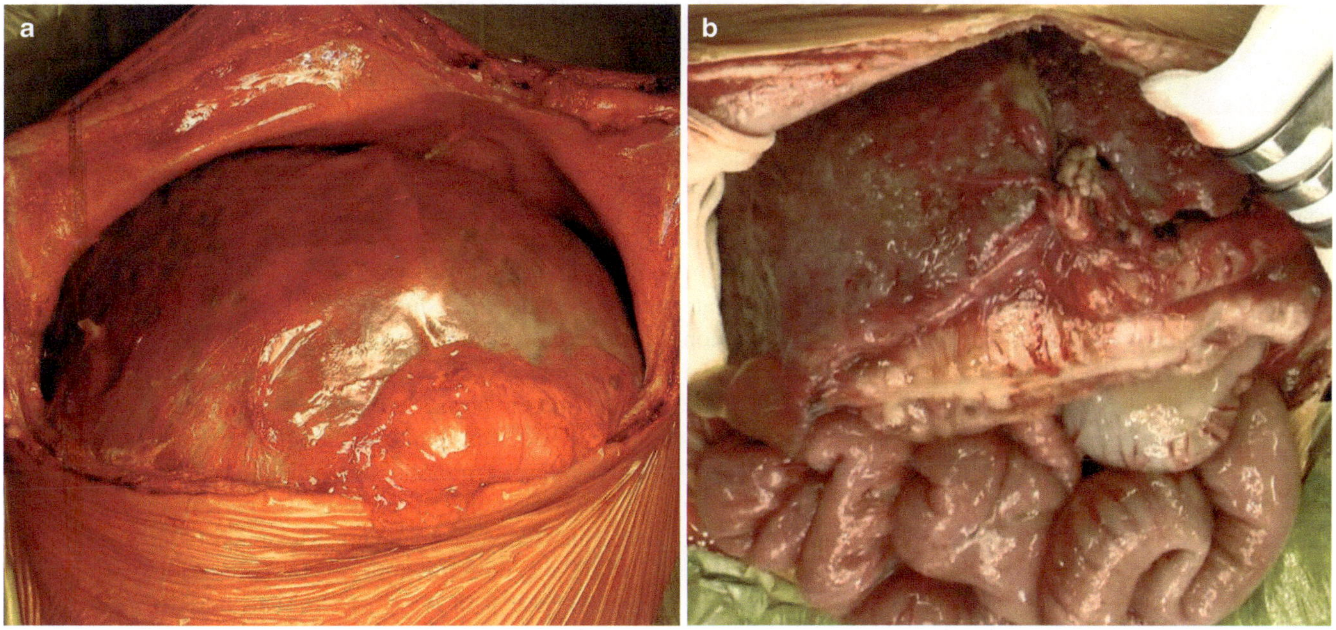


**Fig. 24.14** Intraoperative findings of the biliary atresia patient with open Kasai versus laparoscopic Kasai procedure

ach or intestine to the liver after the Kasai operation, and dissection should be performed carefully close to the liver capsule. Adhesions to the right inferior aspect of the liver are the best-divided approach rather than from the anterior aspect, since the previous Roux-en-Y limb at the time of Kasai operation always runs just above the duodenum. The Roux-en-Y limb should be kept as long as possible because it can be reused for biliary reconstruction.

### 24.3.3 Dissection of Hepatic Hilum

The most important role of hilar dissection in LDLT is to leave the vascular pedicle as long as possible since the graft vasculature is much shorter than those in DDLT. After isolation of Roux-en-Y limb above the duodenum, it is divided high in the porta hepatis and a culture taken of any luminal contents with fine swab (Fig. 24.15). The hepatic arteries are

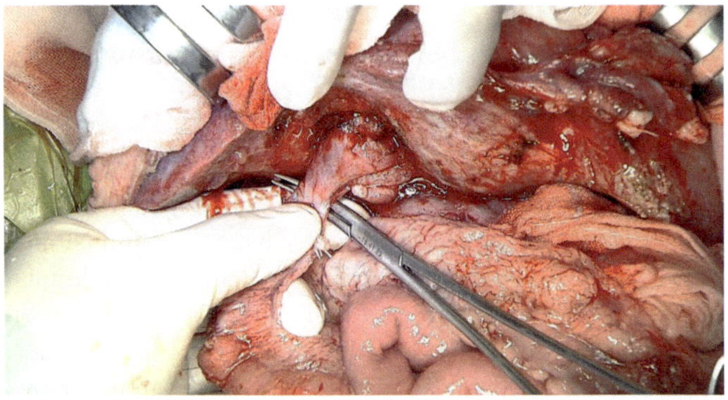

**Fig. 24.15** After isolation of Roux-en-Y limb above the duodenum, it is divided high in the porta hepatis and a culture taken of any luminal contents with fine swab

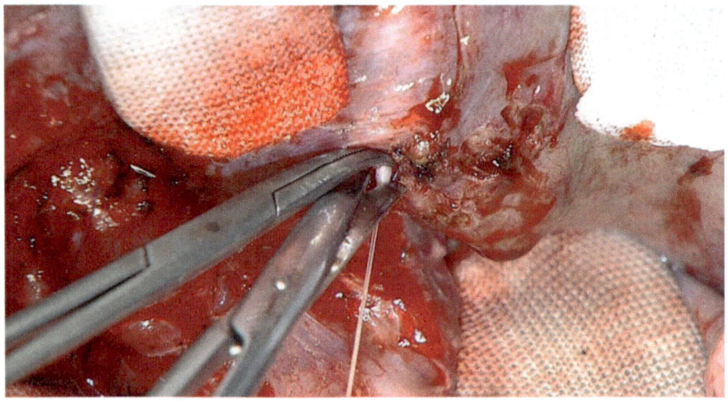

**Fig. 24.16** The hepatic arteries are carefully dissected close to the liver to provide adequate length and enough options for future arterial reconstruction

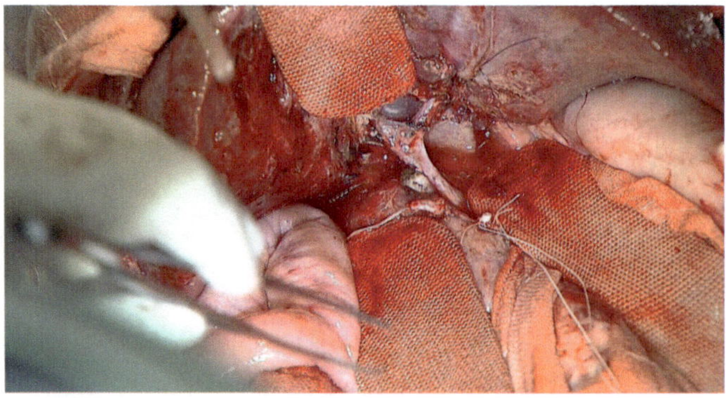

**Fig. 24.17** The portal vein was then dissected from its surrounding tissue and can be divided distal to the main bifurcation in order to obtain enough length for the reconstruction

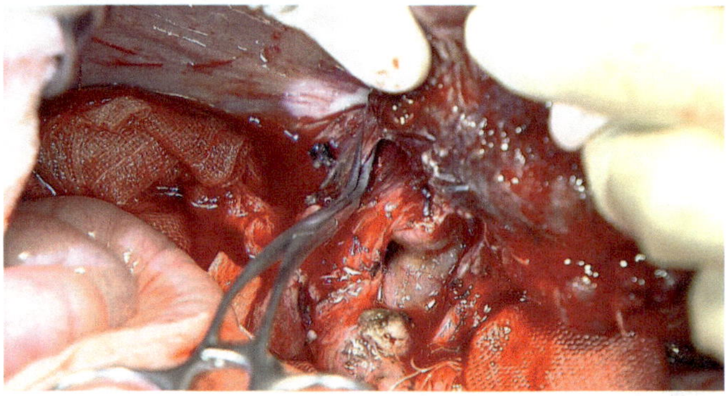

**Fig. 24.18** The triangular ligament (Makuuchi ligament) is suture divided to expose the right side of the inferior vena cava and right hepatic vein

carefully dissected close to the liver to provide adequate length and enough options for future arterial reconstruction (Fig. 24.16). Hepatic artery diameter is enlarged in the patient with BA due to the intimal thickening following the repeated cholangitis and portal hypertension, so that meticulous manipulation should be performed to prevent any intimal injuries during the dissection. Information from the donor team regarding the number, size, and length of the left hepatic artery on the graft is helpful in determining the transection line of the arteries in the recipient. To elongate hepatic artery to facilitate arterial anastomosis and elongate the portal vein, the gastroduodenal artery is almost always dissected.

The portal vein is exposed from the right side of the hilar lesion with removing sentinel/periportal lymph nodes. The portal vein was then dissected from its surrounding tissue and can be divided distal to the main bifurcation in order to obtain enough length for the reconstruction (Fig. 24.17). However, the portal vein in BA patient is attenuated due to repeated cholangitis, and elongation up to the confluence of the superior mesenteric vein and splenic vein should be necessary together with dissecting the left gastric vein. The portal vein can be cut during total hepatectomy in cases with noticeable collateral vessels because it does not increase the portal venous pressure; however, recent, our study revealed preserving the portal flow just before hepatectomy or a temporary portocaval shunt decrease the incidence of intraoperative portal vein thrombosis even in the patient with BA.

Then retracting the liver to the patient's left or cranial side, the triangular ligament (Makuuchi ligament) is suture divided to expose the right side of the inferior vena cava and right hepatic vein (Fig. 24.18). The inferior vena cava is carefully dissected along its anterior surface from caudate to the cranial side, and the short hepatic veins are ligated and transected. Total hepatectomy was completed after side clumping the right hepatic vein and middle/left hepatic vein to maintain caval flow. If there were bowel congestion due to the portal vein obstruction, the portocaval shunt was again initiated temporarily (Fig. 24.19). In the case of right lobe LDLT, the left and middle hepatic veins are sewn over at their junction with running 5-0 Prolene suture because the right lobe graft is generally anastomosed to an extension of the native right hepatic vein orifice. In case the right lobe graft with the middle hepatic vein or V5/8 requires reconstruction, the left and middle hepatic veins should be preserved as long as possible.

### 24.3.4 Implantation of the Graft Liver

#### 24.3.4.1 Hepatic Vein Anastomosis

The liver graft was implanted into the left hepatic cavity after the trimming of the hepatic vasculature orifice (Fig. 24.20). Our standard procedure for left-sided graft implantation is to create one orifice using all of the hepatic veins with total clumping the inferior vena cava, which could make natural triangle orifice on the inferior vena cava. The stomach and intestine are retracted to the caudal side with malleable retractors. This helps to provide a comfortable and correct anastomosis, and good exposure to the surgical field is mandatory for anastomosis. Two stitches with double-armed 5-0 Prolene are placed on the right and left corners of the recipient vein orifice. A stay suture is placed in the middle of the posterior wall for retraction. After the graft placement, both of the inside stitches are passed through the corners of the graft hepatic vein from the inside to the outside. The left corner stitch is ligated, and the right corner stitch is pulled with gentle tension without ligation to guarantee good coaptation. Then continuous intraluminal suture is made to the right corner. During the posterior anastomosis, the anterior wall is pulled gently with peanut forceps to expose the suture line. The anterior wall is sutured with interruption. After the hepatic vein anastomosis another small vascular clamp is placed just proximal to the anastomosis, and total clumping of inferior vena cava is removed.

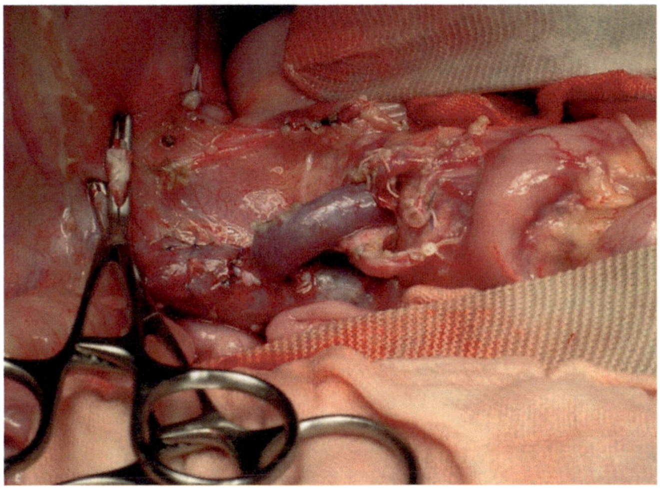

**Fig. 24.19** Temporary proto caval shunt was made, if the recipient shows bowel congestion during total clumping portal vein

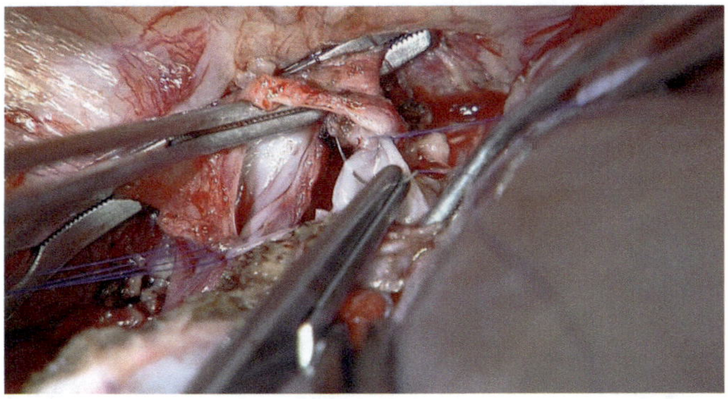

**Fig. 24.20** Hepatic vein reconstruction

#### 24.3.4.2 Portal Vein Anastomosis

Unlike in DDLT, there are restrictions in harvesting vessel graft in LDLT. If there are insufficient portal front flow and/or portal pressure (portal vein pressure should be >25 mmHg prior to implantation), further collateral interruption/devascularization (left gastric vein, spleno-retroperitoneal shunt, paracolic gutter, mesenteric collaterals, and spleno-renal vein) should be applied [31]. If the portal vein looks sclerotic, mural thrombi in intima with diameter less than 4 mm, the interposition vein graft (donor ovarian vein, donor inferior mesenteric vein, native juggler vein, native left renal vein, etc.) should be considered [32] (Fig. 24.21). Due to the retrograde flow to the left gastric vein in patients with severe portal hypertension, spontaneous hypoplasia of the portal vein might have originated from immediately above the termination site of the left gastric vein. Fibrous tissue and lymph nodes around the portal vein are divided. Then the volume of the portal flow should be confirmed by unclumping the portal vein (Fig. 24.22).

For the portal vein reconstruction, various factors in the recipient portal vein, which include the size of the orifice, the length of the pedicle, the quality of intima, and elasticity of

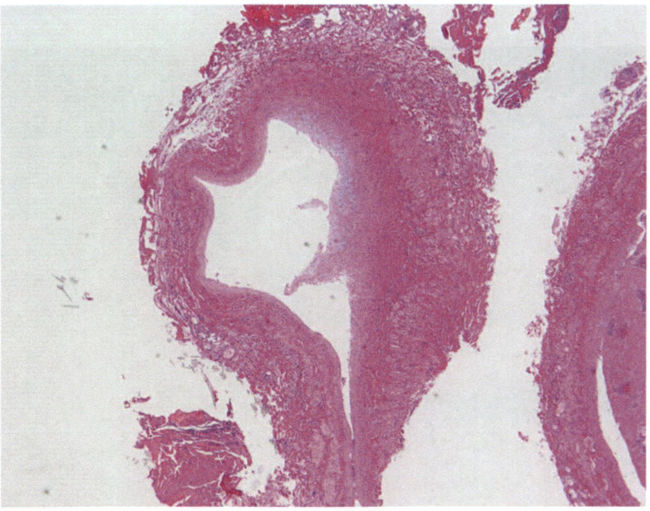

**Fig. 24.21** Mural thrombi of the native portal vein

the lumen, should be checked carefully before anastomosis. The most simple and frequently used technique is the oblique incision of the portal vein trunk and direct anastomosis with graft portal vein, which can prevent redundancy of the anastomosis. If the portal vein wall has sclerosis and less than 4 mm in diameter, it sometimes needs to be replaced by a venous graft (Fig. 24.23).

In portal anastomosis, there should be no redundancy, kinks, twists, or strictures. The vascular clump is opened for just a second and heparinized to remove the possible formation of thrombus, and the portal vein is gently clamped again above the confluence of the superior mesenteric vein and the splenic vein. The two double-armed 6-0 PDS sutures are placed at the right and left corner of the graft portal vein and the both inside needles are passed through the same corner of the recipient portal vein inside out. Both sides are pulled with two mosquito clumps, each in the opposite direction to guarantee good coaptation and extension of the anastomosis.

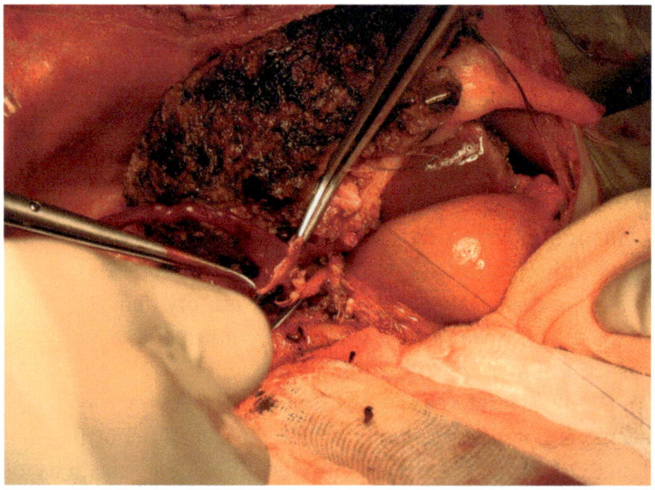

**Fig. 24.22** Sufficient portal front flow after collateral interruption

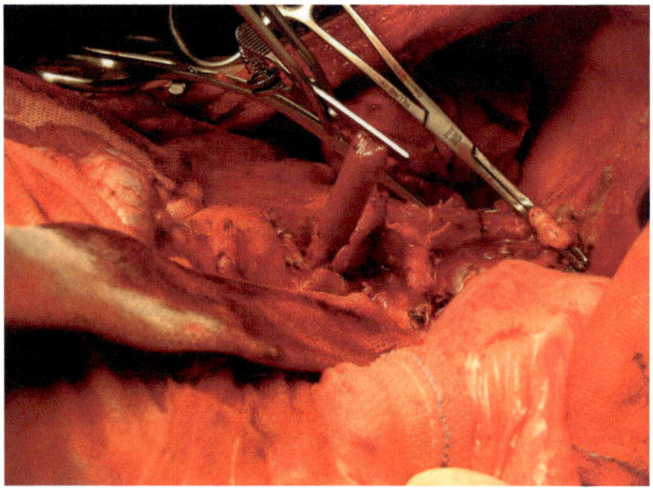

**Fig. 24.23** Portal vein reconstruction using the donor ovarian vein in the patient with attenuated portal vein

Then continuous intraluminal suture is made to the right corner, and 2 ~ 3 mm growth factor is made. During the anastomosis, the suturing stitch should be kept loose to prevent anastomotic stricture. The anterior wall is sutured with interrupted (Fig. 24.24). If adequate portal flow is still not achieved, artery anastomosis should be first conducted.

#### 24.3.4.3 Hepatic Artery Anastomosis

A surgical microscope is used for arterial reconstruction in pediatric LDLT (Fig. 24.25). After securing a good surgical field, both the graft and recipient arteries are clumped using a small vascular clip. The arteries for the anastomosis are selected according to the size and length of both the graft artery and the recipient artery. The position of the artery should also be considered to prevent any twisting, kinking, or over stretching at the anastomotic site. The excellent front flow of the recipient artery is a prerequisite for anastomosis. If the front flow is not enough, the lumen is flushed with heparinized saline, and the flow is checked again. If the flow is still not enough, the artery is dissected further and cut again until the satisfactory flow is obtained. Both arteries are clamped and are dissected out by removing connective tissue

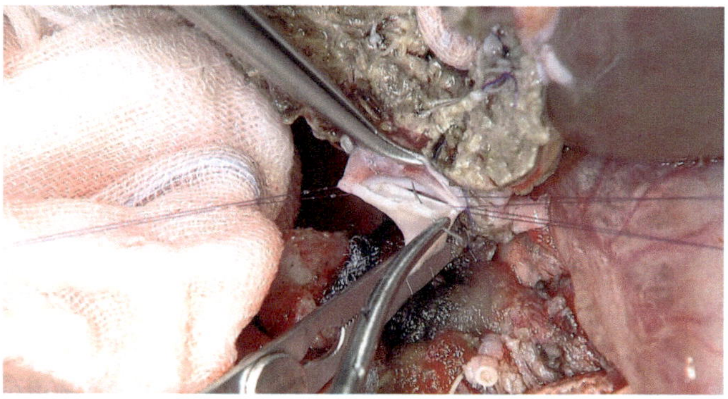

**Fig. 24.24** The portal vein anastomosis

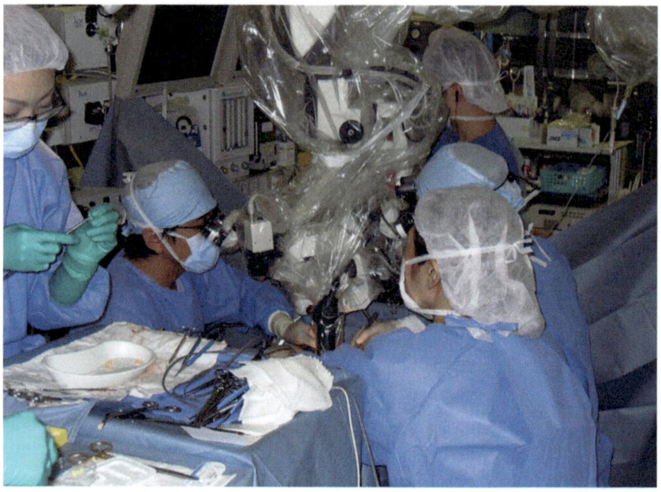

**Fig. 24.25** Hepatic artery anastomosis with surgical microscope

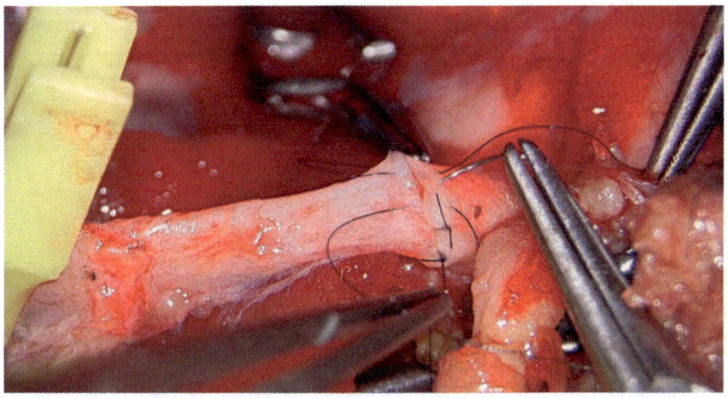

Fig. 24.26 Hepatic artery anastomosis

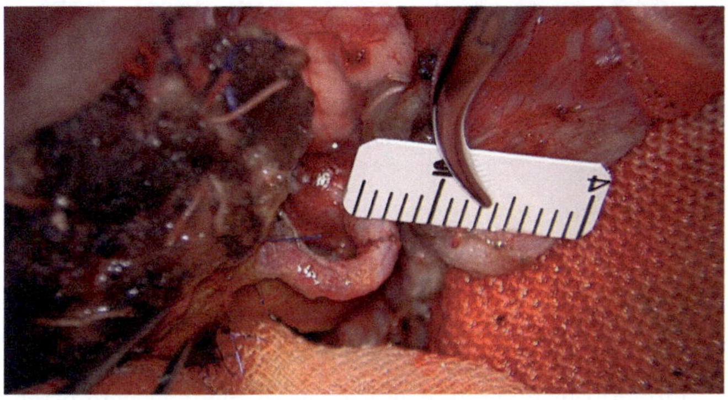

Fig. 24.27 After reperfusion of hepatic artery, the diameter of hepatic artery was 3 mm

slightly with micro scissors until the smooth adventitia surface is reached. The anastomosis is carried out with an interrupted 9-0 Prolene suture. Two stitches are placed and ligated. Depending on the size, 4 ~ 6 stitches are placed on the anterior wall of the anastomosis and are ligated in order. The clamp on the recipient artery is removed first to check for leakage and patency at the anastomosis (Fig. 24.26). In cases of multiple graft arteries, in principle, a larger one is chosen for the anastomosis. A second artery can be ligated as long as the excellent arterial backflow can be observed from its cut end after declumping the first anastomosis.

When the quality of the recipient's hepatic artery is not good enough, non-anatomical arterial anastomosis can be applied using the right gastroepiploic artery, splenic artery turnover, gastroduodenal artery, sigmoid artery interposition, mesentery artery of Roux-en-Y limb, and donor radial artery interposition, etc. (Fig. 24.27).

### 24.3.5 Biliary Reconstruction

The previously created Roux-en-Y limb can be used for the reconstruction in case of post-Kasai BA, if it has not been greatly damaged during total hepatectomy. A small hall (3 ~ 4 mm) is made in the Roux-en-Y limb close to the proximal end. A 4 French polyvinyl alcohol tube is inserted

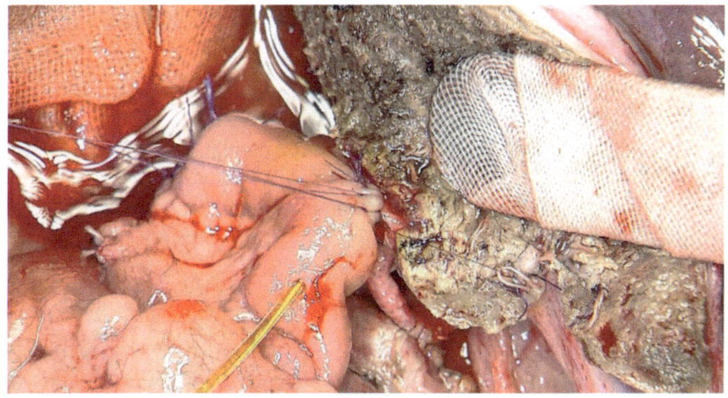

Fig. 24.28 A running suture using the stitch is made first in the posterior wall, and then anterior wall suture was made with interrupted suture

through the hole into the intestinal lumen as an external stent and is led out of the intestinal wall again. Two double-armed 6-0 PDS sutures are placed on the right and left corner of the graft left hepatic duct. A running suture using the stitch is made first in the posterior wall, and then anterior wall suture was made with interrupted suture (Fig. 24.28). After the anastomosis of the posterior wall, the stent tube is inserted into the intrahepatic bile duct (B2) to prevent accidental B2 ligation. The stent tube is secured to the anterior wall of the bile duct. When the orifice of the graft bile duct is too small, an incision is made along the axis on the anterior wall of the bile duct to make it bigger. If there are multiple bile ducts on the graft and are located within the same Glisson's capsule, duct plasty can be possible. However, if there are multiple bile ducts with separate Glisson's capsule, it is better to make multiple hepatic jejunostomy. After the closure of the anterior wall, the stent tube is secured on the intestinal wall with a 6-0 PDS stitch. The tube can be removed around 3 months after LDLT.

## 24.4 Surgical Complications in NCCHD

The National Center for Child Health and Development, Tokyo, Japan, launched the liver transplantation program in 2005, and the Organ Transplantation Center was established in May 2011. We have carried out 600 cases of liver transplantation to date (as of the end of December 2019) (Fig. 24.29). The number of pediatric liver transplantation cases per year is 50–70 cases, accounting for approximately 50–70% of pediatric liver transplantations in Japan. Liver transplantations for cholestatic liver diseases represented by BA at our center accounted for approximately 50%, which is significantly different from the results of national statistics. This is because our center has handled many serious cases, including metabolic liver diseases of 20% occurring immediately after birth and fulminant hepatitis of 20% requiring emergency transplantation as a foundation hospital for pediatric organ transplantation. Although our center treated more

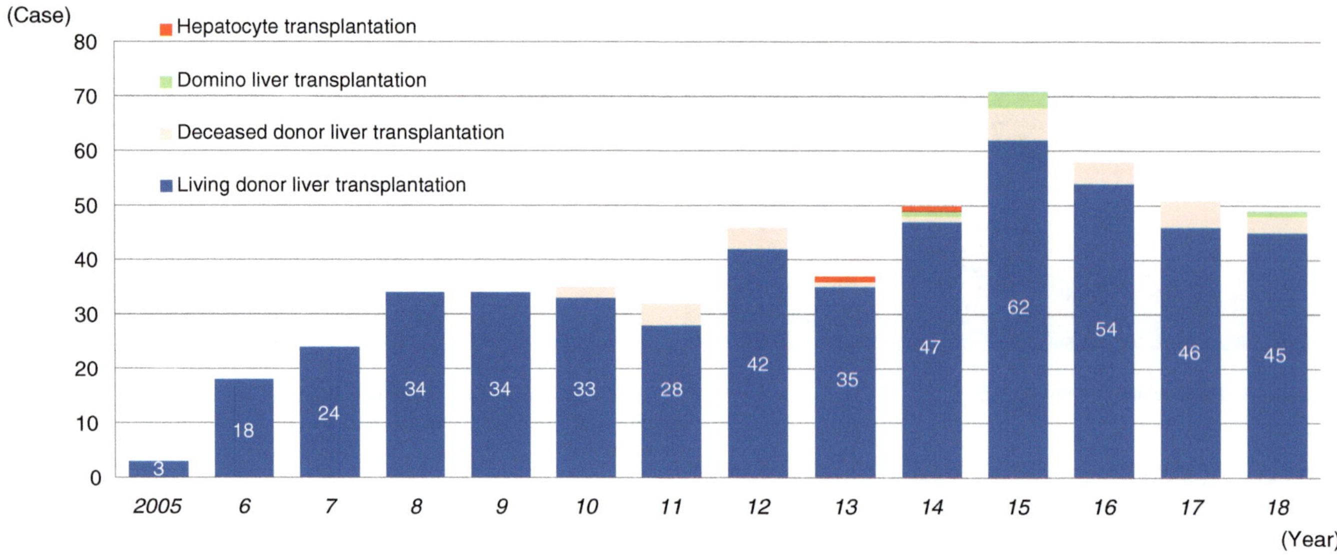


**Fig. 24.29** Pediatric liver transplantation in NCCHD ($N = 600$)

**Table 24.1** Post living donor liver transplantation surgical complications in the national center for child health and development ($N = 600$)

| Surgical complications | | Number | Incidence (%) |
|---|---|---|---|
| Portal vein | Thrombosis | 4 | 0.7 |
| | Stricture | 19 | 3.1 |
| Hepatic vein | Stricture | 5 | 0.9 |
| Hepatic artery | Thrombosis | 1 | 0.2 |
| Bile duct | Leakage | 7 | 1.2 |
| | Stricture | 25 | 4.1 |
| | Accidental ligation of B2 | 5 | 0.9 |

serious patients compared to other institutions, we maintain a relatively high survival rate with a 10-year survival rate following transplantation of 92% (nationwide average 10-year survival rate: 84.4%) along with no serious complications observed in living donors.

Table 24.1 shows surgical complications following LDLT in the National center for child health and development. As a consequence of meticulous donor and recipient technique, vascular and biliary complications are much less than previous reports, and we can achieve 96.6% of the 10-year patient survival after LDLT for BA.

## 24.5 Perspectives of Pediatric LDLT

Currently, pediatric care in Japan has undergone a significant transformation. Because the system that administers anti-infectious vaccinations has improved and a decrease is expected in the number of hospitalizations due to bacterial meningitis, sepsis, dehydration, and respiratory infections, foundation hospitals for pediatric care must appropriately respond to the necessities of highly advanced medical treatments, including the treatment of newborns with complications, maternal therapy, congenital diseases, pediatric cancer, and organ transplantations, etc.

Organ transplantation is a form of medical care established with the intention of providing precious organs to others, so-called "a gift of life." There are very few organ donations from brain dead patients in Japan, and most transplantations for pediatric patients with end-stage organ failure are mainly carried out as living donor transplantations with relatives as donors. In the case of pediatric patients with end-stage organ failure who have small bodies, size mismatches with the organs from living donors are sometimes observed, making it difficult to carry out transplantation. Because there are many pediatric patients whose lives cannot be saved under the present circumstances of organ transplantation dependent on living donors, enlightenment, and promotion of deceased donor organ transplantation are crucial issues in Japan. The National Center for Child Health and Development will humbly accumulate such cases so that the lives of more pediatric patients with end-stage organs can be saved, in addition to developing new transplantation procedures, studies regarding immunosuppressive methods, clinical applications of regenerative medicine, and the development of international medical professionals. We hope that transplantations at our center will help further the development of pediatric care/medical care in Japan.

The pediatric population with end-stage liver disease will possibly remain dependent on not only DDLT but also the additional LDLT program to further reduce the waiting list mortality. Importantly, since the mortality of children on the DDLT waiting list has not entirely disappeared, LDLT should still be considered as an additional option for pediatric candidates, even in DDLT-dominant countries. While we should continue to promote DDLT in Japan, it may also be time to re-explore the outcomes after LDLT in the context of the recent technical and medical improvements in this field with ensured living donor safety.

## References


1. Kasai M, Kimura S, Asakura Y, Suzuki H, Taira Y, Ohashi E. Surgical treatment of biliary atresia. J Pediatr Surg. 1968;3:655–75.
2. Nio M, Miyano T, Saeki M, Shiraki K, Tanaka K. Five- and 10-year survival rates after surgery for biliary atresia: a report from the Japanese biliary atresia registry. J Pediatr Surg. 2003;38:997–1000.
3. Hartley JL, Davenport M, Kelly DA. Biliary atresia. Lancet. 2009;374:1704–13.
4. Karrer FM, Price MR, Bensard DD, Sokol RJ, Narkewicz MR, Smith DJ, Lilly JR. Long-term results with the Kasai operation for biliary atresia. Arch Surg. 1996;131:493–6.
5. Ohi R, Mochizuki I, Komatsu K, Kasai M. Portal hypertension after successful hepatic portoenterostomy in biliary atresia. J Pediatr Surg. 1986;21:271–4.
6. Zagory JA, Nguyen MV, Wang KS. Recent advances in the pathogenesis and management of biliary atresia. Curr Opin Pediatr. 2015;27:389–94.
7. Chen CL, Concejero A, Wang CC, et al. Living donor liver transplantation for biliary atresia: a single center experience with first 100 cases. Am J Transplant. 2006;6:2672–9.
8. Kobayashi H, Stringer MD. Biliary atresia. Semin Neonatol. 2003;8:383–91.
9. Kitajima T, Sakamoto S, Sasaki K, et al. Living donor liver transplantation for post-Kasai biliary atresia: analysis of pre-transplant predictors of outcomes in infants. Liver Transpl. 2017 Sep;23(9):1199–209.
10. Kasahara M, Umeshita K, Inomata Y, et al. Long-term outcomes of pediatric living donor liver transplantation in Japan: an analysis of more than 2200 cases listed in the registry of the Japanese Liver Transplantation Society. Am J Transplant. 2013;13:1830–9.
11. Neto JS, Feier FH, Bierrenbach AL, et al. Impact of Kasai-portoenterostomy on liver transplantation outcomes: a retrospective cohort study of 347 children with biliary atresia. Liver Transpl. 2015;21:922–7.
12. Armon R, Annunziato RA, Willis A, et al. Liver transplantation for children with biliary atresia in the pediatric end-stage liver disease era: the role of insurance status. Liver Transpl. 2013;19:543–50.
13. Barshes NR, Lee TC, Balkrishman R, et al. Orthotopic liver transplantation for biliary atresia: the U.S. experience. Liver Transpl. 2005;11:1193–200.
14. Fouquet V, Alvus A, Branchereau S, et al. Long-term outcome of pediatric liver transplantation for biliary atresia: a 10-year follow-up in a single center. Liver Transpl. 2005;11:152–60.
15. Strong RY, Lynch SV, Ong TH, et al. Successful liver transplantation from a living donor to her son. N Engl J Med. 1990;322:1505–7.
16. Broelsch CE, Emond JC, Whitington PF, et al. Application of reduced-size liver transplants as split grafts, auxiliary orthotopic grafts, and living related segmental transplants. Ann Surg. 1990;212:368–75.
17. Nagasue N, Kohno H, Matsuno S, et al. Segmental (partial) liver transplantation from a living donor. Transplant Proc. 1992;24:1958–9.
18. Yamaoka Y, Washida M, Honda K, et al. Liver transplantation using a right lobe graft from a living related donor. Transplantation. 1994;57:1127–30.
19. Kasahara M, Kaihara S, Oike F, et al. Living donor liver transplantation with monosegments. Transplantation. 2003;76:694–6.
20. Uemoto S, Sugiyama K, Marusawa H, et al. Transmission of hepatitis B virus from hepatitis B core antibody-positive donors in living related liver transplants. Transplantation. 1998;65:494–9.
21. Tokunaga Y, Tanaka K, Fujita S, et al. Living related liver transplantation across ABO blood groups with FK506 and OKT3. Transpl Int. 1993;6:313–8.
22. Egawa H, Umeshita K, Uemoto S. Optimal dosage regimen for rituximab in ABO-incompatible living donor liver transplantation. J Hepatobiliary Pancreat Sci. 2017;24:89–94.
23. Umeshita K, Eguchi S, Egawa H, et al. Liver transplantation in Japan: registry by the Japanese liver transplantation society. Hepatol Res. 2019;49:964–80.
24. Organ Procurement and Transplantation Network [Internet]. Richmond: U.S. Department of Health & Human Services; 2018 July 30. Available from: https://optn.transplant.hrsa.gov/
25. Umeshita K, Fujiwara K, Kiyosawa K, et al. Operative morbidity of living donors in Japan. Lancet. 2003;362:687–90.
26. Kasahara M, Umeshita K, Inomata Y, et al. Long-term outcomes of pediatric living donor liver transplantation in Japan: an analysis of more than 2200 cases listed in the registry of the Japanese Liver Transplantation Society. Am J Transplant. 2013;13:1830–9.
27. Kiuchi T, Kasahara M, Uryuhara K, et al. Impact of graft size mismatching on graft prognosis in liver transplantation from living donors. Transplantation. 1999;67:321–7.
28. Takeda M, Sakamoto S, Uchida H, et al. Technical considerations in liver transplantation for biliary atresia with situs inversus. Liver Transpl. 2019 Sep;25(9):1333–41.
29. Ueda M, Oike F, Kasahara M, et al. Portal vein complications in pediatric living donor liver transplantation using left side graft. Am J Transplant. 2008;8:2097–105.
30. Murase N, Hinoki A, Shirota C, et al. Multicenter, retrospective, comparative study of laparoscopic and open Kasai portoenterostomy in children with biliary atresia from Japanese high-volume centers. J Hepatobiliary Pancreat Sci. 2019;26:43–50.
31. Sakamoto S, Sasaki K, Kitajima T, et al. A novel technique for collateral interruption to maximize portal venous flow in pediatric liver transplantation. Liver Transpl. 2018;24:969–73.
32. Sakamoto S, Uchida H, Kitajima T, et al. The outcomes of portal vein reconstruction with vein graft interposition in pediatric liver transplantation for small children with biliary atresia. Transplantation. 2020;104:90–6.

# Operation Procedure: Deceased Donor Liver Transplantation for Biliary Atresia

# 25

Yoshiyuki Ihara and Koichi Mizuta

**Keywords**

Biliary atresia · Liver transplantation · Deceased donor liver transplantation · Deceased donor · Liver splitting Split liver transplantation · Pediatric liver transplantation

## Abbreviations

BA: biliary atresia
LT: liver transplantation
SLT: split liver transplantation
DBD: donation after brain death
DCD: donation after cardiac death
DDLT: deceased donor liver transplantation
IVC: inferior vena cava
LLS: left lateral segment
ERL: extended right lobe
LL: left lobe
RL: right lobe
LDLT: living donor liver transplantation

## 25.1 Introduction

Biliary atresia (BA) is a progressive cholestatic disease that accounts for nearly 50% of patients referred for liver transplants [1]. Kasai portoenterostomy is the first-line standard treatment for BA and recommended to be performed within 60 days of birth to manage jaundice. However, even if yellowish stool can be eliminated, and a complete correction of the serum bilirubin level to below the normal range can be achieved, then up to half of all BA patients cannot make it through adolescence with their native liver and ultimately require liver transplantation (LT) [2, 3]. Complications of cirrhosis, including portal hypertension, ascites, variceal bleeding, and acute-on-chronic liver failure, are indications for LT [3, 4]. The extrahepatic complications associated with this disease, such as hepatopulmonary syndrome and portopulmonary hypertension, are also indications for LT [4].

Liver transplantation has been used to treat BA since the first clinical liver transplantation was performed in 1963 by Starzl in the United States [5]. After this first case, and up to the 1980s, the only available technical option for pediatric liver transplantation was to transplant the whole liver of a donor with weight as close as possible to that of the recipient. However, the scarcity of size-matched deceased donors has become a major concern and led to innovative surgical techniques, such as split liver transplantation (SLT). In 1989, Pichlmayr was the first to report a case of transplanting one donor liver into two recipients [6]. Since then, SLT has become an important tool to reduce donor organ shortages and mortality among transplant candidates on waiting lists, especially among pediatric patients and small adults [7, 8].

Deceased donor liver grafts are most commonly obtained from donation after brain death (DBD) donors. The blood type should be compatible (or preferably identical) between the donor and recipient. However, another increasingly important source of liver grafts is from donation after cardiac death (DCD) donors. In countries with an active DCD program, such donors account for 5–35% of the total donations [9, 10]. However, DCD donors are generally considered "extended-criteria donors" associated with a risk of primary nonfunction and ischemic cholangiopathy [11, 12]. It has recently been reported that advances in improving the graft quality using donor extracorporeal support and liver machine perfusion have improved the outcomes of DCD grafts [13, 14].

In this chapter, we describe the procedures for graft procurement, liver splitting, and graft implantation in deceased donor liver transplantation (DDLT) for BA.

Y. Ihara (✉) · K. Mizuta
Department of Transplant Surgery,
Saitama Children's Medical Center, Saitama, Japan
e-mail: ihara.yoshiyuki@saitama-pho.jp


M. Nio (ed.), *Introduction to Biliary Atresia*, https://doi.org/10.1007/978-981-16-2160-4_25

## 25.2 Procurement of the Graft Liver

Deceased donor surgery is performed in collaboration with each organ removal team, so it is necessary to reconfirm the method of perfusion, location, and method of drainage, the position of vascular amputation, organ and order of removal, etc., before surgery. The liver procurement method using the standard rapid *en bloc* technique is described below.

Median sternotomy and laparotomy are performed from the upper edge of the sternum to the pubic symphysis, and a large surgical field is secured with a retractor (Fig. 25.1). An intra-abdominal search, including a search for the presence of malignant tumors, and the evaluation of the appropriateness of the organ to be transplanted will be performed by inspection and palpation. Fatty liver is the most commonly encountered abnormality, and suitability is determined based on the liver color during compression and the yellow tone after organ perfusion. A liver biopsy and rapid pathological diagnosis should always be done to ensure the assessment of fatty liver is appropriately performed. Generally, if ≥35% macro steatosis is noted, the organ is not considered suitable for transplantation.

Accessory left hepatic artery branching from the left gastric artery and aberrant right hepatic artery branching from the superior mesenteric artery are often found and should be confirmed. Just above the bifurcation of the common iliac artery, the aorta is encircled twice with cotton tape at the upper and lower points. At this time, operators should be alert for bleeding from the lumbar artery. If atherosclerosis of the aorta is confirmed by palpation, it may be difficult to cannulate, so be careful when selecting the site. The inferior vena cava (IVC) is also encircled in the same way (Fig. 25.2); however, if the thoracic organs are not removed, blood drainage is performed at the supradiaphragmatic IVC, so this procedure is not necessary.

An incision is made in the diaphragm leg just below the diaphragm to expose the aorta, and taping for the aorta is again performed with cotton tape (Fig. 25.3). At this time, be careful not to damage the esophagus. The left cornea and lesser omentum are dissected. If an accessory left hepatic artery is found, it should be encircled and dissected to the vicinity of the celiac artery trunk. An aberrant right hepatic artery can be confirmed by palpation on the right side of the hepatoduodenal mesentery. The common bile duct is ligated and dissected at the upper edge of the pancreas, and the liver side of the common bile duct is left open. An incision is made in the bottom of the gallbladder, and its lumen is thoroughly washed with saline. The bilateral kidneys are fully mobilized from the retroperitoneum.

When the preparation is completed, consult with the anesthesiologist and the chest retrieval team to adjust the timing of cross clamping of the aorta. Systemically administer heparin (400 U/kg) and wait for 3 min. The distal part of the aorta is then ligated, and a 26–28-Fr irrigation catheter is inserted into the aorta with secure fixation. Take care to avoid

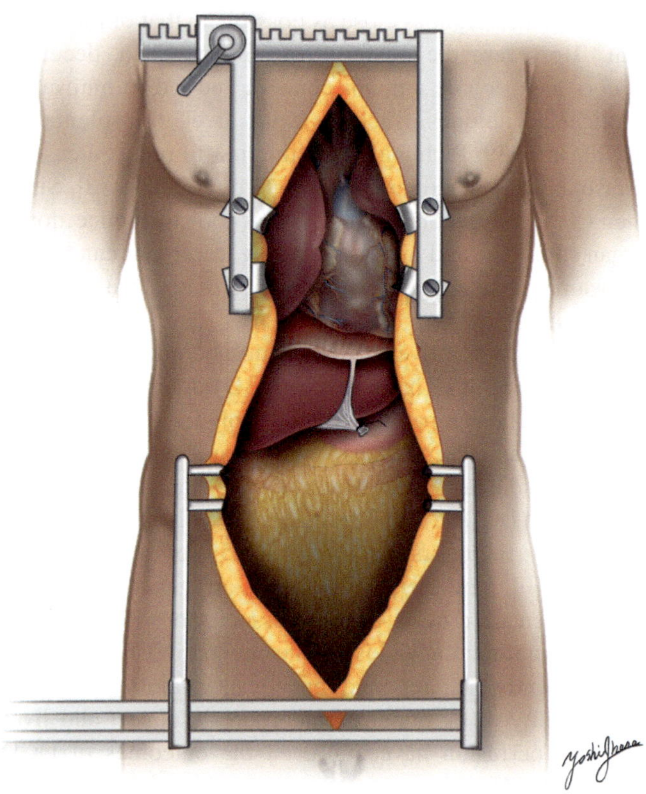

**Fig. 25.1** A median sternotomy and laparotomy from the upper edge of the sternum to the pubic symphysis

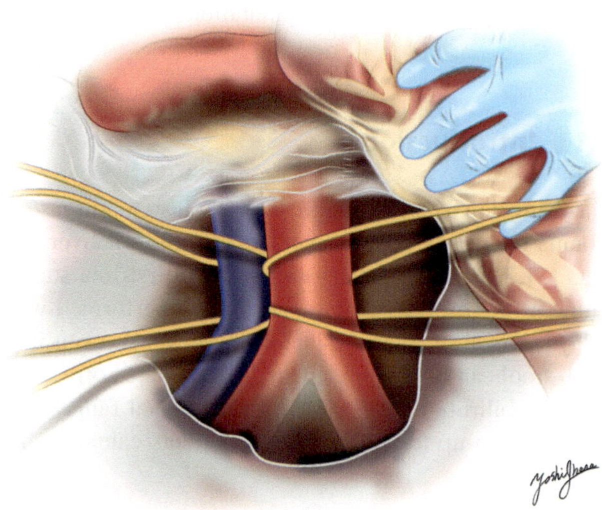

**Fig. 25.2** The aorta and inferior vena cava are taped in each two upper and lower with cotton tapes

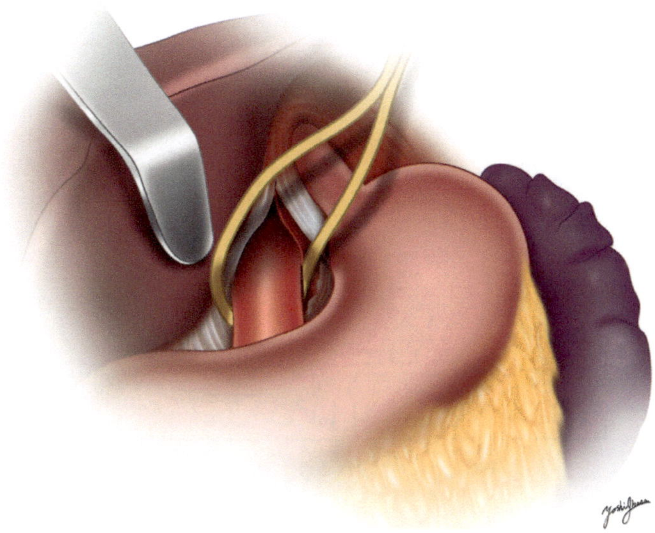

**Fig. 25.3** Taping for the aorta is performed with cotton tape at the site of cross clamping

air contamination at this point. Similarly, ligate the distal site on the IVC and insert a 34–36-Fr irrigation catheter for blood drainage into the IVC, fixing it. The ascending aorta is clamped by the thoracic retrieval team, and at the same time, cross clamping of the abdominal aorta is applied. The catheters inserted into the aorta and IVC are then opened, and organ perfusion with cold UW solution is started. In addition, each organ is sufficiently cooled with crushed ice spread in the abdominal cavity.

If small bowel transplantation is planned, small bowel removal is started first. The superior mesenteric artery and superior mesenteric vein are dissected, and then the ascending colon and jejunum are resected with a surgical stapler. In liver procurement, the gastroduodenal artery is dissected about 5 mm from the branch, and the common hepatic artery is resected as long as possible up to the celiac artery. If there is an aberrant right hepatic artery branching from the superior mesenteric artery, it is resected as long as possible just above the pancreas, taking care to avoid causing pancreatic injury. The portal vein is dissected about 5 mm from the upper edge of the pancreas (Fig. 25.4). An incision is made in the left diaphragm away from the IVC. The upper side of the IVC is dissected just above the diaphragm, and the caudal side is resected above the renal vein bifurcation (Fig. 25.5), after which the liver graft is removed. After pancreatic graft removal and left and right nephrectomy, the internal and external common iliac arteries and veins are collected for the vessel graft, making them as long as possible. The chest and abdominal walls are closed in two layers. The removed liver is then packed and transported under cooling conditions or moved to the liver splitting procedure.

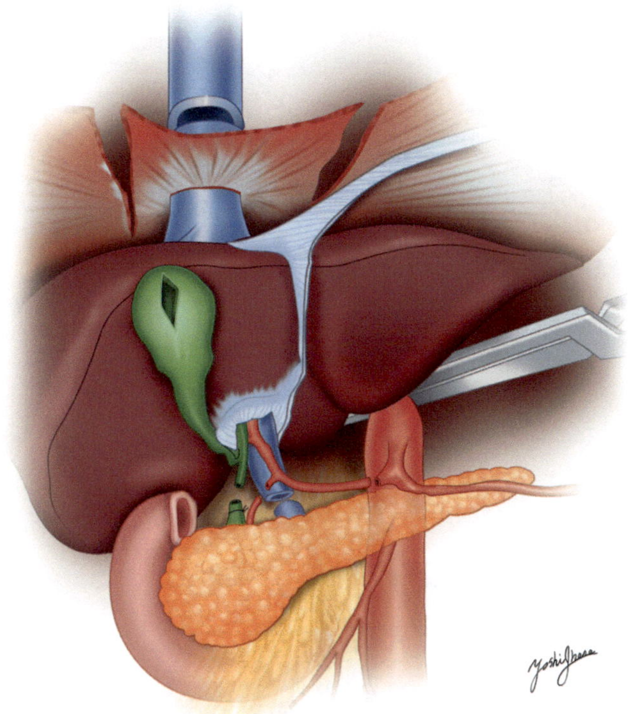

**Fig. 25.4** The graft bile duct, hepatic artery, and portal vein are cut

## 25.3 Splitting of the Graft Liver

### 25.3.1 Donor Selection Criteria for Split Liver Transplantation

As donor selection criteria for split liver transplantation in other countries, the age, body mass index, length of stay in the intensive care unit, liver function, presence or absence of fatty liver, serum sodium level, and presence or absence of vasopressor are considered as factors that can affect the recipient prognosis [8, 15]. Because DBD donors in Japan tend to have a long intensive care unit stay with a stable condition, the intensive care unit stay should be excluded from the selection criteria. Therefore, in Japan, "age under 50 years old, AST/ALT level ≥ 3 times the upper limit of the normal value, and ≤ 1 vasopressor used" have been proposed as guidelines for brain death split liver transplant donor criteria [16].

### 25.3.2 Preparing for Liver Splitting

In a practical situation, in situ graft splitting is rarely selected in multi-organ procurement, as it takes over 2–3 h to finish procurement before aortic cross clamping can be performed. Once sectioning of the parenchyma and vascular supply has been performed in a heart-beating donor, these grafts are ready to use at

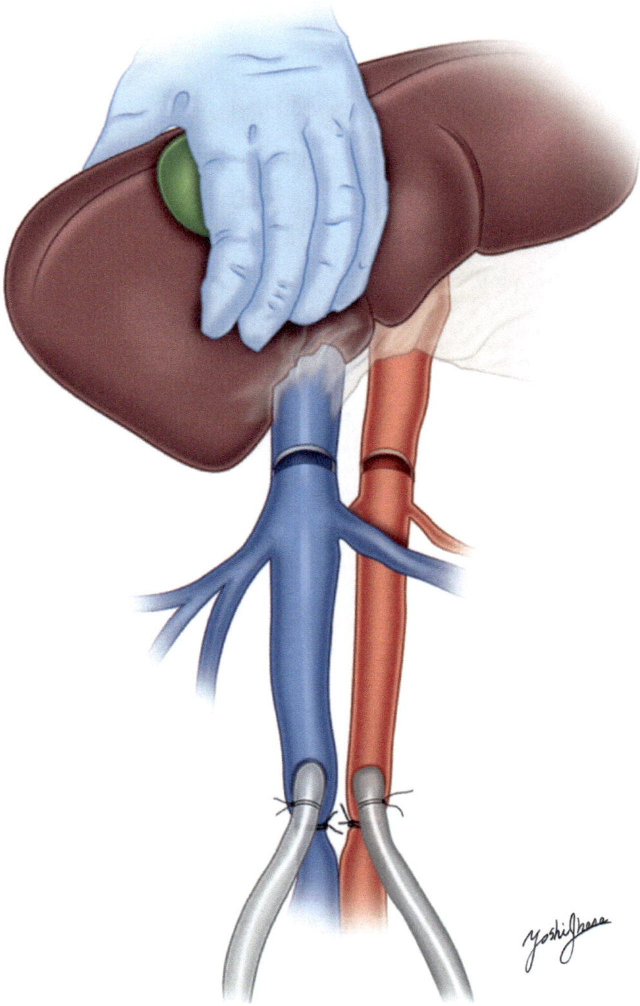

Fig. 25.5 The inferior vena cava is dissected and graft removing

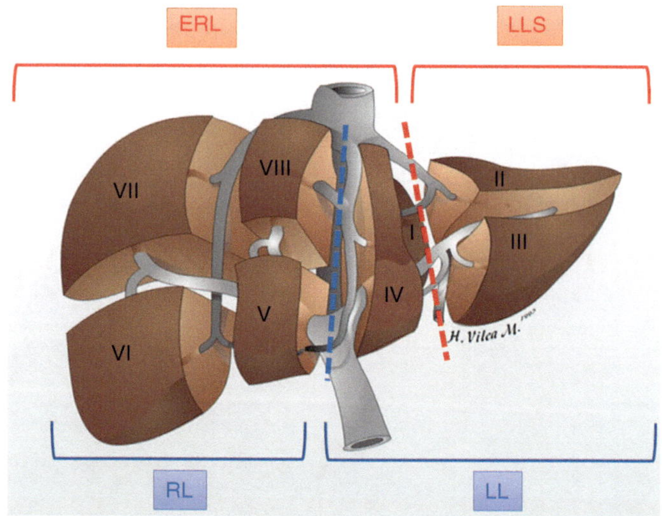


Fig. 25.6 Two types of split liver grafts. (ERL: Extended right lobe, LLS: left lateral segment, RL: right lobe, LL: left lobe)

the end of procurement. Hemostasis of the cut surface is achieved, and all vascular pedicles and the bile duct are dissected. Back-table treatment is limited to preservation solution perfusion [17].

In ex situ situations, splitting preparation and division of the liver takes an additional 2–3 h after liver graft procurement. It is important to maintain the liver graft at a low temperature by using cold preservation solution and surrounding the liver with frozen saline ice. After conventional preservation of the liver, the hepatic artery and bile ducts anatomy must be identified and marked by mini clips. First, the hepatic artery is dissected until the branches for the left lobe and right liver are individualized. It is important to avoid any excessive dissection of the hepatic duct from the right hepatic artery in order to maintain a sufficient blood supply. The portal vein should be freed until its bifurcation is identified for further division. Cholangiography is particularly useful for guiding the division of the left bile duct to ensure a safe procedure [16]. The ideal site for division should be located some distance from the main bile duct confluence and provide a single left bile duct with the left split graft [18, 19].

### 25.3.3 Standard Technique for Liver Splitting

The liver splitting procedure comprises two different entities: adult/child (left lateral segment [LLS] and extended right lobe [ERL]) split liver and adult/adult (left lobe [LL] and right lobe [RL] [20]) split liver. Splitting to LLS and ERL is mainly used for DDLT to a child who weighs under 20 kg (Fig. 25.6) [16]. Splitting to LL and RL is applied for DDLT for BA in older children or adolescents who need a larger graft volume. In this chapter, we mainly discuss the surgical procedure for the division of the LLS and ERL.

The left hepatic vein is dissected from the middle hepatic vein following confirmation of the bifurcation of the left hepatic vein and middle hepatic vein within the cut surface at the IVC (Fig. 25.7). If the umbilical fissure vein or V4 branch influx into the left hepatic vein, then they should be dissected. The IVC and middle hepatic vein are attached to the ERL side. The division line of the parenchyma is typically 5 mm to the right of the falciform ligament from the point where the left hepatic vein is cut to the umbilical fissure. The extent, including segment IV of LLS, may vary depending on the weight of the recipient. After cutting the surface of the liver with a scalpel, the parenchyma is crushed using the forceps fracture method while ligating the major vessels and bile ducts (Fig. 25.8). When the hepatic hilum is reached, the left and right hepatic duct branches are confirmed by inserting a sonde into the bile duct. In addition, cholangiography is performed, and the hepatic hilum plate of the dissection line is marked with 5-0 Proline, and then the bile duct is dissected. In general, the common bile duct is attached to the ERL [21]. The main portal trunk should be attached to the ERL graft, while the appropriate hepatic artery is usually attached to the LLS graft (Fig. 25.9). Leakage from the cut surface of the graft

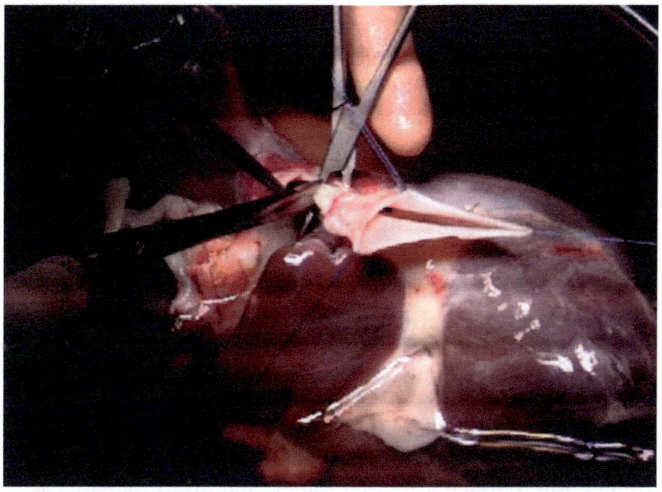

**Fig. 25.7** The left hepatic vein dissection in ex situ situation

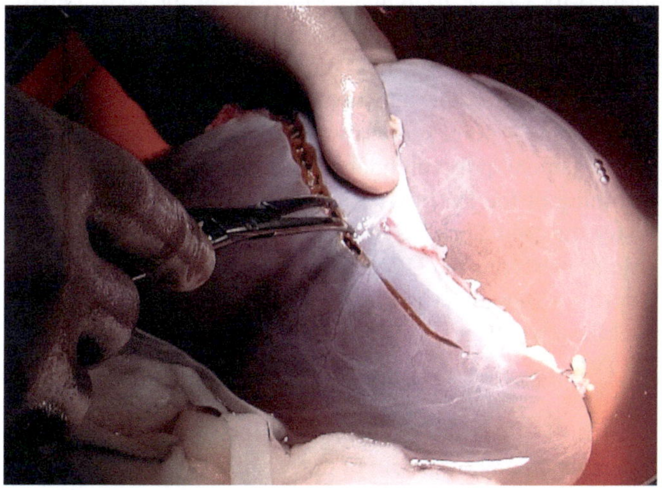

**Fig. 25.8** The parenchyma is crushed using the forceps fracture method

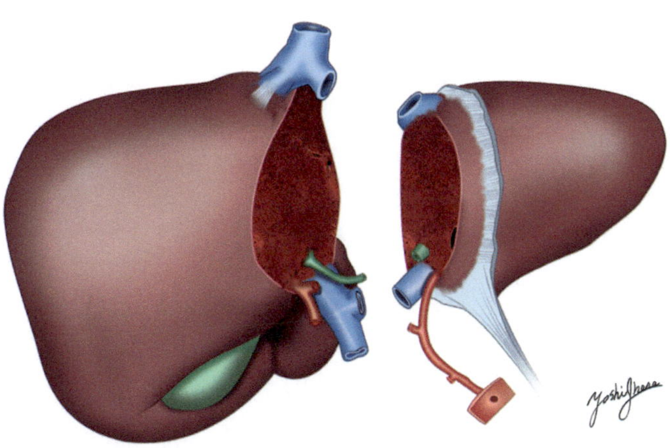

**Fig. 25.9** The division of a left lateral segment graft for a pediatric recipient and an extended right lobe graft for an adult recipient

liver is confirmed after gentle perfusion with cold UW solution (Belzer University of Wisconsin storage solution) via the portal vein and then closed with fibrin sealant and 5-0 proline sutures.

In the case of liver splitting between LL and RL, the middle hepatic vein is generally attached to the LL. The relatively large V5 and V8 veins (>5 mm) in the RL should be reconstructed using a vessel graft at graft implantation. The distribution of the main vessels and bile ducts is generally the same as that for splitting to LLS and ERL, but it should be carefully determined while considering the characteristics and priorities of the two liver transplant recipients [22].

## 25.4 Recipient Operation in DDLT for BA

A recipient operation in DDLT is technically similar to living donor liver transplantation (LDLT). A deceased liver graft has much longer vasculature, and it also contains a useful vascular graft that includes the iliac and cervical veins of the donor. After confirmation of graft liver arrival, which is most important in DDLT, the recipient hepatic vessels should be shut off; this is referred to as the "point of no return." We herein describe a recipient operation using the left lateral segment (Fig. 25.10), which is a common strategy when performing split liver transplantation for BA.

### 25.4.1 Total Hepatectomy

A bilateral subcostal incision or inverted T incision is performed first, and the previous incision for Kasai's procedure is traced as much as possible (Fig. 25.11). Laparotomy should be carefully performed due to the frequent presence

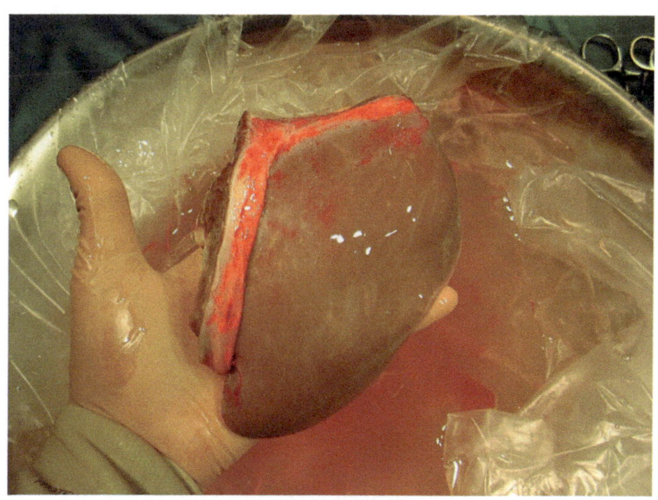

**Fig. 25.10** A left lateral segment graft from an adult donor

of severe adhesion after Kasai's procedure, especially around the portoenterostomy. We usually use an adhesion barrier (Seprafilm®), which facilitates re-laparotomy and prevents bowel injury in Kasai's operation. The round ligament is ligated and divided, the falciform ligament is dissected, and left-to-right dissection is performed. Care is required to avoid injury to the confluence of the hepatic vein and the IVC.

The Roux-en-Y loop should be divided by a linear cutter to leave it as long as possible for biliary tract reconstruction. If bile juice is pooled in the stump of the Roux-en-Y loop, it should be drained with a 4-Fr feeding tube to make it easier to isolate the portal vein. The left and right hepatic arteries are isolated carefully and dissected, keeping them as long as possible for subsequent reconstruction. Dividing the gastroduodenal artery facilitates the dissection of the proper hepatic artery, and it is also a useful option for hepatic artery reconstruction. Taping of the hepatic artery at the time of dissection, which may cause arterial spasm, should be minimized.

The portal vein is then identified and dissected up to the right and left branches. Some caudate branches of the portal vein are divided from the portal vein. The portal vein on the proximal side is dissected down to the level of the pancreas while dividing the left gastric vein. Large lymph nodes around the proximal portal vein should be resected because they may interfere with the portal blood flow after transplantation. If the portal vein pressure is >35 mmHg after the division of the portal trunk, we usually create a temporal portosystemic shunt from the recipient portal vein to the recipient superior vena cava using a heparin-coated catheter (Anti-thrombus tube), in order to prevent severe bowel congestion.

After dissection of the hepatic hilum, the hepatogastric and coronary ligaments on the left side and the coronary ligament on the right side are sectioned free the native liver from its retroperitoneal attachments. The IVC is dissected by carefully ligating the short hepatic vein. Short hepatic veins of ≥2 mm in size are transfixed or sutured to avoid slippage of the ligature. The right IVC ligament is encircled and continuously sutured after division. After ligation of the left IVC ligament and ductus venosus, the right hepatic vein and the confluence of the middle hepatic vein and left hepatic vein are clamped, and then the native liver is removed.

## 25.4.2 Implantation of the Graft Liver

### 25.4.2.1 Hepatic Vein Reconstruction

After total hepatectomy, hemostasis of the abdominal cavity is performed. Before hepatic vein anastomosis, the site of connection between the recipient and graft hepatic vein should be optimized for suitable anastomosis according to the size and location. In infant recipients, the hepatic vein is formed to a large triangular orifice using the right hepatic vein, middle hepatic vein, and left hepatic vein, while dividing the septum (Fig. 25.12). The graft liver is placed into the peritoneal cavity and hepatic vein anastomosis is then performed on a 3-point support with running suture (5-0 Asflex; monofilament polyvinylidene fluoride sutures) under total clamping of the IVC. After posterior wall anastomosis, perfusion of cold Ringer's solution is started from the portal vein to wash out the UW solution. After anastomosis of the anterior wall with a running suture, the graft is perfused with backflow from the IVC by releasing the vascular clamp of the IVC.

### 25.4.2.2 Portal Vein Reconstruction

When the main portal vein of the recipient is not stenotic and has sufficient portal flow, the bifurcation of the right PV and left PV in infants and the main trunk of the portal vein in older children are used for anastomosis. When using a temporary portal bypass, the anti-thrombus catheter is removed

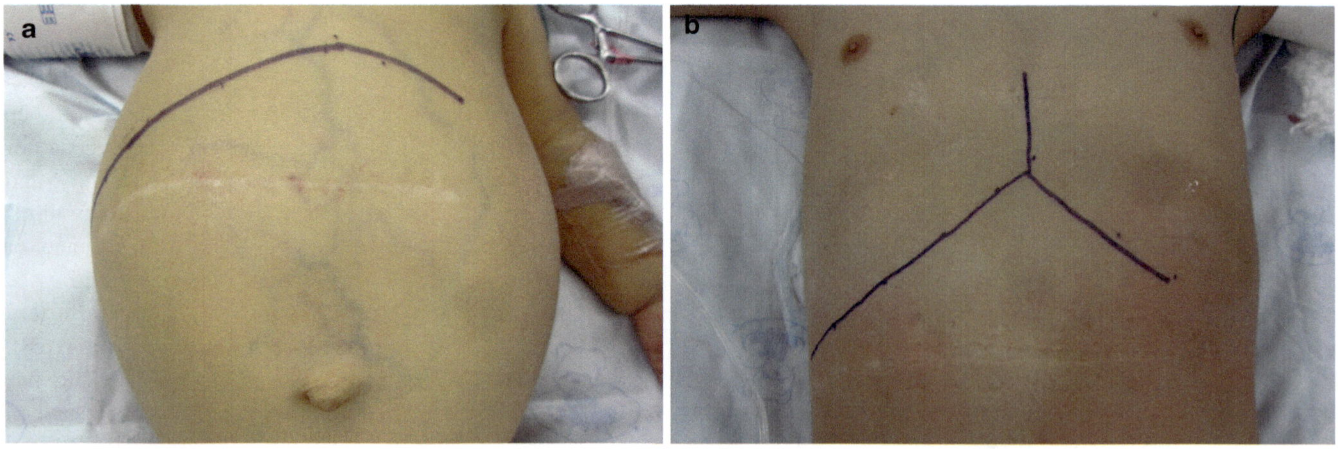


**Fig. 25.11** Skin incision. (**a**): bilateral subcostal incision for infant, (**b**): Mercedes Benz incision for older children

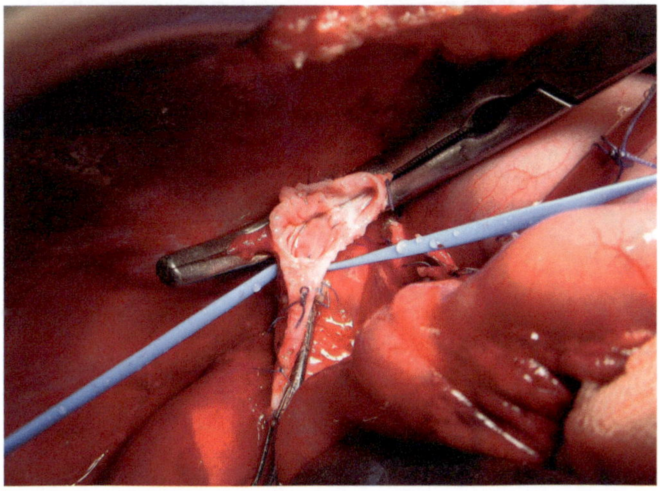

**Fig. 25.12** The recipient hepatic vein is formed to one large orifice for triangular anastomosis to the graft hepatic vein under total clamping of the inferior vena cava

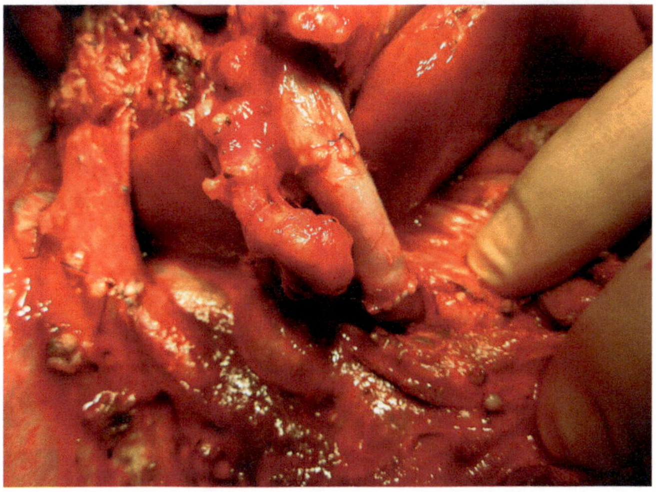

**Fig. 25.13** Portal vein reconstruction using an interposed vascular graft

before starting portal anastomosis. At the time of anastomosis, the graft liver is placed in a natural position, and the alignment of the donor and recipient portal vein are observed to prevent torsion. Portal vein anastomosis is performed on the two-point support with 6-0 absorbable surgical sutures (PDSII) with a running suture. For the prevention of anastomotic stenosis, it is important not to tighten the suture.

Portal vein anastomosis is the most difficult part of implantation in a pediatric recipient with biliary atresia. Graft interposition is chosen in portal vein anastomosis when the recipient's portal vein has become sclerotic, ischemic, or thrombotic. The confluence of the superior mesenteric vein and splenic vein are encircled and then interposed with the deceased donor's vein graft, like the iliac vein (Fig. 25.13). In a small recipient with BA, hepatofugal portal blood flow is sometimes observed due to portal vein steal, which occurs due to the existence of the large gastric coronary vein or retroperitoneal portal vein collateral system after portal vein reconstruction. Ligation of the gastric coronary vein to the gastric esophageal venous plexus or splenorenal shunt vessel and dissection of the retroperitoneal portal vein collateral vessels should be performed to increase portal blood flow. Once the portal vein anastomosis has been completed, the blood flow of the hepatic vein and portal vein should be immediately checked by ultrasound.

#### 25.4.2.3 Hepatic Artery Reconstruction

Hepatic artery anastomosis is performed using the microvascular technique. The graft liver is placed into the left abdominal cavity, and preparation for anastomosis is accomplished by securing the fine surgical area. Generally, a patient with biliary atresia has a compensated thick hepatic artery. Approximately 10–12 stitches of 8-0/9-0 Nylon are required for a single artery reconstruction (Fig. 25.14). If there are two hepatic arteries in the graft liver, we usually reconstruct both of them.

#### 25.4.2.4 Biliary Tract Reconstruction

As the final step of graft implantation, biliary reconstruction is performed by end-to-side anastomosis with the previous or a new Roux-en-Y loop via the retro-colic route. The diameter of the graft bile duct is measured, and an opening of smaller size is made on the jejunum. Anastomosis is performed using running suture in the posterior wall and interrupted suture in the anterior wall of the biliary duct (6-0 PDS). In our institution, a transanastomotic stent tube (4–6-Fr tapered tube) is always inserted into the biliary duct (Fig. 25.15), and placed from the stump of the Roux-en-Y loop to the skin for bile juice drainage to prevent postoperative biliary complications due to anastomotic stricture. If there are two bile ducts that are separated by more than 5 mm in the graft, two anastomoses to the jejunum are made.

### 25.4.3 Abdominal Closure

After taking liver tissue from the transplanted liver (zero biopsy), the abdominal cavity is washed with a sufficient amount of warm saline. Then, hemostasis is carefully performed. In particular, vascular and biliary anastomosis, the liver resection surface, and the area around the IVC should be cautiously observed. Doppler ultrasonography is repeatedly performed to determine the most suitable position of the liver graft. Then the graft is fixed by stitching it to the proper anterior abdominal wall. A closed system abdominal drain is inserted toward the right subphrenic cavity. In the case of the older children, an additional closed system abdominal drain is inserted toward the pouch of Douglas. The abdominal wall

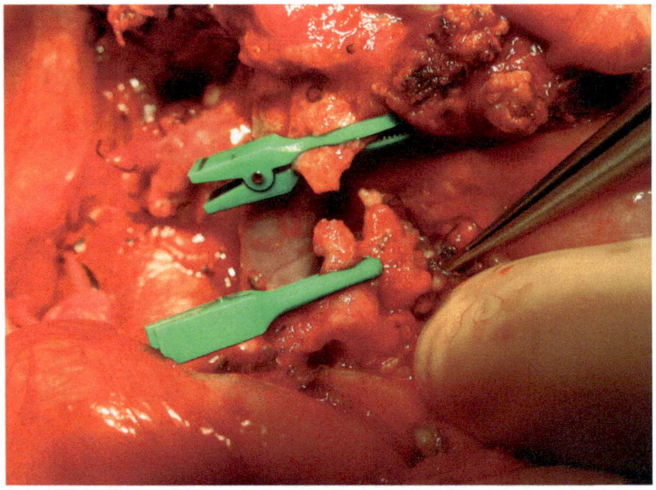

**Fig. 25.14** Hepatic artery anastomosis using the microvascular technique

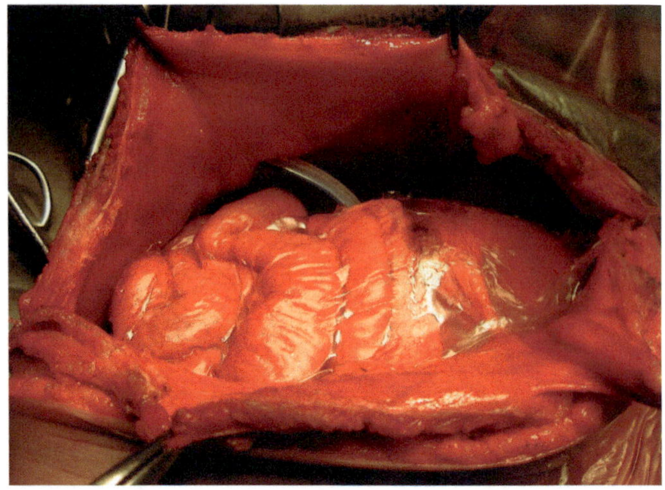

**Fig. 25.16** Seprafilm® is used to prevent abdominal adhesions

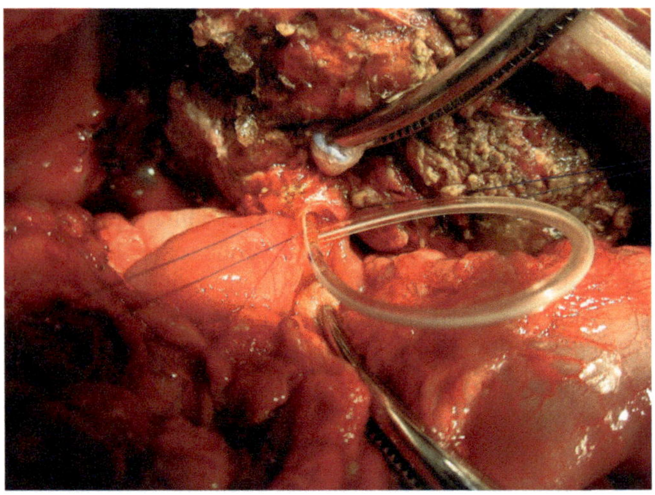

**Fig. 25.15** A transanastomotic stent tube (4–6Fr tapered tube) is inserted from the stump of Roux-en-Y loop at biliary reconstruction

is closed with 1-0 or 2-0 Vicryl after placing an adhesion barrier (Seprafilm®) (Fig. 25.16) in the abdominal cavity. The subcutaneous layer is sutured with 4-0 Vicryl, and the skin is closed with a buried suture.

## 25.5 Perspectives of Pediatric DDLT

In Japan, 20 years have passed since the enforcement of the Organ Transplant Act, and 10 years have passed since the enforcement of the revised Organ Transplant Act. However, the number of organ donations in Japan continues to be extremely low compared to other countries (Fig. 25.17) [23]. In recent years, the number of donated organs from brain death donors is approximately 60 cases per year, and > 90% of liver transplants still rely on LDLT in Japan. In children younger than 18 years of age, approximately 100–120 LDLTs and approximately 5–10 DDLT are performed each year [24].

Among the 2341 patients who underwent LDLT for BA, there were 2102 pediatric patients (90%); this number amounts to approximately two-thirds of the whole pediatric liver transplantation procedures that are performed (3168 cases). The 1-, 5-, 10-, 15-, and 20-year survival rates for patients undergoing LDLT for BA were 92.3%, 90.3%, 88.2%, 86.6%, and 85.0%, respectively, and were better in comparison to other diseases [24]. On the other hand, 30 patients with BA underwent DDLT, and only 13 of these were pediatric patients. However, the 1-, 5-, 10-, 15-, and 20-year survival rates for patients who underwent LDLT for BA were all 85.7% and were comparable to the survival rates of patients who underwent LDLT. Thus, pediatric recipients with biliary atresia should also be given more opportunities to undergo DDLT.

Recently, the Japanese organ allocation system for recipients who are waiting for a deceased donor liver graft has been changed to incorporate the MELD score. Due to these reforms in the transplantation law, severe metabolic diseases, such as neonatal ornithine transcarbamylase deficiency, were therefore moved up to status 1 in the transplantation ranking system, and therefore the chances of receiving a pediatric DDLT were slightly expanded. However, DDLT has shown little benefit in the treatment of BA.

From 2018, the Japanese organ allocation system was modified, so that liver grafts from pediatric deceased donors of <18 years of age are preferentially distributed to pediatric recipients of <18 years of age. Thanks to this "child-to-child rule," in 2019, 15 cases of pediatric DDLT were performed, which is the largest number in Japan to date; however, in 2020, due to the COVID-19 outbreak, the number of DDLT procedures has decreased.

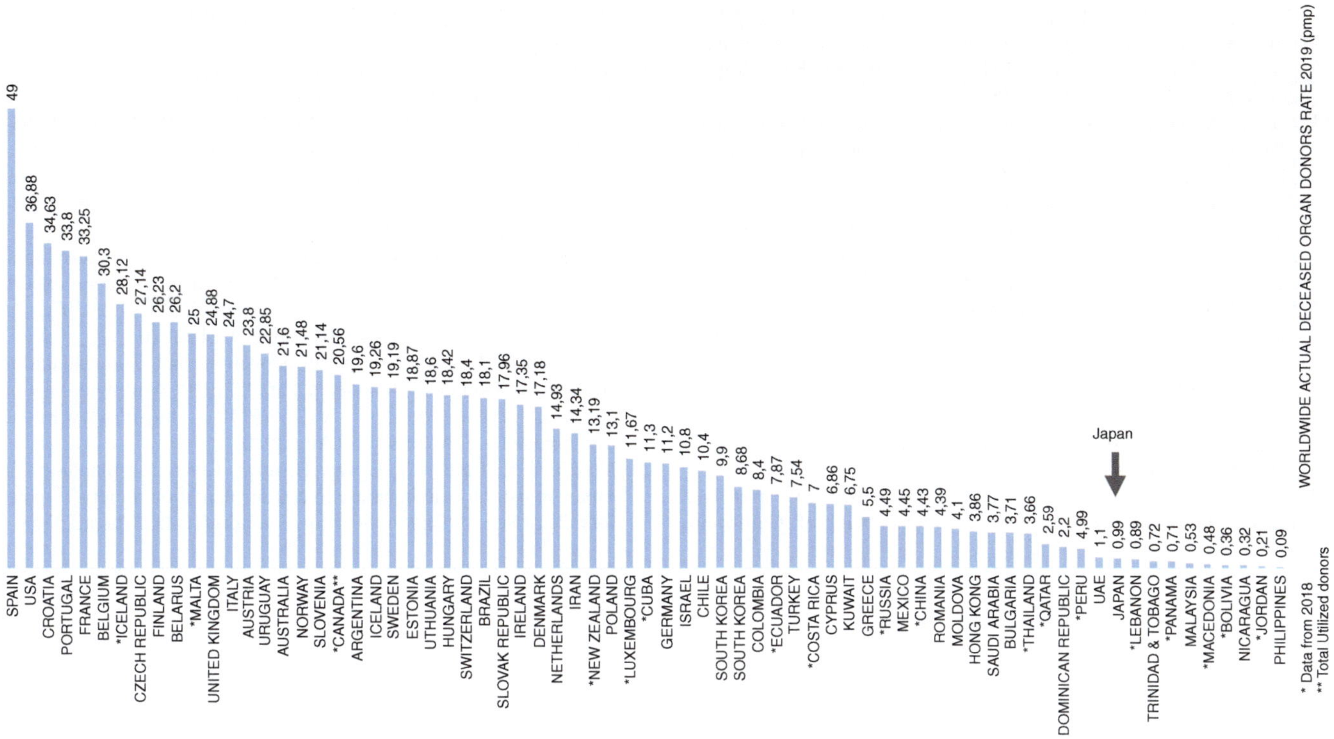


**Fig. 25.17** Worldwide deceased organ donor rate in 2019

Living donor liver transplantation in pediatric patients tends to be considered to be easy in comparison to living donor liver transplantation in adult patients. The reasons for this include "donor stronger voluntary will," "donor younger age," "the donor surgery procedure is simpler," and "more donor candidates:" however, we cannot completely eliminate the risks that are associated with living donor operations. Even in pediatric populations, there is an urgent need for enlightenment activities to increase DDLT and promote split liver transplantation or reformation of the organ distribution system to prioritize pediatric recipients.

## References


1. Vilca-Melendez H, Mieli-Vergani G. Pediatric liver transplantation. In: Klein AA, Lewis CJ, editors. Organ transplantation: a clinical guide. Cambridge, UK: Cambridge University Press; 2011. p. 220–30.
2. Hartley JL, Davenport M, Kelly DA. Biliary atresia. Lancet. 2009 Nov 14;374(9702):1704–13. https://doi.org/10.1016/S0140-6736(09)60946-6.
3. D'Souza R, Grammatikopoulos T, Pradhan A, et al. Acute-on-chronic liver failure in children with biliary atresia awaiting liver transplantation. Pediatr Transplant. 2019 Mar;23(2):e13339. https://doi.org/10.1111/petr.13339.
4. Sundaram SS, Mack CL, Feldman AG, et al. Biliary atresia: indications and timing of liver transplantation and optimization of pretransplant care. Liver Transpl. 2017 Jan;23(1):96–109. https://doi.org/10.1002/lt.24640.
5. Starzl TE, Giles G, Lilly JR, et al. Indications for orthotopic liver transplantation: with particular reference to hepatomas, biliary atresia, cirrhosis, Wilson's disease and serum hepatitis. Transplant Proc. 1971;3:308–12.
6. Pichlmayr R, Ringe B, Gubernatis G, et al. [Transplantation of a donor liver to 2 recipients (splitting transplantation)—a new method in the further development of segmental liver transplantation]. Langenbecks Arch Chir. 1988;373:127–30.
7. Rogiers X, Malagó M, Gawad K, et al. In situ splitting of cadaveric livers. The ultimate expansion of a limited donor pool. Ann Surg. 1996;224:331–9. discussion 339–41
8. Hackl C, Schmidt KM, Süsal C, et al. Split liver transplantation: current developments. World J Gastroenterol. 2018 Dec 21;24(47):5312–21. https://doi.org/10.3748/wjg.v24.i47.5312.
9. Goldberg DS, Karp SJ, McCauley ME, et al. Interpreting outcomes in DCDD liver transplantation: first report of the multicenter IDOL consortium. Transplantation. 2017 May;101(5):1067–73. https://doi.org/10.1097/TP.0000000000001656.
10. Johnson RJ, Bradbury LL, Martin K, et al. Organ donation and transplantation in the UK-the last decade: a report from the UK national transplant registry. Transplantation. 2014 Jan 15;97(Suppl 1):S1–S27. https://doi.org/10.1097/01.TP.0000438215.16737.68.
11. Foley DP, Fernandez LA, Leverson G, et al. Donation after cardiac death: the University of Wisconsin experience with liver transplantation. Ann Surg. 2005 Nov;242(5):724–31. https://doi.org/10.1097/01.sla.0000186178.07110.92.
12. DeOliveira ML, Jassem W, Valente R, et al. Biliary complications after liver transplantation using grafts from donors after cardiac death: results from a matched control study in a single large volume center. Ann Surg. 2011;254(5):716–22.; discussion 722–3. https://doi.org/10.1097/SLA.0b013e318235c572.
13. Ravikumar R, Jassem W, Mergental H, et al. Liver transplantation after ex vivo Normothermic machine preservation: a phase 1 (first-in-man) clinical trial. Am J Transplant. 2016;16(6):1779–87. https://doi.org/10.1111/ajt.13708. Epub 2016 Mar 7

14. Schlegel A, Muller X, Kalisvaart M, et al. Outcomes of DCD liver transplantation using organs treated by hypothermic oxygenated perfusion before implantation. J Hepatol. 2019;70(1):50–7. https://doi.org/10.1016/j.jhep.2018.10.005. Epub 2018 Oct 18
15. Cardillo M, De Fazio N, Pedotti P, et al. Split and whole liver transplantation outcomes: a comparative cohort study. Liver Transpl. 2006 Mar;12(3):402–10. https://doi.org/10.1002/lt.20720.
16. The Japan Society for Transplantation/Brain death split liver transplantation promotion committee project. Brain death split liver transplantation guidelines Ver.1.1, 2018. http://jlts.umin.ac.jp/news/201802_1.html. Accessed 30 Aug 2020.
17. Otte JB, de Ville de Goyet J, Alberti D, et al. The concept and technique of the split liver in clinical transplantation. Surgery. 1990 Jun;107(6):605–12.
18. Renz JF, Emond JC, Yersiz H, et al. Split-liver transplantation in the United States: outcomes of a national survey. Ann Surg. 2004 Feb;239(2):172–81. https://doi.org/10.1097/01.sla.0000109150.89438.bd.
19. Vagefi PA, Parekh J, Ascher NL, et al. Outcomes with split liver transplantation in 106 recipients: the University of California, san Francisco, experience from 1993 to 2010. Arch Surg. 2011 Sep;146(9):1052–9. https://doi.org/10.1001/archsurg.2011.218.
20. Rodriguez-Davalos MI, Arvelakis A, et al. Segmental grafts in adult and pediatric liver transplantation: improving outcomes by minimizing vascular complications. JAMA Surg. 2014 Jan;149(1):63–70. https://doi.org/10.1001/jamasurg.2013.3384.
21. Gundlach M, Broering D, Topp S, et al. Split-cava technique: liver splitting for two adult recipients. Liver Transpl. 2000 Nov;6(6):703–6. https://doi.org/10.1053/jlts.2000.18503.
22. Hashimoto K, Quintini C, Aucejo FN, et al. Split liver transplantation using Hemiliver graft in the MELD era: a single center experience in the United States. Am J Transplant. 2014;14(9):2072–80. https://doi.org/10.1111/ajt.12791. Epub 2014 Jul 10
23. International Registry in Organ Donation and Transplantation (IRODaT). Donation Activity Charts. 2019. Worldwide actual deceased organ donors 2019 (PMP). https://www.irodat.org/?p=database. Accessed 30 Aug 2020.
24. Umeshita K, Eguchi S, Egawa H, et al. Liver transplantation in Japan: registry by the Japanese liver transplantation society. Hepatol Res. 2019 Sep;49(9):964–80. https://doi.org/10.1111/hepr.13364.

# Medical Treatment: Steroids/ Ursodeoxycholic Acid

# 26

Shigeru Ono

## 26.1 Introduction

Kasai hepatic portoenterostomy (HPE) for biliary atresia (BA) has proven acceptable as an initial and standard treatment, with the generally successful outcome of jaundice-free outcomes. However, about 40% of patients who receive initial Kasai HPE, unfortunately, fail to become jaundice-free after the operation, so medical therapies are administered to maintain the bile flow after the Kasai operation. Postoperative medical therapy with choleretic agents, including intravenous 10% dehydrocholic acid, glucagons, prostaglandin E2, ursodeoxycholic acid (UDCA), and corticosteroids is commonly used with good efficacy [1–6].

This chapter describes the medical treatments typically administered after the Kasai operation, with a focus on steroids and UDCA.

## 26.2 Steroids

### 26.2.1 Mechanism of Action

Steroids are well known to exert various effects on biological and physiological activities. However, the details concerning the mechanism by which steroids provide their benefits is unclear.

The beneficial effects of steroids for BA are believed to be choleretic action, immunosuppression, and anti-inflammation. The choleretic effect of steroids involves induction of Na-K adenosine triphosphatase, which increases canalicular electrolyte transport and stimulates bile flow independently of the bile salt concentration [7]. Steroids are also potent anti-inflammatory drugs. There is evidence that there is a marked inflammatory component in at least some infants with biliary atresia. High-dose steroids induce significant anti-inflammatory and immunosuppressive effects, such as decreasing tissue edema and collagen deposition and inhibiting fibrogenesis and migration of infiltrating monocytes and lymphocytes [1]. The titration process has shown that glucocorticoid receptor alfa (GcRa) correlates with the severity of the liver injury and that the required steroids dose is associated with the degree of GcRa expression. Glucocorticoids increase anti-inflammatory and immunosuppressive responses. The mechanism underlying the anti-inflammatory actions of glucocorticoids is mediated through the activation of glucocorticoid receptors (GcRs), which have two isoforms: cytoplasmic glucocorticoid receptor a (GcRa), which mediates the physiological effects, and nuclear-localized glucocorticoid receptor b (GcRb), which acts as a dominant-negative inhibitor of GcRa activity [8].

Steroids also exert profound anti-inflammatory and immunosuppressive effects with reduction of ductal inflammation, edema, and scarring as well as arresting the migration of infiltrating monocytes and lymphocytes [9]. The desired effects of steroid administration are the relief of inflammatory reactions leading to the obstruction of the microscopic ductules and the stimulation of the bile flow to allow the ductules to mature into ducts and form networks to drain bile adequately.

Steroids were first used to augment antibiotic therapy for refractory cases of postoperative cholangitis with a marked decrease or cessation of bile flow after Kasai HPE [10]. The prophylactic use of steroids has since become popularized, with excellent results reported [5]. Lilly et al. categorized the dynamic changes occurring at the PE site after the Kasai procedure as follows: (1) the microscopic communicating ducts open after transection of the fibrous remnant, (2) the microscopic ductules are then replaced by major intrahepatic ducts, and (3) ultimately, autoanastomosis between the duct epithelium and conduit mucosa occurs [11]. The transected microscopic ducts on which postoperative bile flow depends are proposed to be prone to postoperative inflammatory closure [1]. Reports suggest that steroid administration improves

S. Ono (✉)
Pediatric Surgery, Jichi Medical Univesity, Shimotsuke, Japan
e-mail: o-shige@jichi.ac.jp


M. Nio (ed.), *Introduction to Biliary Atresia*, https://doi.org/10.1007/978-981-16-2160-4_26

the outcome of BA by influencing the immunologic and inflammatory components inherent in its etiology.

### 26.2.2 Dosage, Duration, and Efficacy

The overall steroid dose varies according to the initial doses used (high dose or "pulse" or "blast" dose vs. low dose) and length of tapering (fast vs. prolonged) [3–5, 10]. Controversy exists regarding the significance of the difference in outcomes among the different treatment regimens. Prednisone and dexamethasone are used most commonly, with doses ranging from 2 mg/kg per day (low) to 20 mg/kg per day (in pulses). The literature includes various protocols with different doses, periods, and timings of steroid administration for patients following Kasai HPE [1–6].

The majority of Japanese pediatric surgeons use corticosteroids to enhance bile drainage after Kasai HPE for BA. However, there is no clinical evidence to support the efficacy of steroid therapy, and impressions about the results vary. In addition, the ideal dosage, duration, and method of steroid administration vary among institutions.

In 2004, Muraji conducted a national survey on the practice of post-Kasai HPE steroid usage in Japan. He concluded that most pediatric surgeons in Japan use steroids after the Kasai operation, and the jaundice-free survival rate tended to be higher in the steroid group than in the non-steroid group. He also recommended that the initial steroid dose be set at 4.0 mg/kg/day [12]. The Japanese Biliary Atresia Society conducted a multicenter randomized trial of postoperative steroid treatment comparing different doses of prednisolone, including a group starting at 4 mg/kg/day and receiving a total of 52 mg/kg over 30 days and another group starting at 2 mg/kg/day and receiving a total of 29 mg/kg over the same period. They showed that 4 mg/kg/day prednisolone only improved reduced bilirubin levels in the short-term in a subgroup of infants undergoing surgery before 70 days, but it did not improve other liver function test results. And there were no significant complications with either dose of corticosteroids [13].

Karrer and Lilly proposed using "blast"-type (very high dose/short duration) corticosteroids, citing potential choleretic and anti-inflammatory properties that might benefit post-PE BA children with cholangitis. They used methylprednisolone at an initial dosage of 10 mg/kg per day, which was reduced by half and discontinued on the fourth to the seventh day. This suggested that it worked by reducing periductal inflammation to increase bile flow in BA, as there was a marked depletion in lymphocytes in their series [3].

Stringer et al. reported the efficacy of dexamethasone starting at 0.3 mg/kg bd for 5 days with a good outcome of clearance of jaundice compared with patients without steroid treatment [14]. Muraji and Higashimoto reported the use of corticosteroids post-Kasai HPE to ameliorate progressive intrahepatic periportal inflammation. Their initial dosage of 4 mg/kg per day was tapered to 2.5 mg/d over 1–2 weeks, and "pulses" of corticosteroids were given if bile drainage appeared to decrease or if cholangitis ensued [4]. Shimadera et al. reported 23 cases treated with 3–5 mg/kg/day of prednisolone from the seventh postoperative day until jaundice cleared. They found that the mean steroid dose significantly influenced the postoperative jaundice period (shorter postoperative jaundice for higher doses) [15].

Kobayashi et al. provide strong evidence that large-dose prednisolone therapy (20 mg/day) with stool color monitoring of the bile flow has a positive impact on the time taken for patients with BA post-PE to become jaundice-free [2]. Another high-dose regimen of steroids is combined intravenous methylprednisolone (10 mg/kg day 1–5) with a reduced dose of 1 mg/kg from day 6 to 28 [16]. Meyers found that adjuvant therapy using high-dose steroids resulted in the clearance of jaundice in almost 80% of cases. Their protocol of steroids started with a higher initial pulse dose of intravenous methylprednisolone (tapering of 10, 8, 6, 5, 4, 3, 2 mg/kg/day) followed by 8–12 weeks of oral prednisone (2 mg/kg/day) [1].

These authors demonstrated the efficacy of high-dose steroids in combination with ursodeoxycholic acid and intravenous antibiotics, which may accelerate the clearance of jaundice and reduce the need for early liver transplantation after Kasai HPE.

A large retrospective study from Shanghai, China, of 380 infants was published by Dong et al. in 2013, comparing the outcomes of infants receiving a high-dose regimen (intravenously methylprednisolone at 4 mg/kg tapered to completion with oral prednisolone) or a low-dose regimen (starting at 4 mg/kg but tapered quickly for 1–2 weeks). They showed the high-dose steroid protocol could reduce the incidence of cholangitis, increase the jaundice-free rate, and improve two-year survival with native liver after the Kasai operation [17].

The randomized, double-blinded, placebo-controlled study from 2 UK centers used a low-dose and 6-week course of oral prednisolone starting at 2 mg/kg/day [18]. There was a significant reduction in bilirubin levels at 1 month that was more obvious in those who underwent Kasai HPE at <70 days. There was no significant effect on the clearance of jaundice at 6 months or the subsequent native liver survival.

Davenport et al. reported the follow-up study included 44 more infants treated with high-dose prednisolone starting at 5 mg/kg/day and found that there was a significant difference in the clearance of jaundice between the total steroid group (low and high dose) and the placebo group [19]. However, there was no significant improvement in the overall survival or native liver survival between the high-dose steroid and non-steroid groups. This study also found that the bilirubin level, AST level, and AST to platelet index (APRi), but not the GGT were significantly lower in the high-dose steroid group than in the placebo or control group.

The North American START (STeroids in biliary Atresia Randomized Trial) randomized placebo-controlled trial studied the efficacy of a high-dose steroid regimen (intravenously methylprednisolone starting at 4 mg/kg/day on day 1 post-Kasai HPE) for 2 weeks followed by oral prednisolone at 2 mg/kg/day and tapering for 9 weeks in 70 infants [20]. There was a non-significant improvement in the clearance of jaundice at 6 months that was higher in the sub-group receiving Kasai HPE at <70 days than in those receiving it at >70 days.

A meta-analysis report included two randomized controlled trials and five observational studies with a total of 259 cases. There was a significant difference in the clearance of jaundice at 6 months (odds ratio 1.59, 95% confidence interval 1.03–2.45, P = 0.04), in patients treated with high-dose steroids, particularly if <70 days old at surgery [21].

Some current evidence based on the most recent systematic review of published evidence supports the view that high-dose steroids do have a significant benefit in reduction of postoperative bilirubin and clearance of jaundice as the most frequently measured indices of the condition. Tyraskis et al. have shown that other biochemical markers indicating more specific liver injury (i.e., AST, APRi) are also affected by high-dose steroids at least in the first 6 months post-Kasai HPE [22].

### 26.2.3 Protocol of Steroids Administration for Postoperative BA

We herein report a clinical protocol for steroids routinely used after Kasai HPE in our institution. We plan to administer prednisolone with a dose of 4 mg/kg/day intravenously starting on the seventh postoperative day (POD), decreasing to 2 mg/kg/day on POD 9, with oral administration starting at 5 mg/day on POD 11 and tapering gradually to 2 mg/day on POD 13 and 1 mg/day on POD 15. We will perform readministration of steroids according to the same protocol with some revision should the serum bilirubin level increase again in the clinical course of treatment.

There is a consensus that steroids reduce serum bilirubin levels in BA patients after Kasai HPE. Escobar et al. also reported that the clearance of postoperative jaundice was significantly improved, and lower serum bilirubin levels were observed in patients receiving steroids. However, steroids had no effect on the incidence of cholangitis, the need for liver transplantation, or the overall survival [23].

There is level 1A evidence for the beneficial effect of high-dose steroids on increasing rates of the clearance of jaundice by 6 months. However, current evidence does not support the long-term beneficial impact on the native liver survival or overall survival, with only 3B-level evidence supporting the use of steroids.

### 26.2.4 Complications

Most studies have not systematically been reporting complications of steroid treatment for BA. The START trial did systematically report serious adverse events but did not find an overall difference in the number of events in the steroid group compared to the control group [20]. The Japanese Biliary Atresia Society reported in their multicenter randomized trial of postoperative steroid treatment there were no significant complications with use of corticosteroids [13].

### 26.2.5 Conclusion

In conclusion, the usage of adjuvant steroids following Kasai HPE for BA is controversial. Current evidence based on the most recent systematic review of published evidence supports the view that high-dose steroids do have any significant benefit of reducing postoperative bilirubin level or the clearance of jaundice as the most frequently measured indices of the condition. In addition, the Japanese clinical practice guideline of BA cannot confirm the recommendation regarding postoperative steroids therapy for the long-term outcomes of the jaundice-free survival or improvement in the survival rate with native liver [24]. However, a majority of pediatric surgeons tend to use steroids to be intended to increase and to keep the bile flow after Kasai HPE. A prospective, multicenter, randomized, controlled trial is needed to establish the optimal corticosteroid protocols after Kasai HPE.

## 26.3 UDCA

Ursodeoxycholic acid (UDCA) is a hydrophilic physiologic dihydroxy bile acid that was first identified in the bile of a Chinese black bear [25] and is present in humans in approximately 3% of the bile acid pool. It is formed by the 7b-epimerization of primary bile acid chenodeoxycholic acid in the gut by intestinal bacteria [26]. The intake of UDCA in patient with various cholestatic and gall stone diseases was found to increase the bile flow, protect hepatocytes, and dissolve gallstones.

### 26.3.1 Mechanism of Action

The suggested mechanisms underlying the beneficial effects of UDCA in cholestasis include changes in bile acid pool composition, hepatocyte membrane protective effects, immunomodulatory effects, bicarbonate-rich hypercholeresis induced by UDCA, stimulation of impaired hepatocellular secretion, antiapoptotic effects, and potential mediation of cholangiocyte protection [27, 28].

UDCA is a potential candidate for improving choleresis. It is a hydrophilic bile acid that comprises only 1–4% of total bile acids in humans. When used to treat adults with primary biliary cirrhosis, UDCA improves the clinical, biological, and histologic parameters [29]; decreases the need for transplantation; and improves survival. UDCA improves liver function in children after successful surgery for BA, and its biological benefits persist for several years after treatment.

UDCA is frequently used to treat children with BA because of the potential mechanisms by which it exerts its beneficial effects, and it has demonstrated efficacy in several cholestatic liver diseases of adults and children. Furthermore, previous studies have indicated that UDCA has a beneficial effect on patients with BA. Ulrich et al. first administered UDCA to two children in whom the Kasai procedure had failed, causing severe growth retardation.

The functions of bile acids include (1) micelle formation of fat in the intestine to promote the absorption of lipid and fat-soluble vitamins; (2) dissolution of bacterial cell membranes as a surfactant, suppressing bacterial growth in the intestine; (3) excretion of cholesterol; and (4) promotion of the excretion of catabolic substances from the liver.

### 26.3.2 UDCA for Postoperative BA

The secretion of bile acids into the intestinal tract is insufficient in children following biliary atresia surgery due to decreased bile acid production in the hepatocytes and cholestasis, causing impaired absorption of fats and fat-soluble vitamins, suppression of intestinal bacterial growth in the small intestine, and impaired enterohepatic circulation of bile acids.

Therefore, in patients following biliary atresia surgery, the following events are expected by administering UDCA: (1) bile acid is replenished, improving the absorption of fat and fat-soluble vitamins; (2) in the enterohepatic circulation of bile acids, a high proportion of UDCA with low tissue damage replaces bile acids with high tissue damage such as chenodeoxycholic acid, deoxycholic acid, and lithocholic acid, resulting in a reduction of the damaging effects on hepatocytes; and (3) bile acid production is increased and cholangitis reduced due to cholestasis [30–32].

### 26.3.3 Dosage of UDCA Following Kasai HPE

Yamashiro reported that UDCA therapy may be a significant benefit in the treatment of EFA deficiency associated with postoperative BA. The dose of UDCA administration was 15 mg/kg/day [30]. Another report described UDCA at 10–15 mg/kg/day was prescribed to patients with BA for several weeks after Kasai HPE [31]. Willot reported the beneficial effect of UDCA on liver function in children after successful surgery for biliary atresia. All patients were treated with UDCA at a dose of 200 mg/m$^2$ of body area 3 times daily (600 mg/m$^2$ per day) from the time of surgery. The mean dose was 25 mg/kg per day (range: 20–36 mg/kg per day) [33].

On the other hand, in the cohort study of infants with BA, UDCA in a dosage of 20 mg/kg per day for mean duration ± SD of 252.6 ± 544.9 days was not shown to be effective [34]. The UDCA in infants with extrahepatic biliary atresia at 15–30 mg/kg daily dosage was observed to improve biochemical parameters, nutritional status, and, in some cases, with alleviation of pruritus, but not with the inhibition of the progress of the disease. With observed progressing cholestasis, neither an increase of the patients' survival time nor reducing the need for liver transplantation were observed [31, 35, 36].

### 26.3.4 Conclusion

Because UDCA is expected to have effects such as promoting bile acid secretion, improving absorption disorders, and protecting hepatocytes, with no serious side effects having been reported, administration of UDCA following biliary atresia surgery is also recommended in the Japanese clinical practice guideline of BA [37].

## References

1. Meyers RL, Book LS, O'Gorman MA, Jackson WD, Black RE, Johnson DG, et al. High-dose steroids, ursodeoxycholic acid, and chronic intravenous antibiotics improve bile flow after Kasai procedure in infants with biliary atresia. J Pediatr Surg. 2003;38:406–11.
2. Kobayashi H, Atsuyuki Y, Koga H, Okazaki T, Tamura T, Urao M, et al. Optimum prednisolone usage in patients with biliary atresia postportoenterostomy. J Pediatr Surg. 2005;40:327–30.
3. Karrer FM, Lilly JR. Corticosteroid therapy in biliary atresia. J Pediatr Surg. 1985;20:693–5.
4. Muraji T, Higashimoto Y. The improved outlook for biliary atresia with corticosteroid therapy. J Pediatr Surg. 1997;32:1103–7.
5. Dillon PW, Owings E, Cilley R, et al. Immunosuppression as adjuvant therapy for biliary atresia. J Pediatr Surg. 2001;36:80–5.
6. Ohi R, Hanamatsu M, Mochizuki I, et al. Progress in the treatment of biliary atresia. World J Surg. 1985;9:285–93.
7. Miner PB, Gaito JM. Bile flow in response to pharmacologic agents: hepatic DNA as a reference standard. Biochem Pharmacol. 1979;28:1063–6.
8. Tatekawa Y, Muraji T, Tsugawa C. Glucocorticoid receptor a expression in the intrahepatic biliary epithelium and adjuvant steroid therapy in infants with biliary atresia. J Pediatr Surg. 2005;40:1574–80.
9. Haynes RC, Murad F. Adrenocorticotropic hormone; adrenocortical steroids and their synthetic analogs; inhibitors of adrenocortical

steroid biosynthesis. In: Gilman AG, Goodman LS, Gilman A, editors. The pharmacologic basis of therapeutics. 6th ed. New York: Macmillan; 1980. p. 1466–96.
10. Altman RP, Anderson KD. Surgical management of intractable cholangitis following successful Kasai procedure. J Pediatr Surg. 1982;17:894–900.
11. Lilly JR, Karrer FM, Hall RJ, Stellin GP, Vasquez-Estevez JJ, Greeenholz SK, et al. The surgery of biliary atresia. Ann Surg. 1989;210:289–96.
12. Muraji T, Nio M, Ohhama Y, Hashimoto T, Iwanaka T, Takamatsu H, et al. Postoperative corticosteroid therapy for bile drainage in biliary atresia-a nationwide survey. J Pediatr Surg. 2004;39:1803–5.
13. Japanese Biliary Atresia Society, Nio M, Muraji T. Multicenter randomized trial of postoperative corticosteroid therapy for biliary atresia. Pediatr Surg Int. 2013;29:1091–5.
14. Stringer MD, Davison SM, Rajwal SR, McClean P. Kasai portoenterostomy: 12-year experience with a novel adjuvant therapy regimen. J Pediatr Surg. 2007;42:1324–8.
15. Shimadera S, Iwai N, Deguchi E, Kimura O, Fumino S, Ono S. The significance of steroid therapy after hepatoportoenterostomy in infants with biliary atresia. Eur J Pediatr Surg. 2007;17:100–3.
16. Petersen C, Harder D, Melter M, Becker T, Wasielewski RV, Leonhardt J, et al. Postoperative high-dose steroids do not improve mid-term survival with native liver in biliary atresia. Am J Gastroenterol. 2008;103:712–9.
17. Dong R, Song Z, Chen G, Zheng S, Xiao XM. Improved outcome of biliary atresia with postoperative high-dose steroid. Gastroenterol Res Pract. 2013;2013:902431.
18. Davenport M, Stringer MD, Tizzard SA, McClean P, Mieli Vergani G, Hadzic N. Randomized, double-blind, placebo-controlled trial of corticosteroids after Kasai portoenterostomy for biliary atresia. Hepatology. 2007;46:1821–7.
19. Davenport M, Parsons C, Tizzard S, Hadzic N. Steroids in biliary atresia: single surgeon, single centre, prospective study. J Hepatol. 2013;59:1054–8.
20. Bezerra JA, Spino C, Magee JC, Shneider BL, Rosenthal P, Wang KS, et al. Use of corticosteroids after hepatoportoenterostomy for bile drainage in infants with biliary atresia: the START randomized clinical trial. JAMA. 2014;311:1750–9.
21. Chen Y, Nah SA, Chiang L, Krishnaswamy G, Low Y. Postoperative steroid therapy for biliary atresia: systematic review and meta-analysis. J Pediatr Surg. 2015;50:1590–4.
22. Tyraskis A, Davenport M. Steroids after the Kasai procedure for biliary atresia: the effect of age at Kasai portoenterostomy. Pediatr Surg Int. 2016;32:193–200.
23. Escobar MA, Jay CL, Brooks RM, West KW, Rescorla FJ, Molleston JP, et al. Effect of corticosteroid therapy on outcomes in biliary atresia after Kasai portoenterostomy. J Pediatr Surg. 2006;41:99–103.
24. Japanese Biliary Atresia Society, editor. Clinical practice guideline of biliary atresia. Tokyo: Herusu Shuppan; 2018. p. 71–3.
25. Hagey LR, Crombie DL, Espinosa E, Carey MC, Igimi H, Hofmann AF. Ursodeoxycholic acid in the Ursidae: biliary bile acids of bears, pandas, and related carnivores. J Lipid Res. 1993;34:1911–7.
26. Hofmann AF. Pharmacology of ursodeoxycholic acid, an enterohepatic drug. Scand J Gastroenterol Suppl. 1994;204:1–15.
27. Beuers U, Boyer JL, Paumgartner G. Ursodeoxycholic acid in cholestasis: potential mechanisms of action and therapeutic applications. Hepatology. 1998;28:1449–53.
28. Paumgartner G, Beuers U. Ursodeoxycholic acid in cholestatic liver disease: mechanisms of action and therapeutic use revisited. Hepatology. 2002;36:525–31.
29. Poupon RE, Balkau B, Eschwege E, Poupon R. A multicenter, controlled trial of ursodiol for the treatment of primary biliary cirrhosis. UDCA-PBC Study Group. N Engl J Med. 1991;324:1548–54.
30. Yamashiro Y, Ohtsuka Y, Shimizu T, Nittono H, Urao M, Miyano T, et al. Effects of ursodeoxycholic acid treatment on essential fatty acid deficiency in patients with biliary atresia. J Pediatr Surg. 1994;29:425–8.
31. Nittono H, Tokita A, Hayashi M, Watanabe K, Obinata K, Nakatsu N, et al. Ursodeoxycholic acid therapy in the treatment of biliary atresia. Biomed Pharmacother. 1989;43:37–41.
32. Mohanty MK, Gupta SD, Bhatnagar V. Surgical outcome in relation to duct size at porta hepatis and the use of cholagogues in patients with biliary atresia. Trop Gastroenterol. 2010;31(3):184–9.
33. Willot S, Uhlen S, Michaud L, Briand G, Bonnevalle M, Sfeir R, et al. Effect of ursodeoxycholic acid on liver function in children after successful surgery for biliary atresia. Pediatrics. 2008;122:e1236–41.
34. Kotb MA. Review of historical cohort: ursodeoxycholic acid in extrahepatic biliary atresia. J Pediatr Surg. 2008;43:1321–7.
35. Lebensztejn DM. Application of ursodeoxycholic acid (UDCA) in the therapy of liver and biliary duct diseases in children. Med Sci Monit. 2000;6(3):632–6.
36. Ulrich D, Rasting D, Schroter W. Treatment with ursodeoxycholic acid renders children with biliary atresia suitable for liver transplantation. Lancet. 1987;2:1234.
37. Japanese Biliary Atresia Society, editor. Clinical practice guideline of biliary atresia. Tokyo: Herusu Shuppan; 2018. p. 75–7.

# Medical Treatment: Antioxidant Therapy and Kampo Medicine

# 27

Minoru Yagi, Yoshiaki Tanaka, Naoki Hashizume, and Takahiro Asakawa

**Abstract**

Many patients with biliary atresia (BA) continue to suffer from postoperative liver dysfunction, even after undergoing Kasai's hepatic portoenterostomy. Such patients can experience chronic inflammation with or without jaundice. The oxidative stress may exist in postoperative patients with BA. The prevention of progressive liver fibrosis has, therefore, become an important factor to achieve favorable long-term results. For this purpose, a combination of medications that have hepatocyte protective activity has been used routinely in postoperative patients with BA. Catechin originated from green tea and $CoQ_{10}$ is commonly used as anti-oxidative supplementary food in Japan. The herbal medicine Inchinkoto (ICKT) has been commonly used in Japan as an anti-inflammatory, antipyretic, choleretic, and diuretic agent for liver disorders and jaundice. In this chapter, we would like to introduce the presence of oxidative stress and the anti-oxidative effects of green tea catechin, $CoQ_{10}$, herbal medicine ICKT in postoperative patients with BA. After discussing these points, it was shown that all of the oxidative stress markers in the postoperative patients with BA increased in comparison to those in the controls. From these results, green tea catechin, $CoQ_{10}$, ICKT were experimentally and clinically useful for reducing hepatic fibrosis and injury by controlling stellate cell activation with oxidant stress. Furthermore, it was suggested that these agents described above promote clearance of jaundice.

**Keywords**

Antioxidant therapy · Kampo medicine · Catechin · $CoQ_{10}$ · Inchinkoto · Clearance of jaundice

M. Yagi (✉) · Y. Tanaka · N. Hashizume · T. Asakawa
Department of Pediatric Surgery, Kurume University School of Medicine, Fukuoka, Japan
e-mail: yagimi@med.kurume-u.ac.jp

There are many postoperative patients with biliary atresia (BA) who suffer from liver dysfunction such as chronic inflammation, even without jaundice, after a Kasai's hepatic portoenterostomy. This implies that there is continuous inflammation remaining in the liver, such as chronic cytoinfiltration of Glisson's capsules which are identified in biopsied specimens of the liver in the postoperative patients with BA. Baskol et al. reported that oxidative stress contributes to the pathology of adult NASH [1]. The excessive production of active oxygen or radicals is thought to be a worsening factor [1]. However, there have been few reports on oxidative stress in the postoperative patients with BA, except Tiao's report on the measurement of the oxidative stress marker 8-hydroxy-2'-deoxyguanosine (8-OHdG) by immunohistochemistry [2]. There are many postoperative BA patients who suffer from liver dysfunction such as chronic inflammation, even without jaundice, after Kasai's hepatic portoenterostomy. Oxidative stress might be a major factor in liver dysfunction including chronic inflammation. Therefore, it is necessary to perform some options in the peri- and postoperative treatment that provides choleretic or anti-inflammatory activity for the purpose of native liver preservation. From the perioperative period, antioxidant therapy might ameliorate the pathology [3]. In our department, green tea catechin, coenzyme $Q_{10}$ ($CoQ_{10}$), herbal medicine Inchinko-to (ICKT) are used for reducing hepatic fibrosis by suppressing oxidant stress.

In this chapter, we would like to introduce postoperative oxidative stress, antioxidant therapy including Kampo medicine from the viewpoint of our experience.

## 27.1 The Postoperative Patients with BA Are Under Increased Oxidative Stress

We clarified the presence and degree of oxidative stress in postoperative patients with BA [3]. The details are as follows. Twelve outpatients who had undergone a Kasai's hepatic portoenterostomy were evaluated. They were classi-


M. Nio (ed.), *Introduction to Biliary Atresia*, https://doi.org/10.1007/978-981-16-2160-4_27

fied as the BA group ($n$ = 12), seven boys, five girls (mean 5.2 years old), weighing from 10.6 to 33.0 kg (mean 18.6 kg), the control group ($n$ = 6), who were preoperative patients with an inguinal hernia that included 3 boys, 3 girls (mean 4.5 years old), weighing from 8.5 to 30.5 kg (mean 17.2 kg). In 11 of the postoperative patients with BA, jaundice was diminished in 69.5 ± 23.1% (<total bilirubin(TB): 2.0 mg/dl). Hematic, urinary, and hepatic biopsies were obtained after satisfactory informed consent was obtained from the patients and their parents. Besides alanine aminotransferase (ALT), gamma-glutamyl transpeptidase (gamma-GTP), TB, insulin-like growth factor-1(IGF-1), type IV collagen, the following markers were measured: (1) activity level of serum superoxide dismutase (SOD), indicating active oxygen production; (2) serum concentration of antioxygen bioenzymes, such as manganese-superoxide dismutase (Mn-SOD) and copper / zinc-superoxide dismutase (Cu / Zn-SOD); (3) markers of oxidative stress, such as the concentration of urine 8-iso-prostaglandinF2alpha (8-isoprostane) and urine 8-OHdG(8-hydroxy-2'-deoxyguanosine); (4) 8-OHdG immunohistochemical staining of the advancing hepatic disease, in vivo SOD activation was measured by nitrous transformation: Mn-SOD and Cu / Zn-SOD were measured by enzymatic immunoassays: urine 8-isoprostane was also measured by an enzymatic immunoassay: urine 8-OHdG was measured by an enzymatic immunoassay: 8-OHdG was determined by immunohistochemical staining, with anti 8-OHdG monoclonal antibody, using the ABC method. The staining rate was determined in five fields at 400× magnification, reflecting the rate of anti-8-OHdG antibody-positive cells in the pulse regions and the lobules. IGF-1 and type IV collagen were measured by IGF-1 Kit and Type IV collagen Kit, respectively.

In the twelve outpatients, no one showed jaundice except one patient, but all showed chronic liver dysfunction, defined by ALT >50 IU/l or gamma-GTP >50 IU/l. Seven patients showed advance of liver dysfunction, including 5 with portal hypertension, 5 with splenomegaly, 4 with esophageal varix, and 1 with gastric varix. The SOD activity level and Mn-SOD concentration showed extremely high values in 3 patients with extremely low values of IGF-1(normal range in the children below 13 years old: 50–750 ng/ml) and 4 patients with high values of type IV collagen (normal range <6 ng/ml). The SOD activity level in the BA group was significantly higher than those in the control subjects (5.6 ± 1.4 U/mL, normal range: 1.76–3.20 U/mL). The Mn-SOD concentration in 8 of the patients was higher than that in the control (268.3 ± 157.3 ng/mL; normal range <150 ng/ml). Thereafter, liver transplantation was performed in 2 of the 8 patients with an increased Mn-SOD concentration. The Cu/Zn-SOD concentration in 7 patients showed a high value in comparison to that in the control subjects (26.8 ± 15.6 ng/mL, normal range <20 ng/ml). The Cu/Zn-SOD concentration was high (34.9 ± 14.5 ng/ml) in 5 of the 8 patients with an increased Mn-SOD concentration. All of the stress markers in the BA group were significantly higher than those in the controls. There were significant positive correlations between Mn-SOD and ALT, and between Mn-SOD and type IV collagen, and negative correlation between Mn-SOD and IGF-1. Moreover, 8-OHdG immunohistochemical staining was positive in 84 ± 4.8% hepatic cells of the portal area in the BA group.

These results demonstrated that the postoperative patients with BA were under increased oxidative stress, even if their liver dysfunction was mild without jaundice. Antioxidant therapy might be necessary to decrease oxidative stress in the postoperative patients with BA.

## 27.2 Antioxidative Therapy Using $CoQ_{10}$ in the Perioperative Patients with BA

Coenzyme Q, in addition to its function as an electron and proton carrier in mitochondrial and bacterial electron transport linked to ATP synthesis, acts in its reduced form ($CoQ_{10}$) as an antioxidant, preventing the initiation and/or propagation of lipid peroxidation in biological membranes and in serum low-density lipoprotein. The antioxidant activity of $CoQ_{10}$ is independent of the effect of vitamin E, which acts as a chain-breaking antioxidant inhibiting the propagation of lipid peroxidation. $CoQ_{10}$ is the only known lipid-soluble antioxidant that animal cells can synthesize de novo, and for which there exist enzymic mechanisms that can regenerate the antioxidant from its oxidized form resulting from its inhibitory effect of lipid peroxidation. These features, together with its high degree of hydrophobicity and its widespread occurrence in biological membranes and in low-density lipoprotein, suggest an important role of $CoQ_{10}$ in cellular defense against oxidative damage [4].

Hereupon, we evaluated the effect of $CoQ_{10}$ therapy in the postoperative BA patients [5, 6]. The details are as follows. The groups comprised postoperative BA patients administrated with $CoQ_{10}$ ($n$ = 12), and postoperative BA patients administrated without $CoQ_{10}$ ($n$ = 11). $CoQ_{10}$ administration was started at a dose of 3 mg/kg/day (Dose in Adult: 80 mg/day), divided into 3 times, from 6 postoperative days after Kasai's operation. Administrated period was 6 months. We used water-soluble $CoQ_{10}$ as $CoQ_{10}$, which was manufactured in powder form by Taiyo-Kagaku, Co. Ltd, Mie, Japan. Discussed markers were liver function markers (AST, ALT, γ-GTP, TB, DB, IB, TBA), and oxidative stress markers (serum SOD activity, serum Mn-SOD, urine 8-iso-prostane, urine 8-OHdG). Liver biopsies were performed at the points of Kasai's operation and 6 months after $CoQ_{10}$ administration. From the view point of accumulation of oxidation damaged material,

8-OHdG immunohistochemical staining was performed. There were no significant differences in the background factors between the patients with and without $CoQ_{10}$.

Chronological changes of the postoperative stress markers, such as serum SOD and Mn-SOD, in the BA patients administrated with $CoQ_{10}$ were significantly decreased within 6 months after Kasai's operation. Urine oxidative stress markers that showed high values before Kasai's operation such as 8-isoprostane and 8-OHdG were significantly decreased. Although averaged successful clearance days of jaundice were 49.5 days, there were still under oxidative stress in spite of no jaundice. Furthermore, we discussed the effect of postoperative administration with $CoQ_{10}$. We compared with liver function markers, successful clearance days of jaundice in the BA patients with or without $CoQ_{10}$ administration. In the chronological changes of the liver function markers, there were no significant differences except total bilirubin. Total bilirubin was significantly decreased at points of one and three months after Kasai's operation. Direct bilirubin was significantly decreased at point of one month after Kasai's operation. Successful clearance days of jaundice below 2 mg/dL in total bilirubin in the BA patients with or without $CoQ_{10}$ were 27.2 ± 13.4 days, 69.5 ± 23.1 days, respectively. There was a significant difference between them ($p < 0.01$). Furthermore, successful clearance days of jaundice below 1 mg/dL in the BA patients with or without $CoQ_{10}$ were 49.5 ± 29.8 days, 138.0 ± 81.5 days, respectively. There was a significant difference between them ($p < 0.05$). Liver biopsies were performed at the points of Kasai's operation and 6 months after $CoQ_{10}$ administration. From the viewpoint of immunohistochemical staining with anti-8-OHdG antibody, there were approximately 80% positive cells of anti-8-OHdG antibody in the portal area and lobules. Six months after administration of $CoQ_{10}$, there were scarcely rare anti-8-OHdG antibody-positive cells. 8-OHdG is index of accumulation of oxidation damaged material of deoxyguanosine as DNA component factor. From these results, $CoQ_{10}$ may suppress oxidative stress and promote clearance of jaundice [5, 6].

## 27.3 Antioxidative Therapy Using Catechin in the Perioperative Patients with BA

Green tea contains a high level of polyphenol compounds termed catechins. Polyphenol generally refers to a compound with more than two phenolic hydroxyl groups in the same molecule, and catechin is classified as a flavonoid. Flavonoid compounds are involved in physiological regulation, and have anti-oxidative and anti-allergenic functions. The anti-oxidative functions of catechins are reported to be due to the hydroxyl groups on the benzene ring, and to be the strongest in epigallocatechin gallate [7]. Yokozawa et al. reported a decrease of uremia after the administration of green tea polyphenol in rat models of chronic renal failure and renal hypertension [8, 9]. Fujise et al. reported a decrease in anti-oxidative activation after the administration of polyphenols, anti-oxidative vitamins, and chemically intensified anti-oxidative liquid foods in a rat model with invasive surgery [10].

We previously performed bile duct ligation on cholestatic Wistar rats and evaluated the degree of liver dysfunction (fibrosis) [11]. In the study, we investigated the presence and degree of oxidative stress in the hepatic tissues, the anti-oxidative effects of green tea catechin, and the mechanism underlying the suppression of fibrosis by catechin. Bile duct ligation caused hepatic dysfunction in the rats by oxidative stress. Administration of green tea catechin suppressed the degree of fibrosis. After the administration of green tea catechin, we observed decreased rates of staining for 4-HNE (4-hydroxy-2'-nonenal), an indicator of hepatic lipoperoxidation, and 8-OHdG, an indicator of oxidative injuries of deoxyguanosine or a DNA constituent. The staining for 8-OHdG showed a lower number of deeply stained nuclei after catechin administration, thus indicating that the level of oxidative stress had been mitigated. Moreover, there were significant decreases in the following markers: AP-1 m-RNA, TGF beta-1 (a key mediator of inflammatory cytokine activation), alfa-SMA (an indicator of stellate cell activation), and TIMP-1 m-RNA (an indicator of stellate cell activation and fibrosis). Therefore, green tea catechin mixture may have systematically suppressed oxidative stress, transcription factor expression, and stellate cell activation; furthermore, catechin appeared to suppress the accumulation of extracellular matrix by controlling the inhibitors of matrix metalloproteinase, thereby reducing fibrosis [11].

Hereupon, we clinically evaluated the effect of catechin therapy in the postoperative BA patients [5, 12]. The groups comprised postoperative BA patients administrated with catechin ($n = 13$), and postoperative BA patients administrated without catechin ($n = 11$). We used Sunphenon BG3™ as catechin, which was green tea catechin mixture in powder form, which was prepared from green tea by Taiyo-Kagaku, Co. Ltd, Mie, Japan. It was composed mainly of Epigallocatechin gallate (48.8%), Epigallocatechin (21.6%), Epicatechin (6.4%), Epicatechin gallate (3.7%), Catechin (1.3%), Gallocatechin gallate (1.2%), Catechin gallate (48.8%), and Gallocatechin (0%), respectively. Catechin dose was calculated according to the Ivady & Dirner Formula (Dose in adults: 400 mg/day). Catechin administration was started from 6 postoperative day after Kasai's operation, divided into 2 times per day. Administrated period was 6 months. Discussed markers were liver function markers (AST, ALT, γ-GTP, TB, DB, IB, TBA), and oxidative stress markers (serum SOD activity, urine 8-iso-prostane, urine 8-OHdG). These examinations were performed at 1,3,6 months after Kasai's operation. Liver biopsies were performed at the points of Kasai's operation and 3 months after catechin administration. 8-OHdG and 4-HNE (4-hydroxy-2'-nonenal) immunohistochemical staining was performed. There were no significant differences in the background factors between the patients with and without catechin. Preoperatively, stress markers, such as serum SOD, urine 8-iso-prostane, and urine 8-OHdG, in the BA patients administrated with or without catechin showed remarkably high values. Preoperative serum SOD activities (U/mL) with and without catechin were 5.63 ± 1.53, 5.62 ± 1.11, respectively (normal:1.76–3.20 U/mL). Urine 8-iso-prostane (pg/mg-crea) were 1970 ± 662, 1774 ± 650, respectively (normal:<200 pg/mg-crea). Urine 8-OHdG (ng/mg-crea) were 49.8 ± 17.0, 52.2 ± 20.1, respectively (normal:<15 ng/mg-crea). There were no significant differences in these stress markers between postoperative BA patients with and without catechin. Serum SOD activities (U/mL) at 3 and 6 months after operation in the patients with catechin were 4.57 ± 1.04,5.05 ± 2.3, respectively. They were significantly decreased compared with preoperative value ($p < 0.05$). Urine 8-iso-prostane (pg/mg-crea) at 1,3,6 months after operation in the BA patients with catechin were1457 ± 69, 1011 ± 21, 775 ± 449, respectively. They were significantly decreased compared with preoperative value ($p < 0.05$). Urine 8-OHdG (ng/mg-crea) at 6 months after operation in the BA patients with catechin was 42.6 ± 20.8. It was significantly decreased compared with preoperative value ($p < 0.05$). Other stress markers in the BA patients without catechin showed no significant improvement during 6 months after operation. Furthermore, liver function, successful clearance days of jaundice in the BA patients with or without catechin administration were discussed. In the chronological changes of the liver function markers, there were no significant differences except total bilirubin and direct bilirubin in the BA patients with or without catechin during 6 months after Kasai's operation. Total bilirubin (mg/dL) in the patients with or without catechin at one month after Kasai's operation were 2.53 ± 1.7, 6.87 ± 2.8, respectively. There was significant difference between them ($p < 0.05$). Direct bilirubin (mg/dL) in the BA patients with or without catechin at one month after Kasai's operation were 1.4 ± 1.3, 4.87 ± 2.4, respectively. There was significant difference between them ($p < 0.05$). Successful clearance days of jaundice below 1 mg/dL in total bilirubin with or without catechin were 69.7 ± 67.0 days, 138.0 ± 81.5 days, respectively. There was significant difference between them ($p < 0.05$). Liver biopsies were performed at the points of Kasai's operation and 3 months after catechin administration. From the viewpoint of immunohistochemical staining with anti-8-OHdG antibody, there were approximately 80% positive cells of anti-8-OHdG antibody in the portal area and lobules at Kasai's operation. Three months after catechin, there were scarcely rare anti-8-OHdG antibody-positive cells. There were remarkably most 4-HNE positive cells in the portal area and lobules. It was strongly suggested that the liver in the BA patients was under oxidative stress. Three months after catechin administration, there were scarcely rare 4-HNE-positive cells. 4-HNE is index of accumulation of peroxylipid in hepatic cells. Oxidative stress was improved by catechin administration.

From these results, catechin may suppress oxidative stress and promote clearance of Jaundice.

## 27.4 Kampo Therapy (Japanese Traditional Herbal Medicine) Using Inchinkoto in the Postoperative BA Patients

The herbal medicine Inchinkoto (ICKT) has been commonly used in Japan as an anti-inflammatory, antipyretic, choleretic, and diuretic agent for liver disorders and jaundice [13–15]. Inchinkoto (ICKT) is the Kampo medicine formulation, originally described in Shoukanron and Kinkiyouryaku of Chinese herbal medicine about 1800years ago. Recently, ICKT has been reported to have a potent inhibitory effect on hepatocyte apoptosis, induced by transforming growth factor-beta 1 (TGF-beta1), and it inhibits the production of inflammatory cytokines in concanavalin A-induced hepatitis [16, 17]. Furthermore, ICKT has been reported to directly suppress liver fibrosis in vivo [18, 19]. Clinical reports in Japan also suggest that ICKT might be beneficial for the treatment of hepatobiliary diseases in adults [19].

We used TJ-135 as ICKT. TJ-135 is manufactured by Tsumura & Co (Tokyo, Japan) and has been approved as an ethical drug by the Ministry of Health and Welfare of Japan. Seven and one-half grams of this product contains 1.5 g of dried extract obtained from mixed raw herbs in the following ratio; Inchin-ko (Artemisia Capillaries Spike [4.0 g]), San-shishi (JP Gardenia Fruit [3.0 g]), and Daio (JP Rhubarb Rhizome [1.0 g]) [17–20]. The daily amount of TJ-135 is 7.5 g/day in adults. Inchinko and San-shishi are effective for liver disease, and Daio is a laxative and anti-inflammatory agent. Inchinko contains the choleretic agent capillarisin. San-shishi contains genipin, an aglycone converted in the gut from geniposide which has been proven to suppress Fas-induced liver injury in mice [21]. Clinically, administration of ICKT in postoperative BA patients appears to lower the serum levels of markers of fibrosis in the medium term [19, 22, 23]. Hepatic fibrosis may have been inhibited due to a reduction of the hepatic TIMP-1 levels, as a marker of the suppression of matrix metalloproteinase, and thus led to reduction of TGF-beta1 levels. Recently, Nrf2-mediated antioxidant action was reported in cholestatic diseases by administration of ICKT [24] (Fig. 27.1). There are still few reports of its use in the treatment of cholestatic liver disorder [25].

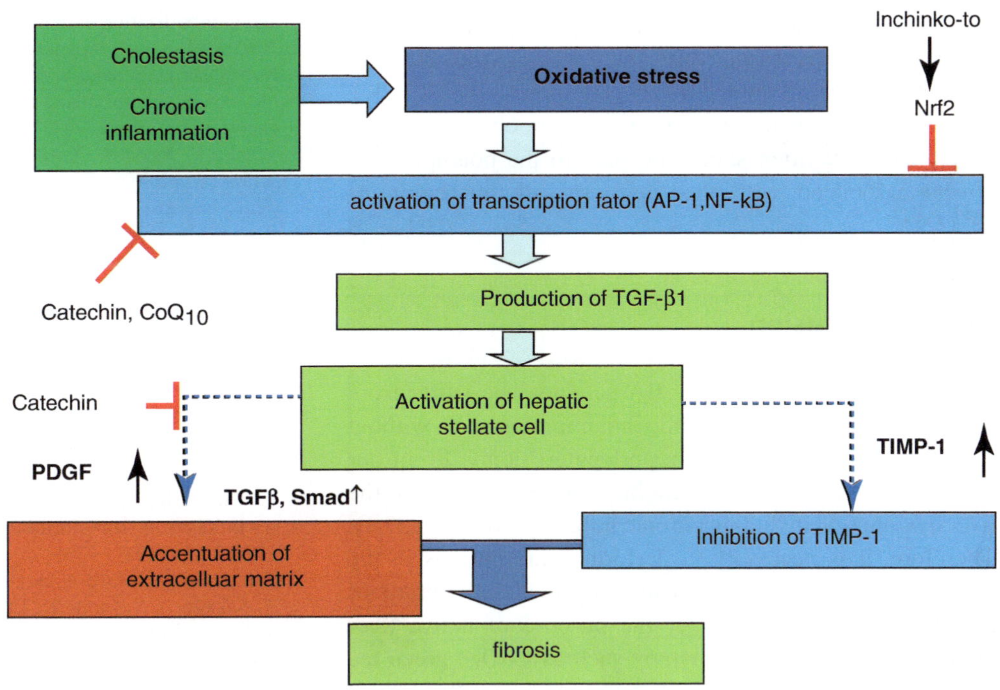


**Fig. 27.1** Mechanism of the liver dysfunction

### 27.4.1 Our Experimental Investigation Concerning ICKT [26]

Hereupon, we discussed whether the administration of ICKT will ameliorate hepatic fibrosis and injury in cholestatic rats. We performed bile duct ligation on 7-week-old male cholestatic Wistar rats and assigned them to one of three groups according to the method of treatment: (1) the SHAM group, (2) the NT-group (nontreatment group), and (3) the T-group (treatment-group). Rats in the T-group were orally administered ICKT (TJ-135) at a dose of 1 g/kg/day and were sacrificed on the 17th postoperative day. We subsequently investigated the levels of fibrosis and various clinical markers through measurement of the following: serum levels of AST and ALT; tissue transforming growth factor-beta 1 (TGF-beta1); tissue inhibitor metalloprotease-1 mRNA (TIMP-1 mRNA) through real-time PCR analysis; and Azan staining and immunohistochemical staining of alfa-smooth muscle actin (alfa-SMA) to evaluate the degree of fibrosis. Results were as following: Serum AST and ALT levels in rats. Serum AST and ALT levels in the NT-group were significantly higher than those in the T-group ($p < 0.05$). Immunohistochemical staining of TGF-beta1. The percentages of positive cells were 22.06 ± 5.4 and 0.97 ± 1.45 % in the NT-group and T-group, respectively. Staining of TGF-beta1 in the T-group was significantly lower than that in the NT-group ($p < 0.05$). Hepatic TGF-beta1 levels. The level of hepatic TGF-beta1 in the NT-group was significantly higher than that in the T-group ($p < 0.05$). Although the relative quantification of hepatic TIMP-1 m-RNA in the T-group was lower than that in the NT-group, there was no significant difference between them. Immunohistochemical staining of alfa-SMA. The rates of positive cells were 47.5 ± 16.4 and 8.4 ± 4.3% in the NT-group and T-group, respectively. The percentage of positive staining areas of alpha-SMA in the T-group was significantly lower than that in the NT-group ($p < 0.05$). The percentages of fibrotic areas were 33.2 ± 8.5 and 11.3 ± 7.1% in the NT-group and T-group, respectively. Staining of Azan in the T-group was significantly lower than that in the NT-group ($p < 0.05$). In spite of the high grade of bridging fibrosis in the NT group, no bridging fibrosis was seen in the T-group.

In conclusion, the herbal medicine ICKT might protect hepatocytes and reduce fibrosis by suppressing hepatic stellate cell activation in a cholestatic rat model.

### 27.4.2 Our Clinical Experience Concerning ICKT (Unpublished Work)

Hereupon, we evaluated the effect of ICKT(TJ-135) therapy in the postoperative BA patients in our department. The groups comprised postoperative BA patients administrated with ICKT ($n = 25$), and postoperative BA patients administrated without ICKT ($n = 5$). ICKT (TJ-135) administration was started at a dose of 0.2 g/kg/day, divided into 3 times, from 6 postoperative day after Kasai's operation. In this series, the discussed marker was total bilirubin. Successful clearance days of jaundice below 1 mg/dL in the BA patients with or without ICKT were 73.9 ± 41.1 days, 126.2 ± 90.5 days, respectively. There was significant difference between them ($p = 0.0463$). The patients with ICKT tolerated TJ-135 well. No side effects were observed in our series, close attention should be paid to the potential side effects associated with the long-term administration of TJ-135.

## 27.5 Conclusion

There are many postoperative BA patients who suffer from liver dysfunction such as chronic inflammation, even without jaundice, after Kasai's hepatic portoenterostomy. From our experience, oxidative stress might be a major factor in the liver dysfunction including chronic inflammation (Fig. 27.1). Therefore, it is necessary to perform some options in the peri- and postoperative treatment that provides choleretic or anti-inflammatory activity for the purpose of native liver preservation. Antioxidant therapy such as $CoQ_{10}$, green tea catechin, herbal medicine ICKT might ameliorate the pathology including successful clearance of jaundice with reducing hepatic fibrosis by suppressing oxidant stress (Fig. 27.1).

## References


1. Baskol G, Baskol M, Kocer D. Oxidative stress and antioxidant defenses in serum of patients with non-alcoholic steatohepatitis. Clin Biochem. 2007;40:776–80.
2. Tiao MM, Lin TK, Kuo FY, Huang CC, Du YY, Chen CL, Chuang JH. Early stage of biliary atresia is associated with significant changes in 8-hydroxydeoxyguanosine and mitochondrial copy number. J Pediatr Gastroenterol Nutr. 2007;45:329–34.
3. Asakawa T, Tanaka Y, Asagiri K, Kobayashi H, Tanikawa K, Yagi M. Oxidative stress profile in the post-operative patients with biliary atresia. Pediatr Surg Int. 2009;25(1):93–7.
4. Ernster L, Forsmark-Andree P. Ubiquinol: an endogenous antioxidant in aerobic organisms. Clin Investig. 1993;71:S60–5.
5. Tanaka Y, Ishii S, Asagiri K, Fukahori S, Saikusa N, Hashizume N, Yoshida M, Komatsuzaki N, Masui D, Higashidate N, Yagi M. Oxidative stress and antioxidant. J Japanese Soc Parenter Enter Nutr. 2016;31(1):3–12. (in Japanese)
6. Tanaka Y, Komori T, Ishii S, Kaida A, Asakawa T, Kobayashi H, Nakamizo H, Akiyoshi K, Asagiri K, Yagi M. Antioxidant effects of Coenzyme $Q_{10}$ on chronic hepatic dysfunction in children with biliary atresia. J Japanese Soc Med Use Funct Foods. 2006;3(4):231–40. (in Japanese)
7. Sugiura K, Okubo T. The feature and functionality of green tea polyphenol. New Food Ind. 2000;42:1–7.
8. Yokozawa T, Hikokichi O, Senji S, Shoichi I, Mujo K. Depressor effect of tannin in green tea on rats with renal hypertension. Biosci Biotechnol Biochem. 1994;58:855–8.
9. Yokozawa T, Chung HY, He LQ, Oura H. Effectiveness of green tea tannin on rats with chronic renal failure. Biosci Biotechnol Biochem. 1996;60:1000–5.
10. Fujise N, Tanaka Y, Tasiro M, Abe S, Nakamura T, Masunaga H. The effect of antioxidant nutrients-rich liquid diet on anti-trauma and antioxidization activity. J Japanese Soc Med Use Funct Foods. 2005;3:53–63. (in Japanese)
11. Kobayashi H, Tanaka Y, Asagiri K, Asakawa T, Tanikawa K, Kage M, Yagi M. Antioxidant effect of green tea catechin ameriolates experimental liver injury. Phytomedicine. 2010;17(3–4):197–202.
12. Tanaka Y, Asakawa T. Effect of antioxidative therapy using catechin in perioperative patients with biliary atresia. J Clin Surg (Rinsyougeka). 2009;64(10):1397–403. (in Japanese)
13. Kiso Y, Ogasawara Y, Hirota K, Watanabe N, Oshima Y, Konno C, Hikino H. Antihepatotoxic principles of Artemisia capillaris buds. Planta Med. 1984;50(1):81–5.
14. Takeda S, Endo T, Aburada M. Pharmacological studies on iridioid compounds. The choleretic mechanism of iridoid compounds. J Pharmacobiodyn. 1981;4:612–23.
15. Okuno I, Uchida K, Nakamura M, Sakurawi K. Studies on choleretic constituents in Artemisia capillaris THUMB. Chem Pharm Bull. 1988;36:769–75.
16. Yamamoto M, Ogawa K, Morita M, Fukuda K, Komatsu Y. The herbal medicine Inchin-koto inhibits liver cell apoptosis induced by transforming growth factor beta 1. Hepatology. 1996;23:552–9.
17. Yamashiki M, Mase A, Arai I, Huang XX, Nobori T, Nishimura A, Sakaguchi S, Inoue K. Effect of the Japanese herbal medicine Inchinko-to (TJ-135) on concanavalin A-induced hepatitis in mice. Clin Sci. 2000;99:421–31.
18. Inao M, Mochida S, Matsui A, Eguchi Y, Yulutuz Y, Wang Y, Naiki K, Kakinuma T, Fujimori K, Nagoshi S, Fujiwara K. Japanese herbal medicine Inchinko-to as a therapeutic drug for liver fibrosis. J Hepatol. 2004;41:584–91.
19. Iinuma Y, Kubota M, Yagi M, Kanada S, Yamazaki S, Kinoshita Y. Effects of the herbal medicine Inchinko-to on liver function in postoperative patients with biliary atresia-a pilot study. J Pediatr Surg. 2003;38:1607–11.
20. Sakaida I, Tsuchiya M, Kawaguchi K, Kimura T, Terai S, Okita K. Herbal medicine Inchinko-to (TJ-135) prevents liver fibrosis and enzyme altered lesions in rat liver cirrhosis induced by a choline-deficient L-amino acid-defined diet. J Hepatol. 2003;38:762–9.
21. Yamamoto M, Miura N, Ohtake N, Amagaya S, Ishige A, Sasaki H, Komatsu Y, Fukuda K, Ito T, Terasawa K. Genipin, a metabolite derived from the herbal medicine Inchin-ko-to, and suppression of Fas-induced lethal liver apoptosis in mice. Gastroenterology. 2000;118:380–9.
22. Kobayashi H, Horikoshi K, Yamataka A, Lane GJ, Yamamoto M, Miyano T. Beneficial effect of a traditional herbal medicine (inchin-ko-to) in postoperative biliary atresia patients. Pediatr Surg Int. 2001;17:386–9.
23. Tamura T, Kobayashi H, Yamataka A, Lane GJ, Koga H, Miyano T. Inchinkoto prevents medium-term liver fibrosis in postoperative biliary atresia patients. Pediatr Surg Int. 2007;23:343–7.
24. Okada K, Shoda J, Kano M, Suzuki S, Ohtake N, Yamamoto M, Takahashi H, Utsunomiya H, Oda K, Sato K, Watanabe A, Ishii T, Itoh K, Yamamoto M, Yokoi T, Yoshizato K, Sugiyama Y, Suzuki H. Inchinkoto, a herbal medicine, and its ingredients dually exert Mrp2/MRP2-mediated choleresis and Nrf2-mediated antioxidative action in rat livers. Am J Physiol Gastrointest Liver Physiol. 2007;292:1450–63.
25. Yokoyama Y, Nagino M. Current scenario for the hepatoprotective effects of Inchinkoto, a traditional herbal medicine, and its clinical application in liver surgery: a review. Hepatol Res. 2014;44(4):384–94.
26. Asakawa T, Yagi M, Tanaka Y, Asagiri K, Kobayashi H, Egami H, Tanikawa K, Kage M. The herbal medicine Inchinko-to reduces hepatic fibrosis in cholestatic rats. Pediatr Surg Int. 2012;28(4):379–84.

# 28 Current Concept About Prevention/Treatment of Postoperative Cholangitis

Kosaku Maeda

**Abstract**

Cholangitis is the most common complication in patients after Kasai portoenterostomy, with an incidence of 30% to 70%. Patients with early bile drainage after Kasai operation are more vulnerable to cholangitis. Early cholangitis and recurrent cholangitis are interrelated and can contribute to reduced overall survival.

The pathogenesis of postoperative cholangitis is still controversial, but one potential cause of cholangitis is ascending intestinal bacteria.

Postoperative cholangitis characterized by fever and acholic stool and positive blood culture is a common and serious complication following Kasai operation for biliary atresia. No modification prevented cholangitis more effectively than the original KP. Consequently, most pediatric surgeons currently use the original KP procedure with a long Rou-en Y loop. Recommendation is to administer the antibiotics intravenously for 2 to 4 weeks after surgery, followed by oral antibiotics.

Individualized treatment considering risk factors for individual BA patients should be strongly considered to prevent cholangitis.

**Keywords**

Biliary atresia · Cholangitis · Kasai portoenterostomy
Jaundice clearance · Long-term outcome · Risk factor

## 28.1 Introduction

Although Kasai's hepatoportoenteric anastomosis-(portoenterostomy) and other perioperative management improved outcomes, many biliary atresia (BA) patients still require liver transplantation for long-term survival [1]. Cholangitis is the most common complication in patients after Kasai operation, with an incidence of 30% to 70%, especially in the first year after Kasai [2]. Patients with early bile drainage after Kasai are more vulnerable to cholangitis. Early cholangitis and recurrent cholangitis are interrelated and can contribute to reduced overall survival.

Cholangitis is a risk factor for poor prognosis in patients after Kasai [3, 4], according to several studies. Nio et al. [5]. assessed the clinical parameters to clarify the early risk factors affecting late-presenting liver failure in BA. They reviewed 92 survived with their native liver for more than 20 years, and 72 continue to survive with their native liver in good condition (Group 1). In 20 patients, persistent jaundice recurred after the age of 20 years (Group 2). As a result, 47% had cholangitis in Group 1, and 74% in Group 2. Cholangitis in the early postoperative period has a significant effect on long-term survivors.

The aim of this chapter is to describe the pathogenesis, clinical manifestations, medical/surgical treatment, and outcome of postoperative cholangitis.

## 28.2 Pathogenesis

The pathogenesis of postoperative cholangitis is still controversial. The etiology of cholangitis remains unknown, but several hypotheses have been established that intestinal bacterial migration and immunoinflammatory responses may be major factors. One potential cause of cholangitis is ascending intestinal bacteria. Biliary stasis and obstruction and poor drainage with bacterial seeding also have been postulated [6].

In addition, cholangitis affects bile excretion, can cause cholestasis, and can accelerate the progression of liver damage and fibrosis. Kasai operation has been performed as a standard surgical procedure for BA, but the bile ducts in the

K. Maeda (✉)
Kobe Children's Hospital, Kobe, Japan


M. Nio (ed.), *Introduction to Biliary Atresia*, https://doi.org/10.1007/978-981-16-2160-4_28

hilum of the liver are so thin that they cannot be seen macroscopically, so it is not possible to perform mucosal/mucosal anastomosis and bile flow.

Early cholangitis is commonly defined as an onset within the first month of post-Kasai and is considered to be an important marker for poor outcomes, including prolonged jaundice clearance and lower native liver survival [3, 7]. Cholangitis patients have a relatively delayed jaundice clearance, while early and recurrent cholangitis may contribute to lower overall survival.

The more episodes of cholangitis (considered as recurrent cholangitis) a patient experiences, the worse liver damage the patient may suffer from. Therefore, recurrent cholangitis is correlated with accelerated development of liver fibrosis and other severe complications [6, 8].

Recurrent cholangitis is associated with earlier cholangitis onsets and can contribute to lower overall survival rates. Cholangitis can cause poor prognosis in patients who have achieved earlier jaundice clearance [9, 10].

## 28.3 Clinical Manifestation

Postoperative cholangitis characterized by fever and acholic stool and positive blood culture is a common and serious complication following Kasai operation for biliary atresia.

The diagnosis of cholangitis is mainly clinical symptoms (fever of unknown cause, recurrent jaundice, acoustic stool) and laboratory tests (increased bilirubin level, increased C-reactive protein (CRP), increased white blood cell (WBC) count) [4].

## 28.4 Risk Factors and Prognostic Effects of Cholangitis After Kasai Operation

Deterioration of liver condition before surgery may be a risk factor for recurrent cholangitis, and preoperative γ-glutamyl transferase levels (γ-GTP) may indicate the development of cholangitis. Therefore, higher γ-GTP prior to Kasai surgery are risk factors for cholangitis.

Older age and increased liver fibrosis score during Kasai surgery are risk factors for recurrent cholangitis. Short use of prophylactic intravenous antibiotics can lead to early cholangitis and can lead to a higher frequency of cholangitis. Recurrent cholangitis is associated with the early onset of cholangitis.

Patients with cholangitis have relatively delayed jaundice clearance, but early recurrent cholangitis may contribute to shorter overall survival.

## 28.5 Postoperative Cholangitis and Antireflux Surgery

Cholangitis is the most serious complication following Kasai operation. Many pediatric surgeons have attempted to prevent development of cholangitis by modifying reconstructive surgery (Fig. 28.1) [11]. However, no modification prevented cholangitis more effectively than the original KP. Consequently, most pediatric surgeons currently use the original KP procedure with a long Rou-en Y loop.

According to the Japanese Biliary Atresia Registry (JBAR2018), 2506 patients underwent the original KP (simple Roux-Y anastomosis), and the remaining 626 underwent the Rou-en Y reconstruction procedure with an antireflux intestinal valve [12, 13]. Jaundice disappearance was 1529 cases (61.8%) in the simple Roux-Y anastomosis and 384 cases (61.3%) in the Roux-Y method with artificial intestinal valve. Although the jaundice clearance rate did not differ significantly between the original KP and intestinal valve procedure, the incidence of cholangitis has recently been reported to be higher in the original KP (42.4%) than in the intestinal valve procedure (34.3%) [12]. Because of the lower incidence of early cholangitis, Nio et al. have used the intestinal valve procedure even in recent era [14].

There are two types of intestinal valves: a spur valve and an intussuscepted valve. Nio et al. [14] currently employed the spur valve, which is technically simple and not associated with any adverse event. The significance of the intestinal valve on the final outcome is still controversial.

The length of the Roux-en Y loop is routinely 55 cm. However, recently performing this procedure on neonates and low-birth-weight infants, who weigh 3 kg or less at surgery. Nio et al. [14]. felt a 55-cm loop was too long for such small infants. Thus, they reduced the length of the Roux-en Y loop to 10 cm/kg/weight in small infants in recent era.

Qiao et al. [1] showed 244 cases those who had surgery in 90 days or more and postoperative cholangitis had a significantly poor prognosis. Since postoperative cholangitis has a poor prognosis, antireflux surgery such as external fistula and artificial intestinal valvuloplasty and administration of antibacterial agents are performed to prevent it. However, there was no difference between the cholangitis incidence rate (33%) of external fistula and the cholangitis incidence rate (32%) of non-external fistula, and the harm associated with the construction of external fistula was pointed out [15]. In recent years, external fistula has not been performed [16].

Sartorelli et al. [17] showed that out of 50 cases of biliary atresia, 38 cases that met the inclusion criteria were divided into two groups with or without artificial intestinal valve and examined retrospectively. As a result, cholangitis developed in all 38 cases, and there was no significant difference in the

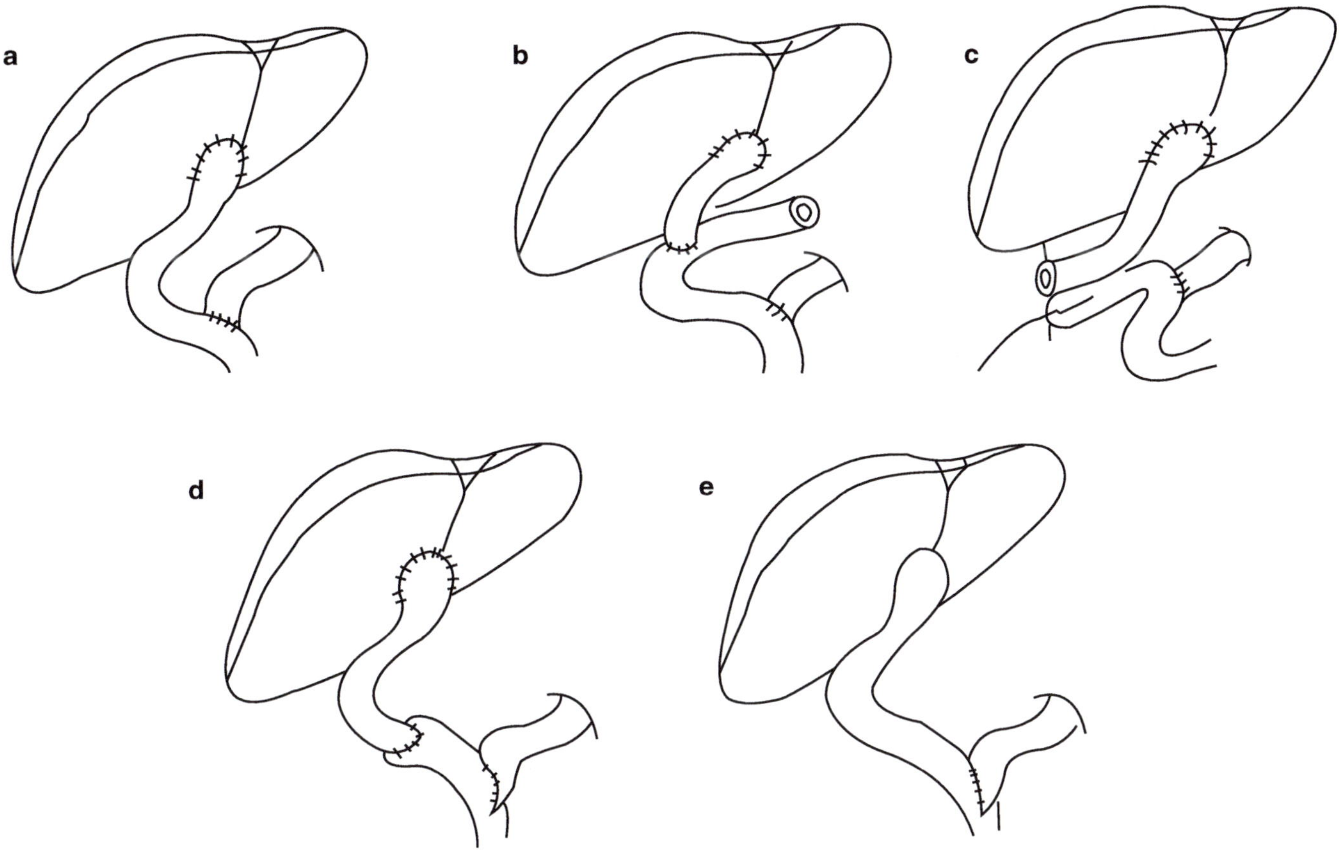


**Fig. 28.1** Modifications of biliary reconstruction. (**A**) Original Kasai (Roux-en Y portoenterostomy); (**B**) Kasai's Double Roux-en Y; (**C**) Suruga II; (**D**) Roux-en Y with intestinal valves (Intussusception and Spur valves); (**E**) Roux-en Y with intestinal valve (Spur valve)

number of cholangitis cases. The disappearance of jaundice was 10/19 (52.6%) in the group with artificial intestinal valve and 9/19 (47.4%) in the group without artificial intestinal valve. There was no significant difference.

Intrahepatic cystic lesion (ICL) is a common complication for biliary atresia post-Kasai portoenterostomy. Patients with ICLs had a high incidence of cholangitis. The prognosis was closely related to the history of cholangitis and the onset time of ICLs. Komuro et al. [18] reviewed their 38 cases of biliary atresia between 1974 and 1999. An intussusception type anti-reflux valve (ARV) was effective in preventing refractory cholangitis without cystic dilatation of intrahepatic bile ducts (CDIB). They suggest that CDIB resulting from the ongoing process of BA could be a potential target of bacterial infection through another route than bilioenteric reflux.

Ogasawara et al. [19], 21 cases of biliary atresia between 1998 and 2001 were non-randomly and prospectively divided into 10 cases with artificial intestinal valve and 11 cases without artificial intestinal valve. As a result, the incidence of cholangitis was 5/10 (50.0%) in the group with artificial intestinal valve and 6/11 (54.5%) in the group without artificial intestinal valve, showing no significant difference between the two groups. The jaundice disappearance rate was 9/10 (90.0%) in the group with artificial intestinal valve and 7/11 (63.6%) in the group without artificial intestinal valve, showing no significant difference between the two groups.

There are two case reports of the harm associated with antireflux surgery. Nichol et al. [20] reported a gallstone ileus formed 20 years after the operation at the intussusceptible valve site, and Ono et al. [21] reported a case of volvulus of the small intestine, which is thought to be caused by an artificial intestinal valve.

The number of facilities is increasing, and the number of reconstruction methods that take Roux-Y legs longer is also increasing. This is considered to be a result of taking into account that part of the Roux-Y leg is excised and shortened when the liver is removed in the case of liver transplantation in the future.

The cause of cholangitis in biliary atresia may be due to a more complex mechanism than simple reflux of enterobacteria.

## 28.6 Can Long-term Intravenous Administration of Antimicrobial Agents Reduce the Incidence of Cholangitis After Surgery?

According to JBAR2018 [12], the incidence of postoperative cholangitis is reported to be 40.4%. Incidence of jaundice and deterioration of liver function is often observed after the onset of cholangitis, but there is no literature that directly states that administration of antibacterial agents reduces the incidence of cholangitis, and the comparative study of antimicrobial administration period was not founded. There is little evidence regarding the type of antibacterial drug and the period of administration regarding prophylactic administration of oral antibacterial drugs.

Regarding the usage of antibacterial drugs, there is a questionnaire survey result on 12 facilities of "Postoperative biliary atresia steroid administration: Multicenter randomized trial working group in Japan" [22]. According to the report, 50% of the facilities receive the first administration of antibacterial drug before and during the operation, and 75% include the facilities that start the administration during the operation. The first antibacterial drug used was 84% of the combination of cephem and aminoglycoside, CMZ was often selected for cephem and AMK for aminoglycoside, and the duration of continuous administration was 1–2 weeks (75%). In 45% of the facilities, the type of antibacterial drug was changed every 1 to 2 weeks on a regular basis and that of infectious disease (suspected). The duration of use of intravenous drug was 36% within 2 weeks and 54% within 3 to 4 weeks, indicating that most institutions completed administration within 4 weeks.

de Vries et al. [23] reported that native liver survival at 4 years postoperatively was 54/127 (43%) with antibiotics and 34/87(39%) without antibiotics, regardless of the type of antibiotics, administration period, and administration method. However, the oral group of prophylactic antibacterial drugs for cholangitis in the postoperative period is included, and it is not clear whether or not the intravenous injection of antibacterial drugs in the early postoperative period contributes to the improvement of the native liver survival rate.

Meyers et al. [24] compared 14 patients in each group with IV steroid + IV antimicrobial agent (8 to 12 weeks) + Ursodeoxycholic acid (UDCA) group and no steroid + IV antimicrobial agent (3 to 4 days) + no UDCA group. The native liver survival rate was significantly high in the group of intravenous steroid + intravenous antimicrobial + UDCA administration (10/14: 1/14). The efficacy of the antibacterial agent alone was not evaluated.

## 28.7 Side Effects of Antimicrobial Administration

Although there are concerns about the emergence of resistant bacteria and the manifestation of fungal infections during the use of antibacterial drugs, there were no literatures evaluating the side effects of antibacterial drugs.

In the questionnaire survey in Japan by Higashimoto et al. [22], 90% of the facilities regularly change the type of antimicrobial agent in consideration of the emergence of resistant bacteria.

Although concerns have been suggested regarding the emergence of resistant bacteria and the manifestation of fungal infections during the use of antibacterial drugs, postoperative cholangitis treatment imposes a heavy burden on patients due to hospitalization.

Recommendation is to administer the antibiotics intravenously for 2 to 4 weeks after surgery, followed by oral antibiotics.

## 28.8 Conclusion

The knowledge on postoperative cholangitis has been increasing in the past 10 years, showing a lower incidence of the disease and better therapeutic results. Cholangitis can cause a poor prognosis for patients who have achieved early jaundice clearance. Therefore, based on these findings, individualized treatment considering risk factors for individual BA patients should be strongly considered to prevent cholangitis, especially early onset, and improve postoperative outcomes.

## References


1. Qiao G, Li L, Cheng W, et al. Conditional probability of survival in patients with biliary atresia after Kasai portoenterostomy: a Chinese population-based study. J Pediatr Surg. 2015;50(8):1310–5.
2. Gunadi GTA, Widiyanto G, et al. Liver transplant score for prediction of biliary atresia patients' survival following Kasai procedure. BMC Res Notes. 2018;11(1):381.
3. Jiang H, Gao PF, Chen HD, et al. The prognostic value of CD8(+) and CD45RO (+) T cells infiltration and Beclin1 expression levels for early postoperative cholangitis of biliary atresia patients after Kasai operation. J Korean Med Sci. 2018;33(30):e198.
4. Koga H, Wada M, Nakamura H, et al. Factors influencing jaundice-free survival with the native liver in post-portoenterostomy biliary atresia patients: results from a single institution. J Pediatr Surg. 2013;48(12):2368–72.
5. Nio M, Wada M, Sasaki H, et al. Risk factors affecting late-presenting liver failure in adult patients with biliary atresia. J Pediatr Surg. 2012;47:2179–83.

6. Muraji T, Tsugawa C, Nishijima E, et al. Surgical management for intractable cholangitis in biliary atresia. J Pediatr Surg. 2002;37:1713–5.
7. Chen SY, Lin CC, Tsan YT, et al. Number of cholangitis episodes as a prognostic marker to predict timing of liver transplantation in biliary atresia patients after Kasai portoenterostomy. BMC Pediatr. 2018;18(1):119.
8. Ernest VHL, Saing H, Tam PK. Cholangitis after hepatic portoenterostomy for biliary atresia: a multivariate analysis of risk factors. J Pediatr. 2003;142(5):566–71.
9. Li D, Wang P, He Y, et al. Intravenous immunoglobulin for the treatment of intractable cholangitis after Kasai portoenterostomy in biliary atresia patients. Pediatr Surg Int. 2018;34(4):399–404.
10. Nakajima H, Koga H, Okawada M, et al. Does time taken to achieve jaundice- clearance influence survival of the native liver in post-Kasai biliary atresia? World J Pediatr. 2018;14(2):191–6.
11. Ohi R, Ibrahim M. Biliary atresia. Semin Pediatr Surg. 1992;1:115–24.
12. Japanese Biliary Atresia Society. Japanese biliary atresia registry 2018. J Jpn Soc Pediatr Surg. 2020;56:219–25. [in Japanese]
13. Nio M, Ohi R, Miyano T, et al. Five-and10-yearsurvivalratesafter surgeryforbiliary atresia: a report from the Japanese biliary atresia registry. J Pediatr Surg. 2003;38:997–1000.
14. Nio M, Wada M, Sasaki H, et al. Technical standardization of Kasai portoenterostomy for biliary atresia. J Pediatr Surg. 2016;51:2105–8.
15. Ando H, Ito T, Nagaya M. Use of external conduit impairs liver function in patients with biliary atresia. J Pediatr Surg. 1996;31:1509–11.
16. Nio M, Sasaki H, Tanaka H, et al. Redo surgery for biliary atresia. Pediatr Surg Int. 2013;29:989–93.
17. Sartorelli KH, Holland RM, Allshouse MJ, et al. The intussusception antireflux valve is ineffective in preventing cholangitis in biliary atresia. J Pediatr Surg. 1996;31(3):403–6.
18. Komuro H, Makino S, Momoya T, et al. Cholangitis associated with cystic dilatation of the intrahepatic bile ducts after antireflux valve construction in biliary atresia. Pediatr Surg Int. 2001;17:108–10.
19. Ogasawara Y, Yamataka A, Tsukamoto K, et al. The intussusception antirefluxvalve is ineffective for preventing cholangitis in biliary atresia: a prospective study. J Pediatr Surg. 2003;38(12):1826–9.
20. Nichol PF, Adzick NS. Gallstone ileus 20 years after a Kasai procedure using a stapled antireflux valve. J Pediatr Surg. 2007;42(1):264–6.
21. Ono S, Nagayasu K, Niwa K, et al. A case of small bowel torsion after biliary atresia operation with intussusception antireflux valve. Nihonfukubukyukyuigakukaizashi. 2011;31(5):807–10. [in Japanese]
22. Higashimoto Y, Saitoh T, Kaneda H, et al. Evidence-based antimicrobial therapy for cholangitis in patients with biliary atresia. Jpn J Pediatr Surg. 2008;40(1):93–101. [in Japanese]
23. de Vries W, de Langen ZJ, Groen H, et al. Biliary atresia in the Netherlands: outcome of patients diagnosed between 1987 and 2008. J Pediatr. 2012;160(4):638–44.
24. Meyers RL, Book LS, O'Gorman MA, et al. High-dose steroids, ursodeoxycholic acid, and chronic intravenous antibiotics improve bile flow after Kasai procedure in infants with biliary atresia. J Pediatr Surg. 2003;38(3):406–11.

# 29 Nutritional Support for Patients with Biliary Atresia

Yuichiro Yamashiro

**Abstract**

Nutritional issues are very common in patients with biliary atresia (BA), from infants to adolescents. Malnutrition is universal in children with BA, even in that post-hepatoportoenterostomy (the Kasai operation), because bile secretion into the intestine may not be sufficient for fat absorption, and the gut microbiota may be aberrant because of the frequent administration of antibiotics, leading to impaired digestibility. Nutritional deficiency or malnutrition includes not only macronutrients such as essential fatty acids, but also fat-soluble vitamins and iron, iodine, zinc, and calcium. Treatment is aimed at reversing the consequences of anorexia, increasing energy needs, and improving associated intestinal malabsorption.

**Keywords**

Biliary atresia · Nutrition · Malnutrition · Bile acids · Fat absorption · Essential fatty acids · Post Kasai operation

## 29.1 Introduction

Nutrition is a prominent and vital part of caring for infants and children. The provision of adequate and balanced nutrition is of greater importance during infancy and childhood. This dynamic phase of life is characterized by rapid growth, development, and developmental plasticity. A sufficient amount and appropriate composition of substrates are of key importance in terms of long-term health and well-being for growth, metabolic programming, and functional outcomes such as cognition and the immune response.

Patients with biliary atresia (BA) suffer from nutritional problems, particularly lipid malabsorption, because of a lack of bile acids in the intestine. However, hepatoportoenterostomy (the Kasai operation) promotes bile secretion into the intestine, resulting in improved absorption, and thereby longer survival rates in recent years. Therefore, nutritional support for patients with BA should take the changing background of treatment results into account.

In this chapter, the fundamental nutritional knowledge required for children's growth and development is first described, followed by nutritional treatment for patients with BA.

### 29.1.1 Characteristics of Nutrition During Childhood

Nutrition exerts a strong regulatory effect during the early stages of life in terms of providing both energy and essential nutrients. Growth is a typical characteristic of childhood and a sensitive indicator of nutritional status. Deviation in growth, especially growth retardation, and excess fat accumulation typical of obesity, are associated with a greater risk of disease in both the short and long run.

#### 29.1.1.1 Nutrition for Infants

##### Milk Feeding

###### Breastfeeding

- Breastfeeding is considered the best choice for infant feeding as it provides optimal nutrition and numerous important non-nutritional benefits for not only the infant, but also the mother. Exclusive or full breastfeeding should be promoted for at least the first 6 months after birth, and exclusive or predominant breastfeeding for approximately 7 months after birth [1, 2].
- Complementary foods (solids and liquids other than breast milk or infant formula) should not be introduced

Y. Yamashiro (✉)
Probiotics Research Laboratory, Juntendo University Graduate School of Medicine, Tokyo, Japan
e-mail: yamasiro@juntendo.ac.jp


M. Nio (ed.), *Introduction to Biliary Atresia*, https://doi.org/10.1007/978-981-16-2160-4_29

within the first 4 months after birth, but should not be delayed beyond 6 months.

- Breastfeeding should be continued by the mother and child for as long as mutually desired and based primarily on considerations other than health outcomes.

#### Supplementation for Breastfed Infants

- Breastfed infants should receive daily vitamin D supplementation regardless of maternal vitamin D status [3].
- Premature and low-birth weight infants, as well as infants with iron deficiency, require early iron supplementation, which can be administered while continuing exclusive breastfeeding [4].
- Vitamin K supplementation is also recommended during the first weeks or months of life to breastfed infants only or all infants [3].

#### Formula Feeding

- Although breastfeeding is the optimal choice for infant feeding, infants who cannot be breastfed (or who should not receive breast milk or for whom breast milk is not available) should receive an infant formula with a composition based on current scientific knowledge.
- Infant formula is required as a substitute for breast milk for infants who are not fully breastfed. Infant formula must satisfy all the nutritional needs of an infant and meet high quality and safety standards. Special infant formulas such as soy protein-based and thickened types should be used according to specific indications [5].

### Complementary Feeding

- Complementary foods (solids and liquids other than breast milk or infant formula) are necessary for both nutritional and developmental reasons and represent an important stage in the transition from milk feeding to family foods.

#### Timing of the Introduction of Complementary Foods

Complementary foods should not be introduced before 5 months after birth, but should not be delayed beyond 7 months [6].

#### Content

- Infants should be offered foods with a variety of flavors and textures, including green vegetables. Continued breastfeeding is recommended alongside complementary foods. Whole cow's milk should not be used as the main drink before 12 months of age (Table 29.1).
- All infants should receive iron-rich complementary foods, including meat products and/or iron-fortified foods. No sugar or salt should be added to complementary foods, and fruit juices or sugar-sweetened beverages should be avoided.
- High protein intake with the consumption of complementary foods may increase the risk of subsequent overweight or obesity, especially in genetically predisposed individuals, and the mean protein-energy ratio should not be >15%. Large volumes of cow's milk are associated with high energy, protein, and fat intake and low iron intake (Table 29.2) [7].
- Long-chain polyunsaturated fatty acids (LCPUFAs), and notably docosahexaenoic acid (DHA), play an important role in brain development. DHA status tends to decline during the complementary foods period, when the intake of breast milk or LCPUFA-supplemented formulas decreases. Therefore, the intake of oily fish (around 10 g/day), DHA, or precursor fatty acids during the complementary foods period may favorably influence DHA status (Table 29.3) [8].

**Table 29.1** Energy requirements of children and adolescents[a]

| Age | Boys | Girls |
|---|---|---|
| 0–5 months | 550 | 500 |
| 6–8 months | 650 | 600 |
| 9–11 months | 700 | 650 |
| 1–2 y | 950 | 900 |
| 3–5 y | 1300 | 1250 |
| 6–7 y | 1550 | 1450 |
| 8–9 y | 1850 | 1700 |
| 10–11 y | 2250 | 2100 |
| 12–14 y | 2600 | 2400 |
| 15–17 y | 2800 | 2300 |

[a]Recommended dietary allowances for Japan, 2020 (Ministry of Health, Labor and Welfare)

**Table 29.2** Protein requirements for infants, children, and adolescents[a]

| Age | Boys | Girls |
|---|---|---|
| 1–2 y | 31–48 | 29–45 |
| 3–5 y | 46–65 | 39–60 |
| 6–7 y | 49–75 | 46–70 |
| 8–9 y | 60–93 | 55–85 |
| 10–11 y | 72–110 | 68–105 |
| 12–14 y | 85–130 | 78–120 |
| 15–17 y | 91–140 | 75–115 |

[a]Recommended dietary allowances for Japan, 2020 (Ministry of Health, Labor and Welfare)

**Table 29.3** LCPUFA requirements for infants, children, and adolescents

| Recommended amounts of $n$–6 LCPUFA | | | Recommended amounts of $n$–3 LCPUFA | | |
|---|---|---|---|---|---|
| Sex | Boys | Girls | Sex | Boys | Girls |
| Age | Target | Target | Age | Target | Target |
| 0–5 months | 4 | 4 | 0–5 months | 0.9 | 0.9 |
| 6–11 months | 4 | 4 | 6–11 months | 0.8 | 0.8 |
| 1–2 y | 4 | 4 | 1–2 y | 0.7 | 0.8 |
| 3–5 y | 6 | 6 | 3–5 y | 1.1 | 1.0 |
| 6–7 y | 8 | 7 | 6–7 y | 1.5 | 1.3 |
| 8–9 y | 8 | 7 | 8–9 y | 1.5 | 1.3 |
| 10–11 y | 10 | 8 | 10–11 y | 1.6 | 1.6 |
| 12–14 y | 11 | 9 | 12–14 y | 1.9 | 1.6 |
| 15–17 y | 13 | 9 | 15–17 y | 2.1 | 1.6 |

**Table 29.4** Examples of adequate amounts of foods to be consumed per day at different ages [10]

| Age, years | 1 | 2–3 | 4–6 | 7–9 | 10–12 |
|---|---|---|---|---|---|
| Total energy, kcal/day | 850 | 950 | 1250 | 1600 | 1900 |
| Recommended foods (90% of total energy) | | | | | |
| Generous | | | | | |
| Beverages, mL/day | 600 | 700 | 800 | 900 | 1000 |
| Vegetables, g/day | 120 | 150 | 200 | 220 | 250 |
| Fruit, g/day | 120 | 150 | 200 | 220 | 250 |
| Potatoes, pasta, rice, etc., g/day | 100 | 120 | 150 | 180 | 220 |
| Moderate | | | | | |
| Milk, milk products, mL or g/day | 300 | 330 | 350 | 400 | 420 |
| Meat, meat products, g/day | 30 | 35 | 40 | 50 | 60 |
| Eggs, n/week | 1–2 | 1–2 | 2 | 2 | 2–3 |
| Fish, g/week | 25 | 35 | 50 | 75 | 90 |
| Sparing | | | | | |
| Oil, butter, margarine, g/day | 15 | 20 | 25 | 30 | 35 |
| Tolerated foods (≤10% of total energy) | | | | | |
| Cake, sweets, jam, sugar, etc., max. Kcal/day | 85 | 95 | 125 | 160 | 190 |

Modified from Alexy et al. [11] according to the most recent dietary reference values

#### Homemade Versus Commercial Complementary Foods

Complementary foods can be homemade or commercially produced. In practice, the relative merits depend on the quality of homemade foods offered.

### 29.1.1.2 Nutrition for Toddlers, Preschoolers, and Schoolchildren

The age range from 1 to approximately 12 years consists of very different phases of development. With increasing motor skills, toddlers—some of whom are still partly breastfed—will eat an increasing variety of foods as part of the family diet. Preschoolers and schoolchildren experience both an increased frequency and variety of social contents outside the home, and thereby, more food and meal choices.

#### Principles of Children's Diets and Eating [9–11]

- Toddlers and schoolchildren participate in family meals.
- Food-based dietary guidelines for children should name basic food groups, give appreciate amounts to be consumed, and provide exemplary recipes according to local habits.
- Nutritional supplements and fortified foods should be used only when indicated, such as in circumstances where nutrient-dense foods are scarce or fortification or supplementation is necessary, particularly with regard to iron, iodine, zinc, and calcium.

#### Examples of Adequate Amounts of Main Foods

- The following main food groups are of high nutrient density: cereals and other starchy foods (e.g., bread, pasta, potatoes), vegetables, fruits and legumes, milk and dairy products, meat, poultry, eggs, oily fish, fats, and oils.
- A list of reference amounts of main food groups, which provide ≥90% of the appropriate energy intake and 100% of practically all micronutrients, is part of an optimal mixed diet (OMD) (Table 29.4) [10].
- The amounts shown in Table 29.4 do not need to be consumed every day; rather, the aim should be to consume an average amount every week.

#### Diet Composition

The OMD shown in Table 29.4 provides about 53% of the energy intake from mostly complex carbohydrates, 33% from fat mostly, of plant origin (saturated fatty acids: 10%; monounsaturated fatty acids: 15%; polyunsaturated fatty acids: 7% of total energy), and 14% from protein. The energy density is about 70 kcal/100 g, fiber density about 17 g/1000 kcal, and water density about 1.2 g/kcal.

#### Preferable Choice of Foods

1. Rice, Bread, Cereals, and Pasta:
   Preferably, these should be whole grain products.
2. Fruits and Vegetables:
   If not served raw, fruits and vegetables should be boiled briefly and in as little water as possible to reduce the loss of vitamins, minerals, and secondary plant substances such as carotenoids, phytosterins, and polyphenols.
3. Vegetables with High Dietary Fiber:
   The intestinal microbiota affects the diet and health of the host, and high-fiber plants containing polysaccharides are particularly important modulators. Dietary

fiber is a source of complex carbohydrates, which are required for the production of short-chain fatty acids (SCFAs) such as acetate, butyrate, and propionate, which are end products of fermentation by the microbiota. SCFAs modulate central metabolism and can signal the host through distinct mechanisms. SCFAs have been implicated as playing diverse roles in obesity and metabolic syndrome [12].

4. Cow's milk and Dairy Products:
   Cow's milk and dairy products are indispensable in children's diets as sources of calcium, vitamins, and other minerals.
5. Meat and Meat Products:
   Meat and meat products are important, particularly for toddlers and young children, because they provide readily available iron and zinc. Moreover, they provide high-quality protein and vitamin B. However, meat products low in fat are preferable.
6. Fish:
   Fish is an important source of long-chain-3 fatty acids (Oily fish is preferable) and iodine and should be eaten at least once a week (Table 29.5).
7. Beverages:
   Sugar-sweetened beverages tend to be overconsumed, which can cause an energy imbalance and overweight.

#### 29.1.1.3 Nutrition for Adolescents [13]

Adolescence (age 10–19 years) is a critical period consisting of remarkable bodily changes, including rapid physical, psychosocial, sexual, and cognitive maturation. Nutrition during this rapid growth period is crucial for ensuring a healthy progression through puberty and final health, bone density, and initiation/continuation of normal menstrual cycles in girls. Hence, nutritional needs are higher in adolescence than at any other time in the life cycle; however, adolescent diets have been found to contain inadequate amounts of calcium, iron, and other essential nutrients.

**Table 29.5** Recommended levels of fish consumption as a source of eicosapentaenoic acid and docosahexaenoic acid

| | |
|---|---|
| High levels of eicosapentaenoic acid and docosahexaenoic acid (>1000 mg per 100 g fish) | Herring (*nishin*) |
| | Mackerel (*saba*) |
| | Salmon (*sake*) |
| | Tuna-bluefin (*maguro*) |
| Medium level (500–1000 mg per 100 g fish) | Flounder (*hirame*) |
| | Tuna-canned white (canned *maguro*, white meat) |
| Low level (300 mg per 100 g fish) | Cod (*tara*) |
| | Catfish (*namazu*) |

### 29.1.2 Nutritional Aspects of Biliary Atresia

Presumably, infants with BA start life with normal nutritional status. However, in the course of BA, a substantial loss of lean body mass can occur because of fat malabsorption. After the Kasai operation, fat malabsorption may gradually improve, depending on whether the postoperative course is smooth or complicated. Most patients with postoperative complications are malnourished because of decreased nutrient intake, which is the result of inhibited bile delivery to the intestine, leading to diminished appetite and fat malabsorption. In addition, children with chronic liver disease show increased energy expenditure, especially when standardized for lean body mass and insufficient energy utilization. As a result, both stunting and wasting are seen. Perturbations in the intake, absorption, and utilization of fuels in patients with BA support the need for nutritional therapy for such children.

## 29.2 Nutritional Assessment

Nutritional assessment of children with BA is critical to health management. Nutritional status is the one prognostic variable that may be amenable to intervention (e.g., liver transplantation). Analyzing growth curves permits the assessment of the degree and duration of growth impairment, which can be a sign of liver failure in patients with BA. Physical examinations allow for a gross assessment of nutritional status, including specific evidence of nutrient deficiency.

| Condition | Nutrient deficiency |
|---|---|
| Areflexia & poor proprioception | Vitamin E |
| Rickets | Vitamin D |
| Xerophthalmia & visual disturbances | Vitamin A |
| Bruising & petechiae (coagulopathy) | Vitamin K |
| Delayed cognitive development | EFA deficiency |

*EFA* Essential fatty acids (e.g., DHA)

## 29.3 Therapy

Malnutrition is universal in children who receive antibiotic therapy after the Kasai operation who develop multiple ascending cholangitis and aberrant gut microbiota (dysbiosis) [14], leading to impaired digestibility. In children who receive antibiotic therapy during the Kasai operation, dysbiosis is inevitable and may affect bile acid metabolism [15]. Therefore, the combined influence of dysbiosis and altered bile acid metabolism may negatively affect fat absorption

**Table 29.6** Nutritional therapy for children with biliary atresia

| | |
|---|---|
| 1. Prevention of or treatment for fat and protein-calorie malnutrition | |
| 2. Vitamin supplementation to prevent deficiency | |
| 3. Improvement in growth and development | |
| Practical points: | |
| 1. Energy: 150% of predicted RDAs[a] based on age and weight | |
| 2. Protein 2–3 g/kg/day | |
| 3. Enteral route preferable | |
| 4. Vitamins (PO doses) | |
| Vitamin A | 3000–10,000 IU/day |
| Vitamin D (25(OH)D) | 400–4000 IU/day |
| Vitamin E (TPGS) | 25 IU/kg/day |
| Vitamin K | 2.5–5 mg/day |

[a]See Table 29.4

postoperatively, although bile secretion improves. Nutritional therapy for children with BA has multiple goals (Table 29.6), and practical dietary therapy is described as follows.

### 29.3.1 Infants

#### 29.3.1.1 Breastfeeding

Breastfeeding should be continued until at least 6 months of age in infants with BA. As breast milk lipase contributes to the improved fat digestibility of human milk, breastfeeding confers benefits to infants with BA.

#### 29.3.1.2 Formula Feeding

Infants who cannot be breastfed for various reasons should be fed formula that satisfies all of their nutritional needs and provides a high intake per kilogram of body weight during this very sensitive period of life.

For infants with BA, whose bile secretion is not sufficient for fat absorption, human milk (from a donor or human milk bank), formulas for preterm infants, or formulas fortified with medium-chain triglyceride (MCT) oil should be supplemented. MCT oil does not require lipolysis or micelles for absorption, but may provide inadequate amounts of essential fatty acids in the case of fat malabsorption.

#### 29.3.1.3 Complementary Foods

Complementary foods provide adequate energy density (minimum 25% fat) and are a good source of protein, iron, and zinc. The European Society for Pediatric Gastroenterology Hepatology and Nutrition Committee on Nutrition recommends that complementary foods should be started by 26 weeks of age [6], by which time the intestinal digestive function has developed sufficiently to be able to accept complementary foods such as rice porridge. Although infants with BA may be hospitalized for postoperative management, complementary foods should be started at around 6 months of age because the second part of the first year of life is the optimal time to acquire masticatory capacity.

For infants in whom bile secretion is impaired, fat-rich animal meats, pork, and beef, which contain high amounts of saturated fatty acids, are poorly absorbed with lower bile acid contents; however, $n - 3$ polyunsaturated fatty acids (PUFAs) such as α-linolenic acid, eicosapentaenoic acid, and DHA, have marginal amounts. Therefore, as shown in Table 29.5, fish products are highly recommended. In addition, red animal meats are good sources of protein and iron. Corn and safflower oils contain large amounts of α-linoleic acid, an $n$–6 PUFA, and are preferred for use in cooking. Soybean oil contains α-linolenic acid and soybeans provide high-quality protein; in addition, tofu is a good food for infants and children with BA. *Natto*, a fermented soybean product, contains vitamin K, a necessary nutrient for such patients as well. Follow-up formula, which contains large amounts of iron, is highly recommended to be introduced to infants at no later than 9 months of age.

### 29.3.2 Toddlers, Preschoolers, and Schoolchildren

Toddlers require more frequent meals than older children. As toddlers with BA tend to have a suppressed appetite, fortification or supplementation becomes necessary, particularly in regard to iron, iodine, zinc, and calcium. Low-sodium varieties of processed foods should be chosen for this purpose. Meat and meat products are indispensable sources of protein, iron, zinc, and B vitamins in all children's diets; however, low-fat products are preferred. Fish is an important source of iodine and $n$–3 LCPUFAs, as described above. Cow's milk and dairy products are very important sources of vitamins, calcium, and other minerals in all children's diets. Appropriate amounts of exposure to sunlight increase vitamin D synthesis. Plants are rich sources of folate and vitamins C, E, and K, so children should be encouraged to consume whole grains, fruits, and green, orange, and yellow vegetables, which are good sources of dietary fiber that produce SCFAs through gut microbiota fermentation. Protein-energy malnutrition leads to decreased insulin-like growth factor 1 synthesis, resulting in muscle wasting and motor developmental delay. To compensate for increased energy needs and anorexia, supplemental nasogastric tube feeding may be helpful. By contrast, schoolchildren can consume school meals without limitations because they tend to enjoy having meals with classmates.

### 29.3.3 Adolescents

Nutritional interventions for adolescents with BA need to be tailored to the hepatic dysfunctional status of each patient.

## 29.4 Conclusion

Nutrition is of particular importance in candidates for potential liver transplantation because malnutrition is the one prognostic variable that may be amenable to interventions [16]. Malnourished patients are associated with increased mortality and morbidity after liver transplantation [17], and the overall benefits of careful nutritional management of patients after the Kasai operation have been reported [18].

Health care professionals who manage the health of patients with BA in accordance with these contents could be expected to contribute to further improvements in nutritional care standards for infants and children with BA.

## References


1. ESPGHAN Committee on Nutrition, Agostoni C, Braegger C, Decsi T, Kolacek S, Koletzko B, et al. Breast-feeding: a commentary by the ESPGHAN Committee on Nutrition. J Pediatr Gastroenterol Nutr. 2009;49:112–25.
2. Section on Breastfeeding. Breastfeeding and the use of human milk. Pediatrics. 2012;129:e827–41.
3. Lo CW. Human milk: nutritional properties. In: Walker WA, Watkins JB, editors. Nutrition in pediatrics. Ontario: B.C. Decker; 1996. p. 436–48.
4. Ziegler EE. Preterm and low-birth-weight infants. In: Koletzko B, et al., editors. Pediatric nutrition in practice. World Rev Nutr Diet, vol. 113. Basel: Karger; 2015. p. 92–6.
5. Codex Alimentation Commission: Standard for infant formula for special medical purposes intended for Codex Alimentarius Commission. 2007;1–21.
6. Agostoni C, Decsi T, Fewtrell M, Goulet O, Kolacek S, Koletzko B, et al. Complementary feeding: a commentary by the ESPGHAN committee on nutrition. J Pediatr Gastroenterol Nutr. 2008;46:99–110.
7. Michaelsen KM, Larnkjaer A, Molgaard C. Early diet, insulin-like growth factor-1, growth and later obesity. Shamir R, et al., editors. Nutrition and growth. World Rev Nutr Diet. Basel, Karger 2013;106:113–118.
8. Krohn K, Demmelmair H, Koletzko B. Macronutrient requirements for growth: fats and fatty acids. In: Duggan C, Watkins JB, Koletzko B, Walker WA, editors. Nutrition in pediatrics. 5th ed. Raleigh, NC: People's Medical Publishing House; 2016.
9. Fewtrell M, Bronsky J, Campoy C, Domellöf M, Embleton N, Fidler Mis N, et al. Complementary feeding: a position paper by the European Society for Pediatric Gastroenterology, Hepatology, and Nutrition (ESPGHAN) committee on nutrition. J Pediatr Gastroenterol Nutr. 2017;64:119–32.
10. Przyrembel H. Toddlers, preschool and school children. In: Koletzko B, et al., editors. Pediatric nutrition in practice. World Rev Nutr Diet. Basel: Karger 2015;118–121.
11. Alexy U, Clausen K, Kersting M. Nutrition of healthy children and adolescents according to the optimized mixed diet concept. Ernährungsumschau. 2008;3:169–77.
12. Yamashiro Y, Nagpal R, Nagata S. Metabolic disease: obesity, malnutrition, and intestinal microbiota. J Pediatr Biochem. 2015;5:65–70.
13. Salam RA, Butta AZ. Adolescent nutrition. In: Koletzko B, et al., editors. Pediatric nutrition in practice. World Rev Nutr Diet. Basel: Karger 2015;122–126.
14. Penders J, Thijs C, Vink C, et al. Factors influencing the composition of the intestinal microbiota in early infancy. Pediatrics. 2006;118:511–21.
15. Ridlon JM, Harris SC, Bhowmik S, Kang DJ, Hylemon PB. Consequences of bile salt biotransformations by intestinal bacteria. Gut Microbes. 2016;7:22–39.
16. Porayko MK, DiCecco S, O'Keefe SJ. Impact of malnutrition and its therapy on liver transplantation. Semin Liver Dis. 1991;11:305–14.
17. Moukarzel AA, Najm I, Vargas J, McDiarmid SV, Busuttil RW, Ament ME. Effect of nutritional status on outcome of orthotopic liver transplantation in pediatric patients. Transplant Proc. 1990;22(4):1560–3.
18. Kelly DA, Davenport M. Current management of biliary atresia. Arch Dis Child. 2007;92:1132–5.

# Protocols of Follow-up Management

# 30

Tatsuro Tajiri and Taizo Furukawa


**Abstract**

Biliary atresia is an intractable disease whose details have yet to be elucidated. Kasai's portoenterostomy (KPE) has been recommended to be performed within 60 days to improve jaundice. After KPE, the rate of jaundice disappearance is said to be 60%–70%. Liver transplantation is required if jaundice does not disappear. Even if jaundice disappears, cholangitis may cause jaundice to recur, and liver fibrosis may progress, necessitating liver transplantation. Cholangitis is common one to two years after surgery. Even if jaundice disappears once, jaundice may relapse, often within one year after surgery. Therefore, it is necessary to perform follow-up with a detailed schedule in the early postoperative period and to monitor the presence of progression of cirrhosis or growth disorders thereafter. We herein report the physical findings, blood test results, and imaging test results for follow-up after KPE. Furthermore, our included figures show how to proceed with examinations according to the clinical course after KPE.



**Keywords**

Biliary atresia · Jaundice-free · Liver cirrhosis · Varix · Hepatopulmonary shunt · Pulmonary hypertension · Liver transplantation


## 30.1 Physical Findings

After KPE, it is important to determine whether or not biliary atresia (BA) patients have a growth disorder, so the height and weight should be measured at the time of the examination. Portal hypertension due to cirrhosis causes the spleen to become stagnant and palpable for splenomegaly, so at the outpatient visit, the attending physician should always check the child for splenomegaly. Postoperative steroids may cause growth disorders in BA children, and growth disorder may occur due to liver dysfunction caused by BA. Liver transplantation may improve growth disorders [1]. However, the long-term administration of steroids after liver transplantation is reportedly a risk factor for growth disorders [2].

## 30.2 Blood Tests

### 30.2.1 Aspartate Transaminase (AST) and Alanine Aminotransferase (ALT)

AST and ALT are enzymes produced by hepatocytes. When the liver is damaged due to liver disorder, these values increase because the amount of blood flowing increases. Since AST is contained in myocardium, skeletal muscle, and blood, it can be increased for reasons other than liver disorder. Since ALT is mainly present in the liver, it increases under conditions of liver injury. These values are elevated in almost all BA children [3] and often exceed 100 U/L in the poor prognosis group after KPE. According to a report delivered to the Japanese Biliary Atresia Society (JBAS) 2018, BA patients with a native liver survival of 25 years had an average ALT of <40 U/L. About half of long-term survivors reportedly have abnormal AST levels [4].

### 30.2.2 Gamma-Glutamyltransferase (GGT)

GGT is a protein-degrading enzyme secreted by the liver and is elevated in blood levels in biliary tract diseases. In BA, GGT is often higher in the poor prognosis group than in patients with a relatively good prognosis and is an important marker to monitor after KPE. When GGT is ≥550 IU/L at 5 months after KPE, the prognosis is reportedly poor, even in jaundice-free (JF) cases [5]. Koga et al. also reported that the


T. Tajiri (✉) · T. Furukawa
Department of Pediatric Surgery, Kyoto Prefectural University of Medicine, Kyoto, Japan
e-mail: taji@koto.kpu-m.ac.jp




M. Nio (ed.), *Introduction to Biliary Atresia*, https://doi.org/10.1007/978-981-16-2160-4_30

GGT was extremely low in patients with a native liver survival who were JF [6]. A high GGT value is also reported to be a risk factor for cholangitis after KPE [7].

### 30.2.3 Albumin

Albumin (ALB) accounts for about 67% of the total protein. It is synthesized only in hepatocytes. When the liver function deteriorates, the ability to synthesize ALB decreases, and the value in blood decreases as well. Generally, ALB decreases as cirrhosis progresses, and hypoalbuminemia is a cause of ascites. The prognosis of children with BA who have ALB <3.5 g/dl is reportedly poor, even if they are JF [8, 9]. ALB is also a marker of the Child Pugh classification, PELD, and BALF score [10].

### 30.2.4 Cholinesterase

Cholinesterase (ChE) is an enzyme that decomposes choline esters into choline and organic acids. ChE is a protein produced by hepatocytes, has a shorter half-life in blood than ALB, and is an indicator of sensitive protein synthesis in the liver. Low ChE levels are caused by a decreased liver function and malnutrition, and levels are low in cases of hepatitis, cirrhosis, severe infections, wasting diseases, and malignant tumors. It can reportedly be used to evaluate the liver function after KPE in children with BA [11]. BA patients with a good prognosis often have ChE values of around 400 U/L. When the ChE value is <200 U/L, liver transplantation is typically necessary.

### 30.2.5 Total Bilirubin

It has been reported that the native liver survival rate is higher when jaundice disappears within 60 days after KPE [6]. Liver transplantation is said to be a smarter choice than redo KPE when jaundice does not ameliorate after KPE. According to the 2018 Japanese guidelines (Japanese), redo should be performed when jaundice is exacerbated again after temporarily disappearing following the first KPE procedure. Re-exacerbation of jaundice is often noted a few months after the first KPE procedure and should be carefully monitored within the first year after surgery. In addition, even if Total bilirubin (T-bil) levels are within the normal range, gastrointestinal bleeding and hepatopulmonary shunt may make the native liver survival impossible. There is also a report that if the T-bil value at 16 years old is ≥21 μmol/L (approximately 1.23 mg/dl), patients will require liver transplantation in the future [12].

### 30.2.6 Bile Acid

Bile acid is synthesized by cholesterol in the liver and excreted in the bile juice. However, most of it is absorbed and returns to the liver via the portal circulation. It is said that more than 99% of bile acid exists in the intestinal circulation. Therefore, normally, the concentration of bile acid in peripheral blood is extremely small. If the secretion of bile acid into the bile canaliculi is impaired, the blood concentration increases [13]. Bile acid is more sensitive than bilirubin and AST/ALT. Even when jaundice disappears, the total level of bile acid may be high. Bile acid levels are often low in patients with a good prognosis.

### 30.2.7 Ca/Vitamin D

Vitamin D is a fat-soluble hormone that is poorly absorbed from the intestinal tract when there is little biliary excretion. After KPE, vitamin D levels may be low during the first year after KP, even after supplementation. In particular, vitamin D levels were found to be low in patients with jaundice after KPE [14]. There are also reports of cases of fracture before and one month after KPE [15]. Even if jaundice disappears, rickets may occur, so supplementation and monitoring of vitamin D are necessary, even after KPE.

### 30.2.8 C-reactive Protein

C-reactive protein (CRP) is a protein synthesized in the liver. When an immune response to any tissue damage, such as infection, occurs, the synthesis of CRP in the liver is promoted, and the plasma concentration is increased. In BA, the CRP level increases when postoperative cholangitis occurs. This is a criterion for diagnosing cholangitis [7]. When inflammation occurs, the CRP level increases with a delay of about one day, as CRP often does not increase on the first day of a fever.

### 30.2.9 Blood Urea Nitrogen

BUN is a waste product produced by the decomposition of proteins in the body. When gastrointestinal bleeding occurs, proteins contained in the secreted blood are decomposed in the intestine to produce ammonia, resulting in an increase in BUN. When gastrointestinal bleeding is small, the BUN may increase before melena is observed. If it is difficult to determine whether or not black stool is melena, the presence or absence of an elevated BUN level may be a good criterion.

### 30.2.10 White Blood Cells

When cholangitis occurs, the white blood cell (WBC) count increases. Bacterial infection causes the production of more neutrophils than lymphocytes, so the count can be used to judge when cholangitis has occurred. The WBC count tends to be >12000 or <4000/μl under conditions of cholangitis [16].

In addition, the WBC is decreased when portal hypertension and pancytopenia progress. There are also reports that a leukocyte count $<4.0 \times 10^9$/L is a diagnostic criterion for hypersplenism [17].

### 30.2.11 Platelets

After KPE, portal hypertension may progress, resulting in splenomegaly. Splenomegaly may occur even when jaundice disappears. Under conditions of splenomegaly, the number of Platelets (Plts) is decreased. In BA patients, a Plt count of $<100 \times 10^9$/L is reportedly a risk factor for variceal hemorrhaging [18]. The Plt count is used as a prognostic marker for BA, including through the Varices Prediction Rule (VPR) and Aspartate Aminotransferase-to-Plt Ratio index (APRI) [19].

### 30.2.12 Prothrombin Time-International Normalized Ratio (PT-INR)

PT is an indicator of blood coagulation factors and the PT-INR is the ratio of the patient's measured PT value to the control value of the laboratory. This ratio is assessed to determine the ability to synthesize vitamin K-dependent coagulation factors. Since coagulation factors are synthesized in the liver, when the liver function declines, the levels of coagulation factors decrease, and the PT-INR is prolonged. The PT-INR is a marker of the Child-Pugh classification [20], which is an index of liver severity. It is also a marker used to determine the PELD, which is used to assess the severity of liver transplant registration patients [21].

### 30.2.13 Aspartate Aminotransferase-to-Plt Ratio Index

The APRI is an index created to evaluate liver fibrosis in patients with hepatitis C [22] and has also been reported useful as an index for evaluating the severity of liver fibrosis in BA patients [23, 24]. Colechhia et al. reported that an APRI of ≥0.96 can predict esophageal varices in BA patients ≥12 years old [25].

### 30.2.14 Biliary Atresia Liver Fibrosis Score

The Biliary Atresia Liver Fibrosis (BALF) score is a liver fibrosis score used for BA patients ≥1-year old [26], while the iBALF is used for patients <1-year old [27]. None of nine previously reported patients with an iBALF score >6 survived with their native liver [27].

## 30.3 Imaging studies

### 30.3.1 Ultrasonography

Ultrasonography is a noninvasive examination that should be performed at each outpatient examination. The presence or absence of ascites, degree of hepatomegaly or atrophy, and size of the bile lake and spleen can be evaluated using ultrasonography. In adult patients with BA, the presence or absence of neoplastic lesions should also be examined.

On ultrasonography, enlargement of the hepatic artery diameter is associated with early liver transplantation [28]. Recently, the evaluation of liver fibrosis by elastography has been performed in children with BA, and liver and spleen stiffness on elastography are reportedly associated with a risk of esophageal varices after KPE [29, 30]. There is also a report that the liver stiffness measurement at three months after KPE can predict the prognosis [31].

### 30.3.2 Computed Tomography

Contrast-enhanced abdominal computed tomography (CT) is useful for the evaluation of portal hypertension in BA patients, but it is accompanied by radiation exposure. Recently, the introduction of multidetector CT (MDCT) has made it possible to conduct observations from multiple directions, making it easier to understand the three-dimensional structure. The imaging time is thus shortened with MDCT, rendering this modality suitable for observing the biliary tract of children. In children with BA, MDCT allows for the detailed observation of the intrahepatic bile duct and collateral circulation [32]. The attending physician should perform imaging examinations while keeping the radiation exposure as low as reasonably achievable (ALARA).

### 30.3.3 Magnetic Resonance Imaging

Magnetic resonance imaging (MRI) is a noninvasive examination without any radiation exposure. The extent and degree of liver fibrosis can be observed in detail. MRI can also evaluate the intrahepatic bile lake that is one of causes cholangitis. MRI is reportedly useful for the morphological evaluation of the liver after KPE [33]. In cases with long-term native liver survival, hypovascular tumors without elevated α-fetoprotein (AFP) levels may be observed, so MRI is useful for the diagnosis [34].

### 30.3.4 Gastrointestinal Endoscopy

In children with BA, portal hypertension may cause esophageal varices. Children with postoperative KPE who have a low Plt count should be regularly examined with gastrointestinal (GI) endoscopy for esophageal varices. When varices are found, they should be observed regularly in order to determine the timing of endoscopic sclerotherapy. Prophylactic endoscopic sclerotherapy for esophageal varices can reportedly lead to better liver transplantation [35]. In cases of failed the first KPE, endoscopy should be performed by the age of six months [36].

### 30.3.5 Technetium 99m-DTPA Galactosyl Human Serum Albumin ($^{99m}$Tc-GSA) Liver Scintigraphy

$^{99m}$Tc-GSA selectively binds to the asialoglycoprotein (ASGP) receptors on hepatocytes [37], and liver scintigraphy using $^{99m}$Tc-GSA can directly and quantitatively measure the hepatic function. Ishii et al. reported that it is also useful for evaluating liver function in children with BA [38]. H/L15 was shown to be correlated with the serum ALB and ChE levels [34]. Nio et al. recommend that even JF patients be monitored regularly using this liver scintigraphy approach [39].

### 30.3.6 $^{99m}$Tc-Labeled Macroaggregated Albumin ($^{99mTc}$-MAA) Scintigraphy

Hepatopulmonary syndrome (HPS) is said to be caused by the expansion of blood vessels in the lungs, although the cause is not well understood. However, it is an indication for liver transplantation. HPS is diagnosed by $^{99m}$Tc-MAA scintigraphy when the shunt rate is ≥10% [40]. There has been a report of a child with BA who developed HPS at 1-year old [40]. Symptoms include dyspnea and shortness of breath. If portal hypertension is advanced, lung perfusion scintigraphy should be conducted annually.

### 30.3.7 Echocardiography

A late complication of BA children is pulmonary hypertension [41], defined as a mean pulmonary arterial pressure of ≥25 mmHg. However, cardiac catheterization is required for the measurement, which is invasive, especially in children. While an accurate diagnosis requires a catheter examination, the pressure can be predicted via echocardiography, as this modality shows right atrium and ventricle enlargement as well as the right ventricular wall thickness. It is a noninvasive test and should be performed regularly in BA patients with advanced portal hypertension, similarly to $^{99mTc}$-MAA scintigraphy for the evaluation of HPS. It can cause sudden death in long-term survivors among children with BA [40]. The average age of the onset of pulmonary hypertension was reported to be 15-years old among children with poor findings after KPE [40].

## 30.4 Protocols Concerning Follow-Up Management

Children with BA require close follow-up after KPE. In BA, jaundice may not decrease even after KPE, and even if it does disappear, cirrhosis may progress, and the continued native liver survival may be difficult. However, with the advent of liver transplantation, the survival rate of BA patients has markedly improved.

It is important for pediatric surgeons to determine the appropriate timing for liver transplantation for children with BA when liver cirrhosis progresses. However, according to the JBAS 2018, about 40% of BA children survive for more than 25 years with their native liver, so pediatric surgeons need to follow them for a long time. Regarding the follow-up, even if jaundice disappears after KPE, it may rise again within a year after the procedure, so follow-up should be conducted carefully. It is therefore desirable to conduct follow-up once a month until one year after KPE.

Postoperative cholangitis is common up to 1-year old. At one year after KPE, the follow-up interval maybe every two to three months, and school-age children may be followed every three to four months. According to The Canadian Biliary Atresia Registry's report, the first outpatient visit after discharge is from one week to one month later and then from one month to half a year later after that, depending on the patient's condition. Blood samples should be collected at every outpatient visit or every three to four months. Ultrasonography was reportedly performed in more than half of the cases [42].

In children with BA, cholangitis is the most common complication after KPE, and an intravenous infusion of antibiotics should be administered as soon as possible in such cases, as the liver is damaged each time cholangitis occurs. Oral antibiotics were reportedly effective for about one and a half years to prevent postoperative cholangitis [43]. Bile lake is a cause of repeated cholangitis, so in such cases, ultrasonography should be performed to check for the presence of a bile lake in detail.

Treating esophageal varices in children with BA is better for liver transplantation [35]. Therefore, GI endoscopy should be conducted regularly if portal hypertension is observed. In adulthood, follow-up about twice a year is suitable for patients with a good clinical course, but the interval should be shortened for cases with portal hypertension. In children with BA and portal hypertension, GI endoscopy should also be performed every six months. In addition, lung perfusion scintigraphy and echocardiography should be performed once a year in order not to miss detecting hepatopulmonary shunt and pulmonary hypertension. In patients with advanced portal hypertension, it is important to consult a transplant surgeon early in order to avoid missing the timing of liver transplantation.

Some women with a long-term native liver survival have been able to give birth. However, in one case, liver failure reportedly occurred about one year after delivery and necessitated liver transplantation [44]. Therefore, it is necessary to pay close attention to female patients with a native liver survival during the perinatal period. In rare cases of a native liver survival, biliary tract cancer or liver cancer may develop, underscoring the need to regularly evaluate tumor markers (CEA, CA19-9, AFP, etc.) and conduct imaging studies into adulthood [45, 46].

Figure 30.1 shows the flow chart of the examination according to the clinical course after KPE. If jaundice disappears early after KPE, only blood sampling and ultrasonography need to be subsequently conducted. However, if jaundice does not disappear, preparations for liver transplantation should be made. If jaundice does not disappear after the first KPE procedure, patients often undergo liver transplantation before the formation of a hepatopulmonary shunt. Attending physicians should pay attention to the formation of esophageal varices in children with BA.

Even in cases of jaundice disappearance, jaundice can rarely but occasionally relapse within a few months after the first KPE procedure. The attending physician should therefore discuss with the family whether or not to perform a redo procedure or liver transplantation. If jaundice does not ameliorate after the redo procedure, liver transplantation should be performed.

Pediatric surgeons should avoid performing KPE many times. Even if jaundice disappears, cirrhosis may progress. When the degree of liver cirrhosis is mild, the native liver may continue to survive, but GI endoscopy should be performed regularly to investigate esophageal varices. After adolescence, lung perfusion scintigraphy and echocardiography should be performed to check for hepatopulmonary shunt and

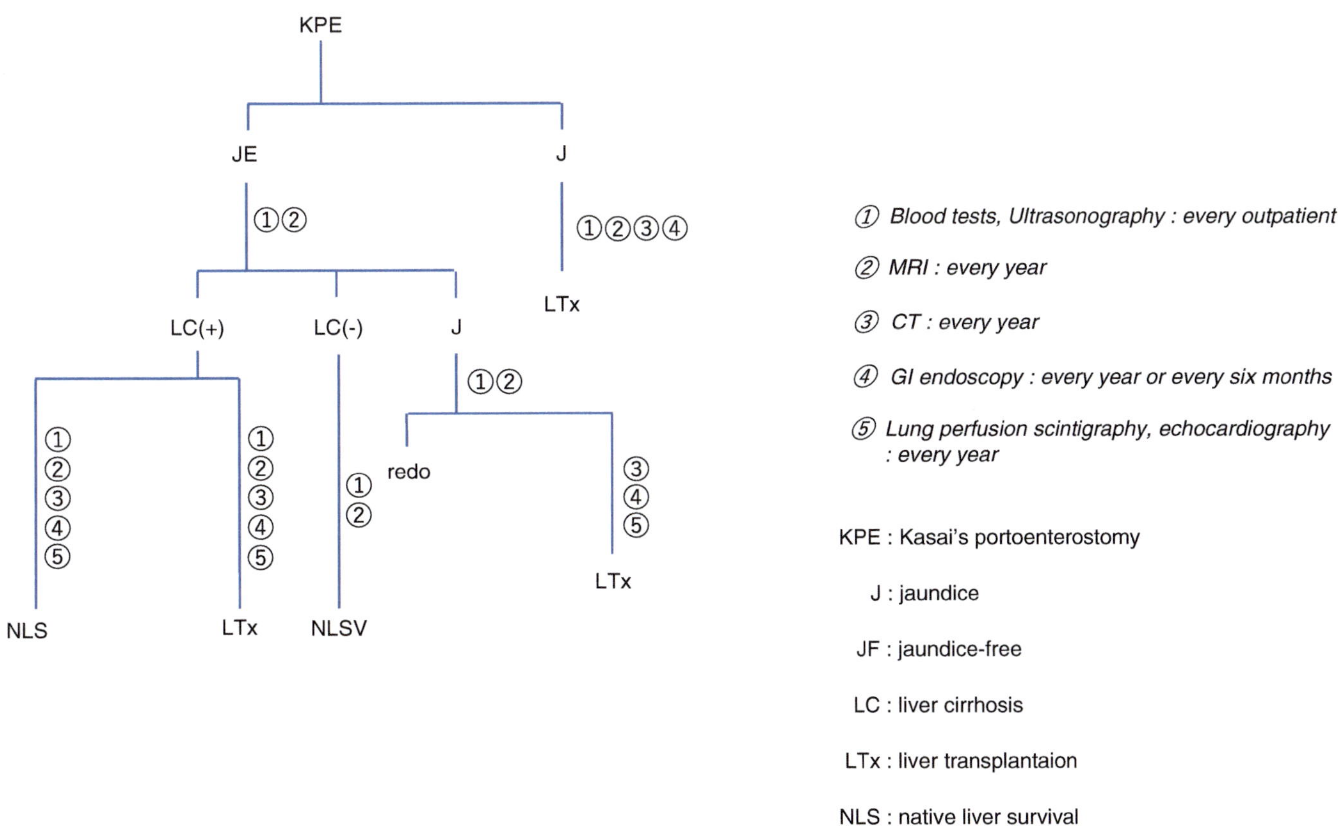


**Fig. 30.1** Follow-up after redo surgery is the same as that after the first KPE, but redo surgery is limited to once

pulmonary hypertension. Even in cases with a long-term native liver survival, liver cirrhosis may worsen, and in such cases, liver transplantation is necessary, as the native liver survival becomes difficult. At that point, lung perfusion scintigraphy and echocardiography should be performed to check for hepatopulmonary shunt and pulmonary hypertension.

## References


1. Alonso G, Duca P, Pasqualini T, et al. Evaluation of catch-up growth after liver transplantation in children with biliary atresia. Pediatr Transplant. 2004;8:255–9.
2. Saito T, Mizuta K, Hishikawa S, et al. Growth curves of pediatric patients with biliary atresia following living donor liver transplantation: factors that influence post-transplantation growth. Pediatr Transplant. 2007;11:764–70.
3. Goda T, Kawahara H, Kubota A, et al. The most reliable early predictors of outcome in patients with biliary atresia after Kasai's operation. J Pediatr Surg. 2013;48:2373–7.
4. Shinkai M, Ohhama Y, Take H, et al. Long-term outcome of children with biliary atresia who were not transplanted after the Kasai Operation: >20-year experience at a children's hospital. J Pediatr Gastroenterol Nutr. 2009;48:443–50.
5. Ihn K, Ho IG, Chang EY, Han SJ. Correlation between gamma-glutamyl transpeptidase activity and outcomes after Kasai portoenterostomy for biliary atresia. J Pediatr Surg. 2018;53:461–7.
6. Koga H, Wada M, Nakamura H, et al. Factors influencing jaundice-free survival with the native liver in post-portoenterostomy biliary atresia patients: results from a single institution. J Pediatr Surg. 2013;48:2368–72.
7. Liu J, Dong R, Chen G, et al. Risk factors and prognostic effects of cholangitis after asai procedure in biliary atresia patients: a retrospective clinical study. J Pediatr Surg. 2019;54:2559–64.
8. Nightingale S, Stormon MO, O'Loughlin EV, et al. Early posthepatoportoenterostomy predictors of native liver survival in biliary atresia. J Pediatr Gastroenterol Nutr. 2017;64:203–9.
9. Ramos-Gonzalez G, Elisofon S, Dee EC, et al. Predictors of need for liver transplantation in children undergoing hepatoportoenterostomy for biliary atresia. J Pediatr Surg. 2019;54:1127–31.
10. Tomita H, Masugi Y, Hoshino K, et al. Long-term native liver fibrosis in biliary atresia: development of a novel scoring system using histology and standard liver tests. J Hepatol. 2014;60:1242–8.
11. Popovic L, Batinica S, Mestrovic T, et al. The value of cholinesterase activity after Kasai operation. Pediatr Surg Int. 2003;19:605–7.
12. Jain V, Burford C, Alexander EC, et al. Prognostic markers at adolescence in patients requiring liver transplantation for biliary atresia in adulthood. J Hepatol. 2019;71:71–7.
13. Fukuoka T, Bessho K, Tachibana M, et al. Total bile acid concentration in duodenal fluid is a useful preoperative screening marker to rule out biliary atresia. J Pediatr Gastroenterol Nutr. 2018;67:383–7.
14. Ng J, Paul A, Wright N, Hadzic N, Daveport M. Vitamin D levels in infants with biliary atresia: pre- and post-Kasai portoenterostomy. J Pediatr Gastroenterol Nutr. 2016;62:746–50.
15. Okada T, Honda S, Miyagi H, et al. Hepatic osteodystrophy complicated with bone fracture in early infants with biliary atresia. World J Hepatol. 2012;4:284–7.
16. Wu ET, Chen HL, Ni YH, et al. Bacterial cholangitis in patients with biliary atresia: impact on short-term outcome. Pediatr Surg Int. 2001;17:390–5.
17. Lee WS, Ong SY, Foo HW, et al. Chronic liver disease is universal in children with biliary atresia living with native liver. World J Gastroenterol. 2017;23:7776–84.
18. Chiou FK, Ong C, Low Y, et al. Non-invasive predictors for the first variceal hemorrhage in children with biliary atresia after Kasai portoenterostomy. J Clin Exp Hepatol. 2019;9:581–7.
19. Isted A, Grammatikopoulos T, Davenport M. Prediction of esophageal varices in biliary atresia: derivation of the "varices prediction rule", a novel noninvasive predictor. J Pediatr Surg. 2015;50:1734–8.
20. Peng Y, Qi X, Gup X. Child–pugh versus MELD score for the assessment of prognosis in liver cirrhosis. Medicine. 2016;95:e2877. https://doi.org/10.1097/MD0000000000002877.
21. Wiensner RH, McDiarmid SV, Kamath PS, et al. MELD and PELD: application of survival models to liver allocation. Liver Transpl. 2001;7:567–80.
22. Wai CT, Greeson JK, Fontana RJ, et al. A simple noninvasive index can predict both significant fibrosis and cirrhosis in patients with chronic hepatitis C. Hepatology. 2003;38:518–26.
23. Grieve A, Makin E, Davenport M. Aspartate Aminotransferase-to-Platelet Ratio index (APRi) in infants with biliary atresia: Prognostic value at presentation. J Pediatr Surg. 2013;48:789–95.
24. Kim SY, Seok JY, Han SJ, et al. Assessment of liver fibrosis and cirrhosis by Aspartate Aminotransferase-to-Platelet Ratio Index in children with biliary atresia. J Pediatr Gastroenterol Nutr. 2010;51:198–202.
25. Colecchia A, Di Biase AR, Scaioloi E, et al. Non-invasive methods can predict oesophageal varices in patients with biliary atresia after a Kasai procedure. Dig Liver Dis. 2011;43:659–63.
26. Tomita H, Masugi Y, Hoshino K, et al. Long-term native liver fibrosis in biliary atresia: development of a novel scoring system using histology and standard liver tests. J Hepatol. 2014;60:1242–8.
27. Tomita H, Fuchimoto Y, Fujino A, et al. Development and validation of a novel fibrosis marker in biliary atresia during infancy. Clin Transl Gastroenterol. 2015;19:e177. https://doi.org/10.1038/ctg.2015.55.
28. Jeon TY, Yoo SY, Kim JH, et al. Serial ultrasound findings associated with early liver transplantation after Kasai portoenterostomy in biliary atresia. Clin Radiol. 2013;68:588–94.
29. Tomita H, Ohkuma K, Masugi Y, et al. Diagnosing native liver fibrosis and esophageal varices using liver and spleen stiffness measurements in biliary atresia: a pilot study. Pediatr Radiol. 2016;46:1409–17.
30. Yokoyama S, Ishigami M, Honda T, et al. Spleen stiffness by 2-D shear wave elastography is the most accurate predictor of high-risk esophagogastric varices in children with biliary atresia. Hepatol Res. 2019;49:1162–8.
31. Hahn SM, Kim S, Park KI, et al. Clinical benefit of liver stiffness measurement at 3 months after Kasai hepatoportoenterostomy to predict the liver related events in biliary atresia. PLoS One. 2013;8:1–6. https://doi.org/10.1371/journal.pone.0080652.
32. Saito T, Hishiki T, Terui AK, et al. Use of multi-detector row CT for postoperative follow-up of biliary atresia patients with sequelae. Pediatr Surg Int. 2011;27:309–14.
33. Takahashi A, Hatakeyama S, Suzuki N, et al. MRI findings in the liver in biliary atresia patients after the Kasai operation. Tohoku J Exp Med. 1997;181:193–202.
34. Wang ZJ, Coakley FV, Ferrell LD, Rosenthal P. CT and MRI of hepatic pseudotumor in long-standing biliary atresia. J Comput Assist Tomogr. 2002;26:444–7.
35. Duche M, Habes D, Roulleau P, et al. Prophylactic endoscopic sclerotherapy of large esophagogastric varices in infants with biliary atresia. Gastrointest Endosc. 2008;67:732–7.
36. Lampela H, Kosola S, Koivusalo A, et al. Endoscopic surveillance and primary prophylaxis sclerotherapy of esophageal varices in biliary atresia. J Pediatr Gastroenterol Nutr. 2012;55:574–9.
37. Ishii T, Nio M, Shimaoka S, et al. Clinical significance of 99mTc-DTPA-galactosyl human serum albumin liver scintig-

raphy in follow-up patients with biliary atresia. J Pediatr Surg. 2003;38:1486–90.

38. Stocket RJ, Morell AG. Hepatic binding protein: the galactose specific receptor of mammalian hepatocytes. Hepatology. 1983;3:750–7.
39. Nio M, Wada M, Sasaki H, et al. Using 99mTc-DTPA galactosyl human serum albumin liver scintigraphy as a prognostic indicator in jaundice-free patients with biliary atresia. J Pediatr Surg. 2018;53:2412–5.
40. Ueno T, Saka R, Takama Y, et al. Onset ages of hepatopulmonary syndrome and pulmonary hypertension in patients with biliary atresia. Pediatr Surg Int. 2017;33:1053–7.
41. Karrer FM, Wallace BJ, Estrada AE. Late complications of biliary atresia: hepatopulmonary syndrome and portopulmonary hypertension. Pediatr Surg Int. 2017;33:1335–40.
42. Stagg H, Cameron BH, Ahmed N, et al. Variability of diagnostic approach, surgical technique, and medical management for children with biliary atresia in Canada—Is it time for standardization? J Pediatr Surg. 2017;52:802–6.
43. Wong KKY, Fan AH, Lan LCL, et al. Effective antibiotic regime for postoperative acute cholangitis in biliary atresia—an evolving scene. J Pediatr Surg. 2004;39:1800–2.
44. Kuroda T, Saeki M, Nakano M, Morikawa N. Biliary atresia, the next generation: a review of liver function, social activity, and sexual development in the late postoperative period. J Pediatr Surg. 2002;36:1709–12.
45. Nio M, Wada M, Sasaki H, et al. Correctable biliary atresia and cholangiocarcinoma: a case report of a 63-year-old patient. Surg Case Rep. 2019;29:185. https://doi.org/10.1186/s40792-019-0748-9
46. Yoon HJ, Yoo SY, Kim JH, et al. Hepatic tumours in children with biliary atresia: single-centre experience in 13 cases and review of the literature. Clin Radiol. 2014;69:e113–9.

# Prognostic Indicators of Outcome in Biliary Atresia

31

Joel Cazares, Hiroyuki Koga, and Atsuyuki Yamataka

**Abstract**

Many variables interplay to influence the outcome in biliary atresia (BA). Even after successful portoenterostomy (PE) and patients are clinically stable, inflammation and fibrosis of the biliary tract can obstruct bile flow and cholestasis can progress to liver cirrhosis that will cause gradual or sudden deterioration in liver function serious enough to require liver transplantation or cause death. In this chapter, factors prognostic for jaundice disappearance (JD) and survival with the native liver (SNL) in BA will be presented and discussed according to stages of treatment for easy reference.

**Keywords**

Biliary atresia · Prognostic factors · Survival native liver · Long-term follow-up · Cholangitis

## 31.1 Preoperative Patient Factors

Associations between biochemical data, radiologic/histologic findings, and clinical status have been investigated extensively in BA patients without reaching any concrete consensus about prognostic value, with some factors persisting to the present day without objective reassessment of consistency as legacies of history and tradition [1, 2].

### 31.1.1 Age at PE

According to the Japanese Biliary Atresia Registry (JBAR) that has a total of 3153 BA patients registered since its inception in 1985, the overall average age at PE is 68.1 days of age, with annual averages ranging from 60 to 75 days with no obvious correlation between earlier surgery and outcome [3]. There is a peak between 46 and 60 days old in the distribution of the age at PE as well as a small peak between 91 and 120 days; this double peak phenomenon is also seen in other countries and its cause has yet to be determined.

Overall, early diagnosis and early surgical intervention were both emphasized by Kasai [4] who reported better outcomes if PE was performed before 60 days of age, giving an impression that every single day that passed after 60 days would be detrimental to success. Thus, the timing of PE has come to be considered the most crucial prognostic factor, and over time, "PE before 60 days of life" has become so ingrained [5, 6], that some surgeons and pediatricians have referred patients directly for liver transplantation (LTx) if a child with BA presents later than 100 days after birth because of their age [7]. Unfortunately, the reality is that PE is performed in some countries when BA patients are much older, for example, more than 120 days of age because of a combination of delayed diagnosis due to denial of illness or inefficient referral services or relying directly on primary LTx for treatment without being realistic about waiting times for donors. There is little argument that BA patients benefit from PE and it should be performed before liver damage is too advanced to cause clinical deterioration.

Nio et al. [8] reported that PE before 60 days of life is correlated with long-term outcome, however, many reports do not conclude categorically if age at PE is correlated with prognosis or not. Nevertheless, the consensus is that PE should be performed promptly before deterioration related to failure to thrive, esophageal varices, or liver failure associated with BA can progress, generally considered to be around 100 days age, although successful outcome has been reported for PE performed in BA patients over 100 days old [9].

J. Cazares
Department of Pediatric General and Urogenital Surgery, Juntendo University School of Medicine, Tokyo, Japan

Department of Pediatric Surgery, Hospital Regional de Alta Especialidad Materno Infantil, Monterrey, Mexico
e-mail: joel@juntendo.ac.jp

H. Koga · A. Yamataka (✉)
Department of Pediatric General and Urogenital Surgery, Juntendo University School of Medicine, Tokyo, Japan
e-mail: h-koga@juntendo.ac.jp; yama@juntendo.ac.jp


M. Nio (ed.), *Introduction to Biliary Atresia*, https://doi.org/10.1007/978-981-16-2160-4_31

Evidence both for and against the age as a prognostic factor has been well documented. A selection of reports supportive of chronological age follows BA patients who underwent PE as neonates have the best rates of JD greater than 70%, with JD remaining essentially stable at around 60% until PE performed by 80 days of age, whereupon JD deteriorate with increasing age at PE [8]. Neto et al. [10] reported that one of the main prognostic factors of PE outcome is the patient's age at the time of surgery, which was at a median of 63 days. There was a positive relation, with statistical significance, to survival with the SNL in BA patients who had PE before 72 days of life, which supports the findings of other studies. Higher success of PE has been documented in multiple studies when patients are 60–90 days old [11, 12] with surgery after 100 days of age regarded as controversial [13]. Wong et al. [14] assessed their 28-year experience of PE by classifying 91 BA patients into 4 groups according to age at PE; group A (PE before 60 days of age; $n = 41$; 45.1%), group B (PE between 61 and 80 days of age; $n = 27$; 29.7%), group C (PE between 81 and 100 days of age; $n = 18$; 19.8%), and group D (PE after 100 days of age; $n = 5$; 5.4%). Their youngest patient had PE when 34 days old and their oldest was 134 days old. Patients over 100 days old typically showed marked evidence of hepatitis and hepatic fibrosis with features of early cirrhosis. In the USA, according to Hopkins et al. [15] the overall median age at PEis 63 days (range: 47–76 days) with no significant change in age at PE during the 12-year period of their study.

On the other hand, a selection of reports that do not support age as a prognostic factor include: Nio et al. [16] who investigated the 5- and 10-year survival rates of 735 patients after PE and found while 505 patients underwent PE at the age of 60 days or younger, the impact of age at PE on bile flow was not evident until 90 days of age, after which bile flow deteriorated but 20 year SNL was significantly correlated with early PE, but not short-term SNL [17]. Chen et al. [18] and Wong et al. [14] reported no histologic differences between the livers of patients who had PE before 60 days old and between 60 and 80 days old, but early evidence of cirrhosis when PE was performed at 90 or 100 days old; and Queiroz et al. [7] who reported if PE was performed after 90 days of life, the chance of bile drainage was less than 25% and if performed after 120 days of life, was only 10% to 20%.

Recently, Nakamura et al. [19] reported conclusive evidence that age at PE was not correlated with outcome as reflected by SNL by comparing age at PE, duration from the first pale stool to PE, and age when the first pale stool was passed. Thus, assessing outcome based on the age at PE is inherently wrong because the premise that age at PE is prognostic is incorrect; duration of BA morbidity from onset of symptoms to PE is more intuitive and logical because it reflects clinical status with respect to time and can be applied to all BA patients irrespective of age; for example, a 60-day-old baby diagnosed with BA when 30 days old will be different from a 60-day-old patient diagnosed with BA at birth and duration reflects this difference nicely.

### 31.1.2 Early Diagnosis

Early diagnosis allows PE to be performed promptly with the best chance for SNL before the liver damage progresses. Factors essential for early diagnosis include caregiver awareness and the use of home diagnosis instruments such as stool color cards. Early diagnosis was recommended by Kasai [4] so PE could be performed with the best possible outcome.

All term infants who remain jaundiced after 14 days of life (and preterm infants after 21 days) must be investigated for causes of persistent jaundice. The simplest investigation is determining the conjugated fraction of bilirubin. Babies fed breast milk who are jaundiced will have increased serum concentrations of unconjugated bilirubin, whereas in jaundice secondary to most liver diseases including BA, conjugated bilirubin is raised [20]. BA may present as persistent jaundice with conjugated bilirubin above 18 μmol/L (1.2 mg/dL) comprising more than 20% of total bilirubin with pale stools and dark urine in term infants with normal birth weights. Babies with BA may not necessarily have pale stools before the disease progresses and stool color cards used routinely in some countries, notably northeast Asia are useful for identifying infants at possible risk for BA [3, 21]. A recent report described a two-stage screening program using a combination of stool color cards and newborn bilirubin levels to identify infants at possible risk for BA before they become symptomatic currently under further investigation to assess feasibility and cost-effectiveness [22].

## 31.2 PRE and Intraoperative Morbidity Factors

### 31.2.1 Types of BA

According to a summary of JBAR data reported by Nio et al. [3, 16], 5 and 10 years survival rates after PE for 3160 BA patients, there were differences according to the type of BA involved; 11.9% had type I atresia of the common bile duct, 2.5% had type II atresia of the hepatic ducts, and 84.1% had type III atresia at the porta hepatis, with significant differences in JD and 5-year SNL rates; type I did best, followed by type II, and worst was type III ($p < 0.0001$). Davenport [23] reported type-related differences in outcome with cystic BA patients having better outcomes than isolated BA patients and BA splenic malformation syndrome and BA patients positive for cytomegalovirus IGM having the worst outcome. Other viral associations have been suggested, with mice inoculated with rotavirus developing jaundice with intrahepatic histology similar to that of BA [13]. Similar findings have been reported in mice with reovirus and cytomegalovirus and patients with exposure to rubella, syphilis, and Epstein Barr virus.

### 31.2.2 Biliary Remnant Histopathology

Microbileductule size has been postulated as a prognostic factor and microscopic examination of transected biliary remnants has identified a variety of residual ductules. Older reports suggested that a better outcome of PE would only be possible if larger diameter ductules (300 μm) were present because there is little likelihood of bile flow if a remnant has only minimal or no ductules [24, 25]. However, one institution [26] reported JD was achieved in 60/79 patients and assessed them by creating two groups: SNL ($n$ = 44) and LTx ($n$ = 16). Microbileductules at transected biliary remnants were similar (SNL: 123 ± 128.1 μm versus LTx: 150.0 ± 100.0 μm) with small ductules less than 100 μm identified in 18/44 (41%) SNL patients and 6/16 (38%) LTx patients. In another study of 12 consecutive non-syndromic type III BA patients who had laparoscopic PE (LPE) between 2009 and 2014 [27], outcome was SNL ($n$ = 8) and LTx ($n$ = 4) with mean microbileductule size being 91.3 μm (range: 0–200 μm) for SNL and 212.5 μm (range: 100–400 μm) for LTx; LTx patients had larger microbileductules at the porta hepatis than SNL patients although the difference was not statistically significant ($p$ = 0.06). Thus, while microbileductule size should be prognostic for postoperative JD theoretically because larger microbileductules should facilitate bile flow which, in turn, will improve bile drainage over a wider area of the liver, the reality is that size of microbileductules does not appear to be a prognostic factor in BA [26, 27].

## 31.3 Other Preoperative Factors

### 31.3.1 Investigations

Harpavat et al. [28] reported a screening test for neonates using a ratio of serum direct:conjugated bilirubin that resulted in earlier detection and treatment (PE at less than 30 days of age) with better JD and SNL compared with patients who had direct bilirubin:total bilirubin ratios of more than 0.2.

### 31.3.2 Medications/Prophylaxis

Double-agent broad spectrum antibiotics (usually a cephalosporin and an aminoglycoside) are commenced at the start of PE surgery and continued postoperatively until C-reactive protein (CRP) is less than 0.3 mg/dL or leukocytosis has resolved [29] to prevent cholangitis.

### 31.3.3 Surgical Skill

Operating surgeon experience and familiarity with BA influences diagnosis and postoperative management with Davenport reporting that experience is correlated with better outcome, with at least 5 PE cases per year being relevant [30]. Nakamura et al. [27] were the first to show that if the level of transection of the biliary remnant is kept shallow, JD is better than after extended deep transection. Similar outcomes were reported by Nio et al. [31] after standardized PE consisting of limited and careful transection of the fibrous remnant at the porta hepatis, a long Roux-en-Y loop with a spur valve, and meticulous anastomosis, were associated with favorable outcomes. They assessed the outcomes of 256 patients with BA who underwent PE between 1972 and 2014 and divided them into four groups: Group 1 (1972–1981; double Roux-en-Y; $n$ = 91), group 2 (1982–1991; Suruga II; $n$ = 80), group 3 (1992–2000; double-valve Roux-en-Y; $n$ = 46), and group 4 (2001–2014; total removal of the extrahepatic biliary remnants at the hepatic capsule and Roux-en-Y reconstruction with a spur valve; $n$ = 39). JD were 65.9%, 77.5%, 63.0%, and 87.2%, respectively; 10-year SNL were 53.8%, 60.1%, 44.1%, and 73.7%, respectively; and 10-year overall survival rates were 55.0%, 72.3%, 86.7%, and 97.3%, respectively. The level of dissection level of the fibrous remnant at the porta hepatis and transection in groups 1 and 2 was shallow (limited dissection), in group 3, dissection was wider and deeper, and transection extended beyond the liver capsule (extended dissection), and in group 4, transection was consistent with the hepatic capsule.

Roux-en-Y biliary reconstruction has been modified by various maneuvers; customizing the length of the Roux-en-Y limb, total diversion of the biliary conduit, creation of an intestinal valve, and the use of a physiologic intestinal valve [32] are performed to combat cholestasis to prevent cholangitis. From experience, customizing the Roux-en-Y limb is effective for reducing bile stasis [33]. The jejunal loop should be placed at the umbilicus and the distal end of the limb brought up to the xiphoid process. If predetermined to be, for example, 30, 40, or 50 cm long, the limb has the potential to cause bile stasis as the patient grows. This maneuver also ensures that the jejunojejunostomy fits naturally into the splenic flexure after anastomosis. The jejunojejunostomy is fashioned end-to-side and several sutures are placed at the junction of the native jejunum and the Roux limb to prevent reflux of contents into the Roux limb itself. An antimesenteric enterotomy, 10 mm in length, is made very near the closed end of the Roux-en-Y limb which does not have the long blind pouch seen in some end-to-side anastomoses, taking care not to create a blind pouch between the closed end of the Roux limb and the PE anastomosis because bile flow is prone to stagnate and induce bacterial overgrowth.

This customized Roux-en-Y technique was also supported by a report by Diao et al. [34] who compared 110 patients with short Roux-loops and 108 patients with conventional predetermined 35–40 cm long Roux-loops. They confirmed that a customized Roux-loop was as effective as a conventional Roux-loop. Recently, Nioet al. [31] reported reducing the length of the Roux-en-Y loop to 10 cm/kg/weight in small infants to reduce cholangitis.

Procedures that may cause stasis of intestinal contents such as stomas and portoduodenostomy are not recommended. The incidence of cholangitis after complex modifications such as Roux-en-Y with an intestinal valve and Suruga II is not less than after an original Roux-en-Y procedure and one reason for the Suruga II procedure being almost abandoned was that a stoma could potentially complicate LTx that might be required later [16]. Reconstruction by duodenostomy may cause leakage from the closure site in the duodenum after LTx, a serious complication because of the high amylase content of leaking fluid. Thus, the Roux-en-Y procedure is preferred because of less risks [35, 36].

LPE has excellent prognosis in Japan because the PE procedure was reworked to be as close to Professor Kasai's original PE as possible by studying intraoperative movies taken of his operations [32]. Overall success of PE (open or LPE) would appear to be related to how closely surgical techniques resemble Kasai's original PE procedure. Results for LPE in Japan are better than for open PE and patients also benefit from numerous advantages of minimally invasive surgery (MIS). Further technical improvements, such as robotic assistance for anastomoses are under assessment and preliminary results suggest that MIS and robotic assistance will decrease surgical stress and improve down time and possibly even enhance bilioenteric fistula formation.

Once liver function begins to deteriorate or cholangitis causes sudden decompensation, LTx is the only option. However, in some countries (notably Japan), availability of cadaveric donors is limited and living donors (usually parents or siblings) may be inappropriate because of advanced age or poor health [37].

## 31.4 Postoperative Patient Factors

### 31.4.1 Cholangitis

Cholangitis is the commonest complication after PE affecting up to 40% within 2 years [29]. It is a serious setback and can occur at any time because of cholestasis which is often compounded in the early postoperative period because bilioenteric fistulae have yet to form and function and must never be underestimated. Patients present initially with fever of at least 38.5°C, decreased quantity and quality of bile excretion with change in stool color from normal to acholic, elevation in serum bilirubin to more than 2.5 mg/dL, leukocytosis, and signs of infection/inflammation. It must be treated by intravenous broad-spectrum antibiotics with Gram-negative coverage administered immediately after blood cultures are taken according to pre-established protocols, to prevent damage to the liver that is cumulative with each attack. Once resolved, prophylactic antibiotics such as sulfamethoxazole/trimethoprim should be administered orally [29]. Prophylactic long-term oral antibiotics are advocated to reduce recurrence, but evidence for their efficacy remains scant with only one randomized controlled trial in a much younger age group in the literature [38].

A severe attack of cholangitis can destroy the liver despite intensive treatment. If a patient remains jaundiced, corticosteroid pulse therapy may be used to improve bile flow, but if stools remain acholic, a decreasing dose regime of corticosteroids should be trialed because they are both choleretic and anti-inflammatory and have been shown to augment antibiotics in BA patients with refractory cholangitis [38]. See "corticosteroids/ursodeoxycholic acid administration" later in this chapter. Occasionally, cholangitis still fails to respond to treatment. Intractable cholangitis is an indication for emergency LTx [39, 40] to prevent progression to liver failure. Late-onset cholangitis can even be fatal in long-term survivors.

### 31.4.2 Intrahepatic Bile Lake Cysts

Intrahepatic Bile Lake Cysts (IBLC) can develop any time after PE and cause recurring attacks of cholangitis [41]. Shimadera et al. [42], reviewed 28 postoperative PE patients who achieved JD. In patients who developed IBLC, liver biopsies taken at the time of PE had more evidence of fibrosis irrespective of their preoperative clinical status or history of postoperative cholangitis. SNL in IBLC patients was significantly lower, with no IBLC patients surviving over the age of 6 with native livers. Postoperative IBLC formation is predictive of poor prognosis, especially if they develop midterm.

## 31.5 Postoperative Morbidity Factors

### 31.5.1 Jaundice Disappearance

JD is correlated with age at PE. Please refer to "age at portoenterostomy (PE)" earlier in this chapter.

### 31.5.2 Survival with the Native Liver

JBAR [16] reported 5-year postoperative survival rates for SNL patients registered in 1989, 1990, 1991, 1992, 1993, and 1994 as being 62%, 64.5%, 61.3%, 59.0%, 58.7%, and 52.7%, and after LTx as being 69.4%, 74.2%, 72.5%, 79.5%, 78%, 78.3%, respectively. Differences in survival after LTx were not statistically significant ($p = 0.1206$). For the 108 patients registered when JBAR was inaugurated, 10-year survival rates were 57/108 (52.8%) for SNL patients and 72/108 (66.7%) for LTx patients. Twenty-year survival rates were 49% for SNL patients and 89% for LTx patients [3]. Compared with other reports, J-BAR 5-year survival rates are better by 24–48% [43–45] with 10-year survival rates exhibiting the same trend (JBAR: 52.8% versus 28-34% in other reports). At last count, 1236 of the 3160 BA patients on the JBAR have had LTx. Only one patient was lost to 10-year follow-up; and further improvement of the 10-year survival rate is expected, because LTx had become widely available in Japan since the early 1990s.

JBAR remains the most comprehensive database for BA patients and is used as a reference worldwide, but results vary. For example, in England and Wales, the 10-year survival rate is nearly 90% [30] and a review of 139 BA patients from a single institution in China [46] treated from January 2009 to December 2012 found the average age at PE was 78.3 ± 22.9 days and 5-year SNL was 75/139 (54.0%). However, by 5 years after PE, 58/139 (41.7%) had died or required LTx; 47/58 (81%) within the first year after PE.

Recently, a retrospective review [47] of 127 patients at multiple centers in Japan with type III BA who underwent open PE ($n = 106$ at 8 centers) and LPE ($n = 21$ at 3 centers) found 1-year SNL was 63% after open PE and 67% after LPE. JD one year after LPE was 71%. JD after PE and LPE were 64% (68/106) and 71% (15/21) of patients, respectively. These figures indicate the potential that LPE has, and while results in Japan are good, it has yet to gain acceptance generally.

Nakamura et al. [19] reviewed 96 BA patients who underwent PE when aged 91 days or older and found SNL was 66.7% (8/12) when the pre-PE duration was less than 60 days after a mean follow-up of 11.8 years (range: 0.16–22.6 years), indicating that favorable SNL is achievable after PE in older patients when duration is not prolonged. Correlation between SNL and duration pre-PE was statistically significant ($p = 0.003$), with the best survival being for when duration pre-PE was 30 days or less, followed by duration of 31–60 days, and worst form duration of 61 days or more.

### 31.5.3 Portal Hypertension

Portal hypertension can develop after PE even in patients with good postoperative bile flow who achieve JD, with livers showing evidence of hepatic fibrosis [48] secondary to the progressive morbidity of BA and is a negative prognostic factor.

The portal system drains the capillaries of the mesenteric and splenic veins and ends in the hepatic capillaries. The portal vein supplies partially oxygenated blood to the liver that supplements the highly oxygenated blood supplied by the hepatic artery; blood from both systems combines within the sinusoids. Any disturbance in perfusion can be offset to a certain degree by increased flow through the other system. Portal hypertension occurs when there is increased resistance and/or increased blood flow in the portal system defined as portal pressure greater than 10 mmHg or hepatic venous pressure gradient (HVPG) greater than 4 mmHg. HVPG greater than 10 mmHg is associated with esophageal varices, hypersplenism, gastropathy, gastric antral vascular ectasia, and ascites. The incidence of a first-time variceal hemorrhage in children with cirrhosis, 22%, increases to 38% over a 5-year period if a child is known to have varices [49, 50]. Bleeding occurs in 15%–25% of patients with BA on long-term follow-up, usually after an episode of fever or cholangitis. Ectopic intestinal variceal bleeding and pulmonary arteriovenous fistulas are sometimes seen in long-term survivors with chronic impaired liver function [51]. The presence of gastroesophageal varices requiring endoscopic injection sclerotherapy is a significant long-term prognostic factor [17].

Over time, the susceptibility to complications from portal hypertension seems to decrease, resulting in reduced frequency and severity of variceal bleeding. This observation is difficult to explain and may be related to improvement in hepatic histology or the development of spontaneous portosystemic shunts that justify a nonsurgical approach to portal hypertension as long as hepatic function is preserved (i.e., the patient remains anicteric with no coagulopathy and normal serum albumin level). However, in the presence of poor hepatic function, complications from portal hypertension are an indication for LTx. Presence of evidence of portal hypertension is a negative prognostic factor.

### 31.5.4 Splenomegaly

Splenomegaly is the second most common finding in children with portal hypertension after gastrointestinal bleeding and in many instances, an enlarged spleen is first discovered on routine follow-up physical examination. Otherwise, clinical manifestations of splenomegaly such as thrombocytopenia, leukopenia, petechiae, or ecchymoses may be identified and splenomegaly confirmed by subsequent investigations. Up to 70% of long-term survivors can show clinical, ultrasonographic, or endoscopic signs of splenomegaly [52]. Size does not correlate well with portal pressure and rarely requires surgical intervention.

### 31.5.5 Hepatopulmonary Syndrome

Hepatopulmonary syndrome is characterized by cyanosis, dyspnea on exertion, hypoxia, and finger clubbing. Diffuse intrapulmonary shunting can occur as a complication of chronic liver disease in children with BA as a result of vasoactive compounds from the mesenteric circulation not being broken down by the liver. It appears to be more prevalent in children with syndromic BA. Hepatopulmonary syndrome only occurs in patients with portal hypertension who have both thrombocytopenia and splenomegaly. According to Shneider [53] in a multicenter study conducted in the USA involving 163 BA patients, 80% with either ascites or esophageal variceal bleeding had both low platelets and splenomegaly. This complication is progressive and can usually be reversed by LTx.

### 31.5.6 Portopulmonary Hypertension

Portopulmonary hypertension is an uncommon complication that can also develop in long-term survivors after PE. The goal of management is to reduce pulmonary pressure to below 35 mmHg [24, 54]. If hepatopulmonary syndrome or portopulmonary hypertension are suspected, LTx should be encouraged actively before symptoms worsen. If pulmonary artery pressure is greater than 35 mmHg at LTx, the outcome is likely to be poor.

## 31.6 Other Postoperative Factors

### 31.6.1 Investigations

Serum biochemistry is highly prognostic of outcome and there are numerous tests that are essential for diagnosis and follow-up that also provide valuable data for predicting prognosis. A transient postoperative decrease in total bilirubin that occurs has been studied extensively. Shneider et al. [55] reported that infants whose total bilirubin did not fall below 2.0 mg/dL within 3 months of PE had a higher risk for early progression of BA, suggesting such patients are indicated for LTx.

Koga et al. [26] reviewed the liver function tests of 76 patients who had PE, comparing results pre- and post-PE with respect to outcome (SNL or LTx). They found aspartate aminotransferase (AST) and gamma-glutamyl transpeptidase ($\gamma$-GT) were both elevated preoperatively in all patients and decreased as total bilirubin levels fell, with both AST and $\gamma$-GT being significantly lower in SNL patients 1, 2, and 3 months after PE compared with patients who eventually required LTx ($p < 0.001$, respectively). Thus, AST (and $\gamma$-GT) would appear to be prognostic for LTx as early as 1 month post-PE. Sun et al. [56] reported preoperative $\gamma$-GT levels were lower in patients who did not do well postoperatively, which confirms that the short-term increase in $\gamma$-GT after PE may be an indicator of poor prognosis. Both Koga and Sun conclude that $\gamma$-GT is prognostic.

Nakamura et al. [19] used AST-to-platelet ratio index (APRI) scores as a noninvasive indicator of fibrosis and cirrhosis for detecting significant liver fibrosis and portal hypertension with good accuracy. Lower APRI scores (less than 0.5) exclude cirrhosis and higher APRI scores (more than 1.5) predict cirrhosis; mid-range values are not particularly relevant. From a meta-analysis of 40 studies, APRI scores greater than 1.0 had a sensitivity of 76% and specificity of 72% for predicting cirrhosis. In addition, an APRI score greater than 0.7 had a sensitivity of 77% and specificity of 72% for predicting significant hepatic fibrosis. For detection of cirrhosis, using an APRI cutoff score of 2.0 was more specific (91%) but less sensitive (46%).

### 31.6.2 Corticosteroids/Ursodeoxycholic Acid Administration

The choleretic effect of corticosteroids involves induction of Na-K-ATPase, which increases canalicular electrolyte transport and stimulates bile flow independent of bile salt concentrations, and when given in high doses, steroids have pronounced anti-inflammatory and immunosuppressive effects, decreasing edema and collagen deposition, inhibiting scarring, and arresting migration of infiltrating monocytes and lymphocytes [57].

We administer prednisolone intravenously in a decreasing dose regime routinely after postoperative CRP falls below 1.0 mg/dL. Each dose is given for 3 days, starting with an initial dose of 4 mg/kg/day, then 3, 2, 1, and 0.5 mg/kg/day. This 15-day cycle can be repeated up to four or five times if there is evidence of clinical benefit (i.e., lower serum bilirubin or improved stool color). However, if there is no evidence of clinical benefit and total bilirubin remains over 2.0 mg/dL, only a maximum of three cycles should be administered, and the patient considered actively for LTx [29, 32]. An important feature of this protocol is that if stools begin to turn pale, the cycle can either be restarted, or the previous dose readministered, depending on clinical circumstances.

The role of corticosteroids and ursodeoxycholic acid is actually unproven despite their widespread usage.

### 31.6.3 Nutrition

Due to the presence of residual hepatic disease, metabolic problems associated with malabsorption of fat, protein, vitamins, and trace minerals can occur postoperatively because of impairment of bile flow to the gut [58]. Essential fatty acid deficiencies and rickets may occur. Growth and development after PE may be poor if hepatic dysfunction persists and should be assessed independently of body weight. Long-term monitoring of growth and development and adequate nutritional supplementation are recommended. Poor nutrition is a negative prognostic factor as a patient is prevented from mounting an effective immune response.

### 31.6.4 Reproductive Health

While not strictly a prognostic factor, as more postoperative BA patients reach adulthood, reproductive health becomes an important issue. In post-PE SNL patients, preterm cesarean delivery at around 34 weeks gestation appears to be reasonable because poor hepatic reserve defines the pregnancy as being high risk. Conversely, delivery at full term may be possible for selected mothers with good liver function [59, 60].

### 31.6.5 Hepatic Malignancy

Rarely, malignant changes (hepatocellular carcinoma or cholangiocarcinoma) can complicate long-standing biliary cirrhosis after PE. A case of hepatocellular carcinoma [61] has been reported in a 19-year-old male post-PEBA patient, indicating the need for a high index of suspicion for the development of carcinoma, even in young patients.

## 31.7 Conclusions

Factors strongly prognostic for successful PE include:

(a) Age at PE
(b) Duration of symptoms pre-PE
(c) JD preserves hepatocyte function and prevents cholangitis postoperatively by diminishing cholestasis and intrahepatic periportal inflammation

Factors strongly prognostic for clinical deterioration include:

(a) Cholangitis
(b) Portal hypertension
(c) High $\gamma$-GT after PE

Other factors to consider include:

(a) Nutrition
(b) Affordable accessible health services
(c) Prompt diagnosis and treatment

Factors considered prognostic for SNL that are inconsistent include:

(a) Age at PE [19]
(b) Microbileductule size
(c) Modifications such as intestinal valves, spur valves, intussuscepted valves at the Roux-en-Y

For successful management of BA:

(a) Early diagnosis
(b) Prompt PE (open or LPE) after diagnosis
(c) Intensive follow-up and monitoring for signs/symptoms of deterioration

## References


1. Balistreri WF. Neonatal cholestasis. J Pediatr. 1985;106(2):171–84.
2. Brough AJ, Bernstein J. Conjugated hyperbilirubinemia in early infancy. A reassessment of liver biopsy. Hum Pathol. 1974;5(5):507–16.
3. Nio M. Japanese biliary atresia registry. Pediatr Surg Int. 2017;33(12):1319–25.
4. Kasai M. Advances in treatment of biliary atresia. Jpn J Surg. 1983;13(4):265–76.
5. Altman RP, Levy J. Biliary atresia. Pediatr Ann. 1985;14(7):481–2. 484–485
6. Nio M, Wada M, Sasaki H, Tanaka H. Effects of age at Kasai portoenterostomy on the surgical outcome: a review of the literature. Surg Today. 2014;45(7):813–8.
7. Queiroz TCN, Ferreira AR, Fagundes EDT, Roquete MLV, Penna FJ. Biliary atresia: evaluation on two distinct periods at a reference pediatric service. Arq Gastroenterol. 2014;51(1):53–8.
8. Nio M, Wada M, Sasaki H, Tanaka H. Effects of age at Kasai portoenterostomy on the surgical outcome: a review of the literature. Surg Today. 2014;45(7):813–8.
9. Davenport M, De Ville de Goyet J, Stringer MD, Mieli-Vergani G, Kelly DA, McClean P, Spitz L. Seamless management of biliary atresia in England and Wales (1999–2002). Lancet (London, England). 2004;363(9418):1354–7.
10. Neto B, Borges-Dias M, Trindade E, Estevão-Costa J, Campos JM. Biliary atresia – clinical series. GE Port J Gastroenterol. 2017;25(2):68–73.
11. Coran A, Adzick NS, Krummel T, Laberge J-M, Shamberger R, Caldamone A. Pediatric surgery. 7th ed. Mosby; 2012. p. 1321–30.
12. de Carvalho E, Ivantes CAP, Bezerra JA. Extrahepatic biliary atresia: current concepts and future directions. J Pediatr (Rio J). 2007;83(2):105–20.
13. Hartley JL, Davenport M, Kelly DA. Biliary atresia. Lancet. 2009;374(9702):1704–13.
14. Wong KKY, Chung PHY, Chan IHY, Lan LCL, Tam PKH. Performing Kasai portoenterostomy beyond 60 days of life is not necessarily associated with a worse outcome. J Pediatr Gastroenterol Nutr. 2010;51(5):631–4.
15. Hopkins PC, Yazigi N, Nylund CM. Incidence of biliary atresia and timing of hepatoportoenterostomy in the United States. J Pediatr. 2017;187:253–7.
16. Nio M, Ohi R, Miyano T, Saeki M, Shiraki K, Tanaka K, Japanese Biliary Atresia Registry. Five- and 10-year survival rates after sur-

gery for biliary atresia: a report from the Japanese Biliary Atresia Registry. J Pediatr Surg. 2003;38(7):997–1000.
17. Sasaki H, Tanaka H, Wada M, Kazama T, Nakamura M, Kudo H, Okubo R, Sakurai T, Nio M. Analysis of the prognostic factors of long-term native liver survival in survivors of biliary atresia. Pediatr Surg Int. 2016;32(9):839–43.
18. Chen G, Zheng S, Sun S, Xiao X, Ma Y, Shen W, Chen L, Song Z. Early surgical outcomes and pathological scoring values of older infants ($\geq$ 90 d old) with biliary atresia. J Pediatr Surg. 2012;47(12):2184–8.
19. Nakamura H, Ara M, Koga H, Miyano G, Okawada M, Doi T, Lane G, Okazaki T, Urao M, Yamataka A. Duration from the first pale stool to portoenterostomy is prognostic in biliary atresia. Comparison with age at portoenterostomy. Clin Res Hepatol Gastroenterol. 2020; (in press)
20. Livesey E, Cortina Borja M, Sharif K, Alizai N, McClean P, Kelly D, Hadzic N, Davenport M. Epidemiology of biliary atresia in England and Wales (1999–2006). Arch Dis Child Fetal Neonatal Ed. 2009;94(6):451–5.
21. Hsiao C-H, Chang M-H, Chen H-L, Lee H-C, Wu T-C, Lin C-C, Yang Y-J, Chen A-C, Tiao M-M, Lau B-H, Chu C-H, Lai M-W, Taiwan Infant Stool Color Card Study Group. Universal screening for biliary atresia using an infant stool color card in Taiwan. Hepatology (Baltimore, MD). 2008;47(4):1233–40.
22. Harpavat S, Garcia-Prats JA, Shneider BL. Newborn bilirubin screening for biliary atresia. N Engl J Med. 2016;375(6):605–6.
23. Davenport M. Adjuvant therapy in biliary atresia: hopelessly optimistic or potential for change? Pediatr Surg Int. 2017;33(12):1263–73.
24. Howard ER, Driver M, McClement J, Mowat AP. Results of surgery in 88 consecutive cases of extrahepatic biliary atresia. J R Soc Med. 1982;75(6):408–13.
25. Tan CE, Davenport M, Driver M, Howard ER. Does the morphology of the extrahepatic biliary remnants in biliary atresia influence survival? A review of 205 cases. J Pediatr Surg. 1994;29(11):1459–64.
26. Koga H, Wada M, Nakamura H, Miyano G, Okawada M, Lane GJ, Okazaki T, Yamataka A. Factors influencing jaundice-free survival with the native liver in post-portoenterostomy biliary atresia patients: results from a single institution. J Pediatr Surg. 2013;48(12):2368–72.
27. Nakamura H, Koga H, Miyano G, Okawada M, Doi T, Yamataka A. Does the level of transection of the biliary remnant affect outcome after laparoscopic Kasai portoenterostomy for biliary atresia? J Laparoendosc Adv Surg Tech A. 2017;27(7):744–7.
28. Harpavat S, Finegold MJ, Karpen SJ. Patients with biliary atresia have elevated direct/conjugated bilirubin levels shortly after birth. Pediatrics. 2011;128(6):e1428–33.
29. Cazares J, Ure B, Yamataka A. Biliary atresia. In: Holcomb GW, Murphy JP, St Peter SD, editors. Ashcraft's pediatric surgery. 7th ed. Amsterdam: Elsevier; 2009. p. 679–94.
30. Davenport M. Biliary atresia: clinical aspects. Semin Pediatr Surg. 2012;21(3):175–84.
31. Nio M, Wada M, Sasaki H, Kazama T, Tanaka H, Kudo H. Technical standardization of Kasai portoenterostomy for biliary atresia. J Pediatr Surg. 2016;51(12):2105–8.
32. Yamataka A, Lane GJ, Cazares J. Laparoscopic surgery for biliary atresia and choledochal cyst. Semin Pediatr Surg. 2012;21(3):201–10.
33. Yamataka A, Kobayashi H, Shimotakahara A, Okada Y, Yanai T, Lane GJ, Urao M, Miyano T. Recommendations for preventing complications related to Roux-en-Y hepatico-jejunostomy performed during excision of choledochal cyst in children. J Pediatr Surg. 2003;38(12):1830–2.
34. Diao M, Li L, Zhang J-Z, Cheng W. A shorter loop in Roux-Y hepatojejunostomy reconstruction for choledochal cysts is equally effective: preliminary results of a prospective randomized study. J Pediatr Surg. 2010;45(4):845–7.
35. Tanaka K, Shirahase I, Utsunomiya H, Katayama T, Uemoto S, Asonuma K, Inomata Y, Ozawa K. A valved hepatic portoduodenal intestinal conduit for biliary atresia. Ann Surg. 1991;213(3):230–5.
36. Shinkai M, Ohhama Y, Take H, Kitagawa N, Kudo H, Mochizuki K, Hatata T. Long-term outcome of children with biliary atresia who were not transplanted after the Kasai operation: >20-year experience at a children's hospital. J Pediatr Gastroenterol Nutr. 2009;48(4):443–50.
37. Bu L-N, Chen H-L, Chang C-J, Ni Y-H, Hsu H-Y, Lai H-S, Hsu W-M, Chang M-H. Prophylactic oral antibiotics in prevention of recurrent cholangitis after the Kasai portoenterostomy. J Pediatr Surg. 2003;38(4):590–3.
38. Luo Y, Zheng S. Current concept about postoperative cholangitis in biliary atresia. World J Pediatr. 2008;4(1):14–9.
39. Chung PHY, Tam PKH, Wong KKY. Does the identity of the bacteria matter in post-Kasai cholangitis? A comparison between simple and intractable cholangitis. J Pediatr Surg. 2018;53(12):2409–11.
40. Ernest van Heurn LW, Saing H, Tam PKH. Cholangitis after hepatic portoenterostomy for biliary atresia: a multivariate analysis of risk factors. J Pediatr. 2003;142(5):566–71.
41. Bu L-N, Chen H-L, Ni Y-H, Peng S, Jeng Y-M, Lai H-S, Chang M-H. Multiple intrahepatic biliary cysts in children with biliary atresia. J Pediatr Surg. 2002;37(8):1183–7.
42. Shimadera S, Iwai N, Deguchi E, Kimura O, Ono S, Furukawa T, Fumino S. Predicting factors on the occurrence of cystic dilatation of intrahepatic biliary system in biliary atresia. Pediatr Surg Int. 2010;26(6):611–4.
43. de Vries W, de Langen ZJ, Groen H, Scheenstra R, Peeters PMJG, Hulscher JBF, Verkade HJ, Netherlands Study Group of Biliary Atresia and Registry (NeSBAR). Biliary atresia in the Netherlands: outcome of patients diagnosed between 1987 and 2008. J Pediatr. 2012;160(4):638–44.
44. Shneider BL, Brown MB, Haber B, Whitington PF, Schwarz K, Squires R, Bezerra J, Shepherd R, Rosenthal P, Hoofnagle JH, Sokol RJ, Biliary Atresia Research Consortium. A multicenter study of the outcome of biliary atresia in the United States, 1997 to 2000. J Pediatr. 2006;148(4):467–74.
45. Chardot C, Carton M, Spire-Bendelac N, Le Pommelet C, Golmard J-L, Auvert B. Prognosis of biliary atresia in the era of liver transplantation: French national study from 1986 to 1996. Hepatology. 1999;30(3):606–11.
46. Wang Z, Chen Y, Peng C, Pang W, Zhang T, Wu D, Shen Q, Li M. Five-year native liver survival analysis in biliary atresia from a single large Chinese center: the death/liver transplantation hazard change and the importance of rapid early clearance of jaundice. J Pediatr Surg. 2019;54(8):1680–5.
47. Murase N, Hinoki A, Shirota C, Tomita H, Shimojima N, Sasaki H, Nio M, Tahara K, Kanamori Y, Shinkai M, Yamamoto H, Sugawara Y, Hibi T, Ishimaru T, Kawashima H, Koga H, Yamataka A, Uchida H. Multicenter, retrospective, comparative study of laparoscopic and open Kasai portoenterostomy in children with biliary atresia from Japanese high-volume centers. J Hepatobiliary Pancreat Sci. 2019;26(1):43–50.
48. Altman RP, Chandra R, Lilly JR. Ongoing cirrhosis after successful portoenterostomy in infants with biliary atresia. J Pediatr Surg. 1975;10(5):685–91.
49. Karrer FM, Price MR, Bensard DD, Sokol RJ, Narkewicz MR, Smith DJ, Lilly JR. Long-term results with the Kasai operation for biliary atresia. Arch Surg (Chicago, IL: 1960). 1996;131(5):493–6.
50. Ryan BM, Stockbrugger RW, Ryan JM. A pathophysiologic, gastroenterologic, and radiologic approach to the management of gastric varices. Gastroenterology. 2004;126(4):1175–89.
51. Agarwal GS, Saxena A, Bhatnagar V. The development of intrapulmonary arteriovenous shunts as a poor prognostic factor following surgery for biliary atresia. Trop Gastroenterol. 2009;30(2):110–2.

52. Lykavieris P, Chardot C, Sokhn M, Gauthier F, Valayer J, Bernard O. Outcome in adulthood of biliary atresia: a study of 63 patients who survived for over 20 years with their native liver. Hepatology. 2005;41(2):366–71.
53. Shneider BL, Abel B, Haber B, Karpen SJ, Magee JC, Romero R, Schwarz K, Bass LM, Kerkar N, Miethke AG, Rosenthal P, Turmelle Y, Robuck PR, Sokol RJ, Childhood Liver Disease Research and Education Network. Portal hypertension in children and young adults with biliary atresia. J Pediatr Gastroenterol Nutr. 2012;55(5):567–73.
54. Karrer FM, Wallace BJ, Estrada AE. Late complications of biliary atresia: hepatopulmonary syndrome and portopulmonary hypertension. Pediatr Surg Int. 2017;33(12):1335–40.
55. Shneider BL, Magee JC, Karpen SJ, Rand EB, Narkewicz MR, Bass LM, Schwarz K, Whitington PF, Bezerra JA, Kerkar N, Haber B, Rosenthal P, Turmelle YP, Molleston JP, Murray KF, Ng VL, Wang KS, Romero R, Squires RH, Arnon R, Sherker AH, Moore J, Ye W, Sokol RJ, Childhood Liver Disease Research Network (ChiLDReN). Total serum bilirubin within 3 months of hepatoportoenterostomy predicts short-term outcomes in biliary atresia. J Pediatr. 2016;170:211–7.
56. Sun S, Zheng S, Lu X, Chen G, Ma Y, Chen L, Dong K. Clinical and pathological features of patients with biliary atresia who survived for more than 5 years with native liver. Pediatr Surg Int. 2018;34(4):381–6.
57. Pang W-B, Zhang T-C, Chen Y-J, Peng C-H, Wang Z-M, Wu D-Y, Wang K. Ten-year experience in the prevention of post-Kasai cholangitis. Surg Infect (Larchmt). 2019;20(3):231–5.
58. Andrews WS, Pau CM, Chase HP, Foley LC, Lilly JR. Fat soluble vitamin deficiency in biliary atresia. J Pediatr Surg. 1981;16(3):284–90.
59. Kuroda, T., Saeki, M., Morikawa, N. and Fuchimoto, Y. (2005). Biliary atresia and pregnancy: puberty may be an important point for predicting the outcome. J Pediatr Surg, 40(12), 1852–1855.
60. Sasaki H, Tanaka H, Nio M. Current management of long-term survivors of biliary atresia: over 40 years of experience in a single center and review of the literature. Pediatr Surg Int. 2017;33(12):1327–33.
61. Hol L, van den Bos IC, Hussain SM, Zondervan PE, de Man RA. Hepatocellular carcinoma complicating biliary atresia after Kasai portoenterostomy. Eur J Gastroenterol Hepatol. 2008;20(3):227–31.

# Long-Term Complication after Portoenterostomy: Gastroesophageal and Gastrointestinal Tract Bleeding

32

Yutaka Kanamori

**Abstract**

One of the most important complications after the portoenterostomy operation (Kasai operation) in patients with biliary atresia is gastrointestinal bleeding. The source of bleeding is variable, and includes esophageal varices, gastric varices, jejunal loop varices, portal hypertensive gastropathy, and colonopathy. Endoscopy is the most important and useful examination for esophageal varices. In pediatric patients, several indexes that predict the presence of esophageal varices have been proposed, but they are suboptimal tools to predict severe esophageal varices in patients with biliary atresia. Bleeding esophageal varices requires urgent treatment, and pharmacological, endoscopic treatment is effective. Injection sclerotherapy was the first endoscopic treatment for bleeding esophageal varices, but recently the band ligation method is preferred. To prevent rebleeding and as primary prophylaxis, repeated endoscopic treatments are recommended. Liver transplantation is the most effective treatment for esophageal varices to reduce portal pressure but the indication of liver transplantation should be evaluated carefully considering the residual function of the liver and other complications.

**Keywords**

Gastroesophageal varices · Injection sclerotherapy · Band ligation · Beta-blocker · TIPS (transjugular intrahepatic portosystemic shunting)

Y. Kanamori (✉)
Division of Surgery, Department of Surgical Specialties, National Center for Child Health and Development, Tokyo, Japan
e-mail: kanamori-y@ncchd.go.jp

## 32.1 Introduction

The most severe and troublesome postoperative complication after portoenterostomy is gastrointestinal (GI) and esophageal bleeding, which is caused by severe portal hypertension. Almost all patients with biliary atresia suffer from liver fibrosis or cirrhosis, and after portoenterostomy portal hypertension progresses rapidly with hepatic inflammation in some patients. According to long-term follow-up reports on patients with biliary atresia [1, 2, 3], about 40% of postoperative patients had esophageal varices and more than 15% of patients experienced variceal bleeding. These data strongly suggest that esophageal varices and bleeding of esophageal varices are an important and significant prognostic factor [4], that should be comparable to repetitive cholangitis, which is another important complication after portoenterostomy in patients with biliary atresia. Patients who have undergone portoenterostomy must be frequently screened to see whether they have portal hypertension or not by obtaining physical findings and performing the proper examinations. Recently, liver transplantation has become widely accepted for the treatment of patients with biliary atresia if the portoenterostomy failed and bile drainage is poor.

In adults, portal hypertension is defined as a pressure greater than 10 mmHg in the portal venous system or a hepatic venous pressure gradient (HVPG) of greater than 5 mmHg [5]. The HVPG is the pressure difference between free and wedged hepatic venous pressure and it should be measured by venous catheterization from the jugular vein. Participants of the recent consensus meeting held in 2016 (which is called the Baveno VI Consensus) announced the importance of stratifying the risk and individualizing the care for patients with portal hypertension [6, 7]. However, in the pediatric field, there are very few studies that show the scientific evidence for proper treatment against portal hypertension, and at the Baveno VI pediatric satellite symposium, consensus was not achieved regarding primary


M. Nio (ed.), *Introduction to Biliary Atresia*, https://doi.org/10.1007/978-981-16-2160-4_32

prophylaxis of varices among endoscopic variceal ligation, sclerotherapy, or nonspecific beta-blockade medication [8]. Although high-quality scientific evidence is scarce for the treatment of portal hypertension in pediatric patients, many studies suggesting an efficient treatment strategy for portal hypertension in children have been reported, and here we present them and discuss the more efficient treatment strategies

## 32.2 Pathophysiology of Portal Hypertension in the Cirrhotic Liver of Patients with Biliary Atresia

In the cirrhotic liver, structural changes increase intrahepatic vascular resistance by direct disruption of sinusoidal blood flow (para-sinusoidal factor). In the cirrhotic liver the vascular tone also increases, which is caused by a relative deficiency of intrahepatic local vasodilators such as nitric oxide [9]. Another factor that increases portal pressure is increased portal blood flow that is caused by nitric oxide-mediated splanchnic vasodilatation and compensatory sodium retention with plasma volume expansion mediated by activation of the renin–angiotensin–aldosterone axis [9].

## 32.3 Development of Portosystemic Collaterals and Varices (Fig. 32.1)

The portal hypertensive change caused by a cirrhotic liver results in the development of collateral vessels in some venous networks and they cause several troublesome clinical consequences. These portosystemic collaterals develop from 1) the coronary vein (left gastric vein) to the esophageal vein, 2) the umbilical veins to the abdominal wall veins, 3) the inferior mesenteric vein to the inferior hemorrhoidal veins, and 4) the gastric, splenic, and adrenal veins to the left renal vein. These collateral vessels result in significant portosystemic shunting and cause several important clinical symptoms such as hyperammonemia, encephalopathy, hepato-pulmonary syndrome, and varices in the luminal surfaces of the esophagus, stomach, and intestine. Esophageal varices are known to occur when the HVPG value becomes greater than 12 mmHg [10]. The cirrhotic liver causes esophageal varices in 40–70% of patients with biliary atresia before the age of five years [11, 12] and the reported mean age at which first bleeding of esophageal varices occurred was 3 years [12]. Considering these data, we must be careful to monitor the progression of portal hypertension and anticipate the presence of esophageal varices by several periodic examinations, which are described later. We must also be aware that gastrointestinal bleeding can be caused not only by esophageal and gastric varices but also by portal hypertensive gastropathy [13] and by varices that develop in the Roux-en-Y jejunal loop [14]. These types of bleeding are very difficult to treat and in some cases emergency living liver transplantation may be needed to rescue the patients.

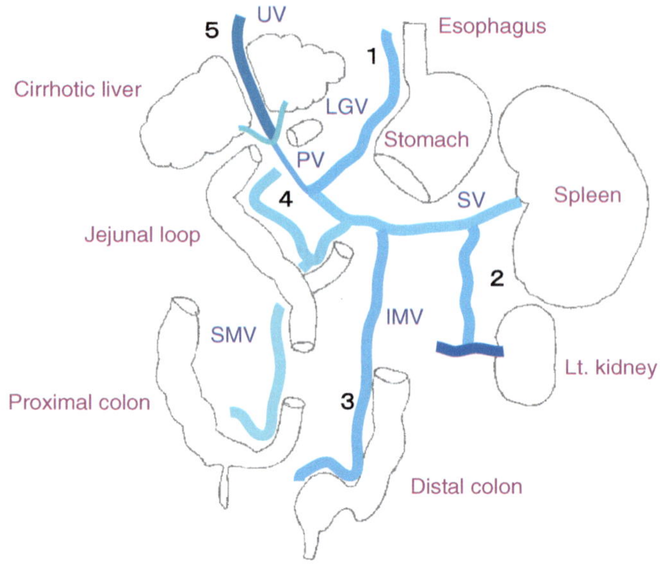


Fig. 32.1 Various portosystemic shunts may form in patients with liver cirrhosis after Kasai operation for the treatment of biliary atresia. Five patterns of portosystemic shunt in patients with liver cirrhosis are illustrated with their associated organs. 1, Left gastric vein to esophageal vein (gastroesophageal varices). 2, Splenic vein to left renal vein (splenorenal varices). 3, Inferior mesenteric vein to lower rectal vein (hemorrhoidal varices). 4, Superior mesenteric vein to raised jejunal loop vein (jejunal loop varices). 5, Umbilical vein to abdominal wall vein (paraumbilical varices). PV: portal vein, SMV: superior mesenteric vein, IMV: inferior mesenteric vein, LGV: left gastric vein, SV: splenic vein, UV: umbilical vein. Lt. kidney, left kidney

## 32.4 Prediction and Diagnosis of Varices and Mucosal Lesions That Have a Bleeding Risk

**4-1.** In adults with esophageal varices, the HVPG value is an excellent barometer that can be used to predict the progression of esophageal varices. However, in pediatric patients its measurement is not practical in the vast majority of cases and alternative methods of predicting the presence of portal hypertension and esophageal varices have been proposed in many reports [15–23]. In these reports the tools to predict portal hypertension are varied (Table 32.1), such as morphological changes in organs and the portal venous system as observed by abdominal ultrasound examination, echo-elasticity measurement of the liver and spleen (transient elastography [15], two-dimensional shear wave elastography [16]), magnetic resonance elastography [17], abdominal contrast-enhanced computed tomography (CT), and the combination of several values obtained by blood tests [APRI,

**Table 32.1** Various indices that have been developed to predict whether portal hypertension and gastroesophageal varices are present in patients with biliary atresia

| | |
|---|---|
| Serum marker panels | APRI (aspartate aminotransferase-to-platelet ratio index)<br>AAR (aspartate aminotransferase-to-alanine aminotransferase ratio)<br>FIB-4 score<br>Fibroindex<br>Forns score<br>VPR (varices prediction rule) |
| Imaging modality | Transient elastography<br>Two-dimensional shear-wave elastography<br>Magnetic resonance elastography<br>LSM (liver stiffness measurement) as determined by Fibroscan[R] |
| Indices that combine serum and imaging parameters | CPR (clinical prediction rule)<br>LSPS (LSM-spleen diameter to platelet ratio score) |

AA ratio, Fib-4 index, Fibroindex, Forns index, varices prediction rule (VPR), etc.] [18, 20, 21]. Furthermore, some reports stressed the efficacy of predicting the presence of varices by a combination of these parameters [clinical prediction rule (CPR), liver stiffness-spleen size-to-platelet ratio score (LSPS)] [19, 22, 23]. These methods are all indirect barometers of indicating the presence of portal hypertension, but they are suboptimal tools to show the possibility of severe bleeding complications in pediatric patients with biliary atresia. The true efficacy of these parameters is not well estimated in patients with biliary atresia, but they are less-invasive parameters compared with endoscopic evaluation and may be useful as the first line of screening. Hence, it is useful for all doctors and caregivers of patients with biliary atresia to keep this strategy in mind.

**4-2.** Endoscopy of the upper gastrointestinal tract is the most efficient examination for detecting the presence of esophageal and gastric varices [24–35, 37–43] and it also reveals other mucosal lesions such as gastric/duodenal ulcer and portal hypertensive gastropathy [13]. Especially in emergency cases where acute bleeding is suspected from the GI tract, endoscopic examination is essential and successive proper treatment must be performed according to the type of mucosal lesion. Endoscopic treatment is also performed periodically to prevent bleeding from varices (primary prophylaxis) and to prevent recurrent bleeding after acute bleeding from esophageal varices. Primary prophylaxis in which periodic endoscopic examinations are performed in patients with biliary atresia who had undergone portoenterostomy, is most effective for preventing GI bleeding from varices, and many institutes treating such patients in Japan have adopted this approach. However, its scientific efficacy has not been proven, repeated general anesthesia procedures may be harmful for the patients, and the cost-performance issue over the long term has been discussed and should be discussed further in the future. As described in the former section, alternative barometers that can predict the progression of portal hypertension and esophageal varices will be adopted widely in the future if they are demonstrated to strictly show the pathophysiological changes in mesenteric/portal venous blood flow that cause esophageal and gastric varices. Endoscopic examination is the gold standard method of diagnosing the presence of varices and makes direct treatment of varices with the least invasion possible. In primary prophylaxis, endoscopic findings of various esophageal varices are empirically classified into three stages [44]: F1 (small straight varices), F2 (enlarged, tortuous varices that occupy less than one-third of the lumen), F3 (large, coil-shaped varices that occupy more than one-third of the lumen). In addition to this criterion, "red-signs" (i.e., red wale marking or red color spot, hematocystic spot, and diffuse erythema, which are believed to have a high risk of bleeding) [44] and severely deteriorated liver function should be considered together to judge the total risk for variceal bleeding.

Portal hypertensive gastropathy is a specific mucosal lesion that is believed to occur in patients with cirrhotic liver but its exact pathophysiological features are not yet apparent. We must keep this lesion in mind if patients show chronic iron deficiency anemia. Acute bleeding from this lesion is uncommon but may occur according to a recent study [ 13].

Another important type of GI bleeding is Roux-en-Y jejunal loop bleeding. After portoenterostomy, the raised jejunal loop may be a focus of bleeding and its anatomical site makes the endoscopic approach difficult. Abdominal contrast-enhanced CT may suggest abnormal dilatation of the superior mesenteric vein. If intractable bleeding occurs in this area, emergency liver transplantation should be considered to rescue the patient.

## 32.5 Treatment of Acute GI Tract Bleeding (Table 32.2)

### 32.5.1 Acute Variceal Bleeding

If a patient with biliary atresia who had undergone portoenterostomy develops acute variceal bleeding, a standard resuscitation method should be rapidly applied to maintain the circulating volume and to protect the airway. It is better to access the central venous route and pressure monitoring should be started. Blood and colloid transfusion must be considered to maintain acceptable circulation. A nasogastric tube is inserted to aspirate gastric contents. If needed, pharmacological therapy should be administered to lower the pressure of the portal venous system such as octreotide, vasopressin, or terlipressin. Once circulation is restored and the hemodynamic state stabilizes, upper GI endoscopy should be performed without delay. If the bleeding is mas-

Table 32.2 Treatment options for esophageal varices

| | | |
|---|---|---|
| **Pharmacological therapy** | | **Beta-blocker**<br>**Nitrates**<br>**Vasopressin**<br>**Terlipressin**<br>**Somatostatin**<br>**Octreotide** |
| **Endoscopic therapy** | **For acute bleeding**<br>**Prevent recurrent bleeding**<br>**Primary prophylaxis** | **Band ligation**<br>**Injection sclerotherapy** |
| **TIPS (transjugular intrahepatic portosystemic shunting)** | | |
| **Shunt operation** | | **Meso-caval shunt**<br>**Spleno-renal shunt** |
| **Liver transplantation** | | |

sive and a stable circulatory state cannot be obtained, balloon tamponade (using the Sengstaken-Blakemore tube) is an option. This method is effective in gaining transient control of bleeding with high probability and makes the successive endoscopic treatment possible.

### 32.5.2 Endoscopic Treatment

To identify the lesion that is responsible for bleeding, it is necessary to perform upper GI endoscopy.

When esophageal variceal bleeding is confirmed, injection sclerotherapy or variceal banding should be performed. Injection sclerotherapy has a long history of about 50 years in pediatric practice and it can be performed in two different ways, intra-variceal and para-variceal injection. The most widely used sclerosant is 5% ethanolamine oleate, which is injected by retractile needles through the operating channel of the fiber. It was reported that control of acute bleeding by this method was quite effective in pediatric patients [24, 26]. Injection sclerotherapy has a longer history, but recently it has been replaced by the variceal banding method because sclerotherapy causes severe esophageal constriction with repetitive therapy and the banding method is safer than sclerotherapy. The variceal banding method was first reported in 1989 [36] and several reports were published that showed its safety and efficacy in pediatric cirrhotic patients [25, 30]. Now the variceal banding method is widely performed in the pediatric field. This method is superior to sclerotic therapy because once bleeding is controlled, visibility of the mucosa dramatically improves. One point that should be kept in mind is that in smaller children, the diameter of the band-loaded apparatus is too large to pass through the esophageal orifice of the patients and sclerotherapy is the only possible method for treatment [30].

Once the variceal bleeding is under control, prophylactic therapy should be planned carefully because the recurrent bleeding rate was reported to be high in pediatric patients [5]. Endoscopic treatments should be scheduled once every 2 to 4 weeks until the varices are eradicated. Long-term follow-up is also needed in these patients.

### 32.5.3 Transjugular Intrahepatic Portosystemic Shunting

In adult patients with cirrhosis who were admitted for acute variceal bleeding, transjugular intrahepatic portosystemic shunting (TIPS) was demonstrated to be a useful tool to reduce portal pressure if endoscopic treatment and/or pharmacologic treatment for hemostasis failed [45]. TIPS has not been performed in many pediatric patients, but a recent report commented about its feasibility and effect in pediatric and adolescent patients as a bridge to liver transplantation [46]. The effectiveness and feasibility of TIPS in pediatric patients should be addressed in the future by a scientific planned study.

### 32.5.4 Liver Transplantation

Liver transplantation is a definitive treatment that restores hepatic blood flow and reduces portal pressure in patients with liver disease [47, 48]. When acute bleeding from the jejunal loop occurs and conservative therapy is not effective, emergency living donor liver transplantation is planned in Japan, where brain-dead cadavers cannot be easily obtained in a short period of time after bleeding [14]. As living donor liver transplantation is a burden to the donor, it should be carefully planned under strict indication criteria. Some reports commented that esophageal bleeding itself was not a strict indicator for liver transplantation. Considering this bleeding complication and residual hepatic functions together, the indication for liver transplantation should be decided carefully. Also, it is still controversial in what situations primary prophylaxis for GI bleeding by endoscopy before liver transplantation is needed and a prospective study to resolve this issue is required in the future [47, 48].

### 32.5.5 Another Shunting Operation

A portosystemic shunt, such as a splenorenal shunt or mesocaval shunt, may be considered in limited cases in order to reduce portal pressure. The indication for portosystemic shunting operation is now limited to main cases with congenital hepatic fibrosis and portal thrombosis/obstruction. Portosystemic shunting operation is the last option to reduce portal pressure in patients with biliary atresia when all other treatments have failed.

## 32.6 Strategy for Preventing Recurrent Bleeding and Primary Prophylaxis for Variceal Bleeding (Table 32.2) [32, 33, 34]

The following strategy was developed based on the fact that the recurrent variceal bleeding rate is very high in pediatric patients [5] and that almost all patients with biliary atresia have liver fibrosis. Some reports showed that portal hypertension was induced within a few years after Kasai operation in patients with poor bile drainage. Pharmacological prophylaxis using a β-blocker is now accepted in adult patients with esophageal varices, but in pediatric patients there are little scientific data reported and the effect of β-blockers should be considered modest [49, 50].

If high-risk varices, such as F3 varices or F2 varices with red sign, are found in pediatric patients with liver cirrhosis and portal hypertension, periodic endoscopic treatments may be safe and effective [25, 26, 28, 33, 34]. Nowadays, band ligation may be the first choice of endoscopic treatment [34].

The idea that all patients with native liver after portoenterostomy should undergo periodic endoscopic examinations to check for the presence of esophageal and gastric varices is controversial. As described earlier, an effective predictor of variceal formation may be useful to screen patients as to whether they have clinically significant varices or not, and selective patients with some risk factors should undergo periodic endoscopic examinations.

Liver transplantation has now become a popular and acceptable treatment for patients who had undergone portoenterostomy with hepatic failure. The risk of variceal bleeding has become less important than before and periodic endoscopic examinations may be essential for transplant candidates to prevent variceal bleeding until the planned date of liver transplantation.

## References


1. Howard ER, Davenport M. The treatment of biliary atresia in Europe 1969-1995. Tohoku J Exp Med. 1997;181:75–83.
2. Sasaki H, Tanaka H, Nio M. Current management of long-term survivors of biliary atresia: over 40 years of experience in a single center and review of the literature. Pediatr Surg Int. 2017;33:1327–33.
3. Parolini F, Boroni G, Milianti S, Tonegatti L, Armellini A, Magne MG, Pedersini P, Torri F, Orizio P, Benvenuti S, De Previde Prato DM, Alberti D. Biliary atresia: 20-40-year follow-up with native liver in an Italian centre. J Pediatr Surg. 2019;54:1440–4.
4. Sasaki H, Tanaka H, Wada M, Kazama T, Nakamura M, Kudo R, Sakurai T, Nio M. Analysis of the prognostic factors of long-term native liver survivors of biliary atresia. Pediatr Surg Int. 2016;32:839–43.
5. McKiernan PJ. Treatment of variceal bleeding. Pediatr Gastrointest Endosc. 2001;11:789–812.
6. De Franchis R. Expanding consensus in portal hypertension. Report of Baveno VI consensus workshop: stratifying risk and individualizing care for portal hypertension. J Hepatology. 2015;63:743–52.
7. Garcia-Tsao G, Abraldes JG, Berzigotti A, Bosch J. Portal hypertensive bleeding in cirrhosis: risk stratification, diagnosis, and management: 2016 practice guidance by the American association for the study of liver diseases. Hepatology. 2017;65:310–35.
8. Shneider BL, de Ville de Goyet J, Leung DH, Srivastava A, Ling SC, Duche M, McKiernen P, Superina R, Squires RH, Bosch J, Groszmann R, Sarin SK, de Franchis R, Mazariegos GV. Primary prophylaxis of variceal bleeding in children and the role of MesoRex bypass: summery of the Baveno VI pediatric satellite symposium. Hapatology. 2016;63:1368–80.
9. Wiest R, Groszmann RJ. Nitric oxide and portal hypertension: its role in the regulation of intrahepatic and splanchnic vascular resistance. Semin Liver Dis. 1999;19:411–26.
10. Garcia-Tsao G, Groszmann RJ, Fisher RI, Conn HO, Atterbury CE, Glickman M. Portal pressure, presence of gastroesophageal varices and variceal bleeding. Hepatology. 1985;5:419–24.
11. Ohi R, Mochizuki I, Komatsu K, Kasai M. Portal hypertension after successful hepatic portoenterostomy in biliary atresia. J Pediatr Surg. 1986;21:271–4.
12. Stringer MD, Howard ER, Mowat AP. Endoscopic sclerotherapy in the management of esophageal varices in 61 children with biliary atresia. J Pediatr Surg. 1989;24:438–42.
13. Rockey DC. Portal hypertensive gastropathy and colonopathy. Clin Liver Dis. 2019;23:643–58.
14. Sanada Y, Mizuta K, Urahashi T, Ihara Y, Wakiya T, Okada N, Yamada N, Egami S, Ushijima K, Otomo S, Sakamoto K, Yasuda Y, Kawarasaki H. Indication of liver transplantation for jaundice-free biliary atresia with portal hypertension. Ann Transplant. 2011;16:7–11.
15. Chongsrisawat V, Vejapipat P, Siripon N, Poovorawan Y. Transient elastography for predicting esophageal/gastric varices in children with biliary atresia. BMC Gastroentorol. 2011;11:41.
16. Yokoyama S, Ishigami M, Honda T, Kuzuya T, Ishizu Y, Ito T, Hirooka Y, Tanaka Y, Tainaka T, Shirota C, Chiba K, Uchida H, Fujishiro M. Spleen stiffness by 2-D shear elastography is the most accurate predictor of high esophagogastric varices in children with biliary atresia. Hepatology Res. 2019;49:1162–8.

17. Yoon H, Shin HJ, Kim MJ, Han SJ, Koh H, Kim S, Lee MJ. Predicting gastroesophageal varices through spleen magnetic resonance elastography in pediatric liver fibrosis. World J Gastroenterol. 2019;25:367–77.
18. Deng H, Qi X, Guo X. Diagnostic accuracy of APRI, AAR, FIB-4, FI, King, Lok, Forns, and FibroIndex scores in predicting the presence of esophageal varices in liver cirrhosis. Medicine. 2015;94:1–12.
19. Isted A, Grammatikopoulos T, Davenport M. Prediction of esophageal varices in biliary atresia: derivation of the "varices prediction rule", a novel noninvasive predictor. J Pediatr Surg. 2015;50:1734–8.
20. Chiou FK, Ong C, Low Y, Chiang LW, Phua KB. Non-invasive predictors for the first variceal hemorrhage in children with biliary atresia after Kasai portoenterostomy. J Clin Exp Hepatol. 2019;9:581–7.
21. Tomita H, Fuchimoto Y, Fujino A, Hoshino K, Yamada Y, Masugi Y, Sakamoto M, Kasahara M, Kanamori Y, Nakazawa A, Yoshida F, Akatsuka S, Nakano M, Kuroda T. Development and validation of a novel fibrosis marker in biliary atresia during infancy. Clin Translat Gastroenterol. 2015;6:e127.
22. Colecchia A, Di Biase AR, Scaioli E, Predieri B, Iughetti L, Reggiani MLB, Montrone L, Ceccarelli PL, Vestito A, Viola L, Paolucci P, Festi D. Non-invasive methods can predict oesophageal varices in petients with biliary atresia after Kasai procedure. Dig Liver Dis. 2011;43:659–63.
23. Hukkinen M, Lohi J, Heikkila P, Kivisaari R, Jahnukainen T, Jalanko H, Pakarinen MP. Noninvasive evaluation of liver fibrosis and portal hypertension after successful portoenterostomy for biliary atresia. Hepatology commun. 2019;3:382–91.
24. Goncalves MEP, Cardoso SR, Maksoud JG. Prophylactic sclerotherapy in children with esophageal varices: long-term results of a controlled prospective randomized trial. J Pediatr Surg. 2000;35:401–5.
25. Celinska-Cerdro D, Teisseyre M, Woynarowski M, Socha P, Ryzko J. Endoscopic ligation of esophageal varices for prophylaxis of first bleeding in children and adolescents with portal hypertension: preliminary results of a prospective study. J Pediatr Surg. 2003;38:1008–11.
26. Duche M, Habes D, Roulleau P, Haas V, Jacquemin E, Bernard O. Prophylactic endoscopic sclerotherapy of large esophagogastric varices in infants with biliary atresia. Gastrointest Endosco. 2008;67:732–7.
27. Duche M, Ducot B, Tournay E, Fabre M, Cohen J, Jacquemin E, Bernard O. Prognostic value of endoscopy in children with biliary atresia at risk for early development of varices and bleeding. Gastroenterology. 2010;139:1952–60.
28. Lampela H, Kosola S, Koivusalo A, Lauronen J, Jalanko H, RintalaR PMP. Endoscopic surveillance and primary prophylaxis sclerotherapy of esophageal varices in biliary atresia. J Pediatr Gastroenterol Nutr. 2012;55:574–9.
29. Duche M, Ducot B, Ackermann O, Baujard C, Chevret L, Frank-Soltysiak M, Jaquemin E, Bernard O. Experience with endoscopic management of high-risk gastroesophageal varices, with and without bleeding, in children with biliary atresia. Gasroenterology. 2013;145:801–7.
30. Kim SJ, Kim KM. Recent trends in the endoscopic management of variceal bleeding in children. Pediatr Gastroenterol Hepatol. 2013;16:1–9.
31. Kim SJ, Oh SH, Jo JM, Kim KM. Experiences with endoscopic interventions for variceal bleeding in children with portal hypertension: a single center study. Pediatr Gastroenterol Hepatol. 2013;16:248–53.
32. Duche M, Ducot B, Ackermann O, Jacquemin E, Bernard O. Progression to high-risk gastroesophageal varices in children with biliary atresia with low-risk signs at first endoscopy. J Pediatr Gastroenterol Nutr. 2015;60:664–8.
33. Duche M, Ducot B, Ackermann O, Guerin F, Jacquemin E, Bernard O. Portal hypertension in children: high-risk varices, primary prophylaxis and consequences of bleeding. J Hepatol. 2017;66:320–7.
34. Jeanniard-Maret O, Duche M, Fabre A. Survey on clinical practice of primary prophylaxis in portal hypertension in children. J Pediatr Gastroenterol Nutr. 2017;64:524–7.
35. Wanty C, Helleputte T, Smets F, Sokal EM, Stephenne X. Assessment of risk of bleeding from esophageal varices during management of biliary atresia in children. J Pediatr Gastroenterol Nutr. 2013;56:537–43.
36. Stiegmann GV, Goff JS, Sun JH, Davis D, Bozdech J. Endoscopic variceal ligation: an alternative to sclerotherapy. Gastrointest Endosc. 1989;35:431–4.
37. Cano I, Urruzuno P, Medina E, Vilarino A, Benavent MI, Manzanares J, Berchi FJ. Treatment of esophageal varices by endoscopic ligation in children. Eur J Pediatr Surg. 1995;5:299–302.
38. Fox VL, Carr-Locke DL, Connors PJ, Leichtner AM. Endoscopic ligation of esophageal varices in children. J Pediatr Gastroenterol Nutr. 1995;20:202–8.
39. Nijhawan S, Patni T, Sharma U, Rai RR, Miglani N. Endoscopic variceal ligation in children. J Pediatr Surg. 1995;30:1455–6.
40. Price MR, Sartorelli KH, Karrer FM, Narkewicz MR, Sokol RJ, Lilly JR. Management od esophageal varices in children by endoscopic variceal ligation. J Pediatr Surg. 1996;31:1056–9.
41. Reinoso MA, Sharp HI, Rank J. Endoscopic variceal ligation in pediatric patients with portal hypertension secondary to liver cirrhosis. Gastrintest Endosc. 1997;46:244–6.
42. Sasaki T, Hasegawa T, Nakajima K, Tanano H, Wasa M, Fukui Y, Okada A. Endoscopic variceal ligation in the management of gastroesophageal varices in postoperative biliary atresia. J Pediatr Surg. 1998;33:1628–32.
43. McKiernan P, Davison SM. A prospective study of endoscopic esophageal variceal ligation using a multi-band ligator. J Pedaiatr Gastroenterol Nutr. 1999;28:583.
44. Howard ER, Stringer MD, Mowat AP. Assessment of injection sclerotherapy in the management of 152 children with esophageal varices. Br J Surg. 1988;75:404–8.
45. Hernandez-Gea V, Procoper B, Giraldez A, Amitrano L, Vilanuera C, Thabut D, Ibanez-Samaniego L, et al. Preemptive-TIPS improves outcome in high-risk variceal bleeding: an observational study. Hepatology. 2019;69:282–93.
46. Bertino F, Hawkins M, Shivaram G, Gill AE, Lungren MP, Reposar A, Sze D, Hwang GL, Koo K, Monroe E. Technical feasibility and clinical effectiveness of transjugular intrahepatic portosystemic shunt creation in pediatric and adolescent patients. J Vasc Interv Radiol. 2019;30:178–86.
47. Hui Ng NB, Karthik SV, Aw MM, Quak SH. Endoscopic evaluation in children with end-stage liver disease-associated portal hypertension awaiting liver transplant. J Pediatr Gastroenterol Nutr. 2016;63:365–9.
48. Angelico R, Pietrobattista A, Candusso M, Tomarchio S, Pellicciaro M, Liccardo D, Basso MS, Grimaldi C, Saffioti MC, Torroni F, Dall'Oglio L, Torre G, Spada M. Primary prophylaxis for gastrointestinal bleeding in children with biliary atresia and portal hypertension candidates for liver transplantation: a single-center experience. Transplant Proc. 2019;51:171–8.
49. Shashidhar H, Langhans N, Grand RJ. Propranolol in prevention of portal hypertensive hemorrhage in children: a pilot study. J Pediatr Gastroenterol Nutr. 1999;29:12–7.
50. Samanta T, Purkait R, Sarkar M, Misra A, Ganguly S. Effectiveness of beta blockers in primary prophylaxis of variceal bleeding in children with portal hypertension. Tropical Gastroenterol 2011;

# Long-Term Complications: Hypersplenism

33

Akira Nishi

**Abstract**

Hypersplenism is often seen as a long-term complication after surgery for biliary atresia (BA). Treatment is based on liver function, platelet count, and complications, current treatment options include partial splenic embolization (PSE) and a liver transplant. Although the results of PSE are good, long-term regular follow-up while considering a liver transplant is necessary.

**Keywords**

Biliary atresia · Hypersplenism · Partial splenic embolization

## 33.1 Epidemiology

Patients with biliary atresia (BA) already have a variable grade of hepatic fibrosis at the time of the hepatoportoenterostomy (HPE). In addition, hepatic fibrosis often progresses in both successful and failed HPE. Consequently, the patient may develop portal hypertension, which is the most serious late complication of HPE, even in jaundice-free survivors of BA. Esophageal varices and hypersplenism are known sequelae of portal hypertension.

Hypersplenism is investigated because of the presence of splenomegaly, thrombocytopenia, or complications from hypersplenism, and during therapeutic intervention, but its definition is not consistent. In long-term survivors of BA, the incidence of portal hypertension varies from 34% to 76% and the incidence of hypersplenism varies from 19.6% to 35% [1–3].

Hypersplenism often appears in early childhood after a HPE, and its incidence tends to increase with the increase in portal pressure at the HPE. In addition, the onset of splenomegaly is greatly influenced by early complications [4].

Many centers now perform liver transplants in infants with BA who have poor bile excretion and severe cirrhosis after a HPE. A liver transplant to treat poor bile excretion early in the case prevents the complication of portal hypertension, resulting in a reduction in the severity of hypersplenism. When liver transplants were not widely performed, hypersplenism was treated in patients with severe cirrhosis caused by BA. Therefore, the criteria, frequency, and results of intervention to treat hypersplenism are different from those in the 1990s.

## 33.2 Pathophysiology

Hypersplenism was formerly considered simply a consequence of passive congestion due to increased portal venous pressure. However, the size of and flow in the splenic artery are actually increased due to the increased splenic blood flow, and oxygen saturation in the splenic vein is high [5] (not low, as if flow to the liver is stagnant). There is a poor correlation between the size of the spleen and the level of portal pressure or the degree of hepatic fibrosis. On the other hand, there is a close correlation between splenic arterial flow and the degree of splenomegaly. Splenic arterial flow increases with the increased demand for blood flow because of splenic hypertrophy. Consequently, visceral flow and portal pressure are increased, resulting in even more splenomegaly.

## 33.3 Diagnosis

A diagnosis of hypersplenism is often based on the presence of splenomegaly or thrombocytopenia and the occurrence of complications, but there are various definitions of hypersplenism.

Many reports [1, 6] define thrombocytopenia as a platelet count of <50,000/μl. Spleen size is evaluated by abdominal

A. Nishi (✉)
Gunma Children's medical center, Department of surgery, Shibukawa, Gunma, Japan
e-mail: anishi@gcmc.pref.gunma.jp


M. Nio (ed.), *Introduction to Biliary Atresia*, https://doi.org/10.1007/978-981-16-2160-4_33

palpation, ultrasonography, and computed tomography (CT), where the latter is more objective but more invasive. The criterion for a diagnosis of splenomegaly in adults is a spleen volume of ≥400 $cm^3$, whereas in children, the diagnosis depends on the physical size of the child. Schlesinger and colleagues [7] calculated the spleen volume from CT images and showed that it has a strong correlation with the body weight of the patient. As a result, they defined the upper limit of the 95% tolerance interval for spleen volume in children as spleen volume ($cm^3$) = [4.5 × weight (kg)] + 150.

Rosenberg and colleagues [8] propose using the vertical length of the spleen on an ultrasound image as a simple assessment. As a result, their guidelines for the upper limit of the normal length of the spleen are as follows: length ≤6 cm at 3 months, 6.5 cm at 6 months, and 7.0 cm at 12 months, 8.0 cm at 2 years, 9.0 cm at 4 years, 9.5 cm at 6 years, 10.0 cm at 8 years, 11.0 cm at 10 years, 11.5 cm at 12 years, 12.0 cm at 15 years or older for girls, and 13.0 cm at 15 years or older for boys.

For an outpatient clinic diagnosis, splenomegaly is suspected when the spleen can be felt 2 cm or more under the left subcostal region.

## 33.4 Treatment

### 33.4.1 Indication

Many authors reported treating splenomegaly when the platelet count was <50,000/μl and there was a tendency toward bleeding [1, 6]. On the other hand, treatment is indicated sometimes by thrombocytopenia alone, even without the tendency toward bleeding, and sometimes when complications due to portal hypertension are relieved by reducing portal pressure. In most cases, indications for the treatment of splenomegaly are relative and determined by careful clinical judgment.

### 33.4.2 Surgery for Hypersplenism

Until about 1990, splenectomy and shunt surgery were the main treatments for hypersplenism. Overwhelming infection is a late complication of splenectomy. A pneumococcal vaccination is recommended to prevent overwhelming infection, which can be fatal, but it cannot completely prevent overwhelming infection. On the other hand, development of encephalopathy is a long-term risk of shunt surgery [9]. The longer the follow-up period, the higher the incidence of both rebleeding and encephalopathy. In addition, the shunt procedure interferes with a subsequent liver transplant. To avoid an overwhelming infection after a splenectomy and encephalopathy after major shunt surgery, the indications for these procedures are limited [1].

Transjugular intrahepatic portosystemic shunt (TIPS) is an alternative shunt treatment for adults. However, its use in infants with BA is extremely limited by the technical difficulties of the procedure due to the size of the infant and the risk of encephalopathy in the long term, as with shunt surgery.

White et al. [10] in 1981 and Stellin et al. [11] in 1982 reported on the use of partial splenic embolization (PSE) in children and its superior results. Currently, PSE is the first choice for the treatment of pediatric hypersplenism when there is good liver function.

The long-term results of a liver transplant to treat end-stage liver disease have improved dramatically, even in children, because of improvements in surgical techniques and postoperative management. The 1-year survival rate for children after a liver transplant is between 75% and 90% [12]. Liver transplantation offers the opportunity for long-term survival and, therefore, alters the therapeutic approach for cases of BA with cirrhosis and complications of portal hypertension.

Although a liver transplant is an ultimate treatment for portal hypertension, relative portal hypertension remains when the transplant is relatively small, in addition to increased blood flow in the spleen. In some cases, the liver transplant does not resolve the hypersplenism. A study of spleen size after a liver transplant found that 44% of the patients had a normal recovery [13]. If necessary, a splenectomy and PSE before and after the liver transplant may be considered. These interventions may control portal blood flow and improve liver function [14, 15].

### 33.4.3 Partial Splenic Embolization

Splenectomy is no longer used to manage secondary hypersplenism because of the recognized hazard of post-splenectomy sepsis in children. Consequently, embolization methods aimed at eliminating hypersplenism while conserving splenic immune function have been developed.

In 1973, Maddison [16] was the first to perform embolization to treat hypersplenism using an autologous blood clot. Improvements in methods and materials have made splenic embolization the treatment of choice for clinically significant hypersplenism in children [10, 11]. In the technique, injected Gelfoam particles embolize into splenic artery radicles until 60%–80% splenic infarction is achieved. Immediate postembolization morbidity, including fever and pain, is significant. In one study, almost all the children had an elevated temperature (38°C or higher) significantly longer than adults (mean of 23.7 days). Lower-left-lobe atelectasis and pleural effusions, a mild increase in amylase, prolonged ileus, and sterile subdiaphragmatic fluid collection were sometimes observed. Major complications such as splenic rupture and splenic abscess were rare but hospitalization was prolonged (average of 16 days). Postsplenectomy sepsis did not develop during long-term follow-up [17].

If PSE is performed in the early stages of hypersplenism, a more aggressive embolization can be avoided and the complications of PSE can be reduced [18]. In addition, PSE is less invasive than a splenectomy and thus can be performed sooner.

PSE is expected to improve blood flow in the spleen, control portal blood flow, improve liver function, and reduce collateral blood flow [15, 19]. In addition, the decrease in endothelin derived from the spleen should cause a decrease in portal pressure [20], and the increase in platelets should improve liver regeneration [21].

## 33.5 Results

Partial splenic embolization is effective in controlling hypersplenism. The beneficial effects of PSE on the blood cell counts and the tendency toward bleeding are evident.

Recurrence of thrombocytopenia after PSE, which depends on the state of liver cirrhosis and portal hypertension, has been reported to be 12.5%–30.6% [18, 22]. The recurrence of thrombocytopenia can be controlled by a second PSE procedure but many cases experience a relapse. Nio et al. [22] reported that there was no significant difference in the volume embolized or the platelet count before PSE between the patients who did and did not have a recurrence of thrombocytopenia, and that the peak platelet count after PSE was significantly lower in the patients who had a recurrence of thrombocytopenia.

According to Sasaki et al. [23], the incidence of hypersplenism after HPE that required intervention until the patient with BA reached 10 years of age was significantly different between 20-year-old patients with and without an autologous liver, but the difference was not a significant prognostic factor in multivariate analysis. Even in cases of BA requiring PSE, long-term survival of the autologous liver is possible with proper control of the cirrhosis if it has not progressed.

The final prognosis of native liver survival in BA patients after HPE depends on liver function and pulmonary complications rather than on hypersplenism. Because pulmonary complications secondary to portal hypertension may change the indication for the use of a liver transplant, early detection and proper control of hypersplenism are required for the correct timing of a liver transplant.

## 33.6 Conclusion

The presence and severity of sequelae due to hypersplenism should be carefully examined to determine what therapeutics are indicated while considering liver function.

## References


1. Ohi R, Nio M. The jaundiced infant: biliary atresia and other obstructions. In: O'Neill JA, editor. Pediatric Surgery, vol. 2. 5th ed. Maryland Heights, MO: Mosby; 1998. p. 1465–81.
2. Ohi R. Biliary atresia. A surgical perspective. Clin Liver Dis. 2000;4(4):779–804.
3. Shneider BL, Abel B, Haber B, et al. Portal hypertension in children and young adults with biliary atresia. J Pediatr Gastroenterol Nutr. 2012;55(5):567–73.
4. Chiba T, Ohi R, Nio M, et al. Late complications in long-term survivors of biliary atresia. Eur J Pediatr Surg. 1992;2(1):22–5.
5. Karrer FM. Portal hypertension. Semin Pediatr Surg. 1992;1(2):134–44.
6. Matsuo S, Suita S, Kubota M, et al. Long-term results and clinical problems after portoenterostomy in patients with biliary atresia. Eur J Pediatr Surg. 1998;8(3):142–5.
7. Schlesinger AE, Edgar KA, Boxer LA. Volume of the spleen in children as measured on CT scans: normal standards as a function of body weight. AJR Am J Roentgenol. 1993;160(5):1107–9.
8. Rosenberg HK, Markowitz RI, Kolberg H, et al. Normal splenic size in infants and children: sonographic measurements. AJR Am J Roentgenol. 1991;157(1):119–21.
9. Hassall E, Benson L, Hart M, et al. Hepatic encephalopathy after portacaval shunt in a noncirrhotic child. J Pediatr. 1984;105(3):439–41.
10. White JJ, Goldman ML, Lepow M. Correction of hypersplenism without splenectomy. J Pediatr Surg. 1981;16(6):967.
11. Stellin G, Kumpe DA, Lilly JR. Splenic embolization in a child with hypersplenism. J Pediatr Surg. 1982;17(6):892–3.
12. Karrer FM. Portal hypertension. Semin Pediatr Surg. 1992;1(2):134–44.
13. Chezmar JL, Redvanly RD, Nelson RC. Persistence of portosystemic collaterals and splenomegaly on CT after orthotopic liver transplantation. AJR Am J Roentgenol. 1992;159(2):317–20.
14. Sockrider CS, Boykin KN, Green J, et al. Partial splenic embolization for hypersplenism after liver transplantation. Transplant Proc. 2001;33(7-8):3472–3.
15. Chikamori F, Kuniyoshi N, Kawashima T, et al. Short-term portal hemodynamic effects of partial splenic embolization for hypersplenism. Hepatogastroenterology. 2007;54(78):1847–9.
16. Maddison FE. Embolic therapy of hypersplenism. Invest Radiol. 1973;8:280–1.
17. Kumpe DA, Rumack CM, Pretorius DH, et al. Partial splenic embolization in children with hypersplenism. Radiology. 1985;155(2):357–62.
18. Petersons A, Volrats O, Bernsteins A. The first experience with non-operative treatment of hypersplenism in children with portal hypertension. Eur J Pediatr Surg. 2002;12(5):299–303.
19. Tajiri T, Onda M, Yoshida H, et al. Long-term hematological and biochemical effects of partial splenic embolization in hepatic cirrhosis. Hepatogastroenterology. 2002;49(47):1445–8.
20. Nagasue N, Dhar DK, Yamanoi A, et al. Production and release of endothelin-1 from the gut and spleen in portal hypertension due to cirrhosis. Hepatology. 2000;31(5):1107–14.
21. Matsuo R, Ohkohchi N, Murata S, et al. Platelets strongly induce hepatocyte proliferation with IGF-1 and HGF in vitro. J Surg Res. 2008;145(2):279–86.
22. Nio M, Hayashi Y, Sano N, et al. Long-term efficacy of partial splenic embolization in children. J Pediatr Surg. 2003;38(12):1760–2.
23. Sasaki H, Tanaka H, Wada M, et al. Analysis of the prognostic factors of long-term native liver survival in survivors of biliary atresia. Pediatr Surg Int. 2016;32(9):839–43.

# Long-Term Complications: Cholangitis/Gall Stones

34

Minoru Kuroiwa

**Abstract**

Long-term survivors after surgery for biliary atresia sometimes develop cholangitis associated with intrahepatic biliary cysts (IBCs). In early adolescence and adulthood, IBCs frequently have biliary calculi (gall stones), which makes cholangitis treatment difficult. Herein, the etiology, pathophysiology, and treatment options for late-presenting cholangitis and gall stones have been discussed.

**Keywords**

Biliary atresia · Complications · Cholangitis · Gallstone · Hepatolithiasis · Intrahepatic biliary cysts · Bile lake

## 34.1 Introduction

The proportion of biliary atresia (BA) survivors with a native liver after the Kasai operation (hepatic portoenterostomy) has been increasing. However, according to a recent report from the Japanese Biliary Atresia Registry [1], approximately 40% of such patients needed liver transplantation (LTx) within the first five years after Kasai operation. The remaining patients survived for five years or longer with a native liver. Although bile flow is restored, and jaundice disappeared after the Kasai operation, some complications can affect the quality of life and prognosis of long-term survivors with a native liver. The most common conditions noted in these patients are cholangitis and portal hypertension. Late-presenting cholangitis can sometimes become a serious and refractory complication for long-term BA survivors after surgery [2]. The development of these complications can lead to hepatic failure and LTx. Herein, we discuss the occurrence of late-presenting cholangitis and gall stones in long-term BA survivors with a native liver and present a literature review.

M. Kuroiwa (✉)
Division of Pediatric Surgery, Toho University Omori Medical Center, Tokyo, Japan
e-mail: mkuro@med.toho-u.ac.jp

## 34.2 Pathogenesis and Etiology

### 34.2.1 Cholangitis

Cholangitis unexpectedly occurs as a common complication after Kasai operation and may affect short- and long-term outcomes, especially in children with BA. However, the pathogenesis of cholangitis is controversial and uncertain. It has been reported that it occurs in 30–60% of postoperative BA patients, most commonly in the first few years after surgery [3]. In contrast, late-onset cholangitis is sometimes seen in a considerable number of adult BA survivors with a native liver, resulting in portal hypertension and liver failure, which may lead to expedited LTx [4].

Cholangitis following a Kasai operation may occur because of the creation of the bilioenteric conduit. Additionally, in most cases, it is ascending in nature (also ascending cholangitis). Other principle mechanisms that have been implicated in its etiology include bacterial translocation through the lymphatic system and hematogenous spread through the portal venous system. These pathogens are derived from the intestinal bacterial flora such as *Escherichia coli*, *Klebsiella pneumoniae*, and *Pseudomonas aeruginosa* [5, 6]. Another report described that the blood culture was positive in 52% of patients with cholangitis, showing *Klebsiella* species as the most common organisms followed by *E. coli*, *P. aeruginosa*, and *Enterococcus*, or *Enterobacter* [7]. Further, it has recently been reported that the proportion of patients with obvious bacterial cholangitis is under 50%, except for one report [8]. Lykavieris et al. showed that overt bacterial cholangitis developed in 30.2% of long-term survivors over a period of 20 years [9].

In addition, fungal infection is also suggested as a possible cause of cholangitis. The same finding was reported in two patients, including a one-year-old child and a 19-year-


M. Nio (ed.), *Introduction to Biliary Atresia*, https://doi.org/10.1007/978-981-16-2160-4_34

old long-term survivor. Cholangitis in both these patients was recurrent and refractory to antibiotic treatment. The adult died of progressive liver failure due to persistent *Aspergillus* infection.

Some reports also suggest that the mechanical obstruction of the Roux-en-Y loop is rarely the cause of late presenting cholangitis. Loop obstruction in patients was initially reported by Gollaway et al. who presented a review of their experience with 15 patients in 1990. Nio et al. reported that 13 adult survivors with late-onset cholangitis and a native liver showing Roux loop pooling in isotope scan only temporarily responded to surgical adhesiolysis [10]. Some case series have reported deterioration of liver function, portal hypertension, and cholangitis during pregnancy or after delivery [11, 12].

Cholangitis occurring in long-term survivors with native livers is occasionally associated with IBCs, which is a condition called "bile lake." Long-time follow-up indicates that IBCs often develop after Kasai operation. Several reports have described a close relationship between IBCs and cholangitis. In addition, cholangitis in long-term survivors with IBCs is sometimes recurrent and refractory to treatment. These conditions (cholangitis and IBCs) are not fully understood in terms of etiology, and there is no consensus on the relationship between these complications. Previous studies have reported an IBC occurrence rate of 6.4% to 26% in patients [13], whereas the incidence of IBCs ranges from 6% to 28%. Inoue et al. [14] reported that patients develop initial BLCs at an average of 25.7 months after the Kasai operation. In addition, the mean interval between the first and second IBCs was 10.8 months. According to Ling et al. [15], the median age for finding IBCs was 1 year 4 months, with age ranging from 8 months to 14 years.

Although the pathophysiology of IBCs remains unclear, some hypotheses regarding the mechanism of IBCs have been explored (1) IBCs are formed secondary to the intrahepatic duct by a fibro-obliterated process; (2) the ongoing inflammatory process leads to intrahepatic biliary obstruction; (3) ductal plate malformation plays a role in cyst formation; (4) damaged bile ducts with calculi and inflammation fuse together, leading to IBCs [16].

IBCs are now detected in an early stage compared to that in the late 1990s due to active ultrasonography monitoring and routine MRIs. The most recent study has reported an incidence of 13%, accounting for a quarter of patients with frequently recurring cholangitis [16]. IBCs may be found in younger infants immediately after the Kasai operation as well as long-term survivors after over 20 years of surgery. Recurrent or sometimes refractory cholangitis has a significant impact on survival and quality of life in patients. Giström et al. [17] reported that the yearly cholangitis rate is significantly correlated with long-term survivors with a native liver, and the total number of cholangitis episodes also has a major impact on survival.

Tainaka et al. [18] suggested that IBCs are of two different types: solitary cysts and continuous beaded cysts, and the former is associated with poor prognosis, whereas the latter may be reversed. In addition, they noted that a differential diagnosis is crucial for determining a treatment strategy. Watanabe et al. [19] divided IBCs into three types according to morphological features including the number and shape of cysts. They also showed that treatment for IBCs is dependent on the association of cholangitis. In these cases, prognosis may be poor or there may be a need for liver transplantation in patients with infected multiple complicated cysts.

### 34.2.2 Gall Stones (Biliary Lithiasis, Intrahepatic Stone, or Hepatolithiasis)

Chronic infection and/or stenosis of the biliary system is the most likely cause of intrahepatic stone formation, as seen postoperatively in patients with congenital biliary dilatation. Because intrahepatic stones, biliary lithiasis, or hepatolithiasis were thought to be rare in BA patients after Kasai operation, these complications were paid little attention. However, pathological and bacteriological evidence from resected livers during LTx has shown that intrahepatic stones are more common than previously thought [20]. In some reports, biliary stones were present in half of the patients examined (8/15, 53%), bacteria in the bile were present in 5 (63%) patients, history of cholangitis was observable in 7 (88%), and in 6 of 10 patients (60%), the location of cholangitis was the porta hepatis. The authors speculate that bile stasis and bacterial infection are important for stone formation. Other reports [21, 22] also documented that biliary stones were frequently found in patients with IBCs.

In addition to intrahepatic stones, gallstones in the intestinal conduit, which is a condition called enterolithiasis, can be found in patients. Gallstones are formed in the Roux-en-Y limb and the interposed ileocecal appendix during hepatic portoduodenostomy. The etiological factors for this rare condition include a stapled antireflux valve in the Roux-en-Y limb, interposition of the ileocecal appendix, and bile congestion due to a gravid uterus.

### 34.2.3 Clinical Symptoms and Diagnosis

Cholangitis is generally characterized by fever, acholic stool, abdominal discomfort, pain with or without jaundice, and a positive blood culture ruling out other causes of infection. Lee et al. [7] defined cholangitis as fever (> 37.5 °C) or clinically worsening jaundice, and elevated transaminase or acholic stool. Liu et al. [2] strictly suggest that cholangitis is diagnosed when a combination of at least one of the following symptoms are present: (1) fever over 38 °C, (2) clinically worsened jaundice, and (3) elevated C-reactive protein. Recently, the measurement of urinary sulfated bile acids (USBA) has been reported as a simple and noninvasive test for cholangitis.

Intrahepatic biliary stones are frequently discovered on imaging examinations for recurrent and/or refractory cholangitis. Most BA patients with cholangitis present with early signs such as dilatation of the intrahepatic bile ducts and bile stasis, which ultimately leads to stone formation. Conventional methods such as diagnostic imaging for gall stones include ultrasound (US) and computed tomography (CT). In rare cases, for hepatolithiasis, cholangiography through double-balloon endoscopy may be performed. However, endoscopic retrograde cholangiography and percutaneous transhepatic cholangiography are invasive. Unlike these cholangiography techniques, magnetic resonance cholangiopancreatography (MRCP) is noninvasive and does not cause complications such as intestinal perforation, cholangitis, and sepsis.

However, CT scan is superior to MRCP for diagnosing intrahepatic biliary stones and enterolithiasis.

### 34.2.4 Treatments

Treatments for bacterial cholangitis include administration of intravenous antibiotics and high-dose steroids. Prompt intravenous administration of broad-spectrum antibiotics is needed to accelerate the clearance of jaundice and to improve long-term survival with a native liver.

Over the last two decades, the protocol for antibiotic treatment has been modified several times. In the early 1980s, second-generation cephalosporins with or without aminoglycosides were used. In the 1990s, third-generation cephalosporins, usually ceftriaxone or cefoperazone, were widely used with administration occasionally combined with aminoglycosides. In the 2000s, the effectiveness of sulfamethoxazole/trimethoprim (SMZ/TMP) or neomycin was reported by Bu et al. [23]. Subsequently, carbapenems (commonly called meropenem) were introduced as potential therapeutic agents for refractory cholangitis. Although we understand that the appropriate selection of antibiotics for cholangitis treatment is essential for good clinical outcomes [24], there is no consensus on a standard treatment regimen with defined drug protocol, duration of treatment, and clinical benefits.

Steroids have been used to augment antibiotic treatment for refractory cholangitis in BA patients for more than 20 years. Its pharmacological benefits include choleretic and anti-inflammatory effects. However, the efficacy of steroids in infants after Kasai operation is controversial and unclear. Additionally, there have been no reports on steroid efficacy in long-term survivors with native livers except for infants who received steroids immediately after the Kasai procedure.

Recurrent and/or refractory cholangitis occurring after many years of infection-free life in BA patients without jaundice indicates IBCs with gall stones, and a possible mechanical problem with the Roux-en-Y loop. BA patients should be fully investigated using US, MRCP, CT, and radionuclide imaging if needed. IBCs with cholangitis are conventionally treated with antibiotic administration and percutaneous transhepatic cholangio-drainage (PTCD). Watanabe et al. divided IBCs into three types based on morphology. Additionally, they emphasized the importance of cholangitis in the treatment for IBCs, predicting poor prognosis for patients with multiple complicated and infected cysts. However, single or multiple simple cysts without cholangitis do not need treatment. On the other hand, a simple cyst with cholangitis may require PTCD if antibiotics fail to improve infection. Multiple complicated cysts cannot be controlled with PTCD or other interventions, ultimately requiring LTx.

For a small number of patients undergoing surgical intervention, Giström et al. [17] recommended operative intestinal drainage for IBC-associated cholangitis, ensuring prolonged jaundice-free survival with a native liver. Hepatectomy, which is another surgical option, was performed in two cases of IBCs associated with intractable recurrent cholangitis [25, 26].

## 34.3 Conclusions

Despite an excellent long-term postoperative course, BA survivors with native livers often develop severe late complications that ultimately require liver transplantation. Cholangitis after Kasai operation is one such complication that can lead to poor prognosis and unexpected transplantation. Although numerous studies have focused on cholangitis in the past decades, its distinct pathogenesis remains unclear. Recurrent and/or refractory cholangitis in adulthood should be fully investigated for IBCs, gall stones, and abnormality of the Roux-en-Y limb using imaging modalities. Immediate treatment with appropriate therapeutic methods is strongly recommended in cholangitis patients with or without gall stones.

## References

1. Nio M. Japanese biliary atresia registry. Pediatr Surg Int. 2017;33:1319–25.
2. Liu J, Dong R, Chen G, et al. Risk factors and prognostic effects of cholangitis after Kasai procedure in biliary atresia: a retrospective clinical study. J Pediatr Surg. 2019;54:2559–64.

3. Ernest van Heurn LW, Saing H, PKH T. Cholangitis after hepatic portoenterostomy for biliary atresia: a multivariate analysis of risk factors. J Pediatr. 2003;142:566–71.
4. Kelay A, Davenport M. Long-term outlook in biliary atresia. Semin Pediatr Surg. 2017;26(5):295–300.
5. Chuang JH, Lee SY, Shieh CS, et al. Reappraisal of the role of the bilioenteric conduit in the pathogenesis of postoperative cholangitis. Pediatr Surg Int. 2000;16:29–34.
6. Wu ET, Chen HL, Ni YH, et al. Bacterial cholangitis in patients with biliary atresia: impact on short-term outcome. Pediatr Surg Int. 2001;17(5):390–5.
7. Lee JY, Lim LTK, Quak SH, et al. Cholangitis in children with biliary atresia: health-care resource utilization. J Pediatr Child Health. 2014;50:196–201.
8. Kumagi T, Drenth JPH, Guttman O, et al. Biliary atresia and survival into adulthood without transplantation: a collaborative multicentre clinic review. Liver Int. 2012;32(3):510–8.
9. Lykavieris P, Chardot C, Sokhn M, et al. Outcome in adulthood of biliary atresia: a study of 63 patients who survived for over 20 years with their native liver. Hepatology. 2005;41:366–72.
10. Nio M, Sano N, Ishii T, et al. Cholangitis as a late complication in long-term survivors after surgery for biliary atresia. J Pediatr Surg. 2004;39:1793–9.
11. Kuroda T, Saeki M, Morikawa N, et al. Management of adult biliary atresia patients: should hard work and pregnancy be discouraged? J Pediatr Surg. 2007;42:2106–9.
12. Shimaoka S, Ohi R, Saeki M, et al. Problems during and after pregnancy of former biliary atresia patients treated successfully by the Kasai procedure. J Pediatr Surg. 2001;36:349–51.
13. Jiang J, Wang J, Lu X, et al. Intrahepatic cystic lesions in children with biliary atresia after Kasai procedure. J Pediatr Surg. 2019;54:2565–9.
14. Inoue Y, Kato Y, Tamura T, et al. Prognostic implications of bile lakes after surgery for biliary atresia. J Pediatr Surg. 2008;43:2165–8.
15. Ling SC. Management of adult survivors of biliary atresia. Clin Liver Dis. 2014;4:86–8.
16. Tainaka T, et al. Histological assessment of bile lake formation after hepatic portoenterostomy for biliary atresia. Pediatr Surg Int. 2008;24:265–9.
17. Giström DA, et al. Biliary atresia-associated cholangitis: the central role and effective management of Bile Lakes. JPGN. 2019;68(4):488–94.
18. Tainaka T, Kaneko K, Seo T, et al. Intrahepatic cystic lesions after hepatic portoenterostomy for biliary atresia with bile lake and dilated bile ducts. J Pediatr Gastroenterol Nutr. 2007;44:104–7.
19. Watanabe M, Hori T, Kaneko M, et al. Intrahepatic biliary cyst in children with biliary atresia who have had a Kasi operation. J Pediatr Surg. 2007;42:1185–9.
20. Tainaka T, Kaneko K, Seo T, et al. Hepatolithiasis after hepatic portoenterostomy for biliary atresia. J Pediatr Surg. 2006;41:808–11.
21. Nio M, Ohi R, Shimaoka S, et al. The outcome of surgery for biliary atresia and the current status of long-term survivors. Tohoku J Exp Med. 1997;181:235–44.
22. Takahashi A, Masuda N, Suzuki M, et al. Evidence for segmental bile drainage by hepatic portoenterostomy for biliary atresia: cholangiographic, hepatic venographic, and histologic evaluation of the liver taken at liver transplantation. J Pediatr Surg. 2004;39:1–5.
23. Bu LN, Chen HL, Chang CJ, et al. Prophylactic oral antibiotics in prevention of recurrent cholangitis after the Kasai portoenterostomy. J Pediatr Sutg. 2003;38:590–3.
24. Gomi H, Solomkin JS, Schlossberg D, et al. Tokyo guidelines 2018: antimicrobial therapy for acute cholangitis and cholecystitis. J Hepatobiliary Pancreat Sci. 2018;25:3–16.
25. Yamanaka J, Iimuro Y, Hirano T, et al. Successful liver resection fore biliary atresia with intrahepatic biliary cysts after Kasai procedure. J Pediatr Surg. 2005;40:E9–E11.
26. Milyano G, Hayashi T, Arakawa A, et al. Left hepatic lobectomy in a long -term biliary atresia survivor. Afr J Pediatr Surg. 2012;9(2):155–6.

# Long-Term Complications: Hepatopulmonary Syndrome

# 35

Takehisa Ueno

## 35.1 Introduction

Hepatopulmonary syndrome (HPS) is a disease of gas exchange caused by intrapulmonary shunting secondary to liver disease-associated intrapulmonary vascular dilation [1]. HPS is characterized by the triad of arterial deoxygenation, intrapulmonary vascular dilatation, and liver disease, all of which occur in the absence of a primary cardiopulmonary anomaly. Liver diseases that are commonly involved include cirrhosis, portal hypertension, and portosystemic shunt [2]. HPS is not correlated with cirrhosis severity and can be caused even by asymptomatic cirrhosis [3]. HPS may also develop in noncirrhotic portal hypertension [4].

HPS is a common complication of biliary atresia (BA), which is characterized by complete obliteration of the extrahepatic bile ducts. Progressive liver fibrosis usually develops in patients with BA [5], leading in most cases to cirrhosis. BA may cause portal hypertension and portosystemic shunt even if it has not yet resulted in cirrhosis. BA generally results in extrahepatic complications, including HPS. The natural history of HPS is not clear, and the majority of BA patients exhibit normal gas exchange and do not progress to HPS. Moreover, it is unknown what factors underlie the development of HPS in BA patients, though the prevalence of HPS has been reported to be approximately 30% in patients with end-stage liver disease [6]. Studies of HPS in BA patients have been limited to case reports or case series [7–11]. However, HPS is an indication for liver transplantation (LT) in BA patients, and therefore timely diagnosis improves the outcome of BA.

LT is the only standard, long-term treatment for HPS. However, severe hypoxemia due to HPS is a relative contraindication for this procedure; therefore, it must be performed early in the disease course. Since HPS can progress rapidly, it is clinically important to diagnose it promptly. Importantly, HPS is associated with poor patient survival and quality of life. Mortality in cirrhosis patients who undergo LT has been shown to be twice as high in those with HPS compared to those without [12].

## 35.2 Pathophysiology

The pathophysiology of HPS in BA has not yet been fully elucidated. Impaired oxygenation in HPS is due to a widened alveolar-arterial oxygen gradient. Diffusely or locally dilated pulmonary capillaries result in inadequate oxygenation of venous flow through the pulmonary circulation [13].

Nitric oxide (NO) has been linked to the development of HPS. Cirrhosis patients with HPS exhibit increased levels of exhaled NO derived from the lungs [14]. Endothelin-1 (ET-1) is both a vasoconstrictor and a vascular smooth muscle mitogen, and its levels in plasma have been reported to correlate with the severity of liver cirrhosis and portal hypertension [15, 16], as well as with the severity of portal hypertension in BA [17].

Most of the current data on the pathophysiology of HPS were derived from animal experiments. Chronic common bile duct ligation in the rat is the only established model that reproduces the physiologic features of human HPS. Model rats demonstrate the increased activity of both endothelial and inducible NO synthase in the pulmonary microvasculature [18]. ET-1 and tumor necrosis factor-alpha play key roles in NO synthase activation [19]. ET-1 enhances the activation of NO synthase and contributes to monocyte accumulation through endothelin B receptor overexpression in the pulmonary vascular endothelium [20]. Bacterial translocation and endotoxemia also contribute to HPS development [21]. Both vascular endothelial growth factor A and increased fractalkine, known as chemokine ligand production, contribute to angiogenesis [22].

Moreover, HPS may overlap portopulmonary hypertension (PoPH). Smooth muscle hypertrophy in the pulmonary arteries may overcome vasodilation and

T. Ueno (✉)
Osaka University, Osaka, Japan
e-mail: ueno@pedsurg.med.osaka-u.ac.jp


M. Nio (ed.), *Introduction to Biliary Atresia*, https://doi.org/10.1007/978-981-16-2160-4_35

intrapulmonary shunt, resulting in an overlap between PoPH and late-stage HPS. HPS and PoPH are not mutually exclusive, and it has been hypothesized that the development of PoPH reverses intrapulmonary vasodilatation and thus interferes with each of the potential causes of hypoxemia in HPS [23].

## 35.3 Diagnosis

Once HPS is diagnosed, in most cases, the only treatment is LT. The timing of LT is very important. BA-associated HPS can develop insidiously and lack symptoms until an advanced stage. If BA patients present with symptoms such as shortness of breath, dyspnea, or palpitations, their HPS is often already very severe and is, therefore, a contraindication for LT, and the opportunity to undergo LT has been lost. Therefore, it is important to identify subclinical HPS in BA patients.

Patients with early-stage HPS may present with dyspnea or even be asymptomatic. Dyspnea upon standing and hypoxemia exacerbated by an upright position are common. Oxygen desaturation during sleep may occur in patients with HPS [24]. Patients with severe, long-term HPS may exhibit digital clubbing and distal cyanosis. Chest radiographs may show bibasilar nodular or reticulonodular opacities, reflecting vascular dilation [25].

The diagnosis of HPS requires the demonstration of both intrapulmonary vascular dilatation and abnormal arterial gas exchange. Diffusion impairment is commonly seen in HPS. Pulmonary function tests typically demonstrate a reduction in the diffusion capacity of carbon monoxide ($D_LCO$) [26]. However, the presence of decreased $D_LCO$ with normal spirometry results is not specific for HPS.

Arterial blood gas (ABG) measurement is a standard procedure that allows for the calculation of the alveolar-arterial (A-a) oxygen gradient P(A-a) $O_2$. Established diagnostic criteria for HPS in adults include P(A-a)$O_2$ > 15 mmHg and a partial pressure of oxygen ($PaO_2$) < 80 mmHg during regular breezing on room air [27]. The severity of HPS can be categorized based on the degree of hypoxemia, as follows: mild ($PaO_2$ > 80 mmHg), moderate ($PaO_2$ 60–79 mmHg), severe ($PaO_2$ 50–59 mmHg), and very severe ($PaO_2$ < 50 mmHg) [28]. These values may not be applicable in children. P(A-a)$O_2$ with age-adjusted cut-off was found to have a very low positive predictive value compared to the existing criterion of P(A-a)$O_2$ > 15 mmHg in adults [29]. The age-appropriate P(A-a)$O_2$ gradient is likely a better option in pediatric patients [30]. A drawback of ABG analysis, however, particularly in children, is the need for an arterial puncture. If patients require gastroesophageal endoscopy under general anesthesia to rule out esophageal varices, ABG can easily be obtained.

Pulse oximetry indirectly measures oxygen saturation ($SpO_2$) in a noninvasive fashion. $SpO_2$ < 96% was shown to be highly sensitive (100%) and specific (88%) for detecting HPS in patients with $PaO_2$ < 70 mmHg who were undergoing LT evaluation [31]. Serial $SpO_2$ measurements may be useful to monitor impaired oxygenation over time in patients with HPS [32].

The utility of pulse oximetry in HPS diagnosis has not been proven in children with cirrhosis [33]. The difference in $SpO_2$ between the supine and standing positions was found to be unreliable as a screening test for HPS [31]. Also, studies using pulse oximetry often fail to diagnose mild HPS, resulting in a lower diagnostic rate than those using ABG-based criteria [34].

Contrast echocardiography is the most useful test for detecting HPS (Fig. 35.1). This procedure is performed by intravenously injecting agitated saline during transthoracic echocardiography, creating sonographically visible microbubbles. These microbubbles are visualized in the right ventricle within seconds after administration, and in the absence of a right-to-left shunt, the microbubbles are absorbed by the alveoli. HPS is characterized by the delayed appearance of microbubbles in the left cardiac chambers, from approximately 3 to 6 beats after injection [35]. Contrast echocardiography can successfully evaluate BA patients with HPS. HPS can lead to life-threatening complications in postoperative BA patients, and contrast echocardiography may be a convenient and useful method to evaluate the degree of HPS and determine the optimal therapeutic strategy [10].

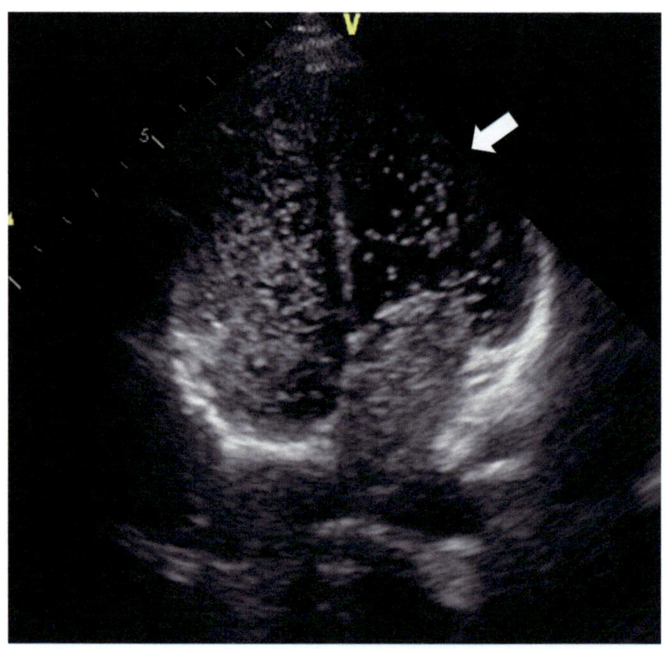

**Fig. 35.1** Contrast echocardiography: The microbubbles are found in the right ventricle (white arrow) within seconds after administration

Radioactive lung perfusion scintigraphy using technetium-99m (Tc-99m)–macroaggregated albumin (Tc-99m MAA) particles is another technique for detecting HPS (Fig. 35.2). During this procedure, 20-μm-diameter Tc-99m MAA particles are injected intravenously, and in healthy individuals, they then become trapped in the pulmonary microvasculature [36]. By contrast, in HPS patients, these particles escape through pulmonary shunts and become localized in downstream capillary beds supplied by systemic arteries. Quantitation of Tc-99m MAA particle distribution in the lungs, and other organs make it possible to calculate the degree of shunting [37].

Tc-99m MAA scintigraphy is less sensitive than contrast echocardiography, does not distinguish intracardiac from intrapulmonary shunting, and has not been properly standardized, making it a less useful screening test for HPS [35]. However, Tc-99m MAA scintigraphy is convenient in BA patients because cardiac abnormalities have usually been ruled out by the time portoenterostomy is performed. It may also serve as a complementary tool to contrast echocardiography to determine whether HPS contributes to hypoxemia in patients with the concomitant obstructive pulmonary disease [38]. Tc-99m MAA was used to show that a shunt (>20%) with very severe HPS ($PaO_2 < 50$ mmHg) was associated with high mortality after LT [39].

Diagnosing severe HPS ($PaO_2 < 60$ mmHg) during LT evaluation is particularly important, because HPS influences whether special perioperative care is needed. One study demonstrated the cost-effectiveness of first screening LT candidates for HPS by $SpO_2$ assessment, followed by contrast echocardiography and ABG if needed [40]. Since HPS develops significantly earlier than other pulmonary complications of BA, patients should receive routine pulse oximetry and contrast echocardiograms to detect HPS in its early stages [41].

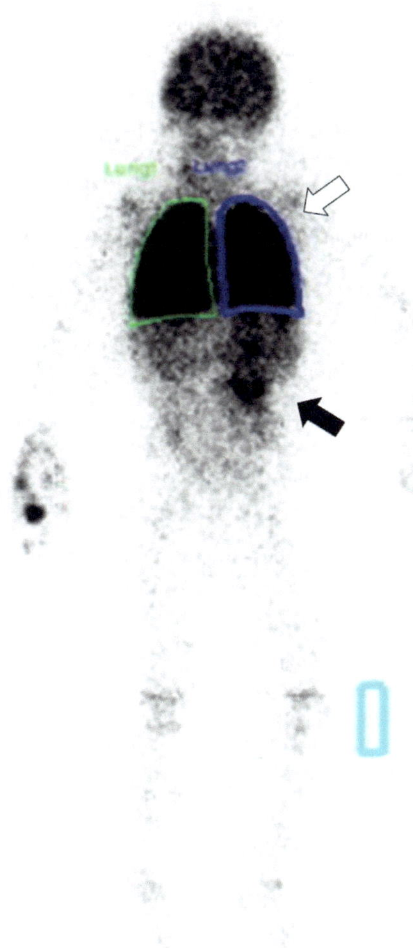

**Fig. 35.2** Radioactive lung perfusion scintigraphy: Technetium-99m macroaggregated albumin (Tc-99m MAA) scintigraphy was shown. Most of Tc-99m MAA particles are trapped in the pulmonary microvasculature (white arrow). Partial particles escaped through pulmonary shunts and were seen in downstream organs (black arrow)

## 35.4 Treatment

There are currently no effective medical therapies for HPS. Small, uncontrolled studies have reported a lack of efficacy using medications [42]. Oxygen supplementation remains a main therapeutic option even though no data exist regarding its efficacy or cost-effectiveness. In patients with $PaO_2 < 60$ mmHg at rest or with exertion, the administration of supplemental oxygen is appropriate. Oxygen supplementation is a low-risk treatment option that may have important benefits.

BA is the most common indication for LT among pediatric liver diseases. LT is an effective therapy for HPS, resulting in significant improvement or complete normalization of gas exchange in over 85% of patients with severe hypoxemia [43]. However, normalization of arterial hypoxemia after LT occurs at various time points and can take more than 1 year. The mortality risk of liver disease was estimated to be twice as high in patients with HPS as in those without [12]. Adult patients with severe HPS who underwent LT had better 5-year survival than those who did not (79% vs. 22%, respectively). [44], and post-LT survival was shown to be 87.5% at 10 years after LT [33]. The treatment effects and impact on candidates for LT require further characterization by well-designed prospective studies before practice guidelines can be suggested [45].

Before the model for end-stage liver disease (MELD) system was introduced in the United States, a prospective study found that the strongest predictor of mortality in patients with HPS was a preoperative $PaO_2 < 50$ mmHg, particularly in combination with a Tc-99m MAA shunt fraction of 20% [39]. Before the introduction of the MELD system, patients with HPS had a 5-year survival rate of 67%

after LT, and this improved to 88% under the MELD system [46]. Moreover, an analysis of the United Network for Organ Sharing (UNOS) data showed that patients with very severe HPS did not have worse survival after LT [43]. In pediatric LT, 60% of severe HPS patients, including those with BA, died within 3 months. LT can be safely performed in patients with mild or moderate intrapulmonary shunts, but in severe cases, LT should be carefully considered because concomitant PoPH may be masked by HPS [47]. The aforementioned findings may reflect recent improvements in HPS management and suggest that appropriately selected patients with very severe HPS may be suitable LT candidates. Overall, the early detection of HPS in BA patients and the regular assessment of hypoxemia in those with HPS who are listed for LT are critical to facilitate LT before the development of very severe hypoxemia.

## 35.5 Summary

Patients with BA may develop various extrahepatic complications. Pulmonary complications of BA are generally the result of portal hypertension. Of these, HPS is the most common and is characterized by impaired oxygenation. Angiogenesis and circulating vasodilators are important pathogenetic mechanisms in HPS. While HPS increases mortality, survival improves dramatically after LT. Pulse oximetry and contrast echocardiography are essential early screening tests for HPS.

## References


1. Rodriquez-Roisin R, et al. Highlights of the ERS Task Force on pulmonary-hepatic vascular disorders (PHD). J Hepatol. 2005;42(6):924–7.
2. Rodriguez-Roisin R, Krowka MJ. Hepatopulmonary syndrome—a liver-induced lung vascular disorder. N Engl J Med. 2008;358(22):2378–87.
3. Krowka MJ, et al. International liver transplant society practice guidelines: diagnosis and management of hepatopulmonary syndrome and portopulmonary hypertension. Transplantation. 2016;100(7):1440–52.
4. Kaymakoglu S, et al. Hepatopulmonary syndrome in noncirrhotic portal hypertensive patients. Dig Dis Sci. 2003;48(3):556–60.
5. Okazaki T, et al. Long-term postsurgical outcome of biliary atresia. J Pediatr Surg. 1999;34(2):312–5.
6. Castro M, Krowka MJ. Hepatopulmonary syndrome. A pulmonary vascular complication of liver disease. Clin Chest Med. 1996;17(1):35–48.
7. Ogawa E, et al. Living-donor liver transplantation for congenital biliary atresia with porto-pulmonary hypertension and moderate or severe pulmonary arterial hypertension: Kyoto University experience. Clin Transpl. 2014;28(9):1031–40.
8. Umeda A, et al. Hepatopulmonary syndrome can show spontaneous resolution: possible mechanism of portopulmonary hypertension overlap? Respirology. 2006;11(1):120–3.
9. Urashima Y, et al. Living related liver transplantation for biliary atresia with portopulmonary hypertension: case report. Transplant Proc. 2004;36(8):2237–8.
10. Sasaki T, et al. Development of intrapulmonary arteriovenous shunting in postoperative biliary atresia: evaluation by contrast-enhanced echocardiography. J Pediatr Surg. 2000;35(11):1647–50.
11. Soh H, et al. Pulmonary hypertension associated with post-operative biliary atresia: report of two cases. J Pediatr Surg. 1999;34(12):1779–81.
12. Fallon MB, et al. Impact of hepatopulmonary syndrome on quality of life and survival in liver transplant candidates. Gastroenterology. 2008;135(4):1168–75.
13. Schraufnagel DE, Kay JM. Structural and pathologic changes in the lung vasculature in chronic liver disease. Clin Chest Med. 1996;17(1):1–15.
14. Rolla G, et al. Exhaled nitric oxide and impaired oxygenation in cirrhotic patients before and after liver transplantation. Ann Intern Med. 1998;129(5):375–8.
15. Matsumoto H, et al. Clinical significance of plasma endothelin-1 in patients with chronic liver disease. Dig Dis Sci. 1994;39(12):2665–70.
16. Uchihara M, et al. Clinical significance of elevated plasma endothelin concentration in patients with cirrhosis. Hepatology. 1992;16(1):95–9.
17. Hasegawa T, et al. Plasma endothelin-1 level as a marker reflecting the severity of portal hypertension in biliary atresia. J Pediatr Surg. 2001;36(11):1609–12.
18. Fallon MB, et al. The role of endothelial nitric oxide synthase in the pathogenesis of a rat model of hepatopulmonary syndrome. Gastroenterology. 1997;113(2):606–14.
19. Luo B, et al. ET-1 and TNF-alpha in HPS: analysis in prehepatic portal hypertension and biliary and nonbiliary cirrhosis in rats. Am J Physiol Gastrointest Liver Physiol. 2004;286(2):G294–303.
20. Ling Y, et al. The role of endothelin-1 and the endothelin B receptor in the pathogenesis of hepatopulmonary syndrome in the rat. Hepatology. 2004;39(6):1593–602.
21. Rabiller A, et al. Prevention of gram-negative translocation reduces the severity of hepatopulmonary syndrome. Am J Respir Crit Care Med. 2002;166(4):514–7.
22. Zhang J, et al. Pulmonary angiogenesis in a rat model of hepatopulmonary syndrome. Gastroenterology. 2009;136(3):1070–80.
23. Mal H, et al. Pulmonary hypertension following hepatopulmonary syndrome in a patient with cirrhosis. J Hepatol. 1999;31(2):360–4.
24. Palma DT, et al. Oxygen desaturation during sleep in hepatopulmonary syndrome. Hepatology. 2008;47(4):1257–63.
25. McAdams HP, et al. The hepatopulmonary syndrome: radiologic findings in 10 patients. AJR Am J Roentgenol. 1996;166(6):1379–85.
26. Martinez GP, et al. Hepatopulmonary syndrome in candidates for liver transplantation. J Hepatol. 2001;34(5):651–7.
27. Borkar VV, et al. Hepatopulmonary Syndrome in children: a comparative study of non-cirrhotic vs. cirrhotic portal hypertension. Liver Int. 2015;35(6):1665–72.
28. Rodriguez-Roisin R, et al. Pulmonary-Hepatic vascular Disorders (PHD). Eur Respir J. 2004;24(5):861–80.
29. Schenk P, et al. Hepatopulmonary syndrome: prevalence and predictive value of various cut offs for arterial oxygenation and their clinical consequences. Gut. 2002;51(6):853–9.
30. Palma DT, Fallon MB. The hepatopulmonary syndrome. J Hepatol. 2006;45(4):617–25.
31. Arguedas MR, et al. Utility of pulse oximetry screening for hepatopulmonary syndrome. Clin Gastroenterol Hepatol. 2007;5(6):749–54.
32. Kochar R, Tanikella R, Fallon MB. Serial pulse oximetry in hepatopulmonary syndrome. Dig Dis Sci. 2011;56(6):1862–8.

33. Warner S, et al. Hepatopulmonary syndrome in children: a 20-year review of presenting symptoms, clinical progression, and transplant outcome. Liver Transpl. 2018;24(9):1271–9.
34. Raevens S, et al. Hepatopulmonary syndrome and portopulmonary hypertension: recent knowledge in pathogenesis and overview of clinical assessment. Liver Int. 2015;35(6):1646–60.
35. Abrams GA, et al. Diagnostic utility of contrast echocardiography and lung perfusion scan in patients with hepatopulmonary syndrome. Gastroenterology. 1995;109(4):1283–8.
36. Wolfe JD, et al. Hypoxemia of cirrhosis: detection of abnormal small pulmonary vascular channels by a quantitative radionuclide method. Am J Med. 1977;63(5):746–54.
37. Abrams GA, et al. Use of macroaggregated albumin lung perfusion scan to diagnose hepatopulmonary syndrome: a new approach. Gastroenterology. 1998;114(2):305–10.
38. Krowka MJ, et al. Hepatopulmonary syndrome: a prospective study of relationships between severity of liver disease, PaO(2) response to 100% oxygen, and brain uptake after (99m)Tc MAA lung scanning. Chest. 2000;118(3):615–24.
39. Arguedas MR, et al. Prospective evaluation of outcomes and predictors of mortality in patients with hepatopulmonary syndrome undergoing liver transplantation. Hepatology. 2003;37(1):192–7.
40. Roberts DN, Arguedas MR, Fallon MB. Cost-effectiveness of screening for hepatopulmonary syndrome in liver transplant candidates. Liver Transpl. 2007;13(2):206–14.
41. Ueno T, et al. Onset ages of hepatopulmonary syndrome and pulmonary hypertension in patients with biliary atresia. Pediatr Surg Int. 2017;33(10):1053–7.
42. Abrams GA, Fallon MB. The hepatopulmonary syndrome. Clin Liver Dis. 1997;1(1):185–200. xiii
43. Gupta S, et al. Improved survival after liver transplantation in patients with hepatopulmonary syndrome. Am J Transplant. 2010;10(2):354–63.
44. Swanson KL, Wiesner RH, Krowka MJ. Natural history of hepatopulmonary syndrome: impact of liver transplantation. Hepatology. 2005;41(5):1122–9.
45. Swanson KL, et al. Survival in portopulmonary hypertension: Mayo Clinic experience categorized by treatment subgroups. Am J Transplant. 2008;8(11):2445–53.
46. Iyer VN, et al. Hepatopulmonary syndrome: favorable outcomes in the MELD exception era. Hepatology. 2013;57(6):2427–35.
47. Hirata Y, et al. Outcomes of 50 cases of pediatric liver transplantation for intrapulmonary shunt while considering the deteriorated prognosis of severe intrapulmonary shunt patients. Transplant Proc. 2019;51(8):2793–7.

# Long-Term Complications: Portopulmonary Hypertension

# 36

Hideaki Okajima

**Abstract**

Porto-pulmonary Hypertension (PPHTN) in patients with biliary atresia (BA) is a rare complication but threatening pulmonary disease. Little is known about the mechanisms of development on pulmonary artery hypertension (PAH) in BA patients with portal hypertension. PPHTN is estimated to occur in 3 to 10% of patients with end-stage liver disease.

PPHTN should be detected within mild PHA because the prognosis of patients with moderate to severe PPHTN, even in patients who received liver transplantation, is extremely poor. Chest X-ray, electric cardiogram, and ultrasound cardiogram are performed as screening modernity. When pulmonary artery pressures are suspected to increase, right heart catheterization which is required for the definitive diagnosis of PPHTN should be performed.

Liver transplantation is the therapeutic option to improve both PPHTN and liver dysfunction with portal hypertension. However, liver transplantation can be indicated in patients with mild PPHTN, because of high intra and postoperative mortality in moderate to severe PPHTN patients. Improvement of therapeutic option in PAH specific therapies, moderate to severe PPHTN patients can be controlled preoperatively, and then liver transplantation can be performed with significantly lower risks.

In BA patients with portal hypertension, the PPHTN should be taken care of and detected within mild PHA. Close monitoring for PPHTN is important in long follow-up BA patients, especially with portal hypertension.

**Keywords**

Biliary atresia · Portal hypertension · Porto-pulmonary Hypertension · Liver transplantation

H. Okajima (✉)
Department of Pediatric Surgery, Kanazawa Medical University, Ishikawa, Japan
e-mail: hokajima@kanazawa-med.ac.jp

## 36.1 Introduction

Porto-pulmonary hypertension (PPHTN) has been considered one of the clinical manifestations in liver cirrhosis patients with portal hypertension. In 1951, Mantz et al. first reported an association between pulmonary hypertension and portal hypertension [1]. The existence of PPHTN in liver transplant candidates with end-stage liver disease due to liver cirrhosis with portal hypertension has been retrospectively assessed by several studies, and it was reported that the prevalence of pulmonary artery hypertension (PAH) in patients with portal hypertension was ranging from 3 to 10% [2–8]. Liver transplantation is a therapeutic option for end-stage liver disease; however, due to high mortality peri-transplantation in patients with PPHTN, PPHTN is considered a contraindication to liver transplantation, especially patients with moderate to severe PPHTN.

Improvement with results after Kasai operation for patients with biliary atresia, the number of patients who achieved adult with native liver has been increasing without jaundice. However, in some of these patients, even without jaundice, liver fibrosis at the periportal area that leads to increasing stiffness of the liver following by portal hypertension has been deteriorating. In these patients, complications regarding portal hypertension, including hypersplenism, gastrointestinal hemorrhage, and pulmonary complications including hepatopulmonary syndrome and porto-pulmonary hypertension are presented, especially in elder children.

This chapter describes PPHTN in patients with biliary atresia as one of the long-term complications.

## 36.2 Ethiology

In biliary atresia patients, PPHTN observes in patients with portal hypertension rather than those with liver dysfunction from cirrhosis. The incidence and prevalence of PPHTN in biliary atresia patients are unknown. Epidemiological studies regarding pulmonary artery hypertension associated


M. Nio (ed.), *Introduction to Biliary Atresia*, https://doi.org/10.1007/978-981-16-2160-4_36

with portal hypertension have been reported; however, the majority of estimates are in patients to evaluate for liver transplantation.

In 1979, Lebrec et al. reported the first case-series description of 9 patients with portal hypertension who had subsequently developed pulmonary artery hypertension [9]; the authors argued that pulmonary artery hypertension was a rare complication of portal hypertension. In a clinical prospective study comprising over 500 hospitalized patients with portal hypertension, but without previously known pulmonary artery hypertension. Hadengue et al. reported that 10 (2%) of them had pulmonary artery hypertension, and of those, six patients were clinically asymptomatic at the time of diagnosis [10]. In a prospective study comprising 165 consecutive patients who were submitted to right heart catheterization at the time of pre-transplant evaluation, 10 (6%) of patients met the criteria for PPHTN [11]. The prevalence of PPHTN among patients with non-cirrhotic portal hypertension remains ill defined; data from the French Referral Center for pulmonary artery hypertension showed that a non-hepatic cause of portal hypertension was present in 11.7% of PPHTN cases [12].

PPHTN is commonly diagnosed in adults several years after the diagnosis of portal hypertension [10, 13, 14]. Symptoms of pulmonary artery hypertension may precede those of portal hypertension [13]. Children with portal hypertension caused by biliary atresia, congenital hepatic fibrosis, extrahepatic portal vein obstruction, and primary sclerosing cholangitis also develop PPHTN [15–17]. A recent retrospective case-control study showed that the presence of large spontaneous portosystemic shunts, in particular splenorenal shunts, was significantly associated with moderate and severe PPHTN and with a lack of response to treatment [18]. Kawut et al. reported that female was independently associated with an increased risk of PPHTN from a multicenter case-control study [19]. Cholestatic liver disease such as primary biliary cirrhosis and another autoimmune liver disease with females showed a trend towards significance. Females have nearly three times the risk of men, and even there are more men affected with cirrhosis [20] Also, the severity of PPHTN is not correlated with the severity of liver dysfunction, as measured by the Child-Turcotte-Pugh or the Model of End-stage Liver Disease (MELD) scores, or the degree of portal hypertension [7, 19, 21].

## 36.3 Pathogenesis

Little is known regarding the pathogenesis of PPHTN because of its low prevalence; the histological picture of PPHTN is indistinguishable from that of idiopathic pulmonary artery hypertension [22], such as pulmonary vascular changes including vascular cell proliferation, concentric intimal fibrosis, plexogenic arteriopathy and *in situ* thrombosis [23]. Several mechanisms of pulmonary artery hypertension in patients with portal hypertension have been proposed with genetic predisposition, pulmonary vascular wall shear stress, and dysregulation of vasoactive, proliferative, angiogenic, and inflammatory mediators.

From hepatic functional points of view, the factors leading to portal hypertension are an increase in portal blood flow at the microcirculation level together with an increased blood flow through the portal venous system due to splanchnic arteriolar vasodilation, both resulting in the characteristic hyperdynamic circulation [24]. This hyperdynamic state may cause higher shear stress on the pulmonary endothelium with resultant vascular remodeling [13, 25]; however other mechanisms must be involved, since not all liver disease patients progress to develop PPHTN [26]. Importantly, as portal hypertension progresses, an extensive network of portosystemic collaterals ensues, allowing the presence of such portosystemic shunts that may expose the pulmonary vasculature to deleterious vasoactive substances from the splanchnic circulation [9, 27]. Up-regulation of several mediators have been implicated in the pathogenesis of PPHTN, such as thromboxane A2, interleukin-1, interleukin-6, glucagon, calcitonin gene-related peptide, serotonin, vasoactive intestinal peptide, and endothelin-1 [22, 28–30]. Endothelin-1 is a potent pulmonary and systemic vasoconstrictor whose production by the cirrhotic liver is increased [31], contributing to hepatic stellate cell contraction and increased hepatic sinusoidal tone, thereby aggravating portal hypertension [26].

The role of endothelin-1 in the pathogenesis of PPHTN was shown in two reports that the levels of endothelin-1 are elevated in cirrhosis patients with PPHTN compared to those without PPHTN [28, 32]. Then treatment with endothelin-1 receptor antagonists leads to a reduction in pulmonary artery pressure in patients with PPHTN [33]. Recently a genetic study showed that variations in estrogen signaling, oxidative stress, and cell growth regulator genes are associated with an increased risk of PPHTN [34].

## 36.4 Clinical Manifestations

Biliary atresia patients with PPHTN are usually asymptomatic during the early phase, such as within mild pulmonary artery hypertension. The clinical manifestations of portal hypertension or of the underlying liver dysfunction may or may not be present. Dyspnea is the most common presenting symptom [14] following by other symptoms, including fatigue, orthopnea, chest pain, and syncope may develop [4, 13, 14, 35]. In very advanced stages, patients may present with hemoptysis. The physical examination findings indicating PAH are usually completely absent, depending on the

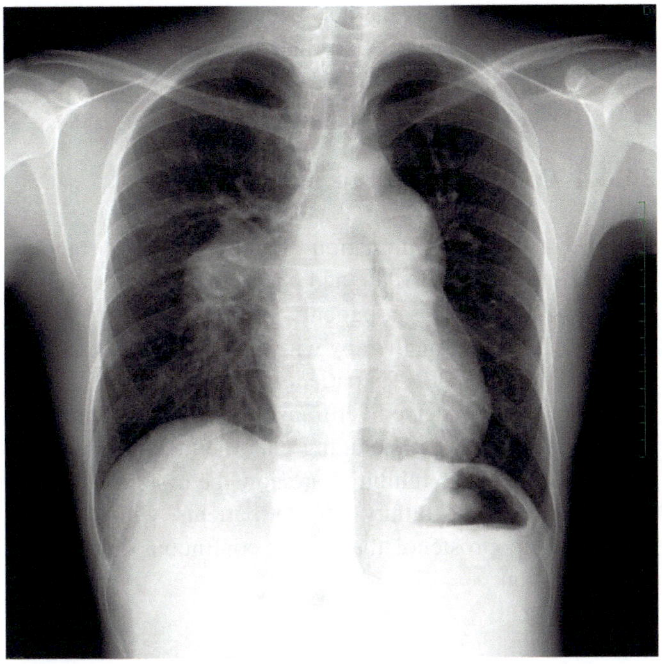

**Fig. 36.1** Chest plain X-ray of 15 years biliary atresia boy with PPHTN (mPAP: 61 mmHg) reveals a prominent main pulmonary artery

severity of the deteriorated liver function and portal hypertension, such as jaundice, coagulopathy, hypersplenism, and ascites.

Chest plain X-ray may reveal a prominent main pulmonary artery, cardiomegaly due to enlarged right cardiac chambers and increased vascularity in the upper lobes (Fig. 36.1). Electrocardiogram (ECG) shows right ventricular hypertrophy and strain [36, 37]. Echocardiographic evaluation is performed to identify as having mild or suspicious pulmonary artery hypertension. When pulmonary artery hypertension is suspected, cardiac catheter studies should be performed.

Measurement of B-type natriuretic peptide (BNP) plasma levels may be of help. BNP, a molecule released from the ventricles in response to their dilation, has been shown to be related to hemodynamic parameters and is suggested to be of prognostic significance in patients with left or right heart failure [38].

## 36.5 Identification

To identify for diagnosis of PPHTN, right heart catheterization (RHC) is required [39]. When performed at experienced centers, RHC is a relatively safe procedure associated with low morbidity and mortality [40]. RHC allows the accurate direct measurement of pulmonary artery pressures as well as the calculation of pulmonary vascular resistance (PVR). The current diagnostic criteria for PPHTN are defined as follows:

(i). Mean pulmonary arterial pressure (mean PAP) > 25 mmHg (20 mmHg for pediatric) and pulmonary capillary wedge pressure < 15 mmHg
(ii). Pulmonary vascular resistance > 120 dynes s/cm5
(iii). Exclusion of congenital cardiac disorders [7, 41–45]

RHC is also important to assess disease severity [41]. According to the mean PAP, PPHTN may be classified into mild, moderate, and severe.

(i). Mild: mean PAP < 35 mmHg
(ii). Moderate: 35 mmHg ≤ mean PAP < 50 mmHg
(iii). Severe: mean PAP ≥ 50 mmHg

This classification has an impact in terms of prognosis, treatment options, and indication of liver transplantation.

In addition to hemodynamic measurements, vasoreactive studies may be performed. In those patients with idiopathic pulmonary artery hypertension who exhibit a positive vasoreactive response, a calcium channel blocker agent is usually initiated [46]. However, in the context of PPHTN, these studies are being done less frequently [47], since patients with end-stage liver disease do not tolerate calcium antagonists as they may exacerbate portal hypertension [48].

## 36.6 Treatment

Recently the cause of PPHTN has been recognized due to liver cirrhosis with portal hypertension in patients with biliary atresia even without jaundice. The gold standard therapeutic option should be considered to recovery from liver cirrhosis and portal hypertension; therefore the most effective therapeutic procedure could be liver transplantation. Although results from several reports regarding to outcome of liver transplantation for patients with mild PPHTN were acceptable, those for patients with moderate to severe PPHTN were poor. Initially, liver transplantation for patients with moderate to severe PPHTN might be considered as a contraindication.

Since the development of treatment for pulmonary artery hypertension, these therapies have also been applied to PPHTN patients. In the past few decades, several advances have been proposed in the treatment of pulmonary artery hypertension. The approval of new therapies has resulted in improvements in morbidity and survival of patients with advanced pulmonary artery hypertension [49]. There are three types of medical treatments: prostanoids, endothelin receptor antagonists, and phosphodiesterase type 5 inhibitors [46].

### 36.6.1 Prostanoids

Prostacyclin derivatives such as epoprostenol are well known as pulmonary and systemic vasodilators. Epoprostenol has been used, and using epoprostenol treatment improves pulmonary artery hypertension in biliary atresia patients with PPHTN [50]. A retrospective study regarding long-term outcomes in pulmonary artery hypertension patients between treated with epoprostenol and not treated with epoprostenol showed that the treated with epoprostenol group had a significant improvement in mean PAP. Unfortunately, regarding survival, there was no difference between the two groups. On the other hand, this therapy has a possibility to become to be able to perform liver transplantation safely [51]. Awdish et al. compared PPHTN patients from one center who had started intravenous prostanoids with PPHTN patients in the REVEAL registry; five-year survival from the time of diagnosis in the treated PPHTN patients was twice as high as that in the control group [52]. To treat with epoprostenol, it is necessary to administer it continuous intravenously. Moreover, there are several side effects, including catheter-related infection and the need for continuous refrigeration of epoprostenol itself. Recently, other prostanoids such as Treprostinil, given as an intravenous or subcutaneous infusion, inhaled iloprost, and oral synthetic prostanoid beraprost, are introduced to improve in patients with PPHTN [53–56]. These agents might also have the possibility of efficacy for biliary atresia patients with PPHTN.

### 36.6.2 Endothelin Receptor Blockers

Endothelin-1 is known as vasoconstrictor molecule and has been shown to be up-regulated in PPHTN patients [28, 31, 32]. Bosentan, an oral endothelin A and B receptor antagonist is used in patients with pulmonary artery hypertension [49]. The efficacy of Bosentan in the PPHTN patients has been reported [33, 57]. Hoeper et al. reported efficacious of 1-year treatment in patients with severe PPTHN [58]. Savate et al. reported the safety and hemodynamic improvements of Bosentan, especially in Child B patients with portal hypertension [59]. A prospective study with a selective endothelin A receptor antagonist ambrisentan showed improvement in mean PAP in patients with PPHTN without adverse effects on hepatic function [60].

### 36.6.3 Phosphodiesterase-5 inhibitors

Sildenafil, an oral phosphodiesterase-5 inhibitor, affects nitric oxide-induced vasodilation of pulmonary vessels. Reichenberger et al. reported the efficacy of sildenafil in patients with moderate to severe PPHTN patients [61]. Sildenafil monotherapy has also been reported with a significant reduction in mean PAP in patients with liver transplant candidates. [62, 63].

### 36.6.4 Combination Therapy

Double or triple combination therapy with prostanoids, endothelin receptor blocker, and phosphodiesterase-5 inhibitor is also effective for patients with moderate to severe PPHTN. Combination therapy with sildenafil, Bosentan, and iloprost for severe PPHTN patients decreases mean PAP and the patient could receive liver transplant safely [64].

Per-oral mediators, including endothelin-1 inhibitor and phosphodiesterase-5 inhibitor, are now the first line of therapeutic options for biliary atresia patients with PPHTN, instead of epoprostenol that needs continuous intravenous administration.

### 36.6.5 Transplantation

#### 36.6.5.1 Liver Transplantation

Prognosis of PPHTN is reported with 5-years survival of less than 30% without liver transplantation. However, moderate to severe PPHTN is considered a contraindication for liver transplantation due to high intra- and postoperative mortality. Various studies have reported improvement in PAH management by means of vasodilation therapy, including prostanoids, endothelin-1 inhibitor, and phosphodiesterase-5 inhibitor, allowing liver transplantation safely [15, 65]. Sussman reported the feasibility and the effects of liver transplantation following vasodilation therapy with epoprostenol resulted in hemodynamic profile improvement in seven of eight severe PPHTN cirrhotic patients. Then liver transplantation can be performed in four of those seven patients who have been doing well after liver transplantation [66]. Ashfeg reported that 16 patients with moderate to severe PPHTN were treated with epoprostenol either alone or in combination with Bosentan. Mean PAP decreased to a level < 35 mmHg in 12 patients, and 11 of these patients were performed liver transplantation with 1- and 5-years survival 91% and 67%, respectively [67]. Living donor liver transplantation in patients with PPHTN was also successfully reported, including biliary atresia patients [50, 68–70]. Now patients with moderate to severe PPHTN receive medical therapy to decrease mean PAP until less than 35 mmHg then they can receive liver transplantation safely [71]. Regarding vasodilation therapy after liver transplantation, 5 of 6 biliary atresia patients with PPHTN have been able to discontinue vasodilation therapy following liver transplantation [50] successfully.

During liver transplantation surgery, it produces acute hemodynamic changes, particularly during the reperfusion of the allograft, and may precipitate acute right ventricular failure. The probability of acute right ventricular failure is much higher in those patients with an already compromised right ventricle function in patients with PPHTN [5, 72, 73]. To assess enough right ventricular function in the presence of acute increases in preload during transplant surgery, acute volume challenge test (AVCT) prior to liver transplantation is recommended [50]. The test involves the injection of normal saline (10 mL/kg body weight) over 6–7 min via a cardiac catheter. AVCT study is performed during the right cardiac catheter study when the mean PAP is < 35 mmHg [74].

#### 36.6.5.2 Combined Lung and Liver Transplantation

Pulmonary artery hypertension is one of the indications for lung transplantation. However, lung transplantation itself huge invasive surgical procedure. So only selected patients with severe PPHTN and end-stage liver disease may be considered for combined lung and liver transplantation in limited institutes [49]. Grannas et al. reported five patients with PPHTN patients performed lung and liver transplantation, and 1-, 3-, and 5-years survival rates were 69%, 62%, and 49%, respectively [75].

## 36.7 Outcome

In multivariate regression analysis, the two factors associated with an increased risk of death were lower cardiac index and higher severity of cirrhosis as assessed by the Child-Turcotte-Pugh score. Causes of mortality are due to complications of cirrhosis and portal hypertension or related to right heart failure and overall survival reported at 1-, 3-, and 5-years were 88%, 75%, and 68%, respectively [12]. Previous studies have demonstrated that 40% of PPHTN patients die within 15 months since diagnosis and that half of the untreated PPHTN patients die within six months since diagnosis [76, 77]. For PPHTN patients who received liver transplantation, 36% of PPHTN patients die during the early post-transplant period because of right ventricular dysfunction, acute respiratory distress syndrome, and cardiovascular collapse [78]. In addition, liver transplantation does not always result in the reversal of PPHTN [79]. Krowka et al. reported the outcome of 36 non-treated PPHTN patients who have undergone liver transplantation showed that the mortality rate of patients with mean PAP > 50 mmHg, <50 mmHg but higher than 35 mmHg, and < 35 mmHg was 100%, 50%, and 0%, respectively [80]. These outcomes after liver transplantation have led that liver transplantation is considered a contraindication in moderate (mean PAP ≥ 35 mmHg) to severe PPHTN (mean PAP > 50 mmHg) patients [81–84]. Swanson et al. reported a 5-year survival was 14% in patients who had not received any treatment, while that in patients receiving pulmonary artery hypertension therapy or pulmonary artery hypertension therapy followed by liver transplantation was 45% and 67%, respectively [72]. There are several studies that after improvement or even resolution of PPHTN following pulmonary artery hypertension therapy with selective pulmonary vasoactive agents, liver transplantation can be performed safely [84–86].

Regarding liver transplantation for biliary atresia patients with PPHTN, Ogawa et al. reported the mean interval period from initial diagnosis of pulmonary artery hypertension to the performance of living donor liver transplantation was 2.5 year (range: 0.2–11.9 year). Continuous intravenous epoprostenol was administered to all patients before living donor liver transplantation, and oxygen was given in five cases. The length of epoprostenol treatment prior to living donor liver transplantation ranged from 3 to 11 months, with a mean of 7.3 months [50]. Catheterization studies performed before living donor liver transplantation showed that six patients had favorite reactions to the loading tests to the AVCT, but two cases reacted poorly to the loading tests and had positive responses to the AVCT. Living donor liver transplantation was postponed in poorly reactive patients. In the six successful cases of preoperative epoprostenol therapy in the study, epoprostenol therapy was able to be withdrawn after living donor liver transplantation. The mean time of epoprostenol withdrawal after living donor liver transplantation was 0.9 year in the successful cases. Regarding epoprostenol treatment, catheter-related infections occurred in four cases. This is one of the adverse factors on epoprostenol therapy, because it must be administered by continuous intravenously. Due to these adverse factors, recently the first choice of pulmonary artery hypertension therapy may be considered with per-oral administer agents such as endothelin receptor inhibitors and/or Phosphodiesterase-5 inhibitors.

Recommended flowchart to management strategies in biliary atresia patients with PPHTN is shown in Fig. 36.2. In biliary atresia patients with mild PPHTN is an indication for liver transplantation. Patients with moderate to severe PPHTN should be performed pulmonary artery hypertension therapy preoperatively to decrease mean PAP less than 35 mmHg to improve the outcome of liver transplantation. It is important in biliary atresia patients with portal hypertension to close monitoring and screening for PPHTN and detect within mild PPHTN.

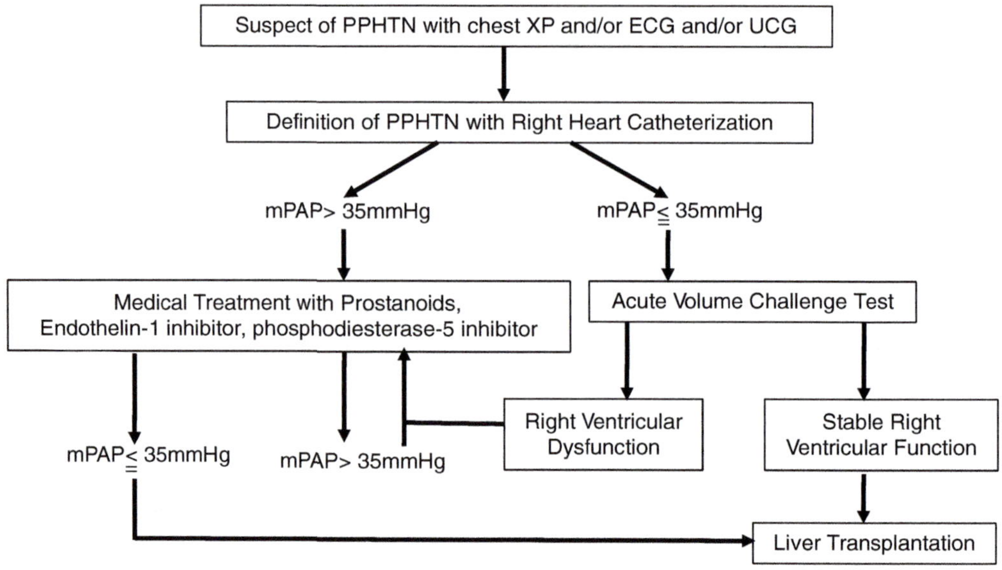


**Fig. 36.2** Flowchart of management for Biliary Atresia patients with PPHTN

## References

1. Mantz FA, Craige E. Portal axis thrombosis with spontaneous portocaval shunt and resultant cor pulmonale. AMA Arch Pathol. 1951;52:91–7.
2. Kuo PC, Plotkin JS, Gaine S, et al. Portopulmonary hypertension and the liver transplant candidate. Transplantation. 1996;6: 1087–93.
3. Chen HS, Xing SR, Xu WG, et al. Porto-pulmonary hypertension in cirrhotic patients: prevalence, clinical features and risk factors. Exp Ther Med. 2013;5:819–24.
4. Yang YY, Lin HC, Lee WC, et al. Porto-pulmonary hypertension: distinctive hemodynamic and clinical manifestations. J Gastroenterol. 2001;36:181–6.
5. Taura P, Garcia-Valdecasas JC, Beltran J, et al. Moderate primary pulmonary hypertension in patients undergoing liver transplantation. Anesth Analg. 1996;83:675–80.
6. Castro M, Krowka MJ, Schroeder DR, et al. Frequency and clinical implications of increased pulmonary artery pressures in liver transplant patients. Mayo Clin Proc. 1996;71:543–51.
7. Ramsay MA, Simpson BR, Nguyen AT, et al. Severe pulmonary hypertension in liver transplant candidates. Liver Transpl Surg. 1997;3:494–500.
8. Torregrosa M, Genesca J, Gonzalez A, et al. Role of Doppler echocardiography in the assessment of porto-pulmonary hypertension in liver transplantation candidates. Transplan- tation. 2001;71:572–4.
9. Lebrec D, Capron JP, Dhumeaux D, et al. Pulmonary hypertension complicating portal hypertension. Am Rev Respir Dis. 1979;120:849–56.
10. Hadengue A, Benhayoun MK, Lebrec D, et al. Pulmonary hypertension complicating portal hypertension: prevalence and relation to splanchnic hemodynamics. Gastroenterology. 1991;100:520–8.
11. Colle IO, Moreau R, Godinho E, et al. Diagnosis of porto-pulmonary hypertension in candidates for liver transplantation: a prospective study. Hepatology. 2003;37:401–9.
12. Le Pavec J, Souza R, Herve P, et al. Porto-pulmonary hypertension: survival and prognostic factors. Am J Respir Crit Care Med. 2008;178:637–43.
13. Herve P, Lebrec D, Brenot F, et al. Pulmonary vascular disorders in portal hypertension. Eur Respir J. 1998;11:1153–66.
14. Robalino BD, Moodie DS. Association between primary pulmonary hypertension and portal hypertension: analysis of its pathophysiology and clinical, laboratory and hemodynamic manifestations. J Am Coll Cardiol. 1991;17:492–8.
15. Losay J, Piot D, Bougaran J, et al. Early liver transplantation is crucial in children with liver disease and pulmonary artery hypertension. J Hepatol. 1998;28:337–42.
16. Laving A, Khanna A, Rubin L, et al. Successful liver transplantation in a child with severe porto-pulmonary hypertension treated with epoprostenol. J Pediatr Gastroenterol Nutr. 2005;41:466–8.
17. Condino AA, Ivy DD, O'Connor JA, et al. Porto-pulmonary hypertension in pediatric patients. J Pediatr. 2005;147:20–6.
18. Talwalkar JA, Swanson KL, Krowka MJ, et al. Prevalence of spontaneous portosystemic shunts in patients with porto-pulmonary hypertension and effect on treatment. Gas- troenterology. 2011;141:1673–9.
19. Kawut SM, Krowka MJ, Trotter JF, et al. Clinical risk fac- tors for porto-pulmonary hypertension. Hepatology. 2008;48:196–203.
20. Taichman DB, Mandel J. Epidemiology of pulmonary arterial hypertension. Clin Chest Med. 2013;34:619–37.
21. Krowka MJ, Swanson KL, Frantz RP, et al. Porto-pulmonary hypertension: Results from a 10-year screening algorithm. Hepatology. 2006;44:1502–10.
22. Farber HW, Loscalzo J. Pulmonary arterial hypertension. N Engl J Med. 2004;351:1655–65.
23. Schraufnagel DE, Kay JM. Structural and pathologic changes in the lung vasculature in chronic liver disease. Clin Chest Med. 1996;17:1–15.
24. Rodriguez-Vilarrupla A, Fernandez M, Bosch J, et al. Current concepts on the pathophysiology of portal hypertension. Ann Hepatol. 2007;6:28–36.
25. Budhiraja R, Hassoun PM. Porto-pulmonary hypertension: a tale of two circulations. Chest. 2003;123:562–76.
26. Al-Naamani N, Roberts KE. Porto-pulmonary hypertension. Clin Chest Med. 2013;34:719–37.
27. Troy PJ, Waxman AB. Porto-pulmonary hypertension: challenges in diagnosis and management. Therap Adv Gastroen- terol. 2009;2:281–6.
28. Pellicelli AM, Barbaro G, Puoti C, et al. Plasma cytokines and porto-pulmonary hypertension in patients with cirrhosis waiting for orthotopic liver transplantation. Angiology. 2010;61:802–6.
29. Egermayer P, Town GI, Peacock AJ. Role of serotonin in the pathogenesis of acute and chronic pulmonary hypertension. Thorax. 1999;54:161–8.

30. Angus PW. Role of endothelin in systemic and portal resistance in cirrhosis. Gut. 2006;55:1230–2.
31. Alam I, Bass NM, Bacchetti P, et al. Hepatic tissue endothelin- 1 levels in chronic liver disease correlate with disease severity and ascites. Am J Gastroenterol. 2000;95:199–203.
32. Benjaminov FS, Prentice M, Sniderman KW, et al. Porto- pulmonary hypertension in decompensated cirrhosis with refractory ascites. Gut. 2003;52:1355–62.
33. Halank M, Miehlke S, Hoeffken G, et al. Use of oral endothelin receptor antagonist bosentan in the treatment of porto- pulmonary hypertension. Transplantation. 2004;77:1775–6.
34. Roberts KE, Fallon MB, Krowka MJ, et al. Genetic risk factors for porto-pulmonary hypertension in patients with advanced liver disease. Am J Respir Crit Care Med. 2009;179:835–42.
35. Pilatis ND, Jacobs LE, Rerkpattanapipat P, et al. Clinical predictors of pulmonary hypertension in patients undergoing liver transplant evaluation. Liver Transpl. 2000;6:85–91.
36. Chan T, Palevsky HI, Miller WT. Pulmonary hypertension complicating portal hypertension: findings on chest radiographs. AJR Am J Roentgenol. 1988;151:909–14.
37. Kuo PC, Plotkin JS, Johnson LB, et al. Distinctive clinical features of porto-pulmonary hypertension. Chest. 1997;112:980–6.
38. Nagaya N, Nishikimi T, Uematsu M, et al. Plasma brain natriuretic peptide as a prognostic indicator in patients with primary pulmonary hypertension. Circulation. 2000;102:865–70.
39. Hoeper MM, Bogaard HJ, Condliffe R, et al. Definitions and diagnosis of pulmonary hypertension. J Am Coll Cardiol. 2013;62:D42–50.
40. Hoeper MM, Lee SH, Voswinckel R, et al. Complications of right heart catheterization procedures in patients with pulmonary hypertension in experienced centers. J Am Coll Cardiol. 2006;48:2546–52.
41. Rodriguez-Roisin R, Krowka MJ, Herve P, et al. Pulmonary-hepatic vascular disorders (PHD). Eur Respir J. 2004;24:861–80.
42. Krowka MJ. Pulmonary hypertension: diagnostics and therapeutics. Mayo Clin Proc. 2000;75:625.
43. Edwards BS, Weir EK, Edwards WD, et al. Coexistent pulmonary and portal hypertension: morphologic and clinical features. J Am Coll Cardiol. 1987;10:1233.
44. Krowka MJ. Hepatopulmonary syndrome versus porto- pulmonary hypertension: distinctions and dilemmas. Hepatology. 1997;25:1282.
45. Barst RJ, Mcgoon M, Torbicki A, et al. Diagnosis and differential assessment of pulmonary arterial hypertension. J Am Coll Cardiol. 2004;43:40S.
46. Galie N, Hoeper MM, Humbert M, et al. Guidelines for the diagnosis and treatment of pulmonary hypertension: the Task Force for the Diagnosis and Treatment of Pulmonary Hyper- tension of the European Society of Cardiology (ESC) and the European Respiratory Society (ERS), endorsed by the International Society of Heart and Lung Transplantation (ISHLT). Eur Heart J. 2009;30:2493–537.
47. Swanson KL, Krowka MJ. Screen for porto-pulmonary hypertension, especially in liver transplant candidates. Cleve Clin J Med. 2008;75:121–122 [125–30, 133 passim].
48. Ota K, Shijo H, Kokawa H, et al. Effects of nifedipine on hepatic venous pressure gradient and portal vein blood flow in patients with cirrhosis. J Gastroenterol Hepatol. 1995;10:198–204.
49. Galie N, Manes A, Negro L, et al. A meta-analysis of randomized controlled trials in pulmonary arterial hypertension. Eur Heart J. 2009;30:394–403.
50. Ogawa E, Hori T, Doi H, et al. Living-donor liver trans- plantation for congenital biliary atresia with porto-pulmonary hypertension and moderate or severe pulmonary arterial hypertension: Kyoto University experience. Clin Transpl. 2014;28(9):1031–40.
51. Fix OK, Bass NM, De Marco T, et al. Long-term follow-up of porto-pulmonary hypertension: effect of treatment with epoprostenol. Liver Transpl. 2007;13:875–85.
52. Awdish RL, Cajigas HR. Early initiation of prostacyclin in porto-pulmonary hypertension: 10 years of a transplant center's experience. Lung. 2013;191:593–600.
53. Sakai T, Planinsic RM, Mathier MA, et al. Initial experience using continuous intravenous Treprostinil to manage pulmonary arterial hypertension in patients with end-stage liver disease. Transpl Int. 2009;22:554–61.
54. Hollatz TJ, Musat A, Westphal S, et al. Treatment with sildenafil and Treprostinil allows successful liver transplantation of patients with moderate-to-severe porto-pulmonary hypertension. Liver Transpl. 2012;18:686–95.
55. Melgosa MT, Ricci GL, Garcia-Pagan JC, et al. Acute and long-term effects of inhaled iloprost in porto-pulmonary hypertension. Liver Transpl. 2010;16:348–56.
56. Kim EJ, Shin MS, Oh KY, et al. Successful management of porto-pulmonary hypertension with beraprost. Eur J Gas- troenterol Hepatol. 2010;22:1503–5.
57. Kuntzen C, Gulberg V, Gerbes AL. Use of a mixed endothelin receptor antagonist in porto-pulmonary hypertension: a safe and effective therapy? Gastroenterology. 2005;128:164–8.
58. Hoeper MM, Halank M, Marx C, et al. Bosentan therapy for porto-pulmonary hypertension. Eur Respir J. 2005;25:502–8.
59. Savale L, Magnier R, Le Pavec J, et al. Efficacy, safety and pharmacokinetics of bosentan in porto-pulmonary hypertension. Eur Respir J. 2013;41:96–103.
60. Cartin-Ceba R, Swanson K, Iyer V, et al. Safety and efficacy of ambrisentan for the treatment of porto-pulmonary hypertension. Chest. 2011;139:109–14.
61. Reichenberger F, Voswinckel R, Steveling E, et al. Sildenafil treatment for porto-pulmonary hypertension. Eur Respir J. 2006;28:563–7.
62. Hemnes AR, Robbins IM. Sildenafil monotherapy in porto- pulmonary hypertension can facilitate liver transplantation. Liver Transpl. 2009;15:15–9.
63. Gough MS, White RJ. Sildenafil therapy is associated with improved hemodynamics in liver transplantation candidates with pulmonary arterial hypertension. Liver Transpl. 2009;15:30–6.
64. Austin MJ, McDougall NI, Wendon JA, et al. Safety and efficacy of combined use of sildenafil, bosentan, and iloprost before and after liver transplantation in severe porto-pulmonary hypertension. Liver Transpl. 2008;14:287–91.
65. Schott R, Chaouat A, Launoy A, et al. Improvement of pulmonary hypertension after liver transplantation. Chest. 1999;115:1748–9.
66. Sussman N, Kaza V, Barshes N, et al. Successful liver transplantation following medical management of porto-pulmonary hypertension: a single-center series. Am J Transplant. 2006;6:2177–82.
67. Ashfaq M, Chinnakotla S, Rogers L, et al. The impact of treatment of porto-pulmonary hypertension on survival following liver transplantation. Am J Transplant. 2007;7:1258–64.
68. Sulica R, Emre S, Poon M. Medical management of porto- pulmonary hypertension and right heart failure prior to living-related liver transplantation. Congest Heart Fail. 2004;10:192–4.
69. Bandara M, Gordon FD, Sarwar A, et al. Successful outcomes following living donor liver transplantation for porto-pulmonary hypertension. Liver Transpl. 2010;16:983–9.
70. Ueno T, Saka R, Takama Y, et al. Onset ages of hepatopulmonary syndrome and pulmonary hypertension in patients with biliary atresia. Pediatr Surg Int. 2017 Oct;33(10):1053–7.
71. Martin P, DiMartini A, Feng S, et al. Evaluation for liver transplantation in adults: 2013 practice guideline by the American Association for the Study of Liver Diseases and the American Society of Transplantation. Hepatology. 2014;59:1144–65.

72. Swanson KL, Wiesner RH, Nyberg SL, et al. Survival in porto- pulmonary hypertension: Mayo Clinic experience categorized by treatment subgroups. Am J Transplant. 2008;8:2445–53.
73. Krowka MJ, Mandell MS, Ramsay MA, et al. Hepatopulmonary syndrome and porto-pulmonary hypertension: a report of the multicenter liver transplant database. Liver Transpl. 2004;10:174–82.
74. Ogawa E, Hori T, Doi H, et al. Living- donor liver transplantation for moderate or severe portopulmonary hypertension accompanied by pulmonary arterial hypertension: a single-centre experience over 2 decades in Japan. J Hepatobiliary Pancreat Sci. 2012;19:638.
75. Grannas G, Neipp M, Hoeper MM, et al. Indications for and outcomes after combined lung and liver transplantation: a single-center experience on 13 consecutive cases. Transplan- tation. 2008;85:524–31.
76. Hadengue A, Benhayoun MK, Lebrec D, et al. Pulmonary hypertension complicating portal hypertension: prevalence and relation to splanchnic hemodynamics. Gastroenterology. 1991;100:520.
77. Robalino BD, Moodie DS. Association between primary pulmonary hypertension and portal hypertension: analysis of its pathophysiology and clinical, laboratory and hemodynamic manifestations. J Am Coll Cardiol. 1991;17:492.
78. Krowka MJ, Mandell MS, Ramsay MA, et al. Hepato- pulmonary syndrome and portopulmonary hypertension: a report of the multicenter liver transplant database. Liver Transpl. 2004;10:174.
79. Ramsay M. Portopulmonary hypertension and right heart failure in patients with cirrhosis. Curr Opin Anaesthesiol. 2010;23:145.
80. Krowka MJ, Plevak DJ, Findlay JY, et al. Pulmonary hemodynamics and perioperative cardiopulmonary-related mortality in patients with porto-pulmonary hypertension undergoing liver transplantation. Liver Transpl. 2000;6:443–50.
81. Ramsay MA, Simpson BR, Nguyen AT, Ramsay KJ, East C, Klintmalm GB. Severe pulmonary hypertension in liver transplant candidates. Liver Transpl Surg. 1997;3:494.
82. Egawa H, Kasahara M, Inomata Y, et al. Long-term out- come of living related liver transplantation for patients with intrapulmonary shunting and strategy for complications. Transplantation. 1999;67:712.
83. De Wolf AM, Scott VL, Gasior T, et al. Pulmonary hypertension and liver transplantation. Anesthesiology. 1993;78:213.
84. Krowka MJ. Portopulmonary hypertension. Semin Respir Crit Care Med. 2012;33:17.
85. Savale L, O'Callaghan DS, Magnier R, et al. Current management approaches to porto-pulmonary hypertension. Int J Clin Pract Suppl. 2011;169:11–8.
86. Laurent S, Manuel G, Nathan E, et al. Portopulmonary hypertension in the current era of pulmonary hypertension management. J Hepatol. 2020;73:130–9.

# Long-Term Complications of Cirrhosis/ Hepatic Encephalopathy

# 37

Tatsuya Suzuki and Takashi Hashimoto

**Abstract**

Postoperative hepatic fibrosis occurring after a Kasai portoenterostomy for biliary atresia is a progressive condition although the severity may differ between cases. Hepatic fibrosis is an important underlying condition with a considerable impact on the postoperative course and development of complications. Advanced hepatic fibrosis is known as cirrhosis. In patients for whom icterus reduction has not been completely achieved after Kasai portoenterostomy, cholestasis is not resolved, which naturally leads to hepatic fibrosis advancement and consequently advanced cirrhosis one to two years after surgery. However, even among patients for whom jaundice has completely disappeared after Kasai portoenterostomy, some will experience gradual hepatic fibrosis and manifest symptoms of cirrhosis after a few years or decades. This chapter offers an overview of cirrhosis as a long-term postoperative complication of surgical treatment for biliary atresia, as well as hepatic encephalopathy, which is a major symptom of cirrhosis. Then, we will also describe the features of cirrhosis and hepatic encephalopathy in post-Kasai portoenterostomy patients whose native liver has developed the condition after reaching adulthood at our institution.

## 37.1 Cirrhosis

### 37.1.1 Concept

Cirrhosis is the terminal phase of any chronic progressive liver disease and, in most cases, is irreversible. Histopathologically, the disease develops as fibrosis, and capillarization of the hepatic sinusoids occurs during the process of necrosis, dropout, and regeneration of hepatocytes. The following can be found in diffuse lesions throughout the whole liver: formation of macroscopic nodules, formation of an interstitial septum connecting the Glisson's capsule and the central veins, and changes in the structure of hepatic lobules (pseudolobule formation) due to the formation of regenerating nodules. Due to hepatocellular dysfunction, patients develop progressive liver dysfunction as well as a chronic liver failure; however, hepatic fibrosis and the formation of regenerative nodules cause an impairment of blood flow, leading to concomitant portal hypertension [1].

T. Suzuki (✉)
Fujita Health University School of Medicine, Toyoake, Aichi, Japan
e-mail: tsuzuki@fujita-hu.ac.jp

T. Hashimoto
Masuko Memorial Hospital, Nagoya, Japan

### 37.1.2 Classification

#### 37.1.2.1 Classification Based on Etiopathogenesis

Depending on the etiopathogenesis, the condition can be classified as viral hepatic, alcoholic, autoimmune, cholestatic, metabolic, congestive, or drug-induced cirrhosis or cirrhosis due to particular infectious diseases, nonalcoholic steatohepatitis, and cirrhosis of unknown etiology. Cirrhosis due to biliary atresia (BA) is a cholestatic cirrhosis.

### 37.1.3 Functional Classification

#### 37.1.3.1 Compensated Cirrhosis

Pathological findings of the liver show cirrhosis but the liver function is well maintained, and clinical symptoms are virtually absent. Even if findings show hepatosplenomegaly, spider hemangiomas, palmar erythema, or esophageal varices, the absence of clinical symptoms indicates compensated cirrhosis.

#### 37.1.3.2 Decompensated Cirrhosis

This is a condition in which hepatic dysfunction and portal hypertension have progressed, and the patient develops


M. Nio (ed.), *Introduction to Biliary Atresia*, https://doi.org/10.1007/978-981-16-2160-4_37

symptoms caused by liver failure, such as hepatic encephalopathy, jaundice, ascites, edema, and a bleeding tendency. Classification is performed in the absence of medical treatment, and patients who become asymptomatic after receiving medical treatment are also considered as having decompensated cirrhosis [2].

### 37.1.4 Diagnostic Guidelines

The definitive diagnosis of cirrhosis is based on a histological diagnosis of liver biopsy specimens. However, because liver biopsies are an invasive diagnostic method, it is not required when the diagnosis of cirrhosis can be established comprehensively based on imaging and blood tests.

Complications such as portal hypertension and hypersplenism are reflected in blood test findings and are accompanied by pancytopenia. Particularly, thrombopenia is important in the evaluation of chronic liver disease progression.

In blood biochemistry tests, serum transaminase levels increase depending on the severity of hepatocellular injury. Biliary enzyme levels are elevated in most post-Kasai portoenterostomy patients. In addition, serum bilirubin and total bile acid levels are elevated as they reflect hepatocellular injury and excretory disorders, but because excretion disorders are the foundation of BA pathogenesis, serum bilirubin and total bile acid levels can also be considerably higher compared to the severity of hepatocellular injury in some patients. In patients whose condition has progressed to liver cirrhosis after receiving surgical treatment for BA, areas with poor bile excretion become atrophic and areas with good bile excretion remain present; as a result, there are patients whose serum transaminase and biliary enzyme levels are within the range of normal values. However, findings show a decrease in the serum levels of albumin, cholinesterase, and cholesterol, which reflects a decrease in hepatocyte synthesis function. In addition, due to impaired synthesis of coagulation proteins, findings show a prolonged prothrombin time. In patients with hepatic encephalopathy, blood ammonia levels are elevated, and both the Fisher's ratio (branched-chain amino acids [BCAA]/aromatic amino acids [AAA]) and BTR (molar ratio of BCAA to tyrosine) are low [3].

Platelet count, hyaluronic acid, and type-IV collagen have conventionally been known as liver fibrosis markers measured in blood tests. Mac-2 binding protein glycosylation isomer (M2BPGi) is a new glycosylation marker that evaluates the progression of hepatic fibrosis. M2BPGi has also shown to be useful owing to its high correlation with the stage of liver fibrosis in post-Kasai portoenterostomy patients [4, 5]. Evaluation of hepatic fibrosis by combining multiple test results such as the Fib-4 index and APRI (aspartate aminotransferase to platelet ratio index) has also been proposed.

Among the imaging tests, ultrasonography (US) is simple, convenient, and provides considerable information. It can show changes in liver morphology (enlargement or atrophy of the liver), irregularities on the liver surface, blunted liver margin, a roughened or heterogeneous liver parenchyma, meandering of the portal vein branches, and poor depiction of the branches of the portal and hepatic vein branches. As extrahepatic findings, US can show ascites, splenomegaly, and portal collateral circulation. US is important for the diagnosis of cirrhosis and as a screening test for the early detection of liver cancers. Like US, computed tomography (CT) and magnetic resonance imaging (MRI) provide findings such as changes in liver morphology and vascular systems, ascites, and splenomegaly. Additionally, CT and MRI are also performed as screening tests for hepatocellular carcinoma and as a means for the qualitative diagnosis of hepatic mass lesions.

Diagnostic US and MRI have recently been used for the measurement of liver stiffness. The US diagnosis of liver stiffness falls roughly into two categories: strain and shear-wave imaging. FibroScan [R], which is currently the most popular ultrasound machine, measures the intrahepatic propagation velocity of mechanical shear elastic waves generated by a probe; for the measurement of liver stiffness (kiloPascal, kPa), it allows for the measurement of liver fibrosis severity in a noninvasive manner. In 2D-shear wave elastography using acoustic pressure, liver stiffness is measured as a color map and in m/second. MRI elastography (MRE), which uses MRI, is a method that quantifies an object's hardness in a noninvasive manner and is highly objective with high reliability in the diagnosis of hepatic fibrosis [6]. In postoperative patients, especially older children, who had received surgical treatment for BA, the measurement of liver stiffness has been reported to be the most accurate method for the diagnosis of cirrhosis [7].

### 37.1.5 Symptoms of Decompensated Cirrhosis

The symptoms of decompensated cirrhosis include indefinite complaints such as bloating, general malaise, fatigue, and loss of appetite, as well as ascites, symptoms caused by edema, and gastrointestinal symptoms due to portal hypertension such as gastrointestinal bleeding, disturbance of consciousness, psychiatric symptoms, and disorientation due to hepatic encephalopathy.

### 37.1.6 Long-term Follow-up Guidelines

In the follow-up of cirrhosis, early detection and therapeutic intervention against the progression of cirrhosis as well as complications such as pleural effusion, ascites, hepatic encephalopathy, esophageal varices, sarcopenia, hepatocellular carcinoma, hepatorenal syndrome, hepatopulmonary syndrome, and spontaneous bacterial peritonitis are imperative. Blood tests including tumor markers and items for the evaluation of the hepatic functional reserve need to be carried out on a regular basis, as well as assessment of the presence or absence of complications. In addition, upper gastrointestinal endoscopy to evaluate varicose vein development and abdominal US, CT, and MRI need to be conducted on a regular basis to assess the presence or absence of coexisting liver cancer.

### 37.1.7 Treatment Guidelines

The treatment of cirrhosis can be roughly divided into several major categories: removal of the cause, nutrition therapy, lifestyle guidance, and the treatment of cirrhosis complications. For cirrhosis patients who are prone to malnutrition, their condition is especially at risk of being complicated with sarcopenia; since the prognosis is likely to be poor, initiation of nutrition therapy at an early stage is important regardless of the cause of cirrhosis, and liver transplantation should also be considered in case of decompensated cirrhosis or comatose acute liver failure.

## 37.2 Hepatic Encephalopathy

### 37.2.1 Concept

Like jaundice, ascites, and edema, hepatic encephalopathy (hepatic coma) is a typical symptom of liver failure. The main causative diseases are fulminant hepatitis, cirrhosis, idiopathic portal hypertension, and congenital errors of amino acid metabolism. Its pathogenetic mechanism is based on an absolute or relative insufficiency of liver function (amount of functional hepatocytes), which metabolizes and neutralizes the so-called encephalopathy-inducing factors such as ammonia. As a result, factors that remain present without being neutralized inhibit central nervous system functions, leading to a disturbance of consciousness [8]. Based on the disease's etiopathology, hepatic encephalopathy can be roughly divided into two types: one that causes an absolute decrease in the amount of functional hepatocytes and another in which the amount of hepatocytes is quantitatively preserved but the portal vein blood flow enters the systemic circulation through a shunt without passing through the liver, rendering the liver ineffective. The clinically most frequent cases of hepatic encephalopathy associated with cirrhosis consist of these two types, combined at various proportions [9].

### 37.2.2 Classification and Diagnosis

The types of hepatic encephalopathy are classified as acute, chronic, or specific. The acute type is represented by fulminant hepatitis, while the chronic type is represented by cirrhosis with developed collateral circulation. The particular type is less frequent, but typical diseases include urea cycle disorder. The term hepatic encephalopathy is used almost as a synonym of hepatic coma, and its severity ranges from a mild to deep coma. Because hepatic encephalopathy is also accompanied by disorientation and psychiatric symptoms, the severity of consciousness impairment or diagnosis of coma is classified using the Inuyama classification instead of the Japan Coma Scale (Table 37.1). However, in most cases, a stage-I coma is particularly difficult to determine in actual clinical settings. Flapping tremors are often seen in encephalopathy cases with a coma stage II or higher. However, the tremors disappear in coma stages IV or higher, when patients reach a comatose state in a more restricted sense of the term. As the coma progresses,

**Table 37.1** Classification of coma severity in hepatic encephalopathy (Inuyama's classification, partially modified)[a]

| Coma severity | Psychiatric symptoms | Reference items |
|---|---|---|
| I | • Reversal of the sleep-wakefulness cycle<br>• Euphoric mood, depression<br>• Sloppy and uncaring attitude | • This condition can only be determined retrospectively in most cases |
| II | • Disorientation, mixing things up<br>• Abnormal behavior<br>• Drowsy state (the patient opens their eyes when being called and can hold a conversation)<br>• The patient follows the doctor's instructions | • No agitated state<br>• No urinary/fecal incontinence<br>• Presence of flapping tremors |
| III | • The patient is often in an agitated state, is delirious, and shows a rebellious attitude<br>• The patient is lethargic (asleep most of the time)<br>• The patient opens their eyes in response to external stimuli but does not or cannot follow the doctor's instructions (the patient responds to simple instructions) | • Presence of flapping tremors (when the patient cooperates)<br>• Orientation is highly impaired |
| IV | • Coma (complete loss of consciousness)<br>• The patient responds to painful stimuli | • The patient shows fending-off movements or frowns in response to stimuli |
| V | • Deep coma<br>• The patient does not respond to painful stimuli | |

[a]The Japan Society of Hepatology (eds) (2019) Treatment guide for chronic hepatitis and cirrhosis. : Liver Cirrhosis 2019 edn. Bunkoudo, Japan, p. 56

patients with hepatic encephalopathy show a symmetrical and diffuse slowing of brain waves, which is useful for the prediction of coma, determination of severity, and estimation of the treatment effect.

### 37.2.3 Acute-on-Chronic Liver Failure

In some cases, heavy alcohol consumption, bacterial infections such as idiopathic bacterial peritonitis, gastrointestinal bleeding, and exacerbation of the underlying disease act as exacerbating factors, which may result in the progression of liver failure within a short period of time. This condition is called "acute-on-chronic liver failure" in order to distinguish it from the chronic decompensation of cirrhosis. As for the diagnostic criteria, a diagnosis of Acute-on-Chronic Liver Failure (ACLF) is established when the aforementioned exacerbating factors are combined with compensated or decompensated cirrhosis with a score of 5–9 points in the Child-Pugh classification, in addition to severe liver dysfunction within a 28-day period and liver damage showing a prothrombin time international normalized ratio $\geq 1.5$, prothrombin activity levels $\leq 40\%$, and total serum bilirubin levels $\geq 5.0$ mg/dl [10].

### 37.2.4 Treatment Guidelines

BCAA infusion formulations have an immediate effect on hepatic encephalopathy complicating cirrhosis. If a cirrhosis patient visits a hospital after developing encephalopathy, the treatment consists primarily of removing the causes of gastrointestinal bleeding and constipation and conducting a parallel administration of BCAA infusion and oral synthetic disaccharides. This treatment alone has been reported to wake up 70–80% of cirrhotic encephalopathy patients within 1–3 days [8]. When the symptoms are stabilized, prevention of recurrence is important. Contributing factors such as excessive protein intake, constipation, dehydration, and infection must be eliminated, while lifestyle guidance is provided and medication is administered. As drug therapy, synthetic disaccharides are administered orally to lower the intestinal pH and inhibit the absorption of ammonia. Next, a poorly absorbed antimicrobial agent (rifaximin) is used to inhibit anaerobic bacterial producers of hepatic encephalopathy-inducing factors. Furthermore, in cirrhosis patients, replacement therapy using orally administered BCAA preparations significantly prevents the onset of liver failure (hepatic encephalopathy, ascites, edema, and jaundice) and has been proven to extend survival.

## 37.3 Features of Cirrhosis and Hepatic Encephalopathy in Patients Who Had Been Operated on for BA and Who Have Reached Adulthood Long After Kasai Portoenterostomy

In BA patients, fibrosis progresses gradually in the liver even in patients whose jaundice disappeared completely after Kasai portoenterostomy. In some cases, the symptoms of cirrhosis become apparent after a few years or decades [11].

The adult patients with post-Kasai portoenterostomy condition visited our institution during the 2019 fiscal year accounted for 28 cases (15 men and 13 women; age range: 20–41 years; median age: 26 years). Jaundice had resolved in 19 cases (68%) but was persistent in 9 cases (32%). Among the 28 cases, cirrhosis was diagnosed in 21 cases (75%), including 11 cases of compensated cirrhosis and 10 cases of decompensated cirrhosis. The blood chemistry test results and CT images of typical cases of compensated and decompensated cirrhosis (33-year-old man vs. 26-year-old woman) are shown in Figs. 37.1 and 37.2, respectively. Blood biochemistry test results varied greatly among cases, and the Model for End-Stage Liver Disease (MELD) score was 7 points in patients with compensated cirrhosis and 15 points in patients with decompensated liver cirrhosis. However, because findings from CT images look similar, the functional severity of cirrhosis cannot be estimated based on CT images alone.

During a one-year observation conducted in 2019, three cases (11%) of hepatic encephalopathy were diagnosed, including two that needed in-hospital treatment. The first patient (26-year-old man) had developed hepatic encepha-

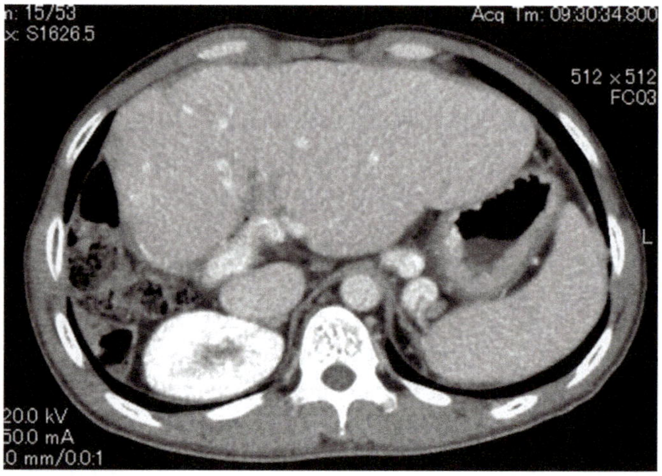


Fig. 37.1 A case of compensated cirrhosis, 33-year-old man with post-Kasai portoenterostomy. MELD 7 point. TB 0.8 mg/dL, DB 0.1 mg/dL, TP 7.3 g/dL, Alb 4.5 g/dL AST 36 U/L, ALT 36 U/L, G-GTP 138 U/L, PT-INR 1.03, CRE 0.6 mg/dL, Na 139 mmol/L

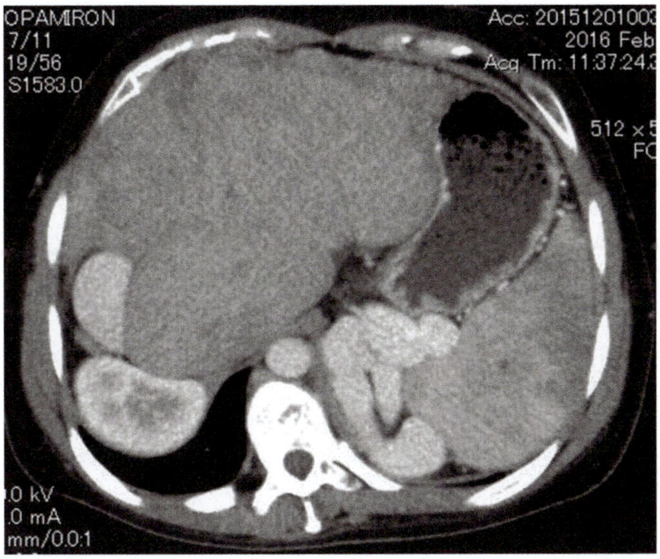


Fig. 37.2 A case of decompensated cirrhosis, a 26-year-old woman with post-Kasai portoenterostomy. MELD 15 points. TB 5.9 mg/dL, DB 2.8 mg/dL, TP 5.7 g/dL, Alb 2.6 g/dL AST 115 U/L, ALT 74 U/L, G-GTP 287 U/L, PT-INR 1.20, CRE 0.35 mg/dL, Na 139 mmol/L. TB; Total bilirubin, DB; Direct bilirubin, TP; Total protein, Alb; Albumin, AST; Aspartate aminotransferase, ALT; Alanine aminotransferase, G-GTP; gamma-glutamyl transpeptidase, PT-INR; Prothrombin Time International Normalized Ratio, CRE; Creatinine, Na; Sodium

lopathy during gastrointestinal bleeding and needed in-hospital treatment. He had a MELD score of 16 points and was waiting for a liver transplant from a brain-dead donor. The patient presented with abnormal behavior and disorientation and was hospitalized after being diagnosed with stage-II hepatic encephalopathy, but immediate improvement was seen after administration of a BCAA infusion preparation. A patient who was hospitalized for cholangitis (34-year-old woman) also had a MELD score of 21 points and was waiting for a liver transplant from a brain-dead donor. The patient presented with abnormal behavior, disorientation, and drowsiness and was hospitalized after being diagnosed with stage-III hepatic encephalopathy. Administration of a BCAA infusion preparation did not lead to a marked improvement, while hepatic dysfunction and thrombocytopenia showed a rapid exacerbation. The patient developed ACLF and was treated with high-efficiency hemodiafiltration in the intensive care unit, which improved hepatic encephalopathy. However, gastrointestinal bleeding and cholangitis relapsed again later, and as a result, the patient developed an ACLF twice in a row. She also developed septicemia, which led to acute respiratory distress syndrome and death. A patient who is actively receiving treatment on an outpatient basis (34-year-old man) was believed to have chronic stage-I/stage-II hepatic encephalopathy and showed signs of liver failure such as jaundice, hypoalbuminemia, thrombocytopenia, gastrointestinal bleeding, and ascites. Therefore, although the patient was unable to work, the patient's condition became stable upon receiving conservative treatment using diuretics, proton pump inhibitors, and oral BCAA supplements.

The symptoms of cirrhosis occurring after Kasai portoenterostomy for BA are diverse, and the intensity of liver fibrosis does not necessarily correlate with the severity of complications (such as gastrointestinal bleeding, hepatopulmonary syndrome, portopulmonary hypertension, or liver failure). However, among patients who had been operated on for BA and reached adulthood without developing jaundice or serious complications during the long-term postoperative course, we recently experienced patients who showed a relapse of jaundice and the development of liver failure after reaching their 20s or 30s. Predictive factors for the early detection of such cases have not yet been established, but regular evaluation of the hepatic functional reserve and the presence or absence of complications is important [12].

Hepatic encephalopathy in post-Kasai portoenterostomy patients is not frequently encountered, but in patients with sarcopenia or hypoalbuminemia, nutritional therapy using oral branched-amino acid supplements is required. Furthermore, intensive care adjusted to the treatment of fulminant liver failure is needed to deal with the onset or aggravation of acute hepatic encephalopathies such as ACLF.

## References

1. The Japan Society of Hepatology (eds) (2019) Treatment guide for chronic hepatitis and cirrhosis.: Liver Cirrhosis 2019 edn. Bunkoudo, Japan, p50
2. The Japan Society of Hepatology (eds) (2019) Treatment guide for chronic hepatitis and cirrhosis.: Liver Cirrhosis 2019 edn. Bunkoudo, Japan, p52
3. The Japan Society of Hepatology (eds) (2019) Treatment guide for chronic hepatitis and cirrhosis.: Liver Cirrhosis 2019 edn. Bunkoudo, Japan, p58
4. Shirabe K, Bekki Y, Gantummur D, et al. Mac-2 binding protein glycan isomer (M2BPGi) is a new serum biomarker for assessing liver fibrosis: more than a biomarker of liver fibrosis. J Gastroenterol. 2018;53:819–26.
5. Ueno T, Kodama T, Noguchi Y, et al. Clinical implications of serum Mac-2 binding protein glycan isomer (M2BPGi) during regular follow-up of patients with biliary atresia. Pediatric Surg. Int. 2018;34:1065–71.
6. Wu JF, Lee CS, Jeng YM, et al. Transient Elastography Is Useful in Diagnosing Biliary Atresia and Predicting Prognosis After Hepatoportoenterostomy. Hepatology. 2018;68:616–24.
7. Hukkinen M., Lohi J, Heikkila P. et.al (2019) Noninvasive Evaluation of Liver Fibrosis and Portal Hypertension After Successful Portoenterostomy for Biliary Atresia. Hepatology Communications 3:382-391

8. Moriwaki H. Treatment system for hepatic encephalopathy. J of the Japanese Society of Gastroenterology. 2007;104:352–6.
9. Kato S, Suzuki K. Hepatic encephalopathy: diagnosis/test. J of the Japanese Society of Gastroenterology. 2007;104:344–51.
10. The Japan Society of Hepatology (eds) (2019) Treatment guide for chronic hepatitis and cirrhosis.: Liver Cirrhosis 2019 edn. Bunkoudo, Japan, pp. 56-57.
11. Bezerra JA, Wells RG, Mack CA, et al. Biliary Atresia: Clinical and Research Challenges for the Twenty-First Century. Hepatology. 2018;68:P1163–73.
12. Kelay A, Davenport M. Long-term outlook in biliary atresia. Seminars in Pediatric Surgery. 2017;26:295–300.

# Long-Term Functional Outcome and Quality of Life After Kasai Operation

38

Masato Shinkai, Norihiko Kitagawa, Kyoko Mochizuki, and Hidehito Usui

**Abstract**

The Japanese Biliary Atresia Registry reported that 10-year and 20-year native liver survival rates were 55% and 49%, respectively. An increasing number of patients with biliary atresia have now survived into adulthood with their native livers, achieving normal physical growth, favorable liver function, near-normal neurodevelopment, and social performances. However, more than half of these patients have had liver-related complications such as portal hypertension and cholangitis, which can be a risk factor for requiring liver transplantation (LT) and impairing health-related quality of life (QOL). Therefore, life-long meticulous follow-up is mandatory in order to promote health and QOL, deal with sequelae and/or complications appropriately, as well as to determine the optimal timing of LT.

**Keywords**

Biliary atresia · Outcome · Native liver survival · Quality of life · Adulthood

## 38.1 Introduction

Biliary atresia (BA) is a chronic inflammatory hepatobiliary disease of unknown etiology which causes a varied degree of destruction and obstruction of the extrahepatic and intrahepatic bile ducts. Since Morio Kasai first reported the effectiveness of hepatic portoenterostomy (HPE) on bile drainage in the patients with "uncorrectable" BA in the 1950s, HPE has eventually been regarded as a standard and sole procedure for rescuing native livers [1]. Nowadays, many BA patients have survived for decades with their native livers. However, HPEs do not always cure BA completely but do alleviate the pathological processes that can induce cholestatic liver cirrhosis. Therefore, insidious hepatic damage may develop even in long-term survivors with native livers and pose a significant risk of sequelae and hepatic deterioration, which does impair the quality of their lives (QOL).

Marked advances in pediatric liver transplantation (LT) have recently achieved a long-term patient survival rate of nearly 90% without major complications, which may raise questions over the role of HPE in BA [2].

In this chapter we will review the long-term outcomes that HPEs have produced and failed to produce in terms of the effect on survival and QOL, which will help in evaluating the role of HPE in BA and shed light on how medical providers can help long-term survivors with BA to promote better health and improve social life.

## 38.2 Survival with Native Livers

Infants with BA will die of liver cirrhosis and failure within 2 years of age if sufficient bile drainage is not established. Due to a shortage of transplant organs, a great deal of effort is continuously being made to save native livers for as long as possible, not only by refinement of HPE surgery, but also by early diagnosis of BA and long-term postoperative management and care.

An increasing number of reports on long-term survival after HPEs have been published in various countries over the past few decades. The survival rates seem to be quite different depending on when and where the HPEs had been done.

In the late 1990s, Altman from the USA already reported 10- and 20-year native liver survival rates of 35% and 21%, respectively [3]. Similar outcomes have also been reported from Western Europe and Canada, with the 10-and 20-year native liver survival rates ranging from 26 to 41% and from 23 to 27%, respectively [4–10]. Furthermore, in East Asia, where BA is more prevalent, HPEs have achieved better outcomes, including 10- and 20-year native liver survival rates ranging from 31% to 60% and from 33% to 51%, respectively [11–16] (Table 38.1).

M. Shinkai (✉) · N. Kitagawa · K. Mochizuki · H. Usui
Kanagawa Children's Medical Center, Yokohama, Japan
e-mail: mshinkai@kcmc.jp


M. Nio (ed.), *Introduction to Biliary Atresia*, https://doi.org/10.1007/978-981-16-2160-4_38

**Table 38.1** Literature review on long-term survival with native livers (SNL) after Kasai operation

| Nation | Authors | Year of Publication | Year of Kasai operation | N of patients after Kasai operation | SNL at 5 year | SNL at 10 year | SNL at 15 year | SNL at 20 year | Reference |
|---|---|---|---|---|---|---|---|---|---|
| USA and Canada | Karrer FM | 1990 | 1976-1989 | 816 | 0.48 | 0.3 | | | 8 |
| Denver, New York | Altman P | 1997 | 1972-1996 | 266 | 0.45 | 0.35 | | 0.21 | 3 |
| UK and Ireland | McKiernan PJ | 2000 | 1993-1995 | 91 | 0.301 | | | | 9 |
| England and Wales, UK | Davenport M | 2011 | 1999-2009 | 424 | 0.46 | 0.4 | | | 5 |
| Netherland | de Vries W | 2011 | 1977-1982 | 49 | | | | 0.2 | 25 |
| | | | 1983-1988 | 55 | | | | 0.32 | |
| France | Lykavieris P | 2005 | 1968-1983 | 271 | | 0.32 | | 0.23 | 4 |
| | Chardot | 1999 | 1986-1996 | 440 | 0.32 | 0.27 | | | 10 |
| | Serinet | 2009 | 1986~2002 | 695 | 0.38 | 0.32 | 0.29 | | 7 |
| Canada | Schreiber RA | 2007 | 1985-2002 | 349 | 0.36 (4-year) | 0.26 | | | 6 |
| Taiwan | Hung | 2006 | 1976-2000 | 185 | 0.347 | 0.305 | | | 15 |
| Hong Kong | Wong | 2018 | 1980-2015 | 141 | | | | 0.51 | 52 |
| Tokyo, Japan | Okazaki T | 1999 | 1968-1985 | 115 | | 0.19 | | | 11 |
| Sendai, Japan | Howard ER | 2001 | 1969-1974 | 52 | 0.39 | 0.39 | | 0.33 | 21 |
| | | 2001 | 1975-1980 | 60 | 0.6 | 0.6 | 0.58 | 0.48 | |
| Yokohama, Japan | Shinkai M | 2009 | 1970-1975 | 27 | | | | 0.32 | 13 |
| | | | 1976-1980 | 29 | | | | 0.43 | |
| | | | 1981-1986 | 24 | | | | 0.58 | |
| | | | total | 80 | 0.63 | 0.54 | | 0.44 | |
| Japan (JBAR) | Nio M | 2003 | 1989 | 108 | 0.62 | 0.528 | | | 16 |
| | | 2017 | 1989-2015 | 3160 | | 0.545 | | 0.49 | 14 |

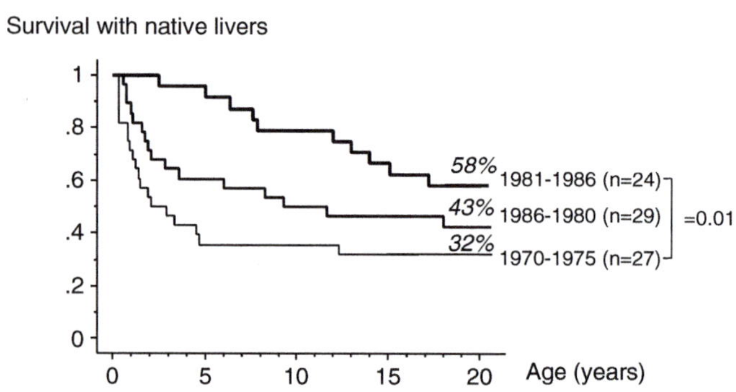


**Fig. 38.1** Improvement of the 20-year survival rates with native livers after the Kasai operation depending on the era of surgery. (Cited from "Fig 3" of Shinkai, M., Ohhama, Y., Take, H., Kitagawa, N., Kudo, H., Mochizuki, K., and Hatata, T., Long-term outcome of children with biliary atresia who were not transplanted after the Kasai operation: >20-year experience at a children's hospital. J Pediatr Gastroenterol Nutr, 2009. 48(4): 443-50.)

It is very difficult to compare the HPE outcomes between institutions based on the literature because native liver survival rates vary depending not only on the institutions performance, but also on the year of the HPE, the year of analysis and publication, patients' background (race, type of BA, age at HPE, genetic disorders associated with syndromic form of BA) and availability of LT.

At present, there is a general consensus that long-term survival with a native liver is significantly better in children who are operated on at an earlier age or children with type I cyst [4, 5, 17, 18]. However, the effect of centralization of centers for BA treatment and the prognostic difference between syndromic and non-syndromic BA have remained controversial [5, 19, 20].

As LT was unavailable in Japan until 1991, many institutions have had no other option but to make great efforts to restore bile flow and salvage native livers by refining HPE surgery and postoperative management during this period. It is noteworthy that great advances in long-term native liver survival rates were achieved in patients operated on during this period in Japan. The 10-year NLS rates improved from 39% to 60% and the 20-year NLS rates from 33% to 48% according to the Sendai group, and similar outcomes were attained in our hospital [13, 21] (Fig. 38.1). During this period, early age at the time of HPE was recognized as the prime requisite for saving native livers. Moreover, the surgical procedures for HPE have various modifications, and was finally standardized to the original Kasai HPE with simple Roux-Y in many institutions in Japan, including our hospital [13, 14, 22] (Fig. 38.2).

As of 2015, the Japanese Biliary Atresia Registry compiled follow-up data on 3160 patients registered between 1989 and 2015 and announced that 10-year and 20-year native liver survival rates were 55% and 49%, respectively [14]. However, subsequent advances in liver transplantation

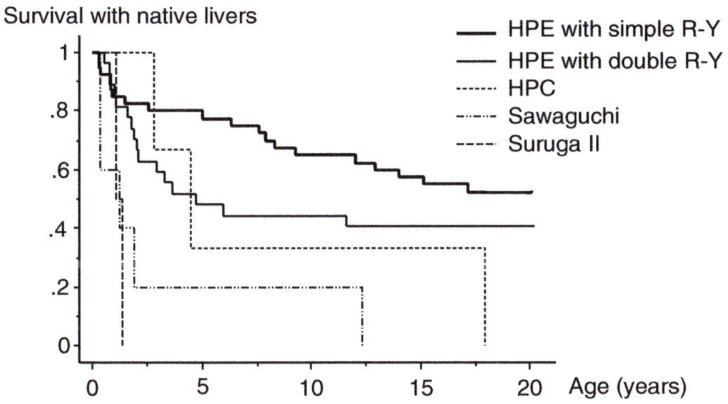


**Fig. 38.2** 20-year survival rates with native livers according to the surgical procedures. (Cited from "Fig 4" of Shinkai, M., Ohhama, Y., Take, H., Kitagawa, N., Kudo, H., Mochizuki, K., and Hatata, T., Long-term outcome of children with biliary atresia who were not transplanted after the Kasai operation: >20-year experience at a children's hospital. J Pediatr Gastroenterol Nutr, 2009. 48(4): 443-50.)

(living and cadaveric donor LT) have remarkably enhanced the overall survival of the patients with BA and broadened the indication and timing of LT, which may affect the length of native liver survival in the future [6].

## 38.3 Functional Outcome of Native Livers

### 38.3.1 Physical Growth

Physical growth is one of the diagnostic indicators of liver function, because end-stage liver disease and cholestasis can cause synthetic dysfunction and nutrient malabsorption.

In the study of 30 adult survivors with native livers in Sendai, normal physical growth, no mental retardation, normal secondary sexual characteristics were obtained in almost all adult survivors [12]. Equivalent outcomes in long-term survivors were confirmed in subsequent studies from various institutions, as long as the patients had no associated disorders, including chromosomal anomalies or intracranial hemorrhage [4, 13, 23]. Additionally, portal hypertension itself was not associated with impaired physical growth when patients with "failed" HPE were excluded [24]. The Bic^etre group reported that all adult females with BA had their first menstrual periods between the ages of 12 and 15 years, and all male patients had achieved pubertal maturation, which was consistent with the above report from Sendai [4].

### 38.3.2 Blood Results

The Sendai group was among the first to report on the hepatic status of adult survivors with native livers [12]. Clearance of jaundice was obtained at least once in all the survivors, 83% of whom experienced no recurrence of jaundice afterward. Blood analyses of 30 patients with a median age of 20.8 years showed near-normal bilirubin and increased gamma-glutamyl transpeptidase (GGT) and aspartate aminotransferase (AST) [21].

The Bic^etre group reported that 75% of adult native liver survivors had a clearance of jaundice at least once, but about a half of them experienced a relapse of jaundice later. Serum transaminase and GGT were normal in 19% of adult survivors. Prothrombin time % and serum albumin levels were below normal only in jaundiced patients [4]. In our own experience, serum levels of total bilirubin were normal in 71% of native liver survivors at the age of 20, and the transaminases' levels were normal in 37% [13]. In the Netherlands, normal serum bilirubin and transaminases were found at age 20 years in 36% of transplant-free patients [25].

A large study from the North American multicenter consortium analyzing 129 patients at median 9.7 [range 5.1-17.9] years of age reported that liver synthetic functions such as total bilirubin, albumin, and prothrombin time-international normalized ratio were normal in 75%, 85%, and 73%, respectively, and the platelet count was >150 x $10^9$/L in 35.6%. However, in this study, liver dysfunction might have been underestimated because those older than age 18 years and those listed for LT were excluded from the study [23].

### 38.3.3 Sequelae and Complications

Although native livers of long-term survivors preserve favorable synthetic function and bile drainage, this does not mean that the livers remain intact. A literature review of 14 articles including 162 adult survivors with native livers described that only 64 (39.5%) had no liver-related complications and that 35 (21.6%) had symptomatic portal hypertension with gastrointestinal bleeding, 98 (60.5%) had cholangitis, and 78 (48.1%) had both cholangitis and symptomatic portal hypertension [26]. Therefore, continued medical follow-up is mandatory for adult survivors with native livers.

#### 38.3.3.1 Cholangitis

Cholangitis soon after HPE surgery has a serious impact on early postoperative outcomes by impeding bile drainage and prompting liver fibrosis during infancy. One literature review revealed that 46% to 66% of adult survivors with native livers experienced and overcame at least one episode of early cholangitis [12, 13, 23, 27, 28]. Nevertheless, late episodes of cholangitis after 20 years of age developed in 21 to 37% of adult survivors and wielded a detrimental impact on the prognosis of their native livers [4, 12, 13, 27]. Some of these adults had developed structural or mechanical abnormalities liable to late cholangitis, including liver fibrosis, intrahepatic bile duct dilatation or biloma, intrahepatic lithiasis, and Roux loop obstruction [4, 27, 29].

In our experience, half of the adult patients who developed late cholangitis eventually lost their native livers [13].

Intrahepatic bile duct pathology is now regarded as a sign of poor prognosis of the native liver [30], although various treatment options including prolonged antibiotic therapy, cholangiodrainage, cholangioplasty, and hepatic resection have been reported to be feasible in selected cases [31–33].

#### 38.3.3.2 Cirrhosis and Portal Hypertension

Clearance of jaundice is an indispensable prerequisite for saving native livers, but that may not be by itself a sufficient condition for preserving the livers intact for the long-term and obviating various degrees of biliary cirrhosis and portal hypertension. As blood tests in adult survivors tend to show subtle abnormalities, imaging tests and upper endoscopy are required to detect liver fibrosis, cirrhosis, or portal hypertension.

The Sendai group and the Bic^etre group reported that portal hypertension represented by esophageal varices or hypersplenism developed in 36.7% and 69.8% of adult survivors with native livers, respectively [4, 12]. Our experience in Yokohama showed that 49% of adult survivors were diagnosed with liver cirrhosis and portal hypertension at age 20 years, because 37% and 26% of them had already undergone endoscopic treatment of varices and partial splenic embolization, respectively [13]. In the Netherlands study, 46% of survivors with native livers had portal hypertension at age 20, and 36% had varices [25].

A recent study from Sendai suggested that regarding jaundice-free patients, gastroesophageal varices requiring sclerotherapy and hypersplenism at 10 year of age might indicate a poor prognosis for 20-year native liver survival [34].

We should bear in mind the possibility that jejunal varices on the Roux-Y loop may develop in long-term survivors who have had gastroesophageal varices eradicated by sclerotherapy or ligation.

Hepatopulmonary syndrome (HPS) and portopulmonary hypertension (PPH) are two important pulmonary vascular complications associated with portal hypertension. Reportedly, HPS and PPH occur in 5-30% and 2-5% of patients with liver cirrhosis, respectively. PPH tends to occur later in life than HPS. Pulse oximetry, electrocardiography, and echocardiography should be done periodically as screening tests because both complications are not easy to diagnose at outpatient clinics until they are advanced [35, 36].

#### 38.3.3.3 Tumors

An increase in long-term survivors with native livers has provided the opportunity of encountering deformed native livers with various kinds of atrophy, hypertrophy, and nodular lesions. In the studies analyzing explanted native livers, our group and the Fukuoka group separately demonstrated that the atrophic area, generally located in the periphery of the liver, was typically cirrhotic, and the hypertrophic or regenerative nodules, located centrally near the hepatic hilum, were composed of a histology of near-normal architecture [37, 38]. The Bic^etre group reported that large regenerative nodules (>6 cm) were found in 5 of 63 adult survivors with native livers [4].

Regarding long-term survivors, we should be very vigilant about the development of malignant tumors, including hepatocellular carcinoma and cholangiocarcinoma, although they are much rarer compared to benign tumors. According to a recent review, malignant tumors were diagnosed at ages ranging from 0.4 to 30 years, and more than half of those evaded image detection and were incidentally found in explanted livers [39]. The longest native liver survivor with a correctable BA in the Sendai series died of cholangiocarcinoma at age 63 years [40].

## 38.4 Prognosis Predictors

Early prognostic factors for infants soon after HPE have been studied vigorously worldwide so as to identify the optimal timing for LT [41, 42]. At least, an early decline in serum bilirubin after HPE is regarded as an important factor for improving native liver survival.

On the other hand, prognostic factors for long-term survivors with native livers have remained unclear. However, this topic is quite relevant not only to patients, pediatricians, and pediatric surgeons, but also to primary care providers, hepatologists, and transplant surgeons for adults, given the present situation that nearly half of all patients with BA survive into adulthood.

Based on retrospective analysis of the outcomes of long-term survivors with native livers, the Sendai group reported age at Kasai, the period required for clearance of jaundice, and early cholangitis as risk factors affecting late-presenting liver failure [43], and recently the group added symptomatic portal hypertension to the list of risk factors [34].

The London group analyzed various parameters of native liver survivors at age 16 years and demonstrated that serum total bilirubin>21 μmol/L (1.2 mg/dl), history of portal hypertension or gastroesophageal varices by age 16 years, and cholangitis in adolescence could be risk factors indicating that LT may be required in adulthood [30]. The same group also pointed out the applicability limit of the MELD (Model for End-Stage Liver Disease) scoring system for young adults with BA [44].

## 38.5 Health-Related Quality of Life

### 38.5.1 Neurodevelopmental Outcome

Recently, HPE alone as well as combination of HPE and LT have achieved excellent non-transplant and transplant survival for patients with BA. Therefore, not only survival rates but also neurodevelopmental outcomes after HPE (and LT) have recently become an active area of research. However, this research is challenging because neurodevelopment depends on a number of influences, including the nature of liver diseases, severity, age at onset, surgical invasiveness, anesthesia, genetic and environmental factors, and associated complications. Various studies on neurodevelopmental outcomes after HPE have been documented in the literature.

Several studies revealed neurodevelopmental delays at 2 years of age, especially after failed HPE [45], developmental deficits in gross motor and/or language skills in young children before LT [46, 47], impairment in verbal intellectual abilities, working memory, mathematical skills, and reading in children waiting too long for LT [48], and high rates of special education, impaired motor outcomes, lower IQs (impaired motor skills, cognition, and behavior) in children (aged 6 to 13) with BA [49]. These deficits are likely to be closely associated with failed HPE and subsequent severe dysfunction of native livers requiring LT.

Importantly, another study showed no marked neurodevelopmental delays in children with BA aged 3 to 12 years, most of whom followed successful HPE. Even in this setting, elevated total bilirubin and GGT and portal hypertension were correlated with lower IQs [50].

### 38.5.2 Social Performance and Competence

In general, adult patients with BA, who survive with native livers, are generally endowed with normal or near-normal liver function, as mentioned above. Therefore, they are expected to have achieved favorable neurodevelopment. In fact, 60-90% of adult survivors have been reported to lead near-normal lives, attending normal schools and building occupational careers [4, 13, 51–53].

### 38.5.3 Pregnancy and Family Planning

Along with favorable social competence, an increasing number of adult survivors with native livers have married and/or had a family. Many female patients have experienced pregnancies and given birth to healthy babies, some of whom may be small for gestation, though [4, 13, 53, 54]. However, a previous history of cholangitis and symptomatic portal hypertension may be risk factors for significant liver-related complications during pregnancy and childbirth [54].

Female patients should be well informed about the risks associated with pregnancy and delivery before planning a family. Continued vigilance is required during gestation, peripartum, postpartum, and child-rearing periods, because deterioration of native livers and variceal bleeding have been experienced during these periods.

Although a study from London proposed MELD scores or UKELD scores to predict clinical outcomes in pregnant women with cirrhosis, the applicability to patients with BA remains unknown [55].

### 38.5.4 Quality of Life

Nowadays, most children with BA have survived with native livers for more than a decade after HPE. Not only how to save their lives but also how to improve their health-related quality of life (HRQOL) have become important issues for medical care providers caring for children as well as for adults with BA.

The literature on HRQOL analysis of patients with BA is heterogeneous in terms of era, patient age, sample size, severity of disease, QOL assessment methods, and study design (cross-sectional or longitudinal). Therefore, the results of analyses have varied considerably, making evaluation very difficult.

The Childhood Liver Disease Research and Education Network studied 221 children with BA at a mean age 9.75 +/- 5.25 years and found significantly poorer HRQOL across all domains, as indicated by poorer physical health, psychosocial health, and total summary HRQOL scores than healthy controls. Scores in school functioning were particularly impaired [56].

On the contrary, in the study from Finland, HRQOLs were similar between BA survivors with native livers (2~18 years of age), BA patients after LT, and matched controls, except in the domain of school functioning [57].

In terms of QOL in adult survivors, the Sendai group demonstrated that 30 Japanese patients ranging in age from 14.2 to 24.4 years were marginally impaired in general health perception and in emotional and physical functioning [21].

A small study from Hong Kong revealed that 16 adult patients with native livers scored significantly lower than disease-free control subjects in Short Forum-36 Health Survey scores, especially in the general health section and the overall physical component [52].

Meanwhile, however, a series of studies from the Netherlands demonstrated that non-transplanted young adult patients with BA (n=25) had an HRQOL similar to an age-matched control group, except that non-transplanted female patients had impaired general health perception [58, 59].

The studies on QOL of long-term survivors with native livers have revealed that adult survivors after HPE thus far obtained a comparable HRQOL to healthy controls. However, those studies dealt with limited numbers of patients accessible, differed from each other in study tools and designs, and were subject to selection or reporting bias. Therefore, it is important to restructure the scheme through a multidisciplinary approach incorporating adult primary care providers, hepatologists, or psychologists and to deal with a larger sample size in a standardized way in order to better evaluate the QOL of long-term non-transplant survivors, to identify risk factors impairing their QOL, to determine the optimal timing of LT in terms of QOL, and finally to promote the QOL of long-term survivors with BA.

## 38.6 Conclusion

Recently, nearly half of the infants with BA have survived into adulthood with native livers after HPE. Those patients are still carrying over intrinsic pathology of the liver typical of BA, which causes various sequelae and complications with adverse effects on their QOL. In this respect, BA might no longer be considered a childhood disease. BA in adult survivors has its characteristic picture that is different from other adult liver diseases, including viral hepatitis, steatohepatitis, or sclerosing cholangitis [44]. Therefore, pediatric surgeons and hepatologists have a role to play as specialists familiar with BA in collaboration with adult primary care providers and hepatologists. It is important to determine the timing for LT for each patient, based on a deep understanding of long-term survivors with BA and the availability of living or cadaveric donors.

## References


1. Kasai M, Watanabe I, Ohi R. Follow-up studies of long term survivors after hepatic portoenterostomy for "noncorrectible" biliary atresia. J Pediatr Surg. 1975;10(2):173–82.
2. LeeVan E, Matsuoka L, Cao S, Groshen S, Alexopoulos S. Biliary-Enteric Drainage vs Primary Liver Transplant as Initial Treatment for Children With Biliary Atresia. JAMA Surg. 2019;154(1):26–32.
3. Altman RP, Lily JR, Greenfeld J. A Multivariable Risk Factor Analysis of the Portoenterostomy (Kasai) Procedure for Biliary Atresia. Ann Surg. 1997;226(3):348–55.
4. Lykavieris P, Chardot C, Sokhn M, Gauthier F, Valayer J, Bernard O. Outcome in adulthood of biliary atresia: a study of 63 patients who survived for over 20 years with their native liver. Hepatology. 2005;41(2):366–71.
5. Davenport M, Ong E, Sharif K, Alizai N, McClean P, Hadzic N, Kelly DA. Biliary atresia in England and Wales: results of centralization and new benchmark. J Pediatr Surg. 2011;46(9):1689–94.
6. Schreiber RA, Barker CC, Roberts EA, Martin SR, Alvarez F, Smith L, Butzner JD, Wrobel I, Mack D, Moroz S, Rashid M, Persad R, Levesque D, Brill H, Bruce G, Critch J, Canadian Pediatric Hepatology Research, G. Biliary atresia: the Canadian experience. J Pediatr. 2007;151(6):659–65. 65 e1
7. Serinet MO, Wildhaber BE, Broue P, Lachaux A, Sarles J, Jacquemin E, Gauthier F, Chardot C. Impact of age at Kasai operation on its results in late childhood and adolescence: a rational basis for biliary atresia screening. Pediatrics. 2009;123(5):1280–6.
8. Kaar FM, Lily JR, Stewart BA, Hall RJ. Biliary Atresia Registry, 1976 to 1989. J Pediatr Surg. 1990;25:1076–81.
9. McKiernan PJ, Baker AJ, Kelly DA. The frequency and outcome of biliary atresia in the UK and Ireland. The Lancet. 2000;355(9197):25–9.
10. Chardot C. Prognosis of Biliary Atresia in the Era of Liver Transplantation: french National Study From 1986 to 1996. Hepatology. 1999;30:606–11.
11. Okazaki T, Kobayashi H, Yamataka A, Lane GJ, Miyano T. Long-term postsurgical outcome of biliary atresia. J Pediatr Surg. 1999;34(2):312–5.
12. Nio M, Ohi R, Shimaoka S, Iwami D, Sano N. The outcome of surgery for biliary atresia and the current status of long-term survivors. Tohoku J Exp Med. 1997;181(1):235–44.
13. Shinkai M, Ohhama Y, Take H, Kitagawa N, Kudo H, Mochizuki K, Hatata T. Long-term outcome of children with biliary atresia who were not transplanted after the Kasai operation: >20-year experience at a children's hospital. J Pediatr Gastroenterol Nutr. 2009;48(4):443–50.
14. Nio M. Japanese Biliary Atresia Registry. Pediatr Surg Int. 2017;33(12):1319–25.
15. Hung PY, Chen CC, Chen WJ, Lai HS, Hsu WM, Lee PH, Ho MC, Chen TH, Ni YH, Chen HL, Hsu HY, Chang MH. Long-term prognosis of patients with biliary atresia: a 25 year summary. J Pediatr Gastroenterol Nutr. 2006;42(2):190–5.
16. Nio M, Ohi R, Miyano T, Saeki M, Shiraki K, Tanaka K. and Japanese Biliary Atresia, R., Five- and 10-year survival rates after surgery for biliary atresia: a report from the Japanese Biliary Atresia Registry. J Pediatr Surg. 2003;38(7):997–1000.
17. Nio M, Sasaki H, Wada M, Kazama T, Nishi K, Tanaka H. Impact of age at Kasai operation on short- and long-term outcomes of type III biliary atresia at a single institution. J Pediatr Surg. 2010;45(12):2361–3.
18. Nio M, Sano N, Ishii T, Sasaki H, Hayashi Y, Ohi R. Long-term outcome in type I biliary atresia. J Pediatr Surg. 2006;41(12):1973–5.
19. Schreiber RA, Barker CC, Roberts EA, Martin SR. and Canadian Pediatric Hepatology Research, G., Biliary atresia in Canada: the effect of centre caseload experience on outcome. J Pediatr Gastroenterol Nutr. 2010;51(1):61–5.
20. Nio M, Wada M, Sasaki H, Tanaka H, Watanabe T. Long-term outcomes of biliary atresia with splenic malformation. J Pediatr Surg. 2015;50(12):2124–7.
21. Howard ER, MacLean G, Nio M, Donaldson N, Singer J, Ohi R. Survival patterns in biliary atresia and comparison of quality of life of long-term survivors in Japan and England. J Pediatr Surg. 2001;36(6):892–7.
22. Nio M, Wada M, Sasaki H, Kazama T, Tanaka H, Kudo H. Technical standardization of Kasai portoenterostomy for biliary atresia. J Pediatr Surg. 2016;51(12):2105–8.
23. Ng VL, Haber BH, Magee JC, Miethke A, Murray KF, Michail S, Karpen SJ, Kerkar N, Molleston JP, Romero R, Rosenthal P, Schwarz KB, Shneider BL, Turmelle YP, Alonso EM, Sherker AH, Sokol RJ, Childhood Liver Disease, R., and Education, N. Medical status of 219 children with biliary atresia surviving long-term with their native livers: results from a North American multicenter consortium. J Pediatr. 2014;165(3):539–46. e2
24. Shneider BL, Abel B, Haber B, Karpen SJ, Magee JC, Romero R, Schwarz K, Bass LM, Kerkar N, Miethke AG, Rosenthal P, Turmelle Y, Robuck PR, Sokol RJ, Childhood Liver Disease, R., and Education, N. Portal hypertension in children and young adults with biliary atresia. J Pediatr Gastroenterol Nutr. 2012;55(5):567–73.
25. de Vries W, Homan-Van der Veen J, Hulscher JB, Hoekstra-Weebers JE, Houwen RH, Verkade HJ, Netherlands Study Group of Biliary Atresia, R. Twenty-year transplant-free survival rate among patients with biliary atresia. Clin Gastroenterol Hepatol. 2011;9(12):1086–91.
26. Bijl EJ, Bharwani KD, Houwen RH, de Man RA. The long-term outcome of the Kasai operation in patients with biliary atresia: a systematic review. Neth J Med. 2013;71(4):170–3.

27. Nio M, Sano N, Ishii T, Sasaki H, Hayashi Y, Ohi R. Cholangitis as a late complication in long-term survivors after surgery for biliary atresia. J Pediatr Surg. 2004;39(12):1797–9.
28. Kumagi T, Drenth JP, Guttman O, Ng V, Lilly L, Therapondos G, Hiasa Y, Michitaka K, Onji M, Watanabe Y, Sen S, Griffiths W, Roberts E, Heathcote J, Hirschfield GM. Biliary atresia and survival into adulthood without transplantation: a collaborative multicentre clinic review. Liver Int. 2012;32(3):510–8.
29. Houben C, Phelan S, Davenport M. Late-presenting cholangitis and Roux loop obstruction after Kasai portoenterostomy for biliary atresia. J Pediatr Surg. 2006;41(6):1159–64.
30. Jain V, Burford C, Alexander EC, Sutton H, Dhawan A, Joshi D, Davenport M, Heaton N, Hadzic N, Samyn M. Prognostic markers at adolescence in patients requiring liver transplantation for biliary atresia in adulthood. J Hepatol. 2019;71(1):71–7.
31. Watanabe M, Hori T, Kaneko M, Komuro H, Hirai M, Inoue S, Urita Y, Hoshino N. Intrahepatic biliary cysts in children with biliary atresia who have had a Kasai operation. J Pediatr Surg. 2007;42(7):1185–9.
32. Yamanaka J, Iimuro Y, Hirano T, Kosaka H, Fujimoto J. Successful liver resection for biliary atresia with intrahepatic biliary cysts after Kasai procedure. J Pediatr Surg. 2005;40(2):E9–11.
33. Weidner M, Mitchell S, Schwarz K. Percutaneous Transhepatic Cholangioplasty to Treat Multiple Intrahepatic Biliary Strictures After Hepatoportoenterostomy. J Pediatr Gastroenterol Nutr. 2017;64(2):200–2.
34. Sasaki H, Tanaka H, Wada M, Kazama T, Nakamura M, Kudo H, Okubo R, Sakurai T, Nio M. Analysis of the prognostic factors of long-term native liver survival in survivors of biliary atresia. Pediatr Surg Int. 2016;32(9):839–43.
35. Karrer FM, Wallace BJ, Estrada AE. Late complications of biliary atresia: hepatopulmonary syndrome and portopulmonary hypertension. Pediatr Surg Int. 2017;33(12):1335–40.
36. Ueno T, Saka R, Takama Y, Yamanaka H, Tazuke Y, Bessho K, Okuyama H. Onset ages of hepatopulmonary syndrome and pulmonary hypertension in patients with biliary atresia. Pediatr Surg Int. 2017;33(10):1053–7.
37. Ijiri R, Tanaka Y, Kato K. Clinicopathological study of a hilar nodule in the livers of long- term survivors with biliary atresia. Pathol Int. 2001;51:16–9.
38. Matsuura T, Kohashi K, Yanagi Y, Saeki I, Hayashida M, Aishima S, Oda Y, Taguchi T. A morphological study of the removed livers from patients receiving living donor liver transplantation for adult biliary atresia. Pediatr Surg Int. 2012;28(12):1171–5.
39. Yoon HJ, Jeon TY, Yoo SY, Kim JH, Eo H, Lee SK, Kim JS. Hepatic tumours in children with biliary atresia: single-centre experience in 13 cases and review of the literature. Clin Radiol. 2014;69(3):e113–9.
40. Nio M, Wada M, Sasaki H, Tanaka H, Hashimoto M, Nakajima Y. Correctable biliary atresia and cholangiocarcinoma: a case report of a 63-year-old patient. Surg Case Rep. 2019;5(1):185.
41. Ohhama Y, Shinkai M, Fujita S, Nishi T, Yamamoto H. Early prediction of long-term survival and the timing of liver transplantation after the Kasai operation. J Pediatr Surg. 2000;35(7):1031–4.
42. Nightingale S, Stormon MO, O'Loughlin EV, Shun A, Thomas G, Benchimol EI, Day AS, Adams S, Shi E, Ooi CY, Kamath BM, Fecteau A, Langer JC, Roberts EA, Ling SC, Ng VL. Early Posthepatoportoenterostomy Predictors of Native Liver Survival in Biliary Atresia. J Pediatr Gastroenterol Nutr. 2017;64(2):203–9.
43. Nio M, Wada M, Sasaki H, Tanaka H, Okamura A. Risk factors affecting late-presenting liver failure in adult patients with biliary atresia. J Pediatr Surg. 2012;47(12):2179–83.
44. Samyn M, Davenport M, Jain V, Hadzic N, Joshi D, Heneghan M, Dhawan A, Heaton N. Young People With Biliary Atresia Requiring Liver Transplantation: a Distinct Population Requiring Specialist Care. Transplantation. 2019;103(4):e99–e107.
45. Ng VL, Sorensen LG, Alonso EM, Fredericks EM, Ye W, Moore J, Karpen SJ, Shneider BL, Molleston JP, Bezerra JA, Murray KF, Loomes KM, Rosenthal P, Squires RH, Wang K, Arnon R, Schwarz KB, Turmelle YP, Haber BH, Sherker AH, Magee JC, Sokol RJ, Childhood Liver Disease Research, N. Neurodevelopmental Outcome of Young Children with Biliary Atresia and Native Liver: results from the ChiLDReN Study. J Pediatr. 2018;196:139–47. e3
46. Caudle SE, Katzenstein JM, Karpen SJ, McLin VA. Language and motor skills are impaired in infants with biliary atresia before transplantation. J Pediatr. 2010;156(6):936–40. e1
47. Wayman KI, Cox KL, Esquivel CO. Neurodevelopmental outcome of young children with extrahepatic biliary atresia 1 year after liver transplantation. J Pediatr. 1997;131(6):894–8.
48. Afshar S, Porter M, Barton B, Stormon M. Intellectual and academic outcomes after pediatric liver transplantation: relationship with transplant-related factors. Am J Transplant. 2018;18(9):2229–37.
49. Rodijk LH, den Heijer AE, Hulscher JBF, Alizadeh BZ, de Kleine RHJ, Verkade HJ, Bruggink JLM. Long-Term Neurodevelopmental Outcomes in Children with Biliary Atresia. J Pediatr. 2020;217:118–24. e3
50. Squires JE, Ng VL, Hawthorne K, Henn LL, Sorensen LG, Fredericks EM, Alonso EM, Murray KF, Loomes KM, Karpen SJ, Cavallo LA, Molleston JP, Bezerra JA, Rosenthal P, Squires RH, Wang KS, Schwarz KB, Arnon R, Magee JC, Sokol RJ, Childhood Liver Disease Research, N. Neurodevelopmental Outcomes in Preschool and School Aged Children With Biliary Atresia and Their Native Liver. J Pediatr Gastroenterol Nutr. 2020;70(1):79–86.
51. Nio M, Ohi R, Hayashi Y, Endo N, Ibrahim M, Iwami D. Current status of 21 patients who have survived more than 20 years since undergoing surgery for biliary atresia. J Pediatr Surg. 1996;31(3):381–4.
52. Wong CWY, Chung PHY, Tam PKH, Wong KKY. Long-term Results and Quality of Life Assessment in Biliary Atresia Patients: a 35-Year Experience in a Tertiary Hospital. J Pediatr Gastroenterol Nutr. 2018;66(4):570–4.
53. Kuroda T, Saeki M, Morikawa N, Watanabe K. Management of adult biliary atresia patients: should hard work and pregnancy be discouraged? J Pediatr Surg. 2007;42(12):2106–9.
54. Sasaki H, Nio M, Hayashi Y, Ishii T, Sano N, Ohi R. Problems during and after pregnancy in female patients with biliary atresia. J Pediatr Surg. 2007;42(8):1329–32.
55. Westbrook RH, Yeoman AD, O'Grady JG, Harrison PM, Devlin J, Heneghan MA. Model for end-stage liver disease score predicts outcome in cirrhotic patients during pregnancy. Clin Gastroenterol Hepatol. 2011;9(8):694–9.
56. Sundaram SS, Alonso EM, Haber B, Magee JC, Fredericks E, Kamath B, Kerkar N, Rosenthal P, Shepherd R, Limbers C, Varni JW, Robuck P, Sokol RJ, Childhood Liver Disease, R., and Education, N. Health related quality of life in patients with biliary atresia surviving with their native liver. J Pediatr. 2013;163(4):1052–7. e2
57. Lampela H, Pakarinen MP, Jahnukainen T, Jalanko H, Kosola S. Quality of Life and Parental Worrying in a National Cohort of Biliary Atresia Children Living With Their Native Livers. J Pediatr Gastroenterol Nutr. 2017;64(6):883–7.
58. Lind RC, de Vries W, Keyzer-Dekker CM, Peeters PM, Verkade HJ, Hoekstra-Weebers JE, van der Steeg AF, Hulscher JB. Health status and quality of life in adult biliary atresia patients surviving with their native livers. Eur J Pediatr Surg. 2015;25(1):60–5.
59. de Vries W, Lind RC, Sze YK. Overall quality of life in adult biliary atresia survivors with or without liver transplantation: results from a National Cohort. Eur J Pediatr Surg. 2016;26:349–56.

# Long-Term Results and Deformities of Intrahepatic Bile Ducts

# 39

Takashi Hashimoto and Tatsuya Suzuki

**Abstract**

The morphology of the intrahepatic bile ducts was studied and evaluated using magnetic resonance (MR) cholangiography images of patients with biliary atresia who survived long-term with their native liver. The study included thirteen survivors aged 24 to 50 years and one patient who died at the age of 40 years.

In type I cases, bile duct branching to the liver segment was normal; however, many segmental intrahepatic bile ducts showed fusiform and/or cystic dilatation. In type II and III cases, multiple ductal structures were found in the segmental intrahepatic bile duct. Some bile ducts had a luminal structure; however, in many cases, small cystic bile ducts had a rosary bead appearance and were connected to the intestine at the site of the Kasai anastomosis.

We speculated that the prognosis would be favorable when the bile ducts were well distributed to the periphery of the liver, and each segmental (bile) duct flowed into the anastomotic intestine. Cholangitis developed when there were few bile ducts at the Kasai anastomosis, and cholelithiasis was found in the intrahepatic bile duct in the patient who died at the age of 40 years. Moreover, when the bile ducts were not widely distributed in the liver, the patient suffered from biliary cirrhosis and portal hypertension.

**Keywords**

Biliary atresia · Long-term survivors · MR cholangiography · Intrahepatic bile duct · Morphology · Clinical study

T. Hashimoto (✉)
Masuko Memorial Hospital, Nagoya, Aichi, Japan
e-mail: htakashi@fujita-hu.ac.jp

T. Suzuki
Fujita Health University School of Medicine, Toyoake, Aichi, Japan

## 39.1 Introduction

An increasing number of patients with biliary atresia (BA) now survive with their native liver for more than 20 years due to improvements in postoperative management and modifications that have been made to the Kasai procedure [1]. However, while some long-term survivors show no complications, many live with disorders such as cholangitis and/or progression of cirrhosis resulting in the need for regular and ongoing medical treatment. The prognosis of BA is primarily affected by the morphological condition of the intrahepatic bile duct. However, because of the small physique of infants and the specificity of the disease, using standard imaging modalities to clarify the features of the intrahepatic bile duct is very difficult in BA patients. Morphological studies of the intrahepatic bile duct in preoperative BA have only been reported in the following cases: preoperative percutaneous transhepatic cholangiography (PTC) [2, 3] and intraoperative cholangiography from a cyst at the hilum of the liver (1-cyst) [4]. Thus, BA has been traditionally classified based on the morphology of the extrahepatic biliary tract.

The fact that there are long-term survivors with their native livers after the Kasai procedure indicates that there is a communication of the biliary tract from the hepatocytes to the anastomosed intestine at the hilum of the liver to excrete the bile and that there is always a patent bile duct in the liver. Features of the intrahepatic bile duct structure are not well known because of the limited literature; Weidner et al. [5] reported on three adult patients who underwent PTC as part of their treatment. In addition, Yokoyama [6] et al. and Hyun et al. [7] reported cases with endoscopic retrograde cholangiography (ERC).

In long-term survivors with good activities of daily living (ADL), direct cholangiography, like in PTC or endoscopic cholangiography, is usually unfavorable to obtain the image of the intrahepatic bile duct considering the invasion and subsequent complications. Omar [8] and Héctor A et al. [9] have published case reports involving magnetic resonance (MR) cholangiography. MR cholangiography can be a useful


M. Nio (ed.), *Introduction to Biliary Atresia*, https://doi.org/10.1007/978-981-16-2160-4_39

modality to investigate the structure of the intrahepatic bile duct, as it is non-invasive and relatively easy to apply.

In this chapter, we will describe intrahepatic bile duct morphology using MR cholangiography along with its characteristics and pathological conditions.

## 39.2 MR Cholangiography

MR cholangiography was first reported in 1991 by Wallner et al. [10] and indirectly shows bile duct morphology based on the presence of bile in the bile duct. This method is almost non-invasive, does not impair the patient's quality of life (QOL), and has been reported to have good resolution compared to ERC and/or drip-infusion cholangiography-computed tomography (DIC-CT). It has also been applied for the diagnosis of the morphological degree of PSC (primary sclerosing cholangitis), which has intrahepatic bile duct lesions similar to those in BA [11–13]. In addition, long-term survivors have been shown to be positive with regards to ADL and are often employed. Therefore, it is necessary to avoid excessive surgical invasion and complications. As a direct cholangiography in postoperative cases, there are reports of PTC [8, 9] and ERC from the anastomosis [6]. These imaging methods, however, are associated with possible impairments due to bleeding because of punctures or increased intrabiliary pressure and biliary tract infections. DIC-CT examinations also include the risk of radiation exposure. In both cases, side effects due to contrast agent allergies are also a concern. Therefore, MR cholangiography is a very suitable method for the determination of intrahepatic bile duct morphology in long-term survivors following the Kasai procedure. In the MR cholangiography method, the biliary tract morphology is visualized by a maximum intensity projection method using 1.5T or 3.0T MR imaging.

## 39.3 Cases with MR Cholangiography

MR cholangiography provided a clear image in the following 14 cases: one case of a patient who died from liver failure due to cholangitis with obstructive jaundice at 40 years of age and 13 cases involving long-term surviving patients aged between 24 and 50 years (Table 39.1). The 14 cases included the following BA types: type I (2 cases), type II (2 cases), and type III (10 cases). Both type I cases and one type II case included female patients. Type III cases included one male who died at the age of 40 and two male and seven female long-term survivors. The MR examinations were performed between January 2015 and May 2020 as part of a regular follow-up examination or diagnostic examination for cholangitis-like fever or liver dysfunction.

## 39.4 Features of MR-Cholangiogram

Although case 1 involved a type I cyst, the patient underwent the Kasai procedure. The branch of the intrahepatic bile duct showed almost normal branching to the liver segments. However, fusiform and/or cystic dilation was noted in the bile duct in the anterior segment of the liver, and there was stenosis on the hilum side that, at first glance, appeared to be anastomotic stenosis. There was, in fact, a distance of a few

**Table 39.1** Long-term survived cases with MR cholangiography

| | | | | | | Recent episode of complication and/or past history | | | |
|---|---|---|---|---|---|---|---|---|---|
| Type of BA | CASE | Gender | Age | Operative Procedure | ADL | Cholangitis | Cirrhosis | GI Bleeding | Delievry |
| I- Cyst | 1 | F | 24 | Modified Kasai | Good | 1-2/year | No | No | / |
| | 2 | F | 45 | Hepaticporto duodenostomy | Excellent | No | mild | Hassab operation | 2 |
| Type II | 3 | M | 24 | Modified Kasai | Excellent | Rare | No | No | / |
| | 4 | F | 30 | Modified Kasai | Excellent | Rare | No | No | 2 |
| Type III | 5 | M | 33 | Suruga II | Excellent | No | No | No | / |
| | 6 | F | 40 | Modified Kasai | Excellent | No | No | No | 3 |
| | 7 | F | 41 | Kasai with anti-reflux valve | Excellent | No | mild | History | 2 |
| | 8 | M | 41 | Modified Kasai | Good | No | Moderate | 1/1-2 years | / |
| | 9 | F | 41 | Modified Kasai | Excellent | No | Splenectomy | history | / |
| | 10 | F | 42 | Modified Kasai | Excellent | Rare | Mild | No | 2 |
| | 11 | F | 42 | Modified Kasai | Excellent | Rare | No | No | / |
| | 12 | F | 49 | Kasai | Excellent | No | No | No | / |
| | 13 | M | 50 | Kasai | Excellent | Rare | No | No | / |
| | 14* | M | 40 | Modified Kasai | Died | Often | Mild | No | / |

Type I cyst: atresia of the common bile duct with a cystic structure which communicates with the intrahepatic bile ducts
Type II: atresia of the hepatic duct-Criteria of ADL in this table
Type III: atresia of the bile duct at porta hepatis-Good; need some medical treatment /year
Modified Kasai ;Our original modification for Kasai procedure-Excellent; free from medical treatment

centimeters between the actual anastomosis and the cystic dilatation. The patient then underwent percutaneous transhepatic dilation at the age of eight years. However, the biliary stenosis remained in the same site, and not only was the main bile duct dilated, but many stricture-like features were also found in the peripheral bile duct. In addition, there were cystic or fusiform dilations in the bile ducts corresponding to B3 and B5. In cholangitis cases, characteristic cholangitis develops, with the usual symptoms of fever, abdominal pain, and jaundice. However, in this case, whole-body computed tomography (WCT) confirmed only partial development of cholangitis, with no observation of jaundice or elevation of liver enzymes (Fig. 39.1).

Case 2 underwent surgery in which the hilum of the liver and the duodenum were anastomosed. This patient had a previous history of bleeding from esophageal varices and underwent Hassab surgery [13] in her 20s. Fortunately, after that, she had two successful pregnancies without any complaints of esophageal varices or cholangitis. In this patient, intraoperative cholangiography was performed at the time of the Kasai procedure, but the clear main branching of bile ducts in the liver and the biliary duct expanding into the liver were not successfully visualized on the operative cholangiography (Fig. 39.2).

In type I patients, the bifurcation of the branching of the intrahepatic bile duct is of an almost normal anatomical form, but there are also cystic or fusiform dilated bile ducts in the liver. These abnormalities should not be considered a result of caudal bile duct stenosis. It was speculated that the bile ducts in long-term survivors with type I BA may have a tendency to form multiple cystic and/or fusiform dilatations. Bile duct dilation also occurs in extrahepatic and intrahepatic bile ducts, as is the case in Caroli disease [14]. It was also suggested that the expansion of the bile ducts might become clear with the passage of time.

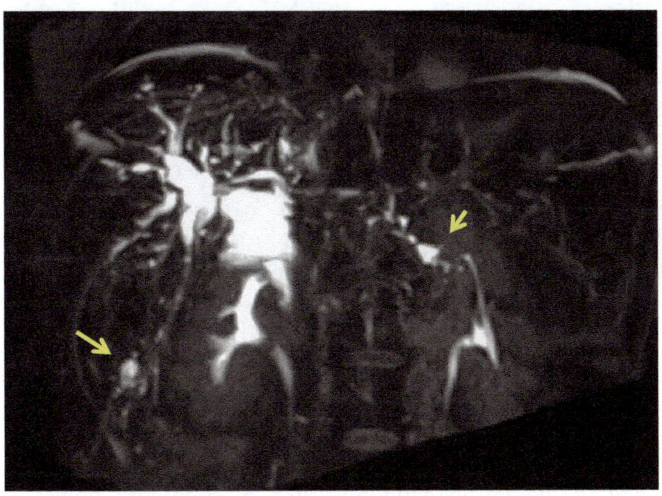

**Fig. 39.1** MR-cholangiogram of case1. The arrow shows cystic dilatation of the peripheral bile duct(in S3 and S5)

Although rare, both type II cases experienced sudden jaundice relapse because of the onset of cholangitis. In both cases, the left and right intrahepatic bile ducts were found to flow into the anastomotic intestine due to the Kasai procedure. In case 3, almost all the bile ducts were widely distributed in the liver and presented with a rosary bead appearance. The bifurcation of these intrahepatic bile ducts seemed to almost coincide with the anatomical area. Duplicated findings of the bile duct were not observed in the vicinity of the anastomosis; instead, they were observed in the periphery. Small cystic-shaped bile ducts appeared like rosary beads and seemed to be connected to the anastomosed intestine at the porta hepatis (hepatic hilum) (Fig. 39.3). In case 4, although branching of the main segmental bile duct was clear, the characteristic finding was the presence of duplicated bile ducts that should usually exist as a single bile duct in a normal individual. In addition, the wall of the bile duct appeared to be irregular, with stenosis and continuing mild dilatation. Small cystic bile ducts, similar to those in case 3, were also observed in the periphery.

Cases 5 to 14 are of type III. Cases 5 and 6 (Fig. 39.4) are of patients who are currently alive and have made good progress with treatment. It was observed that the tubular bile ducts continued near the anastomosis and that the bile ducts could be traced at the periphery and were widely spread in the liver, although in the small cystic form.

In cases 7 and 8 (Fig. 39.5), the tubular bile ducts were located near the anastomosis, but there was a difference in bile duct distribution in the liver between the cases. Case 7 is now a housewife who has successfully delivered two healthy babies but also has splenomegaly and a platelet count of approximately 100,000/mm3.

In case 8, the small cystic bile duct in the periphery was not clearly visible. Although the patient does not currently have jaundice and is usually able to work, he has strong portal hypertension. This leads to cirrhosis-induced bleeding from esophageal varices, which requires treatment every few years. Similar to other cases of portal hypertension, bile ducts visible during MR cholangiography did not appear to be widely distributed in the liver. These characteristics were also observed in case 9 (Fig. 39.6), and the same findings were observed in preoperative PTC. In this case, bifurcation of the segmental bile duct was almost normal, but multiple bile ducts were observed at each segmental bile duct and at dilated bile ducts. Furthermore, many small, cystic rosary-bead-shaped ducts were found to be communicating with the main bile ducts.

The intrahepatic biliary structures of cases 10 and 11 showed similar intrahepatic bile ducts. Case 10 patient is currently able to lead a normal life without any problems (Fig. 39.7). In contrast, although the patient in case 11 has given birth to two children, cholangitis has occurred once during the past two years, and jaundice has recurred. Fortunately, cholangitis was relieved by the administration

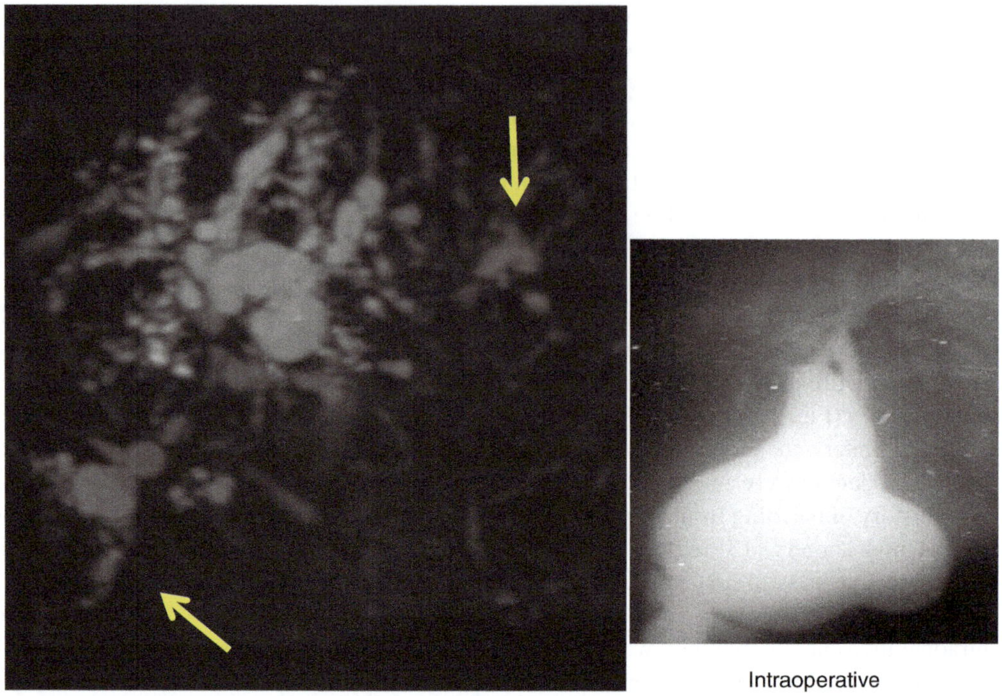


**Fig. 39.2** MR-cholangiogram of case 2. Right side photo is intraoperative cholangiography from the extrahepatic cyst. Allows showed cystic dilatation of the peripheral bile ducts (in S3 and S5)

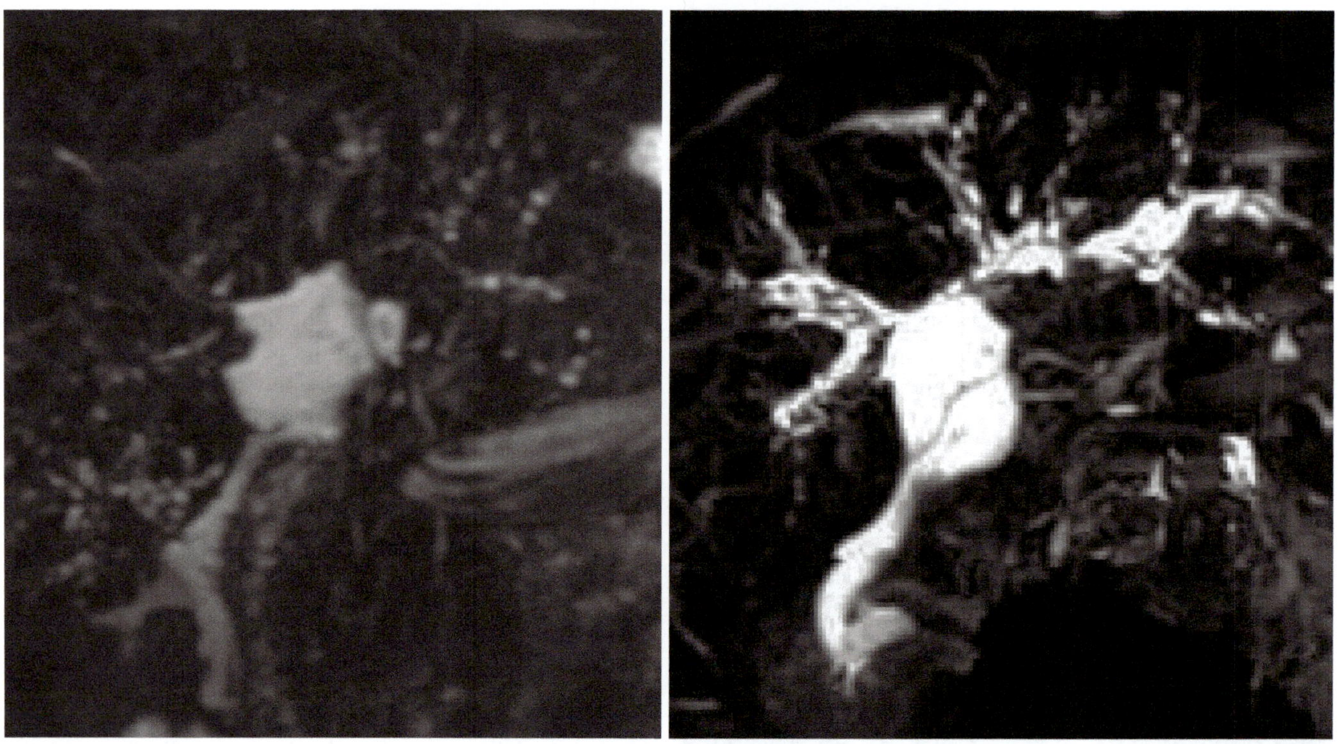

**Fig. 39.3** MR-cholangiogram of case 3 and 4. Small cystic-shaped bile ducts appears like rosary beads and seems to be connected to the anastomosed intestine at the porta hepatis (hepatic hilum). The characteristic finding is the presence of duplicated bile ducts that should usually exist as a single bile duct

of antibiotics, and the jaundice disappeared after approximately one month. Furthermore, her liver function test results have also improved. Both patients are currently alive without any difficulties with regard to ADL. Comparing the images of these two cases, there was no significant difference in the intrahepatic bile duct morphology; however, there were a greater number of bile ducts anastomosed to the hilum of the liver in case 10.

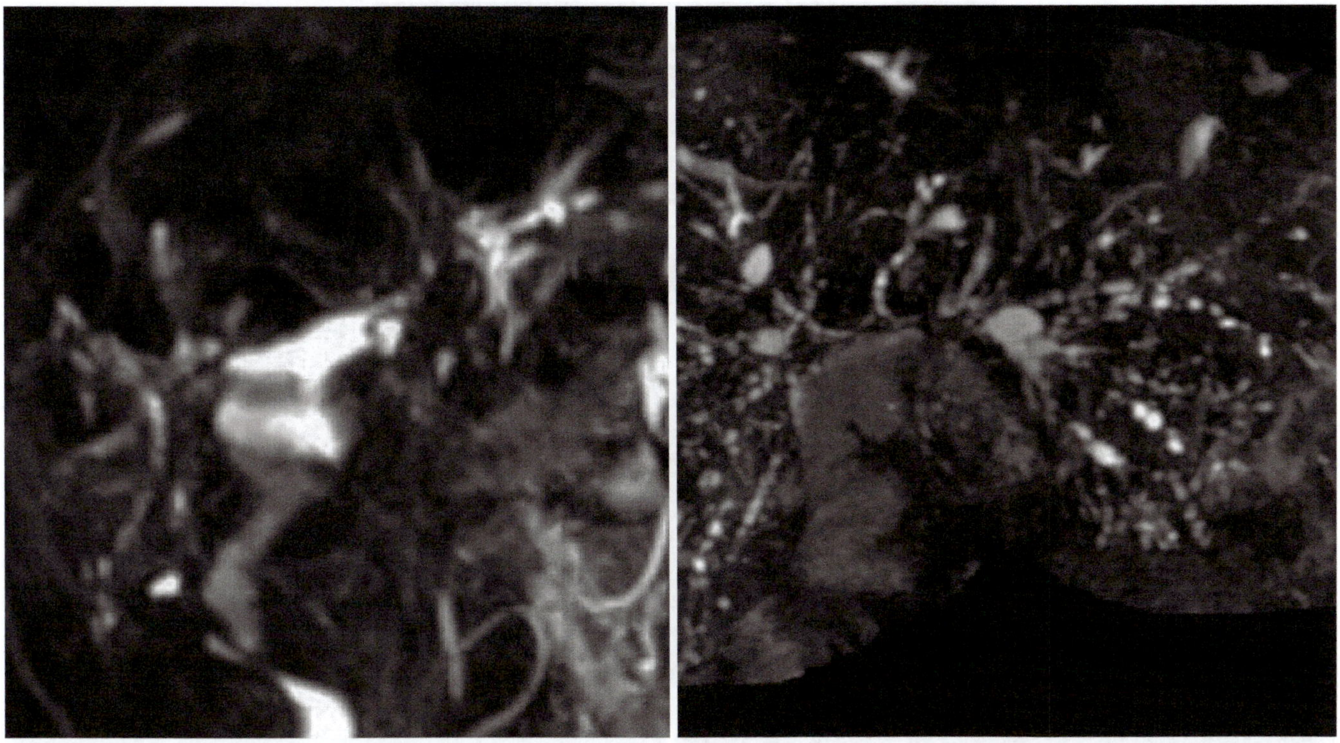

**Fig. 39.4** MR-cholangiogram of case5 and 6. This cholangiogram shows the tubular bile ducts continued near the anastomosis and that the bile ducts could be traced at the periphery and were widely spread in the liver, although in the small cystic form

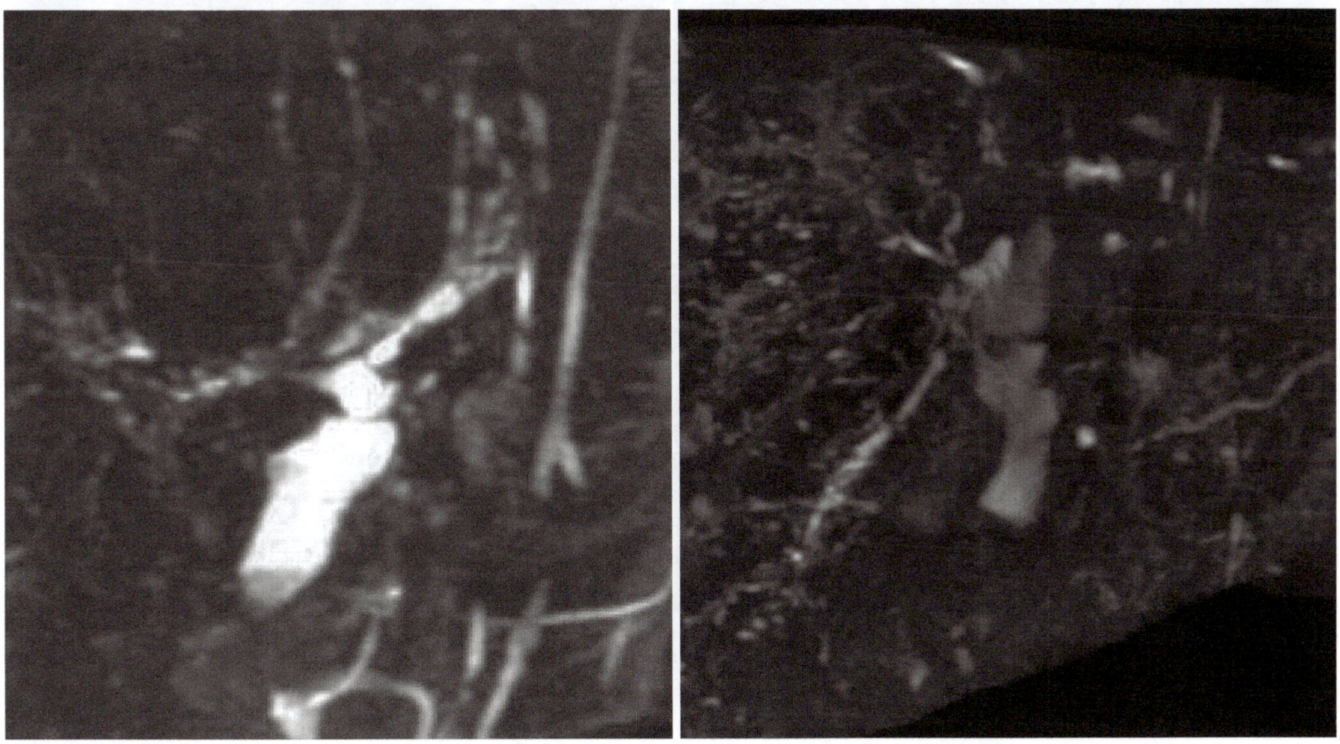

**Fig. 39.5** MR-cholangiogram of cases 7 and 8. The tubular bile ducts were located near the anastomosis, but there was a difference in bile duct distribution in the liver between the cases

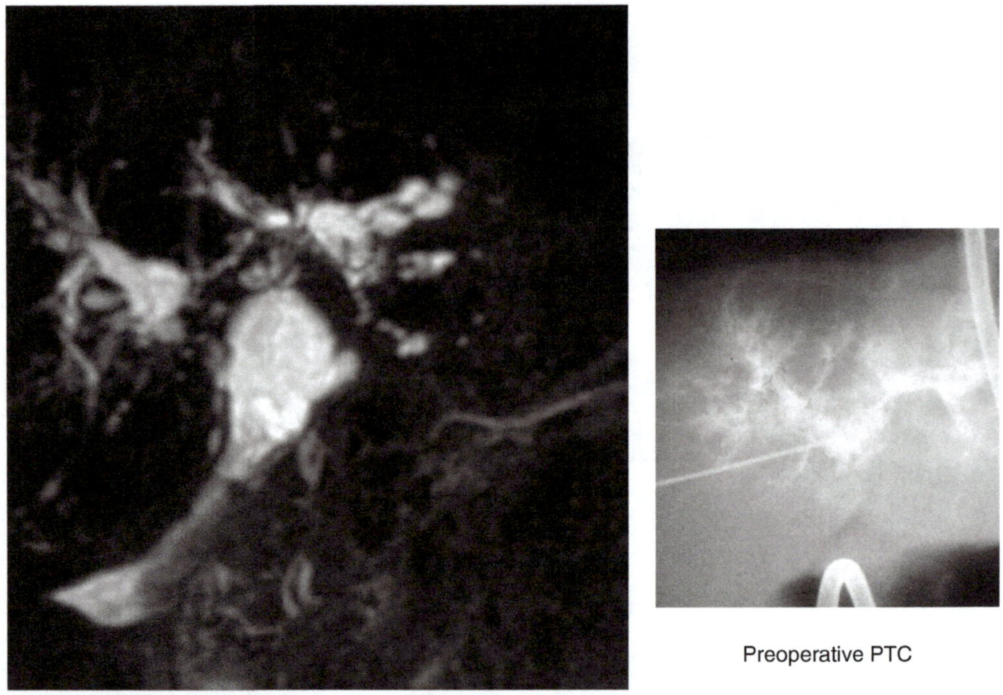


**Fig. 39.6** Cholangiogram of case 9. Left side photo shows MR cholangiography at the age of 4, and preoperative PTC (right side)

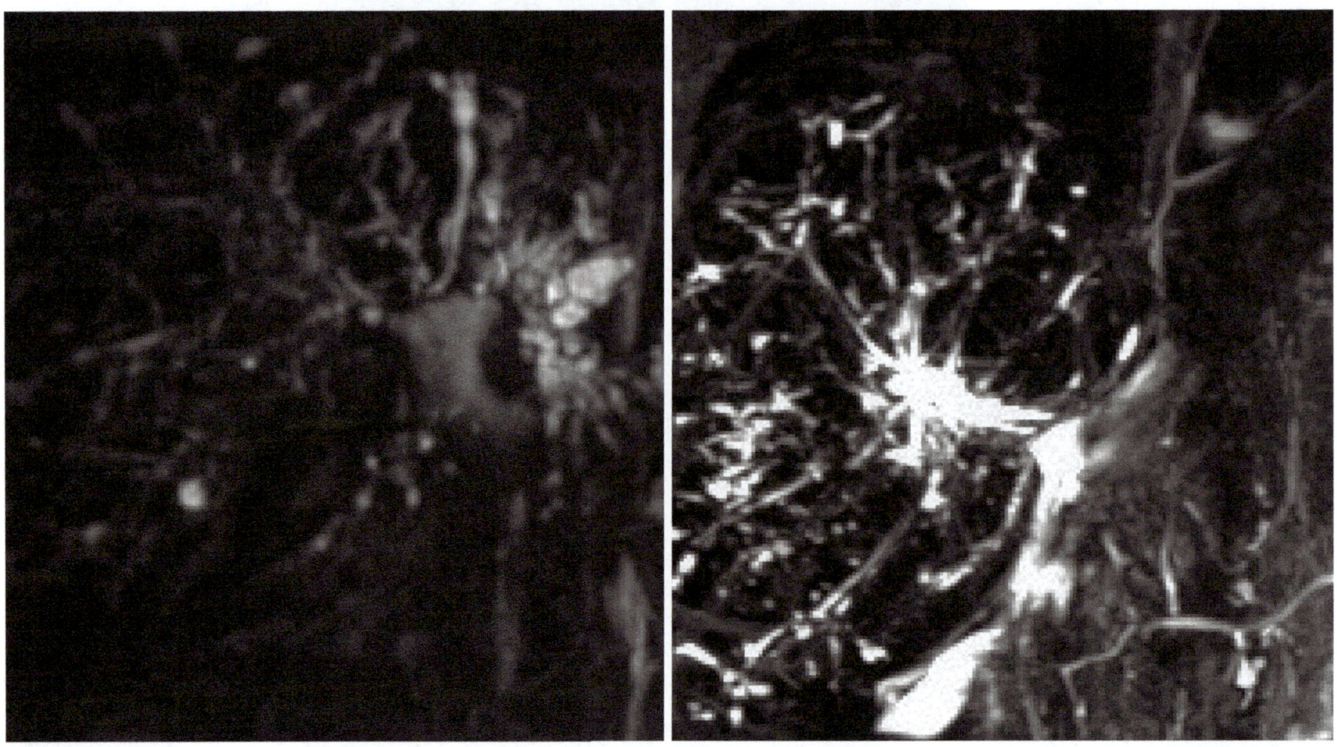

**Fig. 39.7** MR-cholangiogram of case10 and 11. There are a greater number of bile ducts anastomosed to the hilum of the liver in case 10 compared with case 11

Case 12 is a female patient with excellent outcomes with regards to ADL. The patient currently displays no signs of cholangitis or cirrhosis. Her cholangiography image indicated that the intrahepatic bile duct was very characteristic of a dendritic branched bile duct. Her intrahepatic bile ducts showed a series of continued small cystic bile ducts, which followed a rosary bead pattern and appeared to branch normally. They were also connected to the intestine, anastomosed by the Kasai procedure at the hepatic hilum (Fig. 39.8). Even if no obvious luminal structure was apparent, the anas-

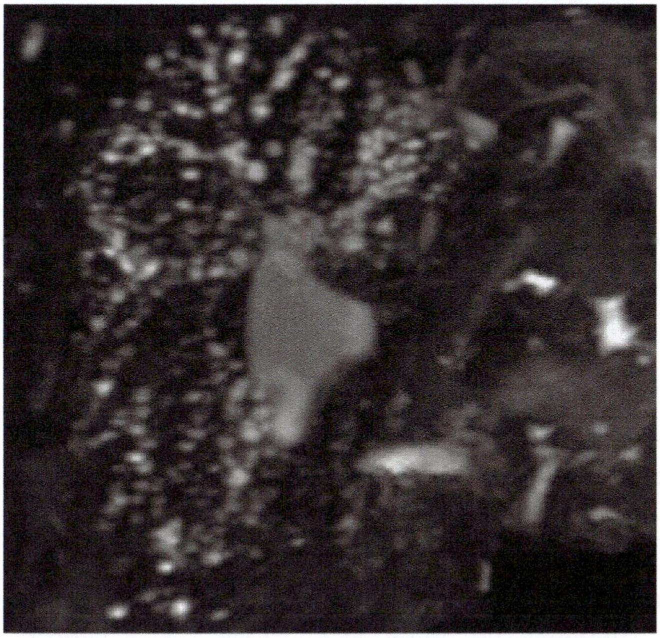

**Fig. 39.8** MR-cholangiogram of case 12. This case has a most favorable prognosis. This cholangiography image shows a dendritic branched bile duct, and a series of continued small cystic bile ducts, which followed a rosary bead pattern

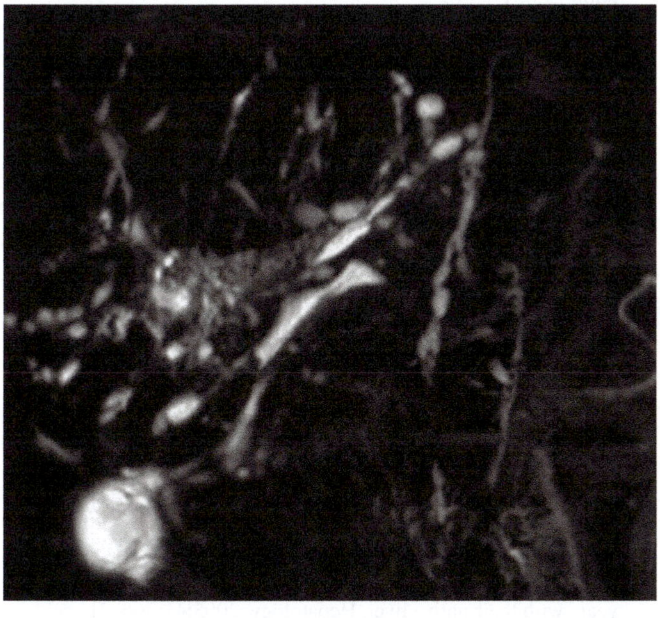

**Fig. 39.9** MR-cholangiogram of case13. This photo shows a characteristic collection of small cysts at the hilum, but irregular dendritic branches in the left lobe of the liver

tomosed part certainly showed continuity, and the wall of each small cystic duct seemed to be smooth, which may have helped maintain the bile outflow.

Case 13 is the oldest surviving male with type III BA (Fig. 39.9) and showed a characteristic collection of small cysts at the hilum but irregular dendritic branches in the left lobe of the liver. Furthermore, bifurcations of the bile duct showed stenosis in some places. A series of small cystic bile ducts were also observed in the atrophied right lobe. This case developed cholangitis 5 years prior to admission and was successfully treated. Currently, he is employed and working without suffering from jaundice and/or any other liver problems.

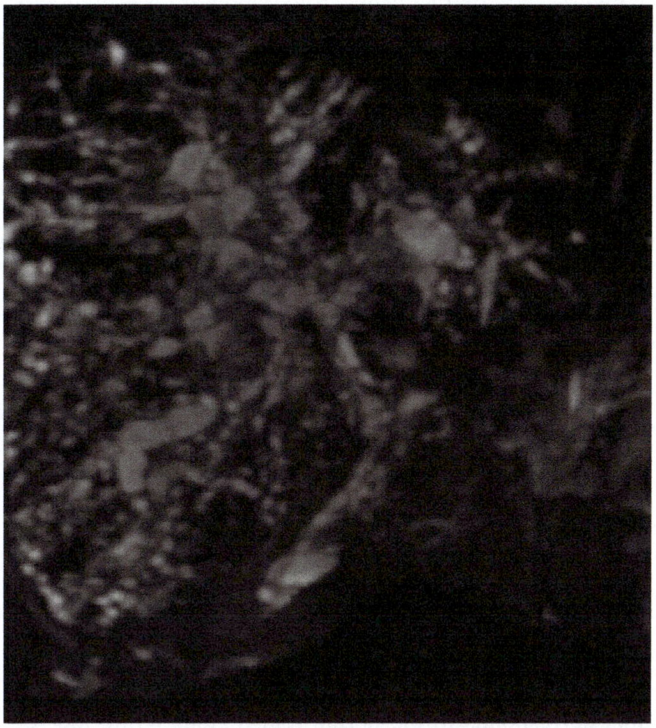

**Fig. 39.10** MR-cholangiogram of case 14. This patient died at 40 of age. The morphology of the beaded bile duct looks very similar to that of case 12. However, the segmental bile duct dilated incrementally, and the lumen is filled with bile sludge

In case 14 (Fig. 39.10), the morphology of the beaded bile duct looked very similar to that of case 12 who had a good prognosis. However, cholangitis developed after three years, the segmental bile duct dilated incrementally, and the lumen was filled with bile sludge. Imaging revealed cholelithiasis-like findings. Such intrahepatic stones are found in a third of cholangitis cases [15]. The patient died at the age of 40 years due to liver failure associated with obstructive jaundice, without having the opportunity to receive a liver transplant.

## 39.5 Summary

In infantile intrahepatic bile duct morphology in BA, direct cholangiography is performed preoperatively or intraoperatively [2–4]. The cholangiogram at the corrective operation, in which the contrast medium is introduced in a retrograde manner, was divided by Nio et al. into three types: cloudy, treelike, and mixed [4]. Furthermore, Yokoyama K et al. [6]

described the feature as a "fire-like" appearance on ERC in the case after the Kasai procedure. The image findings seen in these reports are considered to result from the contrast agent leaking from the bile duct lumen near the surrounding periphery area of the intrahepatic bile duct.

The findings of MR cholangiography showed that the characteristic morphological features of the intrahepatic bile duct (partial cystic dilatation, rosary beads -shaped bile ducts, and duplicated bile ducts) in the long-term surviving cases may have been modified during the continuous bile excretion following the Kasai procedure. The characteristics of intrahepatic bile duct morphology in the cases that survive for a long time with their native livers can be broadly divided into two patterns. This is similar to the findings obtained by PTC in a study by Hashimoto et al. [2]. In the basic type I cyst, biliary branching in the liver maintains the regionality of the liver, but there is fusiform or cystic dilatation at some places. These dilated bile duct lesions are sometimes focal for the development of partial cholangitis; in such cases, this dilation differs from the so-called solitary cysts [16]. In types II and III, the bifurcation morphology of the intrahepatic bile duct corresponds to the portal vein region. While the segmental bile duct is usually visualized as a single lumen, the findings of our study noted that duplicate bile ducts were also observed in some regions.

In addition, there were some cases that displayed a single tubular shape similar to that of a normal bile duct, but most displayed a beaded shape with continuous small cysts. This finding is similar to that of Weidner et al. [5], who reported an irregular intrahepatic ductal system with multiple irregular branches coursing down toward the porta hepatis. Cases with a good prognosis (few complications and/or mild liver damage) were observed when their intrahepatic bile duct was rosary bead-shaped, small cystic bile ducts were widely distributed in the liver, and many segmental bile ducts were opened in the anastomosis. The occurrence of jaundice associated with cholangitis was remarkable in cases where anastomotic orifices were small in number. It is speculated that the formation of intrahepatic stones may cause irreversible damage, resulting in a poor prognosis. These results will provide suggestions for future Kasai procedures in BA patients. The existence of microcystic bile duct morphology seems to be consistent with the results of the examination of liver cysts following the Kasai procedure [16–18]. The morphology of the intrahepatic bile duct in long-term survivors is completely different from that of normal individuals, and the stricture of the bile duct is similar to that of IgG4-related sclerosing cholangitis [19]. To investigate whether this type of abnormality persists or worsens will require further studies.

## References


1. Sasaki H, Tanaka H, Nio M. Current management of long-term survivors of biliary atresia: over 40 years of experience in a single center and review of the literature. Pediatr Surg Int. 2017;33:1327–33.
2. Hashimoto T, Yura J. Percutaneous Transhepatic Cholangiography (PTC) in Biliary Atresia With Special reference to the Structure of the Intrahepatic Bile Ducts. J Pediatr Surg. 1981;16:22–5.
3. Ito T, Horisawa M, Ando H. Intrahepatic bile ducts in biliary atresia—a possible factor determinating the prognosis. J Pediatr Surg. 1983;18:124–30.
4. Nio M, Sano N, Ishii T, et al. Long-term outcome in type –I biliary atresia. J Pediatr Surg. 2006;41:1973–5.
5. Weidner M, Mitchell S, Schwarz K. Percutaneous transhepatic cholangioplasty to treat multiple intrahepatic biliary strictures after hepatoportoenterostomy. J Pediatr Gastroenterol Nutr. 2017;64:200–2.
6. Yokoyama K, Hatanaka H, Inoue M, Yano T, et al. Multiple orifices and cholangiography with a "fire-like" appearance after Kasai hepatoportoenterostomy for biliary atresia. J Pediatr Surg. 2016;51:1574–6.
7. Hyun JJ, Irani SS, Kozarek RA. Endoscopic retrograde cholangiopancreatography in adult patients with biliary atresia. PROCESS-compliant case series. Medicine. 2018;97:1–4.
8. Omar H, Siglin S, Laurie T, Kavin H. 26-Year-Old Survivor of Kasai Procedure With Native Liver. ACG Case Rep J. 2016;3:221–3.
9. Héctor A, González B, Ponciano-Rodríguez G, et al. A 25 years old women after Kasai operation for biliary atresia. Ann Hepatol. 2008;27:381.
10. Wallner BK, Schumacher KA, Weidenmaier W, et al. Dilated Biliary Tract: Evaluation With MR Cholangiography With a T2-weighted Contrast-Enhanced Fast Sequence. Radiology. 1991;181:805–8.
11. Ogawa M, Ozawa Y, Ohta K, et al. Usefulness of 3D Balanced Turbo-Field-Echo MR Sequence Evaluating the Branching Pattern of the intrahepatic Bile Ducts: Comparison With Drip Infusion. CT Cholangiography. Abdom Radiol (NY). 2017;42:1888–95.
12. Holzknecht N, Gauger J, Sackmann M, et al. Breath-hold MR cholangiography with snapshot techniques: prospective comparison with endoscopic retrograde cholangiography. Radiology. 1998;206:657–64.
13. Selvaraj EA, Culver EL, Bungay H, et al. Evolving Role of Magnetic Resonance Techniques in Primary Sclerosing Cholangitis. World J Gastroenterol. 2019;14:644–58.
14. Hassab MA. Gastro-esophageal decongestion and splenectomy GEDS (Hassab), in the management of bleeding varices. Review of literature. Int Surg. 1998;83:38–41.
15. Miller WJ, Sechtin AG, Campbell WL, et al. Imaging findings in Caroli' s disease. Am J Roentgenol. 1995;165:333–7.
16. Lykavieris P, Chardot C, Sokhn M, et al. Outcome in adulthood of biliary atresia: A study of 63 patients who survived for over 20 years with their native liver. Hepatology. 2005;41:366–71.
17. Goda T, Kubota A, Kawahara H, et al. The clinical significance of intrahepatic cystic lesions in postoperative patients with biliary atresia. Ped Surg Int. 2012;28:865–8.
18. Jiang J, Wang J, Lu X, et al. Intrahepatic cystic lesions in children with biliary atresia after Kasai procedure. J Pediatr Surg. 2019;54:2565–9.
19. Tanaka A. IgG4-Related Sclerosing Cholangitis and Primary Sclerosing Cholangitis. Gut Liver. 2019;13:300–7.

# Long-Term Results of Liver Transplantation for Biliary Atresia

# 40

Yukihiro Inomata

**Abstract**

Long-term survival of biliary atresia (BA) patients significantly depends on the outcome of liver transplantation (LT), which is needed at least 50% of the patients. Liver transplantations for BA are commonly undergone within 2 years of age but also done later in various generations for different kinds of indications. Most patient loss after LT occurs within 6 months, and long-term mortality is not common. Twenty-year graft survival after LT for BA is now around 75%, and some the graft loss can be saved by re-transplantation. Because there is no fear of recurrence of BA after LT, in the long-term follow-up after LT, specific problems for BA are limited. As other organ transplantation, lifetime immunosuppression is necessary, although some selected patients can be weaned off from any drugs with meticulous follow-up. In addition to basic drugs like calcineurin inhibitors and steroids, mycophenolate mofetil (MMF) and mammalian target of Rapamycin (mTOR) inhibitors are available as immunosuppressants for rejections, especially for antibody-mediated ones. In surgical complications after LT for BA, portal vein thrombosis or occlusion has a big impact on the graft and patient survival in the long term. Pediatric recipients can achieve a favorable growth unless growth failure is too advanced at the time of LT due to the preceding protein-calorie malnutrition. Physicians and surgeons who follow the recipients should have a wide perspective not to focus on the liver itself. Formation of the team with assists from specialists of various fields under the leadership of the responsible main doctor is also very important. With the increase of long survivors after LT for BA, quality of life should have been more cared for in every phase of their life.

Y. Inomata (✉)
Prof. Emeritus, Department of Pediatric Surgery and Transplantation, Kumamoto University, Director, Kumamoto Rosai Hospital, Yatsushiro, Japan
e-mail: yino@kuh.kumamoto-u.ac.jp

**Keywords**

Biliary atresia · Liver transplantation · Indication
Pediatric · Prognosis · Complication · Growth
Development · Immunosuppression · Re-transplantation
Rejection

## 40.1 Introduction

Biliary atresia (BA) is the leading indication for liver transplantation (LT) in the pediatric age group. Recurrence of BA after the liver transplant has not been reported ever. This means that the new life with a transplanted graft starts after the LT, and recipients can be free of BA-related illness. However, the most drastic change is that the new life should need the lifetime continuing immunosuppression and may have possible medical/surgical complications for this. Some patients undergo even after decades with the native liver, and morbidity with the native liver may have significant consequences after the transplantation. Pediatric recipients, if the transplant is undergone in their early life, should have a phase of growth and development after the transplant. Longer life expectancy is waiting the pediatric recipients than adults. For the team of the long-term care, parents of patients should be incorporated from the beginning of the treatment, with enough explanation of the prognosis, including the liver transplant. In this chapter, long-term outcomes after liver transplantation, both specific and non-specific for biliary atresia, will be described.

## 40.2 Fact of LT for BA in Japan and Other Countries

In Japan, living-donor liver transplantation (LDLT) has been the dominant way of liver transplantation, although deceased donor liver transplantation (DDLT) increased a little after 2010 when the organ transplant law was reformed. In DDLT


M. Nio (ed.), *Introduction to Biliary Atresia*, https://doi.org/10.1007/978-981-16-2160-4_40

from 1999 to 2018 in Japan, BA occupied 13 of 51 pediatric patients and 17 of 365 adult patients. In LDLTs done at the same time, BA occupied 2102 of 3168 (66.3%) pediatric, and 239 of 5741 (4.2%) adult patients. Totally, in Japan, 2371 BA patients (25.4%) have been transplanted in 9325 LTs from 1989 to 2018 [1]. Changes in annual number of DDLT and LDLT after the reform of organ transplant law in pediatric and adult age group in each are shown in Fig. 40.1 (a–d). In the cumulated number of pediatric LDLT until 2018, the percentage of BA patients (66.3%) is much more than 38.4% in the USA that was registered between 2011–2018 [2]. In the USA, metabolic disease, tumor, and fulminant hepatic failure have been more common than those in Japan. In the European registry from 1968 to 2016, 5232 patients in the total of 127,851 LTs, or only 4%, were transplanted for BA [3]. In the same registry, in 8666 children (<=18 yo), LDLT and split LT occupied 36.6% and 46.6%, respectively. Because of the scarcity of organ donations from pediatric donors in Japan, split LT has also been done in pediatric DDLTs [4]. In Korea, DDLT has been increasing much more than in Japan. In 2015, a total of 456 DDLTs were done in contrast to 942 LDLTs, although only 20 were for BA [5].

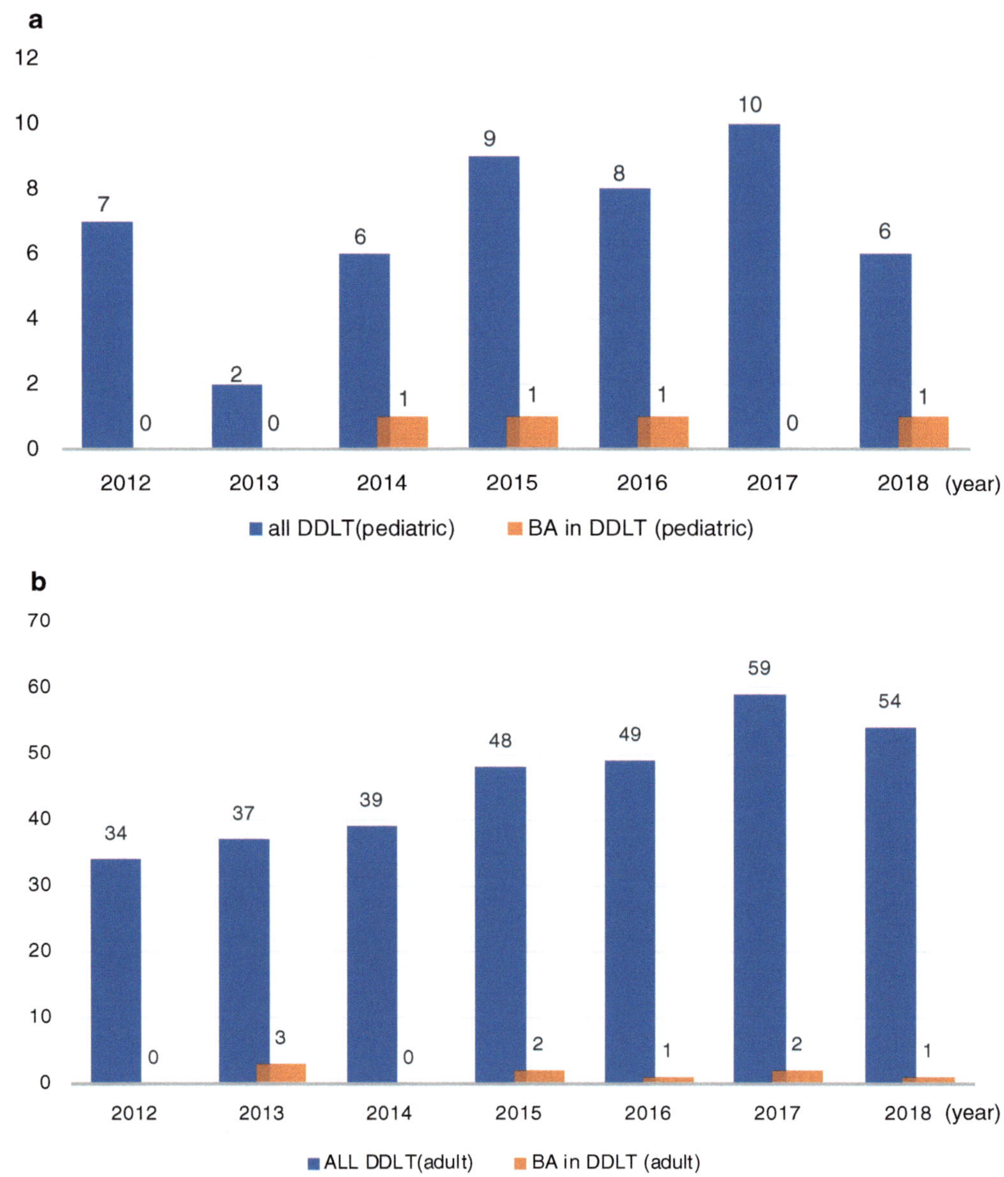


**Fig. 40.1** (**a**) Annual number of all the pediatric DDLT and BA in Japan (Japanese Liver Transplantation Society 1989–2018) pediatric: age < 18yo. (**b**) Annual number of all the adult DDLT and BA in Japan (Japanese Liver Transplantation Society 1989–2018) adult: age > = 18yo. (**c**) Annual number of all the pediatric LDLT and BA in Japan (Japanese Liver Transplantation Society 1989–2018) pediatric: age < 18yo. (**d**) Annual number of all the adult LDLT and BA in Japan (Japanese Liver Transplantation Society 1989–2018) adult: age > = 18yo

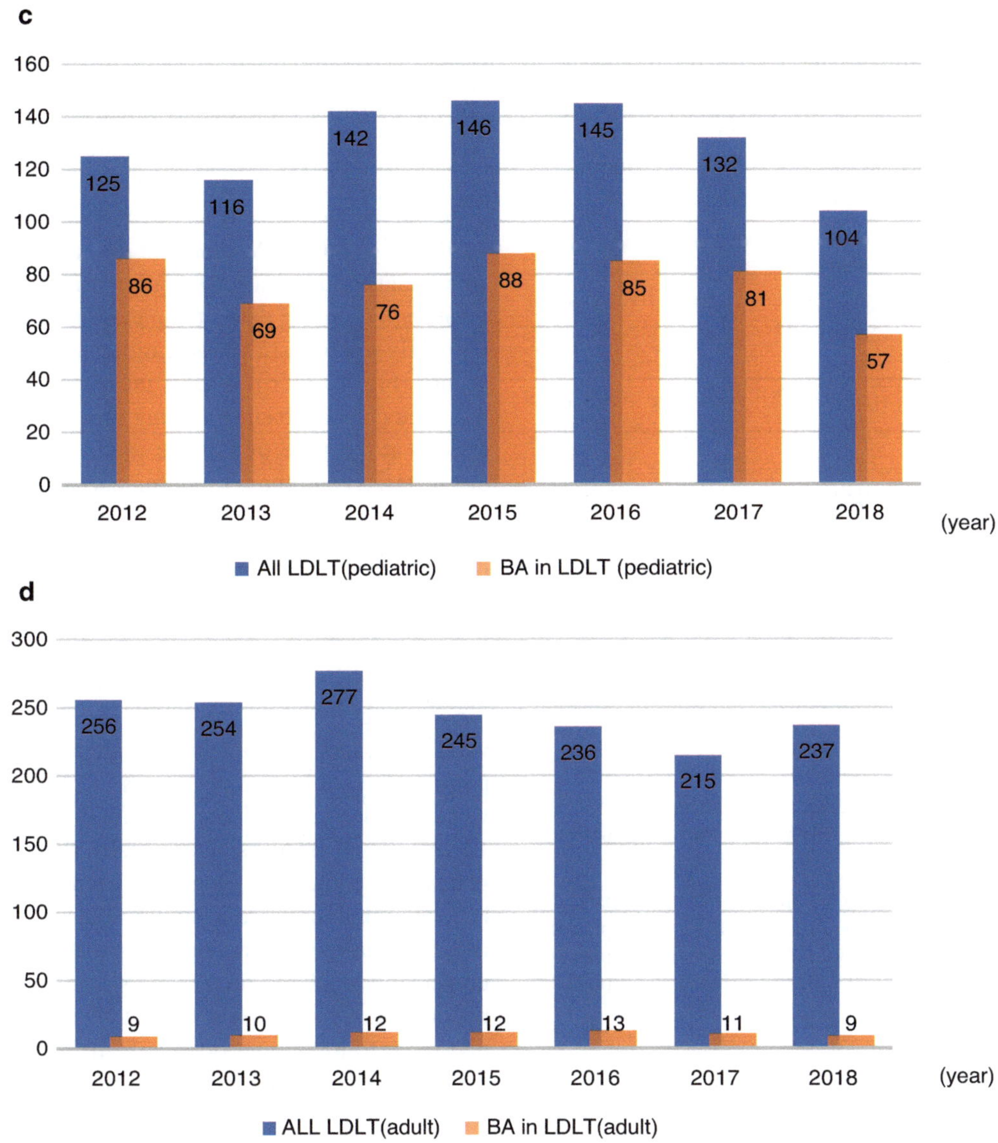


**Fig. 40.1** (continued)

## 40.3 Long-Term Survival after Liver Transplantation for Biliary Atresia

In the registry of the Japanese Liver Transplantation Society (JLTS), 20- and 25-year patient survival after LDLT for biliary atresia has been improving during the time from 1989 to 2018, and in 2018 it is 85.0% and 83.0%, respectively (Table 40.1). Such improvement in Japan, where the graft source has been only the living donor, might be contributed by technical innovations, standardization of nutritional and medical care, and better management of immunosuppressants, in addition to an earlier reference to transplantation. Improvement of the long-term survival mainly depends on that of the short post-transplant phase, but long-term care, including meticulous modulation of immunosuppression based on the findings of protocol biopsy, is also contributing. The history of previous Kasai operation does not affect post-transplant survival. Long-

**Table 40.1** LDLT for biliary atresia Improvement of post-transplant patient survival 1998 → 2010 → 2014 → 2018

| | Cumulative Number of pts. from 1989 | cum. Patient survival(%) | | | | | | |
|---|---|---|---|---|---|---|---|---|
| | | 1y | 3y | 5y | 10y | 15y | 20y | 25y |
| 1998 | 489 | 83.8 | 81.8 | 79.4 | 71.3 | — | — | — |
| 2010 | 1616 | 90.6 | 89.6 | 88.7 | 85.9 | 83.6 | — | — |
| 2014 | 1985 | 91.2 | 90.1 | 89.3 | 86.5 | 84.9 | 84.2 | — |
| 2018 | 2341 | 92.3 | 91.0 | 90.3 | 88.2 | 86.6 | 85.0 | 83.0 |

Japanese Liver Transplantation Society 1989–2018

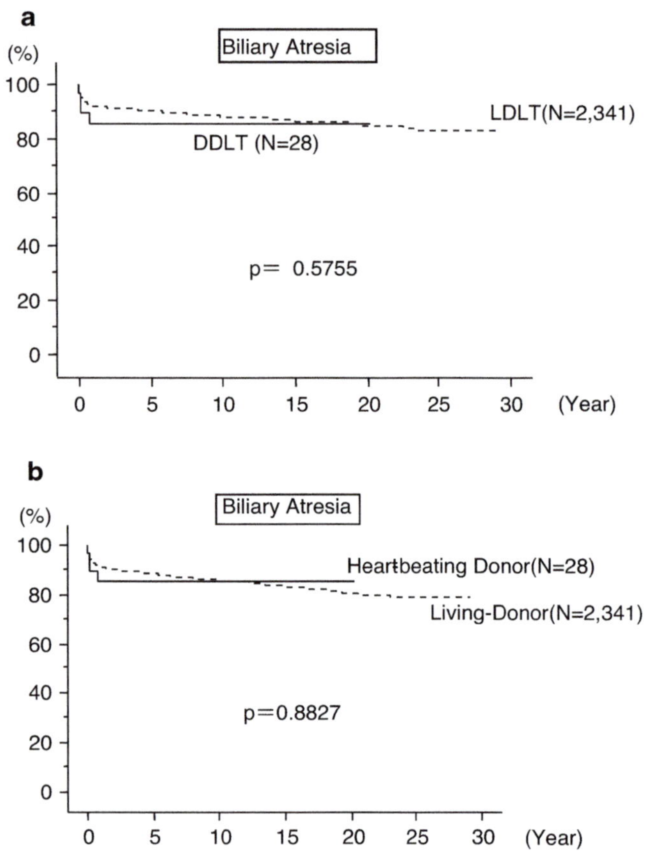


**Fig. 40.2** A: Patient Survival Following Liver Transplantation for Biliary Atresia—DDLT vs. LDLT (Japanese Liver Transplantation Society 1989–2018). B: Graft Survival Following Liver Transplantation for Biliary Atresia—DDLT vs. LDLT—Japanese Liver Transplantation Society 1989–2018

term patient and graft survival of DDLT for BA in Japan is comparable to that of LDLT, although the number is still limited (Fig. 40.2a, b). The patient survival after LT for BA is quite good in recent reports in the world as well. According to the data in ELITA, 20 years of patient and graft survival for BA is 76% for 149 exposed patients [3]. In the data of the SPLIT (Studies of Pediatric Liver Transplantation, which is now incorporated into the Society of Pediatric Liver Transplantation), the overall outcomes of patients receiving LT for patients with BA have improved since 2002 despite evidence of increased disease severity at the time of transplant, probably due to the improvement of post-transplant care [6]. In Korea, in the analysis of 534 recipients (<=18 yo), including 308 BA recipients, who were transplanted between 1998 and 2010, patient and graft survival rates were better in patients transplanted after 2003 [7].

Graft loss can be saved by the re-transplantation in selected patients, and this is why the patient survival is better than the graft survival, although the difference is not so big in Japan (Table 40.2). Predicting factors for graft survival after living-donor liver transplantation for biliary atresia analyzed for huge data of JLTS registry included donor BMI, ABO incompatibility, graft type, recipient age, center experience, and the transplant era [8]. In the report from USA, significant variables for patient survival by multivariate analysis included re-transplantation and donor type, and variables for graft survival included deceased technical variant vs. whole liver and the donor age (0–5 m vs. 10–17 ys) [6]. In the analysis of LDLT for BA, recipient age at the transplant has a significant influence on the long-term graft and patient survival, based on the data of Japanese LDLT. They were significantly worse in 12 years or older groups than the younger groups (Fig. 40.3a, b). What is the reason for such difference has been controversial for a long time. Extrahepatic complications at the time of LT like the hepatopulmmonary syndrome (HPS) and the portopulmonary hypertension (PoPH), the persistence of biliary-related infection for a long time, and prolonged protein-calorie malnutrition would have bad effects. In addition, more tough adhesion due to the previous Kasai procedure and more formation of portosystemic collateral vessels than in infants cause massive bleeding or operative injury during the operation. Kasahara already reported that BA recipients with ages between 12 and 18 had worse graft survival than the younger and the older. Crossing point of the adolescent recipients (12 to <18) turning to be worse in the survival curve than the older adult was at 12 years after the transplant [8]. As other solid organ transplants, this adolescent group in LT tends to have less adherence to immunosuppressants [9]. But in Japan, where easy and financially-supported access to the medical system is universally available for all civils, and transplant surgeons, pediatricians, hepatologists, and transplant coordinators can give close follow-up services, only the non-adherence cannot explain the cause of the poor outcome in that generation. More meticulous consideration for each case is necessary by the team consisting of multi-professionals.

From these findings in LDLT, the indication of LT in younger children is recommended when the possibility of LT is highly estimated. In LDLT, suitable timing of LT can be selected. However, the risk of the live donor cannot be avoided, and incidence of the marginal donors might be higher than DDLT due to the limitation of donor selection in family members. Technical challenges for the limited availability of vascular grafts or difficulty in graft size selection in LDLT are also necessary more than DDLT. About the DDLT, analysis of post-transplant outcome according to the age at the transplant should wait for more accumulation of cases (Fig. 40.4). DDLT for the pediatric patient is a little increasing in Japan, and split liver graft from an adult donor is a significant source. Long-term survival after split DDLT in Japan is satisfactory, although the number of patients, especially that of biliary atresia, is limited [10]. Although technical variation should be considered for pediatric usage of the adult donor, DDLT in Japan should be more enhanced to resolve the negative factors of LDLT.

**Table 40.2** Differences of survival rate (%) between the graft and the patient after the liver transplantation in Japan (JLTS) (For all the first liver transplants undergone in Japan since 1989, regardless to the age and the original diseases)

| | Number of patients | | 1y | 3y | 5y | 10y | 15y | 20y | 25y |
|---|---|---|---|---|---|---|---|---|---|
| DDLT | 504 | Patient | 89.0 | 85.7 | 82.8 | 75.7 | 67.0 | 61.4 | |
| | | Graft | 88.4 | 85.1 | 82.2 | 75.1 | 66.5 | 60.9 | |
| LDLT | 9136 | Patient | 85.2 | 81.2 | 78.7 | 73.5 | 68.8 | 65.9 | 64.7 |
| | | Graft | 84.4 | 80.2 | 77.6 | 71.8 | 66.6 | 63.3 | 62.0 |

DDLT: deceased donor liver transplantation
LDLT: living-donor liver transplantation
(Japanese Liver Transplantation Society 1989–2018)

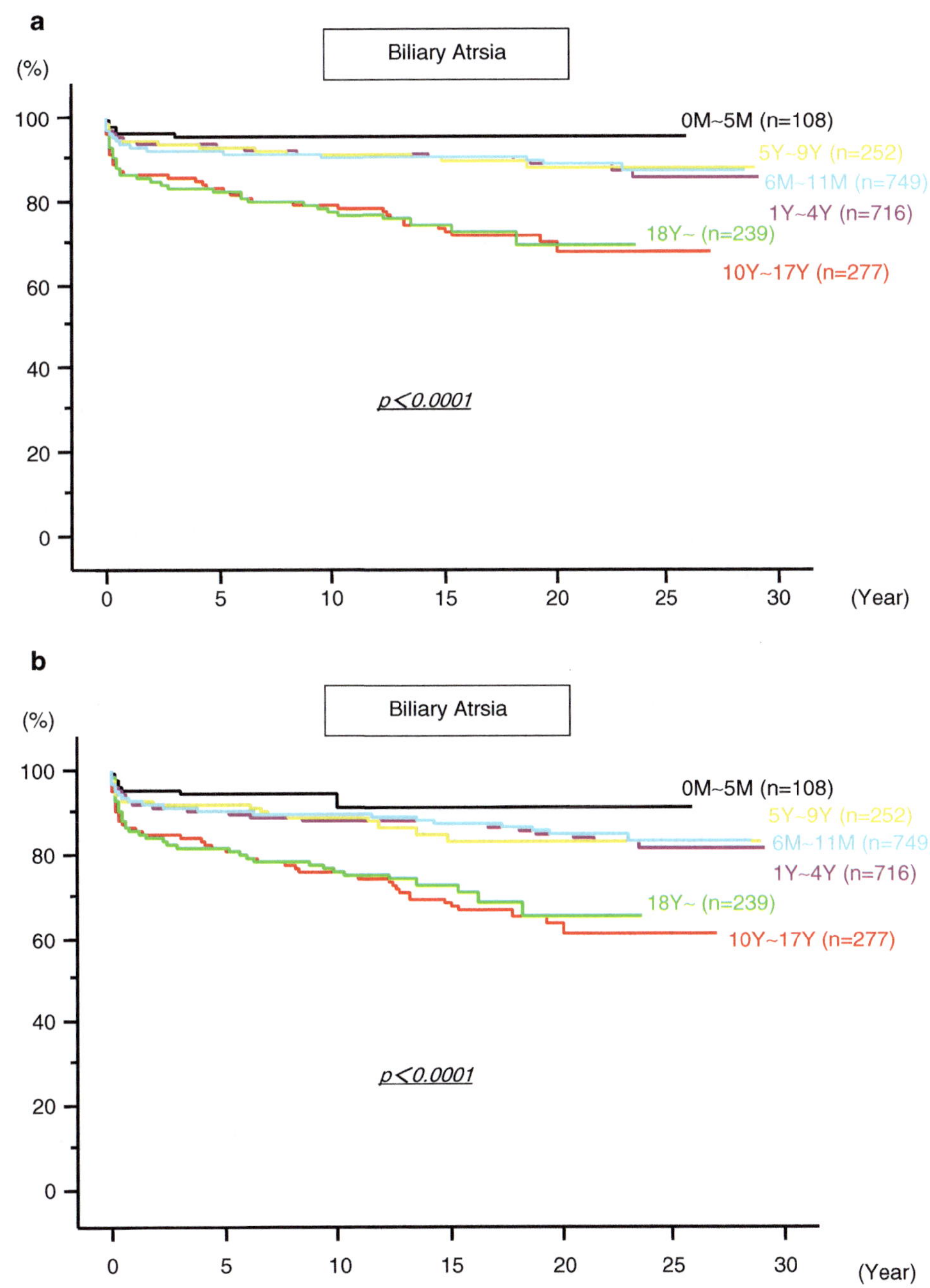


**Fig. 40.3** (**a**) Patient Survival Following Living-donor Liver Transplantation for Biliary Atresia—Age of Recipient—Japanese Liver Transplantation Society 1989–2018. (**b**) Graft Survival Following Living-donor Liver Transplantation for Biliary Atresia—Age of Recipient—Japanese Liver Transplantation Society 1989–2018

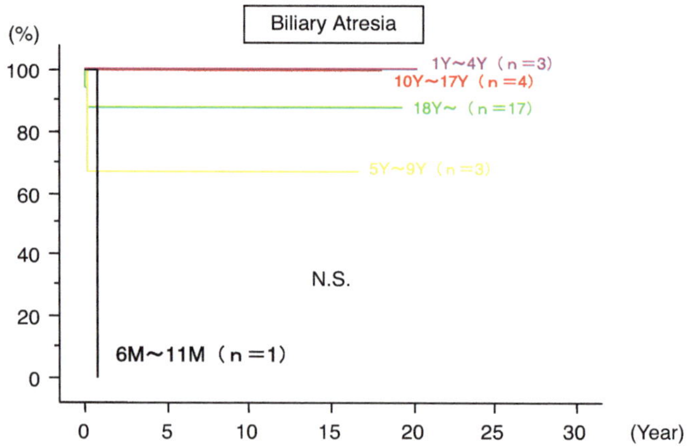


**Fig. 40.4** Graft Survival Following DDLT for Biliary Atresia—Age of Recipient—(Japanese Liver Transplantation Society 1999–2018)

**Table 40.3** Causes of morbidity in the long term after LT for BA

| Graft | | Systemic (extrahepatic) |
|---|---|---|
| Surgical | Medical | |
| •vascular complications (PVT, HV stenosis)<br>•biliary stenosis | •chronic and acute rejections (AMR, TCMR, plasma cell rich-rejection)<br>•De novo HB hepatitis<br>•metabolic disorders (steatosis, NASH, alcoholic) | •infection (viral, fungal, bacterial)<br>•renal dysfunction and hypertension<br>•metabolic disorders (diabetes mellitus, dyslipidemia)<br>•neuro- and cardiovascular events<br>•De novo malignancies (PTLD, solid organ cancer)<br>•growth and developmental delay |

PVT: portal vein thrombosis, HV: hepatic vein. AMR: antibody-mediated rejection, NASH: non-alcoholic steatohepatitis
TCMR: T-cell-mediated rejection. HB: hepatitis B. PTLD: post-transplant lymphoproliferative disorder

## 40.4 Causes of Patient and Graft Loss after Long Term

Except for unexpected accidents or suicides, causes of deaths in the long term are attributed to graft and systemic morbidities (Table 40.3). The cause of death or graft failure usually cannot be explained by a solitary reason, and many factors may correlate comprehensively. For example, a serious infection may be triggered by the treatment of rejection or related to bile duct complications. Infection may be fatal when it is accompanied by graft failure. De novo malignancies, cardio-, or neurovascular events as the consequences of metabolic abnormalities and renal dysfunction may be partly related to the adverse effects of immunosuppression in longer survivors. Even if the graft function has been without any clinical problems over ten years, graft failure due to rejection may happen suddenly, with or without any trigger events.

For graft failure, re-transplantation is indicated if the condition is curable by that procedure and the systemic condition is tolerable [11]. If the original graft was from a living donor, another live donor might not be available in many families in Japan. In that case, registration for DDLT can be another option. In Japan, until 2018, re- and re-re-transplantation occupy 18.1% of all DDLTs, in contrast to 2.5% in total LDLTs [1]. In my institution, 19 patients underwent re-LT after the initial transplant for BA, and only one was done with DDLT after 18 years from the original LDLT (unpublished data). Including this, thirteen were transplanted after 5 years from the initial transplant. Causes for those re-transplantations were immunological events (chronic rejection) in 6, portal vein thrombosis (PVT) in 6, and biliary cirrhosis due to biliary complication in one. Each PVT had a variable length of time after the onset, but most had been recognized within one year. In the treatment of complications, even if it may occur in the short term, the foresight of the prognosis according to the kind of complications is quite important to prevent future graft loss or prepare for the possible re-transplant.

## 40.5 Surgical Complications Long Term after LT for BA

Surgical complications are related to the reconstruction of vessels and bile ducts. In biliary atresia, portal vein reconstruction is the key to the success of the operation, especially in infants or smaller children, because the portal vein in BA tends to be hypoplastic or sclerotic. Incidence of portal vein complications is around 6% in the USA and 7% in the LDLT for small children in Japan [6, 12]. Portal vein complications include stenosis, thrombosis, and both. The onset of PVT is commonly quite soon after the transplant, even in the immediate postoperative days. However, it is common that patients are asymptomatic even with good graft function until it is diagnosed. Persistent portal vein thrombosis or occlusion may cause portal hypertension, and then, variceal bleeding, hypersplenism, and pulmonary complications can follow. Symptoms and findings in the long term are gastrointestinal (GI) bleeding, ascites, persistent thrombocytopenia, hypoalbuminemia, and exertional dyspnea. Doppler ultrasonography (US) study is convenient for check-up of the portal flow. Dynamic enhanced contrast tmography (CT) can detect portal vein complications and collateral vessels. PVT should be treated as soon as possible. For PVT that is diagnosed in the long term, balloon dilatation and stenting by interventional radiology are commonly done through the percutaneous route or via ileocecal vein with small laparotomy. However, if the guidewire cannot pass the thrombotic or occluded part, this interventional treatment is not possible.

Hepatic vein stenosis also occurs usually in the early postoperative period. Incidence is around 7%. It is usually at the site of the anastomosis, but rarely, it occurs in the intrahepatic portion. Symptoms and findings are ascites, hepatomegaly, hypoalbuminemia, and thrombocytopenia. US and CT can diagnose this complication. Catheterization from the IVC side or transhepatic approach followed by balloon dilatation or stent placement is used for definite diagnosis and treatment [13]. The necessity of repeated treatment is common. Incomplete treatment or recurrence may cause graft loss due to the congestion of the graft.

Late-onset hepatic arterial thrombosis is reported to be a causative factor for re-transplantation, but it is rarely reported after LDLT in Japan [14].

Biliary stricture is one of the common surgical problems even in the long-term follow-up. Onset of these complications is usually within 2 years from the transplant, but this may be found even after 5 years. In biliary atresia, reconstruction of the bile duct in the transplant operation is exclusively bilio-enteric anastomosis. The most common pattern is a bilio-jejunal end to side anastomosis using the Roux-en-Y procedure. Stricture is usually at the site of anastomosis, but non-anastomotic stricture may happen. Reported predicting factors for biliary complications are; biliary leakage in the early postoperative days, hepatic arterial thrombosis, long ischemia time, episodes of recurrent rejection, and history of CMV infection. Symptoms are manifested with recurrent cholangitis or persistent graft dysfunction. Abnormalities of the biochemical blood test, like elevation of direct bilirubin, transaminases, gamma glutamyl transpeptidase (GGTP), and bile acids, are clues for diagnosis. Those may be found only at the time of cholangitis and subside soon after the active infection. Routine US can reveal the dilatation of intrahepatic bile ducts, but this is not necessarily positive in all cases, especially after the long term. Hepatobiliary scintigram, MR cholangiography, and drip infusion cholangiography (DIC)-CT are helpful for the diagnosis. Direct cholangiography is definitive for diagnosis. Percutaneous approach may be difficult and invasive if there is no dilatation of the intrahepatic bile duct (IHBD). Retrograde cholangiography using the double-balloon jejunoscope can be an alternative [15]. Balloon dilataion and stenting are the treatment procedures commonly used. If radiological intervention is not effective, surgical revision is necessary. Incomplete resolution of the stricture may cause biliary cirrhosis, which is one of the reasons for re-transplantation.

## 40.6 Medical Complications Long Term after LT for BA

### 40.6.1 Rejection in the Long Term

Rejection after liver transplantation can be diagnosed with biochemical abnormalities in blood chemistry and confirmed with an allograft biopsy. Subjective symptoms are rare, although small children may have a fever and inflammatory signs. Increased levels of transaminases, GGTP, and bilirubin are common findings. Needle biopsy is done for a definite diagnosis, but pathological diagnosis is sometimes comprehensive. There is an international consensus panel, called Banff Working Group on Liver Allograft Pathology, discussing to make guidelines and consensus criteria for the diagnosis of liver allograft pathology. The updated outcome of the Banff Working Group has been published serially, and the latest one is in 2016 [16]. Rejection has several varieties, according to the timing of the onset and possible pathogenicity. Since the establishment of Banff criteria, there were several changes in the terminology for rejections (Table 40.4). The terminology regarding the timing of the episodes has been commonly expressed as "acute" or "early" and "chronic" or "late." Late or chronic are usually used for events after 6 months from the transplant. Most idiopathic post-transplant hepatitis in pathology are now categorized as late T cell-mediated rejection (TCMR) and/or chronic antibody-mediated rejection (AMR) in donor-specific antibody (DSA) -positive patients [16]. De novo autoimmune hepatitis in older terminology, or plasma cell rich-rejection, was recognized and reported in pediatric recipients, including BA [17]. However, specificity to biliary atresia has not been well confirmed. Measurement of DSA may provide additional information for pathogenesis in case of abnormal graft function after excluding the possibility of other causes, although the clinical significance of DSA has not reached to the consensus level. DSA will be beneficial for the modulation of immunosuppressive therapy. Because of increasing recognition as the cause of graft failure, AMR should be more paid attention than TCMR. AMR can be categorized as acute and chronic. Acute AMR usually occurs within the first several weeks. However, although confusing, late-onset acute AMR and mixed AMR/TCMR can happen in sub-optimally immunosuppressed recipients with persistent DSA. If the biopsy is done, deposition of complement component 4d (C4d) is recommended to be checked by immunochemical staining, although again, the significance in the diagnostic meaning has not been fully understood [18]. Now anti-donor antibody as the anti-donor HLA antibody can be measured under the insurance coverage in Japan.

**Table 40.4** Changes of the terminology of rejections in allograft pathology (Demetris et al. from Banff Working Group) (Am J Transpl 2016)

| Older(discouraged) terminology | Newer (preferred) terminology |
|---|---|
| Humoral rejection | Antibody-mediated rejection (AMR) |
| (acute) cellular rejection | T cell-mediated rejection (TCMR) |
| De novo autoimmune hepatitis<br>Plasma cell hepatitis | Plasma cell rich-rejection |

## 40.7 Immunosuppressants in the Long Term

Commonly used basic immunosuppressants for maintenance after LT has been calcineurin inhibitor (CNI), corticosteroid and mycophenolate mofetil (MMF) [19]. They are all given orally. Calcineurin inhibitor is the basal drug, mainly suppress the T-cell-mediated rejection by inhibiting the production of interleukin 2 (IL-2). There are two kinds of CNIs, tacrolimus, and cyclosporin. One of them is used for almost all recipients unless there is a reason that it may cause serious adverse effects. One can be converted to the other if there is any special reason. There is no absolute policy for usage of these drugs, and selection of the drug depends on the preference of institutions or surgeons, degree of adverse effects, and potency of immunosuppression unless there is any reason to avoid a specific drug. The difference of the immunosuppressive potency has been controversial, although cyclosporin is sometimes converted to tacrolimus at the treatment of rejection. Cyclosporin is used as a type of microemulsion for oral administration. Blood level of cyclosporin in the long time after LT is usually set around 100 ng/ml, which is measured at the timing just before the next intake of the drug (trough level, or Co monitoring). Measurement of the blood level 2 hours after the administration (C2 monitoring) is another way for monitoring for cyclosporin. Tacrolimus is usually given twice a day to keep the blood level, like cyclosporin. There is tacrolimus in a sustained-release capsule available for once a day administration. Tacrolimus twice a day will be switched to the sustained-release capsule when the graft function is stable. Once a day administration is effective for better adherence. Trough level is used for monitoring for dose adjustment, and around 5 ng/ml is the targeted level in the long term. In the case with stable liver function, even lower than 4 ng/ml of tacrolimus is effective and not has to be increased. Both CNIs have possibility of interaction with many drugs or foods mainly due to the competition to the degradation enzymes. Most well-known food in such materials is the citrus-like grapefruit. Usually, this fruit is forbidden for intake after the transplant.

In case of rejection or abnormal findings in the protocol biopsy, the dose should be modified with closer observation. If there is an active infection, the drug should be reduced or temporarily stopped. Stop of CNI for only several days usually does not cause acute rejection. If the prescription is done under the suggestion of transplant surgeons/physicians of another center, intimate communication should be maintained about not only the dose itself but also instructions to patients or caretakers. CNI has various kinds of side effects, like nephropathy, neurotoxicity, metabolic dysregulation, and vasculopathy. In the long-term follow-up, such adverse effects should be remembered and checked [20].

Corticosteroid is not commonly used after 1 year from the transplant, especially in the pediatric generation. In the case with instable graft function or pathological findings suggesting rejection, the corticosteroid is added to CNI. If steroid pulse therapy (several days of steroid bolus administration) was given as the treatment of rejection, the corticosteroid is given orally and tapered gradually in the following days or weeks. Because of the possible side effects, the corticosteroid should not be given for a long term unless there is a definite indication.

As one of the antimetabolite drugs, MMF in place of azathioprine is commonly used as the additional drug for maintenance of immunosuppression. Expecting the efficacy for prevention of antibody-mediated rejection, MMF is used with CNI if graft pathology shows some progression of fibrosis or persistent and mild inflammation. Combination of CNI and MMF, without the steroid, is common. Because of the possible teratogenicity, this should be withdrawn for women with the possibility of pregnancy. This drug is commonly used for supplementation to decrease CNI, especially in case of renal dysfunction. Monotherapy with MMF can be considered in case of severe renal dysfunction [21].

In addition to the above three kinds of drugs, mammalian targets of Rapamycin (mTOR) inhibitors, like everolimus and sirolimus, have joined to the drugs for maintenance. Everolimus is the derivative of sirolimus and commercially available in Japan. Due to the expected antiproliferative effects, this kind of drug is used after the transplant for malignant diseases. Also, this drug can be used for attenuation of renal dysfunction due to CNI [22]. Because the mechanism of immunosuppression is different from that of CNI and MMF, this drug can be added as another weapon for intractable rejection.

## 40.8 Operational Tolerance

Maintenance of good graft function after complete withdrawal of immunosuppressant (IS) is called immunological tolerance and has been tried especially for pediatric recipients of LT. Tolerance obtained through intentional induction is called operational tolerance. It is usually started with stepwise reduction of IS [23]. Unavoidable withdrawal of IS, like in case of Epstein-Barr (EV) virus infection, is another trigger for inducing tolerance. Because of various kinds of adverse effects of IS, tolerance is the goal for the best quality of life (QOL) of recipients. However, subclinical progression of liver fibrosis has been reported under incomplete immunosuppression that was retrospectively evaluated [24]. Antibody-mediated rejection is considered to be associated with such progression of fibrosis. Meticulous follow-up with timely protocol biopsy is strongly recommended for such recipients undergoing operational tolerance. Trial to induce the operational tolerance is now done with more careful judgment for possibility, but still, it is the fact that significant number of recipients can maintain their graft function without ISs for a long time [14] (Fig. 40.5). Studies to find potential biomarkers for tolerance have been continuingly conducted [25].

## 40.9 Renal Dysfunction and Hypertension in the Long Term

From the report of western countries, the prevalence of chronic kidney disease (CKD) after pediatric LT was reported to be 25–34% by 5–10 years [26]. The main causative factor of CKD after organ transplant is CNIs. Hypertension may occur in posttransplanted patients with or without renal dysfunction. Prevalence of hypertension was observed in BA patients regardless of the transplanted or non-transplanted status, but the transplanted patients had significantly reduced renal function, which continued to decrease over years [27]. Interstitial fibrosis and hyaline arteriopathy is the pathological findings of the kidney due to CNIs, but IgA nephropathy is reported after LT for BA [28]. Reduction or withdrawal of CNIs should be considered according to the severity of renal dysfunction. MMF or mTOR inhibitor can be used to reduce or stop CNI. Calcium channel blockers, angiotensin-converting enzyme inhibitors, and angiotensin receptor blockers are drugs that are selected for the management of hypertension [29]. Cooperation with a pediatrician or nephrologist is recommended in the follow-up of such complications.

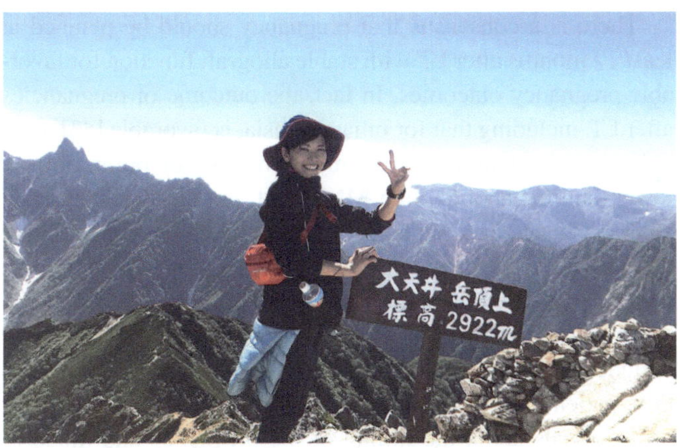


**Fig. 40.5** A lady, forty years old, enjoying mountains in Japan, after 28 years from LDLT at 12 years old. She has been without any immunosuppressants for the last 20 years. (With permission of the patient)

## 40.10 Metabolic Disorders

Diabetes mellitus and dyslipidemia are metabolic disorders seen after the LT. Bodyweight, glucose, transaminases, tiglyceride, cholesterol, and GGTP should be checked routinely. In metabolic disorders after LT, de novo diabetes mellitus is the most common. Effects of ISs, like CNIs and steroids are causative factors, but lifestyle, including diet and exercise, has an influence on the onset as non-transplanted persons. There is a report about the higher incidence of diabetes mellitus in post-transplant pediatric patients than the non-transplanted, and diabetes may influence the long-term mortality after solid organ transplants in children [30]. Teenage is the most common period for the onset, and transitional care is necessary for the management of this complication. Bodyweight, physical activity, and alcohol consumption related to the recipients' social activities should be monitored for the prevention of metabolic disorders in addition to the graft function in the long term [31]. Nurses and coordinators are expected for care in this aspect.

## 40.11 De Novo HB Hepatitis

In living-donor liver, HBs-Ag negative but HBs-Ab and HBc-Ab positive donor can be selected. Hepatitis B virus (HBV) genome remains in the graft from such a donor. After recognition of this fact, prophylaxis for reactivation of HBV in the recipient has been tried. Lifetime maintenance of HBs-Ab above certain level, usually at least 100 IU/L, by repeated administration of hepatitis B immunoglobulin (HBIG) has been recommended. However, this needs much cost and is not effective in all the recipients, especially in cases with escape mutant. Aggressive vaccination for HBV has been tried and confirmed to be effective [32]. Nucleic acid analogs (NA) are used for the treatment of de novo hepatitis, but it is also used for prophylaxis with relatively cheaper cost [33]. Consultation with a hepatologist is recommended because there are several drugs in NA with different possibilities of mutant generation and adverse effects.

## 40.12 De Novo Malignancy

The most common malignancy after pediatric LT has been malignant lymphoma as the post-transplant lymphoproliferative disorder (PTLD). PTLD, especially in pediatric recipients, is caused by persistent infection of Epstein-Barr virus (EBV). However, with surveillance by the EBV-polymerase chain reaction (PCR) of the peripheral blood and timely modulation of immunosuppression, incidence of EBV-infection that can cause

PTLD decreased in these days [34]. Onset of PTLD after pediatric LT is relatively rarer after 1 year, but some occur in the long term. Most PTLD can be treated by decrease or withdrawal of immunosuppression. In B-cell lymphoma, Rituximab is effective, and chemotherapy may be necessary for more severe forms. After successful treatment of PTLD, immunosuppression should be re-started with smaller dose, but in selected cases, immunosuppression can be completely withdrawn forever, as in cases with operational tolerance.

Solid organ malignancies have been sporadically found after LT for biliary atresia. I personally experienced hepatocellular carcinoma, breast cancer, and gastric cancer. Even in the younger generation, in 20 or 30 years, the possibility of malignancy should be kept in mind. Regular check-ups, yearly or every two years according to the age of the recipients, focusing on the non-hepatic abnormalities, including endoscopy for gastrointestinal tracts, screening by tumor markers, breast check for females, and general imaging studies, are recommended.

## 40.13 Opportunistic Infections

Under the immunosuppressive state, patients after LT are theoretically immunocompromised, even though the blood concentration level of IS after long time is quite low. As the viral infections, cytomegalovirus (CMV) and EBV are most commonly watched. In the long term, if there is an episode of fever with origin unknown, screening examination for these viruses should be done. Antigenemia assay for CMV and real-time (RT)-PCR for EBV DNA is common methods. For other epidemic viral infections, vaccination and suitable treatment using antiviral drugs if available, should be given under the instructions of specialists. Reduction or temporary stop of IS are usually applied. It can be re-started after 2 days of afebrile period. Such principles should be taught to parents or caretakers.

Under usual immunosuppression after LT, prophylactic use of antifungal and antiviral drugs is stopped before 1 year after the transplant. Invasive treatment like surgical operations or dental procedure, prophylactic use of antibiotics is recommended for at least 2 days prior to the procedure. I have a case of liver abscess after 16 years without any problems under the level of 5 ng/ml trough level of tacrolimus (Fig. 40.6). Surgery for knee injury before 5 months was suspected as the origin.

Overwhelming post-splenectomy infection (OPSI) is well known and should be kept in mind in cases with splenectomy. Vaccines for pneumococcus, hemophilus influenzae b (Hib), and meningococcus are available. The effect of prophylactic use of antibiotics has not reached the consensus. Education for patients and family members about the fear of such serious infections is necessary [35].

## 40.14 Vaccination

Live attenuated vaccination has been contraindication in post-solid organ transplant patients. However, in these days, the concept is changing [36]. In Japan, too, selected recipients with stable graft function and minimum IS without recent episodes of rejection can undergo live attenuated vaccinations. Inactivated vaccines like that for flu can be injected under any situation and should be given to minimize the infection-associated complications after liver transplantation. There have been no documented reports about higher incidence of rejection episodes after vaccination [37].

## 40.15 Growth, Development, Life Events, and Quality of Life Long Term after LT

Physical and mental growth, social activity, and reproducing activity are especially important for pediatric recipients with long life expectancy. These issues are influenced by many factors, like duration of the illness before the transplant, age and the status at the transplant, and post-transplant immunosuppression and complications. About the physical growth, there is a consensus that earlier transplant before the prominent growth failure becomes apparent is preferable [38, 39]. To obtain linear growth after the pediatric liver transplantation, avoiding advanced growth failure before the transplant and long steroid exposure is beneficial. About the neurodevelopmental outcome, one data described 31% of the recipients suffered from a delayed school performance after 10 years follow-up [40]. Whether the timely liver transplantation has a positive impact on neurodevelopment is not conclusive yet [41]. The neurocognitive outcome depends on the pretransplant nutritional status [42].

There is a consensus that pregnancy should be planned at least 12 months after LT with stable allograft function for favorable pregnancy outcomes. In fact, the outcome of pregnancies after LT, including that for biliary atresia, is favorable [43]. CNI should be kept minimum to make the risk of pre-eclampsia lower. Antimetabolites like MMF and anti-HBV nucleic acid analogs should be stopped for the possible teratogenicity, and taking other means and close watching of the graft function are mandatory. For women after adolescence, counseling should be given to teaching the issues related to pregnancy and delivery. It includes; pregnancy can be possible even after liver transplantation, patients should follow the instruction given by transplant professionals about the timing of the pregnancy and mode of delivery, safe delivery has been documented in many previous cases, and there are some drugs that should be stopped for a possible pregnancy. Pregnancy and delivery should be followed by a multidisciplinary team including transplant surgeons, obstetricians, and coordinators.

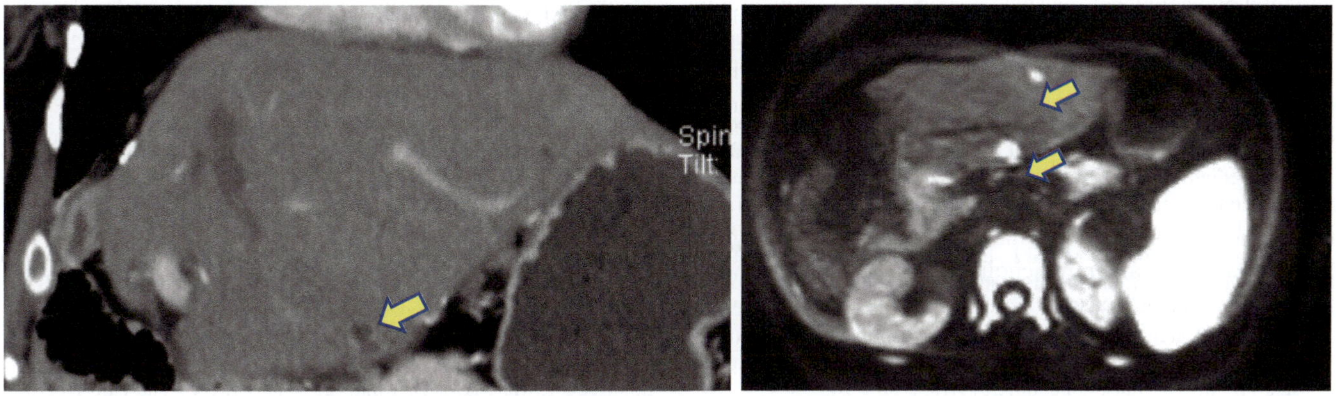

Enhanced CT MRI

**Fig. 40.6** Liver abscess of 21 years old female after 16 years from her LT for BA. She had been doing well without any problems except knee injury that needed surgery 5 months before. She had a mild epigastralgia and fever. Transaminases elevated slightly within the normal range, but C-reactive protein (CRP) increased to 5 mg/dl/. Arrow heads indicate the small multiple abscesses by the imaging studies. The lesion disappeared, and she recovered without any sequelae after 1 week of intravenous antibiotics. CT: computed tomography MRI: Magnetic resonance imaging

## 40.16 How to Manage Recipients Long Term after LT for BA

Regular check-up in the outpatient clinic should include assessment of graft function, renal function, metabolic condition for diabetes mellitus or dyslipidemia, and level of IS by blood test. If the patient was transplanted at the distant transplant center, routine check-up and prescription of routine drugs could be done in the nearby clinic or hospital. In that case, it is preferable that the data is shared with the transplant center. Blood pressure should be checked. The interval of such examinations should be less than 3 months, even when any disorder is not found. Levels of transaminases should be within normal limits. If it is persistently beyond the normal range, liver biopsy is recommended for confirmation of the pathology. Once there are any pathological findings positive in the biopsy, modification of the treatments should be considered. The pathological findings should be followed every one or two years by the protocol biopsy. However, if there were no pathological findings in the biopsy, and there has been no change of immunosuppression without any abnormalities of graft function since the previous biopsy, the next one can be postponed 5 years or later. Donor-specific antibody or anti-HLA antibody can be checked if there are any events about the graft function. Ultrasonography of the liver should be done at the visit of the outpatient clinic for check-up of the vasculature of the graft and for screening of biliary complications and possible tumors. Imaging studies like CT or MRI should be done at least once a few years. For recipients over 40 years, de novo malignancy should be screened by some general measures like endoscopic studies every 2 years. Instead of complete evaluation at the clinic for post-transplant follow-up, voluntary undergoing of regular medical check-up every one or two years is strongly recommended in elderly patients.

## References


1. The Japanese Liver Transplantation Society. Liver transplantation in Japan -registry by the Japanese liver transplantation society. Ishoku. 2019;54:81–96.
2. Elisofon SA, Magee JC, Ng VL, et al. Society of pediatric liver transplantation: current registry status 2011-2018. Pediatr Transpl. 2019;24:e13605. https://doi.org/10.1111/petr.13605.
3. Adam R, Karam V, Cailliez V, et al. Annual report of the European liver transplant registry (ELTR) – 50-year evolution of liver transplantation. Transplant Int. 2018;31:1293–317.
4. Nishimura N, Kasahara M, Ishikura K, et al. Current status of pediatric transplantation in Japan. J Intensive Care Journal of Intensive Care. 2017;5:48. https://doi.org/10.1186/s40560-017-0241-0.
5. Kim SR. The current status of deceased donor liver transplantation in Korea. Kanzo. 2017;58:310–8.
6. Taylor SA, Venkat V, Arnon R, et al. Improved outcomes for liver transplantation in patients with biliary atresia since pediatric end-stage liver disease implementation: analysis of the Society of Pediatric Liver Transplantation Registry. J Pediatr. 2020;219:89–97.
7. Kim JM, Kim KM, Yi NJ, et al. Pediatric liver transplantation outcomes in Korea. J Korean Med Sci. 2013;28:42–7.
8. Kasahara M, Umeshita K, Sakamoto S, et al. Living donor liver transplantation for biliary atresia: an analysis of 2085 cases in the registry of the Japanese liver transplantation society. AM J Transpl. 2018;18:659–68.
9. Foster BJ, Dahhou M, Zhang X, et al. High risk of liver allograft failure during late adolescence and young adulthood. Transplantation. 2016;100:577–84.
10. Sakamoto S, Kasahara M, Ogura Y, et al. And Japanese liver transplantation society. Current status of deceased donor split liver transplantation in Japan. J Hepatobiliary Pancreat Sci. 2015;22:837–45.
11. Miura K, Sakamoto S, Shimata K, et al. The outcome of pediatric liver transplantation from a living donor: a 17-year single center experience. Surg Today. 2017;47:1405–14.

12. Sakamoto S, Uchida H, Kitajima T, et al. The outcomes of portal vein reconstruction with vein graft interposition in Pediatric liver transplantation for small children with biliary atresia. Transplantation. 2020;104:90–6.
13. Shimata K, Sugawara Y, Honda M, et al. Efficacy of repeated balloon venoplasty for treatment of hepatic venous outflow obstruction after pediatric living-donor liver transplantation: a single-institution experience. Pediatr Transplant. 2019;23:e13522. https://doi.org/10.1111/petr.13522.
14. Martinelli J, Habes D, Majed L, et al. Long term outcome of liver transplantation in childhood: a study of 20-year survivors. Am J Transpl. 2018;18:1680–9.
15. Sanada Y, Katano T, Hirata Y, et al. Biliary complications following Pediatric living donor liver transplantation: risk factors, treatments, and prognosis. Transplantation. 2019;103:1863–70.
16. Demetris AJ, Bellamy C, Hubscher G, et al. 2016 comprehensive update of the Banff working group on liver allograft pathology: introduction of antibody-mediated rejection. Am J Transpl. 2016;16:2816–35.
17. Kerkar N, Hadzic N, Davies ET, et al. De-novo autoimmune hepatitis after liver transplantation. Lancet. 1998;351:409–13.
18. Miyagawa-Hayashino A, Yoshizawa A, Uchida Y, et al. Progressive agraft fibrosis and donor-specific human leucocyte antigen antibodies in pediatric late liver allografts. Liver Transpl. 2012;18:1333–42.
19. Tasdogan BE, Ma M, Simsek C, et al. Update on immunosuppression in liver transplantation. Euroasian J Hepato gastroenterol. 2019;9(2):96–101.
20. Youssef D, Niazi A, Alkhouri N. Long term complications in Pediatric liver transplant recipients: what every Pediatrician should know. Curr Pediatr Rev. 2016;12(3):209–21.
21. Ueno T, Kodama T, Noguchi Y, et al. Serum trough concentration and effects of mycophenolate Mofetil based on pathologic findings in infants after liver transplantation. Transplant Proc. 2020;52(6):1855–7.
22. Ganschow R, Ericzon BG, Dhawan A, et al. Everolimus and reduced calcineurin inhibitor therapy in pediatric liver transplant recipients: results from a multicenter, prospective study. Pediatr Transplant. 2017;21(7):1. https://doi.org/10.1111/petr.13024.
23. Takatsuki M, Uemoto S, Inomata Y, et al. Weaning of immunosuppression in living donor liver transplant recipients. Transplantation. 2001;72:449–54.
24. Egawa H, Miyagawa-Hayashino A, Haga H, et al. Non-inflammatory centrilobular sinusoidal fibrosis in pediatric liver transplant recipients under tacrolimus withdrawal. Hepatolo Res. 2012;42:895–903.
25. Tran L, Humar A. Tolerance studies in liver transplantation: are we fooling ourselves? Curr Opin Organ Transplant. 2020;25:151–7.
26. Matloff RG, Arnon R, Saland JM. The kidney in pediatric liver transplantation Pediatr. Transplantation. 2012;16:818–28.
27. Matloff RG, Diamond R, Weinberg A, et al. Biliary atresia is associated with hypertension. J Pediatr Gastroenterol Nutr. 2015;61:182–6.
28. Kar PM, Yi D, Kar SM. Looking beyond the obvious: IgA nephropathy in a liver transplant recipient. Indian J Nephrol. 2010;20:97–9.
29. Najeed SA, Saghir S, Hein B, et al. Management of hypertension in liver transplant patients. Int J Cardiol. 2011;6(152):4–6.
30. Chachlani R, Kim SJ, Dixon SN, et al. Incidence of new-onset diabetes mellitus and association with mortality in childhood solid organ transplant recipients: a population-based study. Nephrol Dial Transplant. 2019;34:524–31.
31. Chambers JH, Zerofsky M, Lustig RH, et al. Diet and exercise in Pediatric liver transplant recipients: Behaviors and association with metabolic syndrome. J Pediatr Gastroenterol Nutr. 2019;68:81–8.
32. Lin CC, Chen CL, Concejero A, et al. Active immunization to prevent de novo hepatitis B virus infection in pediatric live donor liver recipients. Am J Transplant. 2007;7:195–200.
33. Ueda Y, Marusawa H, Kaido T, et al. Efficacy and safety of prophylaxis with entecavir and hepatitis B immunoglobulin in preventing hepatitis B recurrence after living-donor liver transplantation. Hepatol Res. 2013;43:67–71.
34. Seo E, Kim J, Oh SH, et al. Epstein-Barr viral load monitoring for diagnosing post-transplant lymphoproliferative disorder in pediatric liver transplant recipients. Pediatr Transplant. 2020;24(4):e13666. https://doi.org/10.1111/petr.13666.
35. Tahir F, Ahmed J, Malik F. Post-splenectomy sepsis: a review of the literature. Cereus. 2020 Feb;12(2):e6898. https://doi.org/10.7759/cureus.6898.
36. Suersh S, Upton J, Green M, et al. Live vaccines after pediatric solid organ transplant: proceedings of a consensus meeting, 2018. Pediatr Transpl. 2019;23(7):e13571. https://doi.org/10.1111/petr.13571.
37. Suzuki M, Torii Y, Kawada J, et al. Immunogenicity of inactivated seasonal influenza vaccine in adult and pediatric liver transplant recipients over two seasons. Microbiol Immunol. 2013;57:715–22.
38. Sundaram S, Mack CL, Feldman AG, et al. Biliary atresia: indications and timing of liver transplantation and optimization of pretransplant care. Liver Transpl. 2017;23:96–109.
39. Mohammad S, Grimberg A, Rand E, et al. Long-term linear growth and puberty in pediatric liver transplant recipients. J Pediatr. 2013;163:1354–60.
40. Fouquet V, Alves A, Branchereau S, et al. Long-term outcome of pediatric liver transplantation for biliary atresia: a 10-year follow-up in a single center. Liver Transpl. 2005;11:152–60.
41. Rodijk L, Heijer AE, Hilscher JB, et al. Neurodevelopmental outcomes in children with liver diseases: a systematic review. J Pediatr Gastroenterol Nutr. 2018;67:157–68.
42. Sun Y, Lili J, Yu H, et al. The effect of pediatric living donor liver transplantation on neurocognitive outcomes in children. Ann Transpl. 2019;24:446–53.
43. Yu K, Kondoh E, Kawasaki K, et al. Pregnancy outcomes in liver transplant recipients: a 15-year single-center experience. J Obstet Gynecolo Res. 2016;42:1476–82.

# 41 Pregnancy and Delivery in Adult Survivors of Biliary Atresia

Tatsuo Kuroda

**Abstract**

Although the number of adult survivors of biliary atresia has increased considerably in recent decades, pregnancy and delivery remain challenging for female patients. Many key issues, including the appropriate criteria for approving attempts to become pregnant, the selection of a delivery mode, and a maternal monitoring plan during the gestational and postpartum period, have yet to be established. Biliary atresia patients potentially carry metabolic complications such as the impaired synthesis of cholesterol and sexual hormones. Artificial impregnation can be very dangerous for patients with amenorrhea caused by liver-related metabolic disorders. Transvaginal delivery after a full gestational term is safe in patients with an adequate hepatic reserve, but candidacy can be difficult to predict using a single parameter and instead requires comprehensive approval. Close monitoring of the deterioration of biological parameters after puberty is essential to identify patients at risk for sudden hepatic insufficiency caused by the gestational burden on the maternal body. For the patients with a poor hepatic reserve, liver transplantation should be completed prior to pregnancy. A Cesarean section at around the gestational week of 34 should be considered for the borderline cases, especially in cases with fetal growth restriction. In the present chapter, the current concept of pregnancy and delivery in patients with biliary atresia is discussed based on our experience and a literature review.

**Keywords**

Biliary atresia · Biochemical parameters · Cholesterol metabolism · Fertility · Pregnancy · Delivery · Safety instruction · Transplantation

T. Kuroda (✉)
Department of Pediatric Surgery, Keio University, School of Medicine, Tokyo, Japan
e-mail: kuroda-t@keio.jp

## 41.1 Introduction

More than half a century has passed since the successful Kasai operation for biliary atresia was first reported in the English literatures. At that time, the Kasai operation was the only successful surgical treatment available for biliary atresia. In the 1990s, liver transplantation was established as a curable treatment for patients with biliary atresia. Thus, the number of adult survivors of biliary atresia with either their native liver or a transplanted graft has increased drastically. Several studies had reported that 11%–20% of BA patients would be able to survive until adulthood with their native livers [1–7], and that liver transplantation further enhanced long-term survival of BA patients [8–11] already in the first decade of this century. With the number of adult survivors of biliary atresia increasing, ensuring stability and the quality of adult life has become the highest priority. Pregnancy and delivery in female patients who have undergone a Kasai operation are challenging even in the current era of treatment. The feasibility of pregnancy and delivery in patients with biliary atresia has been reported in several series, including our own. However, practical guidelines for the pregnancy and delivery in patients with biliary atresia have not yet been established, including important issues such as the safety criteria for pregnancy, maternal management, the selection of a delivery mode, and a perinatal follow-up protocol. Decisions regarding a suitable timing for liver transplantation are of great importance in terms of maternal safety during pregnancy and delivery. In this chapter, the current consensus on how pregnancy and delivery should be managed in patients with biliary atresia is discussed based on our own experience and a literature review.


M. Nio (ed.), *Introduction to Biliary Atresia*, https://doi.org/10.1007/978-981-16-2160-4_41

## 41.2 Biochemical Aspects of Pregnancy in Patients with Biliary Atresia

### 41.2.1 Overview

The major underlying pathophysiology in adult patients with biliary atresia who have survived with their native liver is essentially the progressive cholestatic liver cirrhosis and insufficient excretion of bile juice to some extent. Although the hepatic function seems well decompensated and quite asymptomatic under normal conditions, some events, such as pregnancy and delivery, can induce a considerable metabolic burden, potentially leading to liver deterioration and even liver insufficiency as the gestational week advances. Assessing the hepatic functional reserve based on biochemical parameters alone is difficult. Recently, several scoring systems, including our own [12], have been proposed to predict the clinical risk arising from potential hepatic insufficiency. Generally, protein synthesis is a good predictor of a deterioration in the hepatic functional reserve. A reduction in maternal protein synthesis can directly affect directly fetal growth, resulting in intrauterine fetal growth restriction (FGR). Insufficient bile excretion is frequently seen in patients who have undergone a Kasai operation, even though recognizable hyperbilirubinemia is not observed. Poor bile juice drainage is associated with a disturbance in cholesterol metabolism and also deficiencies in lipid-soluble vitamins, such as vitamin K and Vitamin D. Coagulopathy can also occur, either because of the hypo-absorption of vitamin K or a disturbance in coagulative protein synthesis.

On the other hand, the patients with the transplanted liver grafts face different problems. Pregnancy can mimic the maternal immune activity; therefore, reductions in the dosage of immunosuppressant agents, such as cyclosporin and tacrolimus, should be considered, since a high trough level of these calcineurin inhibitors can lead to the development of irreversible renal damage.

### 41.2.2 Natural Course of Biochemical Parameters in the Patients with the Native Liver

According to our previous study [13] examining 182 patients with biliary atresia, including 47 patients over the age of 20 years, 33 patients with their native livers exhibited favorable liver function at the age of 20 years. Of these 33 patients, 6 (18.2%) developed liver dysfunction after performing hard physical work or becoming pregnant. These six patients were considered to have the potential hepatic insufficiency and could not endure excessive physical burden; in these patients, however, only the choline-esterase (Ch-E), which is considered to be the biochemical parameter that is most closely correlated with the hepatic reserve, revealed significantly abnormal values at the age of 20 years, compared with the values in the remaining 27 stable patients (239.5 ± 42.6 vs. 285.8 ± 47.5, $P = 0.0216$). No significant differences in the alanine aminotransferase (ALT), aspartate aminotransferase (AST), or total protein levels at the age of 20 years or in any of the biochemical parameters at the age of 15 years were observed. Of the 14 patients who had undergone transplantations, 5 who underwent transplantation after the age of 20 years had relatively uneventful courses prior to the age of 20 years; however, their biochemical parameters had already shown significant deterioration at the time of puberty. These observations suggested that an elevation in hepatic enzyme levels and a decrease in protein synthesis ability at puberty may indicate the potential breakdown of hepatic function within the next several years, predicting a need for liver transplantation during adolescence or as a young adult. Identifying a cohort of patients with the potential to develop hepatic insufficiency who may experience a sudden deterioration in liver function after the age of 20 years, despite showing almost normal biochemical parameters, is important for ensuring patient safety during pregnancy and delivery. The close monitoring of biochemical parameters, especially the cholinesterase level, after puberty may be useful for predicting the risk of potential hepatic insufficiency.

### 41.2.3 Disturbance of Cholesterol Metabolism

Cholesterol is excreted in bile juice once in the forms of cholic acids synthesized by the liver cells or in the form of cholesterol itself; thereafter, it is re-absorbed in the small intestines during digestion and transferred to the liver once again in a process known as enterohepatic circulation that is essential for the maintenance of the hepatic and intestinal function. The enterohepatic circulation of cholesterol is disturbed to varying degrees in patients with biliary atresia, especially those with a poor hepatic reserve. Hypercholesteremia is often observed in patients with biliary atresia, reflecting a decrease in cholesterol excretion into bile juice. The disturbance of cholesterol metabolism is highly associated with more critical symptoms after puberty. Since sex hormones are basically synthesized from cholesterol, disturbed metabolism of cholesterol in patients with biliary atresia is considered to be strongly associated with the maldevelopment of secondary sexual characteristics. Actually, a lack or delay in secondary sexual maldevelopment is often observed in patients with biliary atresia and a poor hepatic reserve. According to our survey, a cohort of female patients developed amenorrhea after their first normal menstruation. We have previously reported that the cholinesterase level was significantly lower in the patients with menses abnormalities compared with normal controls [14]. Thus, menstruation abnormalities should also be highlighted as a clinical feature that is significantly associated with a poor hepatic reserve.

## 41.3 Fertility in Patients with Biliary Atresia

The above-mentioned conditions regarding sexual maldevelopment can result in infertility in both male and female patients. Interestingly, infertility observed at the end-stage of biliary atresia seems to be reversible, since several reports have described the birth of a baby in both fathers and mothers with biliary atresia after liver transplantation. In our initial series of pregnancy and delivery in patients with biliary atresia, hormone therapy was successful at enabling the impregnation of a female patient with amenorrhea. This patient developed rupture of esophageal varices and intrauterine fetal death during the third trimester of her first pregnancy and subsequently developed hepatic insufficiency requiring an urgent liver transplantation immediately after delivery during her second pregnancy, which had been induced using hormone therapy. Artificial pregnancy induced by the replacement of sexual hormones in a patient with biliary atresia and amenorrhea because of a poor hepatic reserve is extremely dangerous and is obviously not recommended [14].

## 41.4 Safety Considerations for the Approval of Pregnancy

Guidelines for safe pregnancy in patients with biliary atresia have not been established. Important problems such as the criteria for approving pregnancy, the selection of a delivery mode, and a suitable timing for delivery are all remained unanswered. No large clinical studies addressing these problems have been reported.

As a general consensus, maternal safety must be given the highest priority when considering pregnancy and delivery in female patients with biliary atresia. Since maternal safety has a higher priority than fetal life, the pregnancy should be terminated if the maternal life is in danger. Pregnancy and delivery are not acceptable for patients endangered by the gestational burden to the maternal body.

Biliary atresia patients with an adequate hepatic reserve in their native livers and unimpaired protein synthesis are capable of safely tolerating full term of gestation and transvaginal delivery. Unfortunately, a reliable means of predicting the risk associated with pregnancy and delivery in patients with a potentially poor hepatic reserve has not been established as described above. In our previous analysis, no significant difference in liver function parameters was observed between patients who underwent pregnancy and delivery uneventfully and non-pregnant patients with uneventful courses who did not require transplantation. In contrast, the ALT, AST, and cholinesterase levels were significantly better maintained at the age of pregnancy in a maternal group, compared with age-matched patients who had experienced recurrent episodes of cholangitis or jaundice. We previously proposed a trial of risk classification in which adult biliary atresia patients were divided into four risk groups according to biological parameters measured after puberty [13]. According to this risk classification, the cohort of patients with elevated liver enzymes and total cholesterol levels and decreased protein synthesis and cholinesterase levels at the time of puberty were considered to have a high risk of liver failure requiring liver transplantation within the next 5 years. Liver transplantation should be performed before pregnancy in patients belonging to this cohort. Meanwhile, the patients with an uneventful course but exhibit a mild deterioration in parameters correlated with protein synthesis, such as choline-esterase, after the age of 20 years are considered to carry a moderate risk. Pregnancy prior to liver transplantation seems to be acceptable in these patients with a moderate risk; however, close monitoring is essential for these patients, since these patients can potentially develop sudden-onset and progressive liver insufficiency during the gestational and puerperal period.

More recently, the regulations regarding pregnancy and delivery in patients with biliary atresia have been gradually relaxed because of the accumulation of clinical experience. The latest experience at our institution reported in 2016 is summarized in Table 41.1. The MELD (Model for End-stage Liver Disease) score and the cholinesterase level, which is a representative biological parameter of the hepatic reserve, of the five patients are plotted with delivery mode in Fig. 41.1. Pregnancy and delivery might be dangerous in patients with either a serum cholinesterase level less than 50 IU/ml or a MELD score over 13, since a patient who met these criteria experienced a rupture of maternal esophageal varices and subsequent fetal death as plotted as the case 5. Liver transplantation should be performed prior to the approval of pregnancy in this cohort, since the termination of pregnancy might otherwise need to be considered. At present, however, only living-related liver transplantations are ethically acceptable for the purpose of enabling pregnancy.

## 41.5 Practical Safety Instructions for Pregnancy and Delivery

Based on our single institutional experience and a literature review, our recommendations for the practical management of pregnancy and delivery in patients with biliary atresia patients are summarized below.

**Table 41.1** Latest experience in pregnancy and delivery in the biliary atresia patients in Keio University Hospital

| | | | Maternal issues | | | Delivery | | | |
|---|---|---|---|---|---|---|---|---|---|
| Case # | Maternal age (y.o.) | Liver | Cholinesterase level (IU/l) | complications | therapy | Gestational age | Delivery mode | Neonatal birth weight (g) | Outcomes |
| 1 | 32 | Native | 144 | Cholangitis (24th G.W.~) | Antibiotics | 36w5d | Transvaginal | 2578 | Alive |
| 2 | 35 | Native | 39 | Esophageal varix rupture (25th G.W.) | EVL | 30w0d | Caesarean section | 842 | Fetal death |
| 3 | 39 | Native | 133 | Cholangitis (21st G.W.~) | Antibiotics | 36w5d | Transvaginal | 2590 | Alive |
| 4 | 40 | Native | 92 | Cholangitis, Esophageal varix (25th G.W.~) | EVL | 37w3d | Caesarean section | 2690 | Alive |
| 5 | 31 | LTx. Graft | 205 | None | | 38w4d | Transvaginal | 2762 | Alive |

The table summarizes complications during the gestational period and delivery in the five patients with biliary atresia who underwent pregnancy and delivery at Keio University Hospital for the last 10 years are plotted

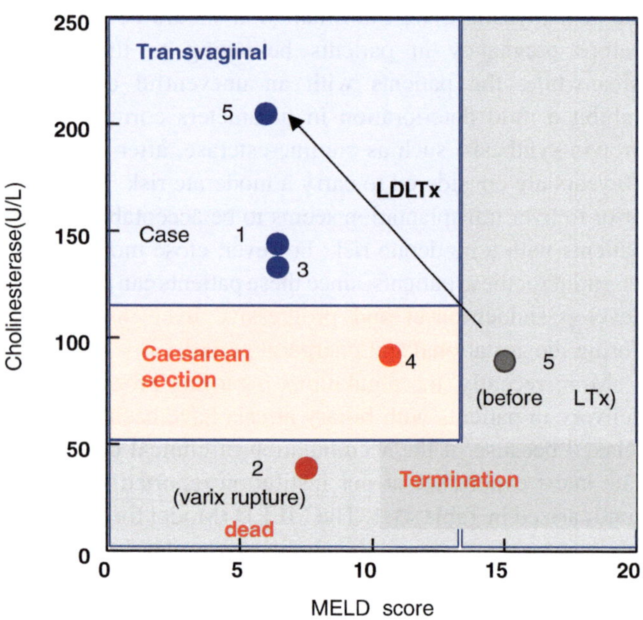


**Fig. 41.1** Delivery mode and hepatic reserve. The MELD scores and the serum cholinesterase levels in the five patients with biliary atresia who underwent pregnancy and delivery at Keio University Hospital for the last 10 years are plotted with delivery mode

### 41.5.1 Maternal Management and Follow-Up Protocol during Pregnancy

#### 41.5.1.1 Monitoring and Management of Esophageal Varices

The rupture of esophageal varices is one of the most common complications seen in survivors with biliary atresia [15–17] and often results in intrauterine fetal death during the pregnancy in patients with biliary atresia. Esophageal varices drastically deteriorate during the early third trimester and can become lethal levels, even in patients with a lower grade of esophageal varices and especially in patients with a poor hepatic reserve. The endoscopic monitoring of esophageal varices at the early third trimester is highly recommended, especially in the patients who show signs suggesting a potentially poor hepatic reserve before pregnancy, such as a low serum level of cholinesterase, mild hypoproteinemia, and a mild elevation of transaminase. Middle-grade esophageal varices should be endoscopically ligated in a prophylactic manner.

#### 41.5.1.2 Avoidance of Physical Overload

Excessive work and physical overload should be avoided during the early gestational period [13]. We experienced a patient who developed gestational toxicosis immediately after an elongation of her working hours, including night duties, even though the patient had shown normal biological parameters before pregnancy. This patient was successfully treated by admitting her for a long hospitalization enabling complete rest.

#### 41.5.1.3 Management of Recurrent Cholangitis

Cholangitis triggered by excessive physical burden is often observed [16–20], especially during the gestational period. In Table 41.1, recurrent cholangitis began at 21 ~ 25 gestational weeks in three of the four patients with their native livers who delivered a baby. The long-term intravenous administration of antibiotics was required to control pregnancy-related cholangitis.

### 41.5.2 Delivery Mode

In our initial series of 6 patients reported in 2002, all the babies were delivered by cesarean section, since the safety of transvaginal delivery was considered to be questionable in those days. Thereafter, the number of biliary atresia patients who underwent transvaginal delivery increased in parallel with the accumulation of experience and knowledge. In our latest series examined in 2016, transvaginal delivery was successfully achieved in two of the four patients with their native livers. Transvaginal delivery can be offered even for patients with a potentially poor hepatic reserve, according to the results of our recent series shown in Table 41.1. This patient cohort also appears to be capable of tolerating a full term of gestation. On the other hand, cesarean section is indicated for patients with obviously less hepatic reserve. Unfortunately, no indices or criteria have been established to predict an insufficiency of the hepatic reserve as cited above. Comprehensive decision must be made based on changes in biological parameters, the maternal general condition, and fetal growth comprehensively.

### 41.5.3 Indication for Cesarean Section

The indications for a cesarean section should also be decided based on a comprehensive consideration. For mothers is in a critical state and in eminent danger, urgent termination is required. Figure 41.1 shows that a cesarean section should be selected for patients who show a decrease of cholinesterase level to less than 100 IU/ml in our series. Even if the maternal condition is stable, fetal growth restriction (FGR) may suggest an insufficiency of maternal hepatic reserve and the need for a cesarean section at suitable timing. In our initial experience, the birth weight seemed to be inversely related to the mother's age at delivery ($r = -0.718$). In our latest series, however, the birth weight of the babies from mothers with biliary atresia, a high cholinesterase level and a low MELD score was normal. These observations appear to suggest that fetal growth is restricted by a decrease in protein synthesis ability and hepatic reserve arising from maternal aging. Therefore, it may be dangerous to continue gestation until the full term in these cases showing FGR. At present, we consider the 34 th gestational week to be a suitable timing for cesarean section in cases with a mild to moderate grade of FGR or maternal abnormality. At this gestational week, the respiratory function of the newborn baby is expected to have matured sufficiently to live on their lungs.

### 41.5.4 Postpartum Follow-Up Point

According to our previous analysis [21], while the serum albumin, total protein, and cholinesterase levels dropped during the third trimester, the ALT, AST levels were slightly elevated during late gestation, though the changes were not statistically significant. The serum albumin, total protein, and cholinesterase levels recovered to the previous levels within one month after delivery, whereas the ALT and AST remained high during the postpartum period, even in patients with a good hepatic reserve. A prolonged elevation of transaminase and bilirubin levels indicates that the patient has a borderline hepatic reserve during recovery from the postpartum state and the patient may require urgent transplantation.

### 41.5.5 Pregnancy and Transplantation

Since 2000, several reports have described favorable results of pregnancy and delivery after liver transplantation, including some cases with multiple deliveries [22–24]. At the same time, several complications, including preeclampsia, hypertension, mild renal failure, elevated liver enzyme levels, preterm labor, and a low birth weight, have been reported to be relatively common [25, 26]. In order to avoid renal dysfunction caused by the nephrotoxicity of immunosuppressive agents during the late post-transplantation period [27], lower trough levels of the immunosuppressive agents may be preferable to preserve renal function during pregnancy. Even though calcineurin inhibitors and other immunosuppressive agents are known to have teratogenic potential, few reports have described visceral malformation in newborns from mothers with biliary atresia and transplanted liver grafts. Consideration should also be given to the timing of pregnancy after transplantation. Usually, contraception should be attempted at least 2 years after liver transplantation.

### 41.5.6 Back-Up Transplantation

For pregnant patients with a borderline hepatic reserve, a back-up transplantation should be prepared in case that the patient requires urgent transplantation because of sudden liver failure during the gestational or postpartum period. In the case of living-related transplantation, the spouse and the siblings of the mother are generally considered as donor candidates. The identification of a donor can be difficult from both medical and social aspects and sometimes takes a long time. Therefore, a deterioration in the maternal condition may occur before the selection of a donor has been completed. We generally start the processing of identifying a potential donor immediately after a diagnosis of pregnancy or if the patient exhibits physical findings of liver insufficiency or some abnormality in a biochemical parameter, such as a mild elevation of bilirubin, a prolonged and significant elevation of liver enzymes, or a decrease in cholinesterase.

The above instructions regarding the management of pregnancy and delivery in patients with biliary atresia should be verified and furthermore revised in future studies.

**Acknowledgments** The author deeply thanks Dr. Nobuhiro Takahashi for preparing the original figure shown in this chapter.

## References


1. Nio M, Ohi R, Hayashi Y, et al. Current status of 21 patients who survived more than 20 years since undergoing surgery for biliary atresia. J Pediatr Surg. 1996;31:381–4.
2. Karrer FM, Price MR, Bensard DD, et al. Long-term results with the Kasai operation for biliary atresia. Arch Surg. 1996;131:493–6.
3. Lopez-Santamaria M, Gamez M, Murcia J, et al. Long-term follow-up of patients with biliary atresia successfully treated with hepatic portoenterostomy. The importance of sequential treatment. Pediatr Surg Int. 1998;13:327–30.
4. Matsuo S, Suita S, Kubota M, et al. Long-term results and clinical problems after portoenterostomy in patients with biliary atresia. Eur J Pediatr Surg. 1998;8:142–5.
5. Kuroda T, Saeki M, Nakano M, Morikawa N. Biliary atresia, the next generation: a review of liver function, social activity, and sexual development in the late post-operative period. J Pediatr Surg. 2002;37:1709–12.
6. Hadzic N, Davenport M, Tizzard S, et al. Long-term survival following Kasai portoenterostomy: is chronic liver disease inevitable? J Pediatr Gastroenterol Nutr. 2003;37:430–3.
7. Lykavieris P, Chardot C, Sokhn M, et al. Outcome in adulthood of biliary atresia: a study of 63 patients who survived for over 20 years with their native liver. Hepatology. 2005;41:366–71.
8. Inomata Y, Oike F, Okamoto S, et al. Impact of the development of a liver transplant program on the treatment of biliary atresia in an institution in Japan. J Pediatr Surg. 1997;32:1201–5.
9. Chardot C, Carton M, Spire-Bendelac N, et al. Prognosis of biliary atresia in the era of liver transplantation: French national study from 1986 to 1996. Hepatology. 1999;30:606–11.
10. Fouquet V, Alves A, Branchereau S, et al. Long-term outcome of pediatric liver transplantation for biliary atresia: a 10-year follow-up in a single center. Liver Transpl. 2005;11:152–60.
11. Uchida Y, Kasahara M, Egawa H, et al. Long-term outcome of adult-to-adult living donor liver transplantation for post-Kasai biliary atresia. Am J Transplant. 2006;6:2443–8.
12. Tomita H, Masugi Y, Hoshino K, et al. Long-term native liver fibrosis in biliary atresia: development of a novel scoring system using histology and standard liver tests. J Hepatol. 2014;60:1242–8.
13. Kuroda T, Saeki M, Morikawa N, et al. Management of adult biliary atresia patients: should hard work and pregnancy be discouraged? J Pediatr Surg. 2007;42:2106–9.
14. Kuroda T, Saeki M, Nakano M, et al. Biliary atresia, the next generation: a review of liver function, social activity,and sexual development in the late postoperative period. J Pediatr Surg. 2002;37:1709–12.
15. Biji EJ, Bharwani KD, Houwen RH, et al. The long-term outcome of the Kasai operation in patients with biliary atresia: a systematic review. Neth J Med. 2013;71:170–3.
16. Kumagi T, Drenth JP, Guttman O, et al. Biliary atresia and survival into adulthood without transplantation: a collaborative multicenter clinic review. Liver Int. 2012;32:510–8.
17. O'Sullivan OE, Crosby D, Byrne B, et al. Pregnancy complicated by portal hypertension secondary to biliary atresia. Case Rep Obstet Gynecol. 2013;2013:421386.
18. Ng VL, Haber BH, Magee JC, et al. Medical status of 219 children with biliary atresia surviving long-term with their native livers: results from a north American multicenter consortium. J Pediatr. 2014;165:539–46. e2
19. Chiba T, Ohi R, Nio M, et al. Late complications in long-term, survivors of biliary atresia. Eur J Pediatr Surg. 1992;2:22–5.
20. Sasaki H, Nio M, Hayashi Y, et al. Problems during and after pregnancy in female patients with biliary atresia. J Pediatr Surg. 2007;42:1329–32.
21. Kuroda T, Saeki M, Morikawa N, et al. Biliary atresia and pregnancy: puberty may be an important point for predicting the outcome. J Pediatr Surg. 2005;40:1852–5.
22. Fouquet V, Alves A, Branchereau S, et al. Long-term outcome of pediatric liver transplantation for biliary atresia: a 10-year follow-up in a single center. Liver Transpl. 2005;11:152–60.
23. Jain AB, Reyes J, Marcos A, et al. Pregnancy after liver transplantation with tacrolimus immunosuppression: a single center's experience updated at 13 years. Transplantation. 2003;76:827–32.
24. Nagy S, Bush MC, Berkowitz R, et al. Pregnancy outcome in liver transplantation recipients. Obstet Gynecol. 2003;102:121–8.
25. Miller JC, Mastrobattista JM, Katz AR. Obstetrical and neonatal outcome in pregnancies after liver transplantation. Am J Perinatol. 2000;17:299–302.
26. Carr DB, Larson AM, Schmucker BC, et al. Maternal hemodynamics and pregnancy outcome in women with prior orthotopics liver transplantation. Liver Transpl. 2000;6:213–21.
27. Avitzur Y, De Luca E, Cantos M, et al. Health status ten years after pediatric liver transplantation—looking beyond the graft. Transplantation. 2004;78:566–73.

# Biliary Atresia and Malignancy

# 42

Tsugumichi Koshinaga

**Abstract**

Liver fibrosis caused by cholestasis progresses even after the Kasai portoenterostomy in biliary atresia. The development of a malignant tumor is one of the late complications of biliary atresia.

Hepatocellular carcinoma is the most common malignant tumor. Before the era of the Kasai portoenterostomy, three cases of hepatocellular carcinoma in the postmortem examination had been reported since 1965.

In the explanted liver at the time of transplant surgery, hepatocellular carcinomas have been frequently reported since 1994. All the patients notably have been alive since liver transplantation. During the follow-up period after portoenterostomy, on the other hand, a total of 18 patients were clinically diagnosed as having hepatocellular carcinoma, of whom eleven patients were diagnosed before the teenage. The age at the Kasai portoenterostomy and outcome of jaundice were not associated with malignant development. However, at more than 16 years of age, four out of seven patients underwent alternative treatments other than liver transplant surgery, suggesting that older patients may have a progressive change of hepatocellular carcinoma development in the cirrhotic liver. Posttransplant prognosis is relatively good in patients who are early diagnosed during the follow-up period after the Kasai portoenterostomy.

Cholangiocarcinomas were found in seven biliary atresia patients, older than those of hepatocellular carcinoma. The prognosis of cholangiocarcinoma is worse than that of hepatocellular carcinoma. Six patients died, despite aggressive adjuvant chemotherapy for recurrent and metastatic disease.

Hepatoblastomas were found in four biliary atresia patients before five years of age. The relationship remains unknown between hepatoblastoma and biliary atresia. Hepatoblastoma was found in the explanted liver on the liver transplantation in two patients and found clinically during the follow-up period in the rest two patients. Three patients underwent liver transplantation with good results.

**Keywords**

Biliary atresia · Malignancy · Hepatocellular carcinoma Cholangiocarcinoma · Hepatoblastoma · Malignant tumor · Liver tumor

In patients with biliary atresia, liver fibrosis caused by the cholestasis progresses even after the Kasai portoenterostomy. The development of the malignant tumor is well-recognized as a late complication of biliary atresia. The hepatic tumors include hepatocellular carcinoma, cholangiocarcinoma, and hepatoblastoma. Hepatocellular carcinoma (Fig. 42.1) is the most common malignant tumor. Cholangiocarcinoma (Fig. 42.2) and hepatoblastoma are rare tumors in the biliary atresia, and the causative relations with biliary atresia remain uncertain. The English literature was reviewed through the PubMed from 1965 to 2020.

## 42.1 Hepatocellular Carcinoma Found at Autopsy

In 1965, Okuyama [1] described the first autopsy case on the development of hepatocellular carcinoma in the biliary atresia liver (Table 42.1), which was thought inevitable natural history of the specific disorder in those days. The postmortem examination revealed hepatocarcinoma developed in the right lobe of the advanced cirrhotic liver with pulmonary metastasis. This report first states that biliary cirrhosis is associated with carcinoma in even children, although the mechanism is unknown [1]. Since then, two more case reports were found at autopsy leading to death before the era of the Kasai portoenterostomy.

T. Koshinaga (✉)
Department of Pediatric Surgery, Nihon University School of Medicine, Tokyo, Japan
e-mail: koshinaga.tsugumichi@nihon-u.ac.jp


M. Nio (ed.), *Introduction to Biliary Atresia*, https://doi.org/10.1007/978-981-16-2160-4_42

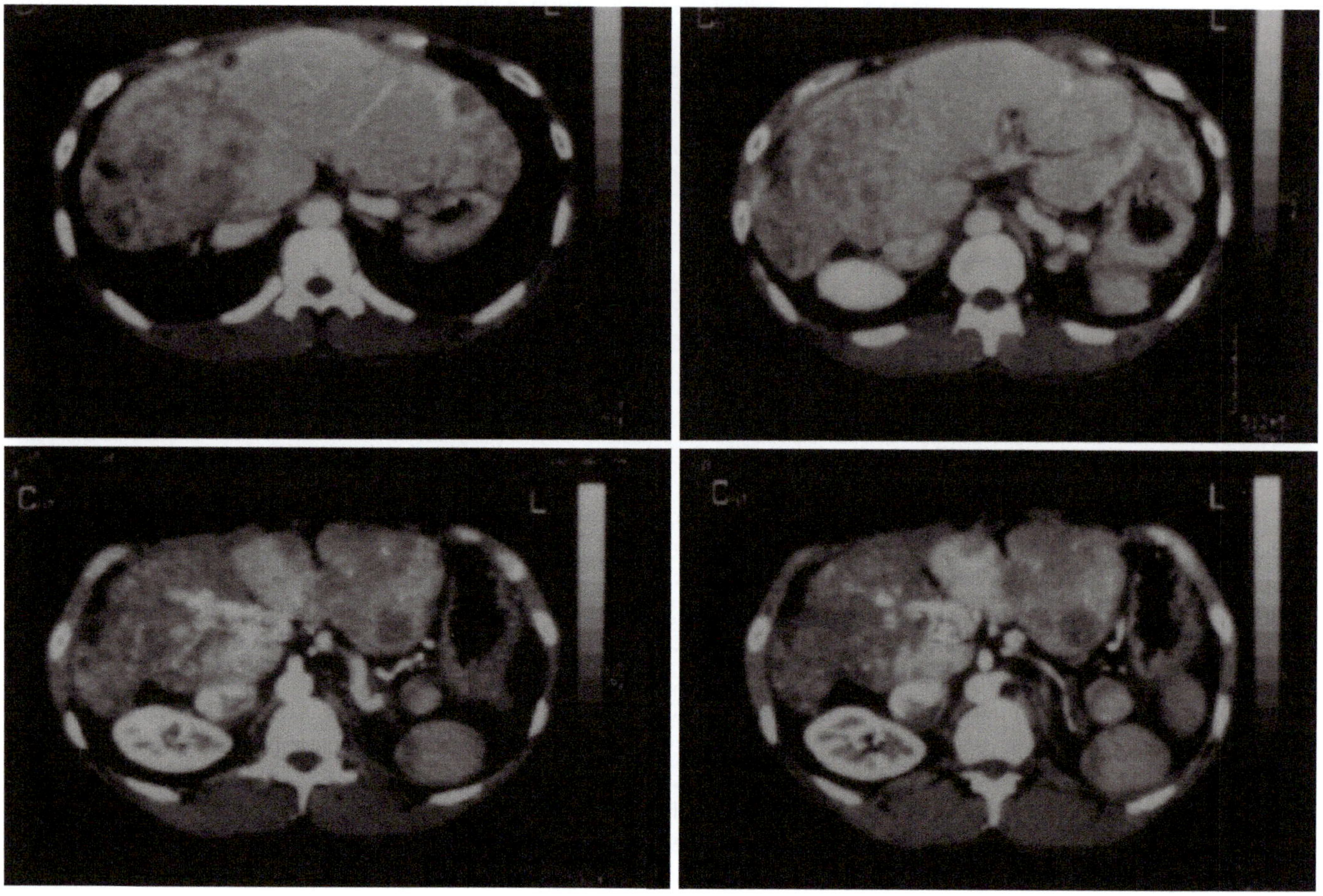


Fig. 42.1 Postcontrast CT findings of multiple tumors of hepatocellular carcinoma developed in a 20-years-old male with biliary atresia after the Kasai portoenterostomy

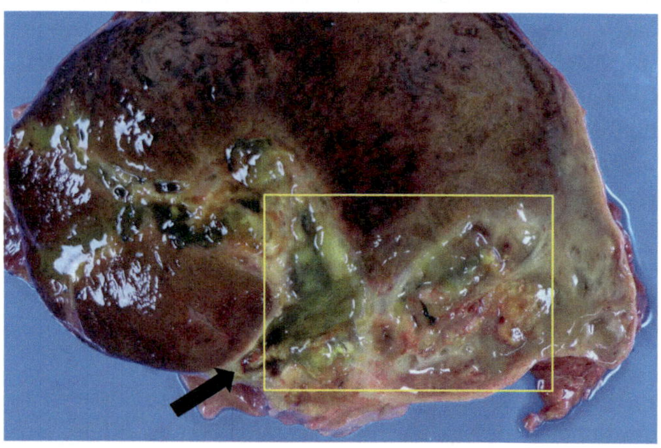

Fig. 42.2 The macroscopic finding of the postmortem examination of 34 years-old female with biliary atresia had undergone the Kasai portoenterostomy. Cholangiocarcinoma extends from the anastomosis site of the portoenterostomy (arrow) along with the extensive region of the intrahepatic ducts (square)

## 42.2 Hepatocellular Carcinoma Incidentally Diagnosed in the Explanted Liver for Transplantation

Since 1994, hepatocellular carcinomas have been often found in the explanted liver at the time of transplant surgery (Table 42.2). Six (Table 42.2, patients no. 1 to 6) patients underwent Kasai portoenterostomy, and the rest of the three (Table 42.2, patients no. 7 to 9) did not have surgery for biliary atresia before transplantation. The size of the tumors ranges from 5 mm to 25 mm in the patients undergoing the Kasai Portoenterostomy. The adult one (Table 42.2, patient no. 7) having a large tumor of 180 mm in size. All the patients notably have been alive since liver transplantation.

**Table 42.1** Hepatocellular carcinoma found at autopsy before the era of Kasai portoenterosotomy

| No. | 1 [1] | 2 [2] | 3 [3] |
|---|---|---|---|
| Publication year | 1965 | 1966 | 1968 |
| Age at hepatic tumor diagnosis | 3 years | 2 years | 6 years |
| Gender | M | M | F |
| Mode of diagnosis | Autopsy | Autopsy | Autopsy |
| Tumor size (cm) | n/a | n/a | n/a |
| Location | Right lobe | n/a | Entire liver |
| Treatment | None | None | None |
| Survival period after treatment | – | – | – |
| Outcome | Dead | Dead | Dead |

*LT* Liver transplantation, *LRLT* Living-related liver transplantation

## 42.3 Hepatocellular Carcinoma Clinically Diagnosed During the Follow-Up Period after Portoenterostomy

From1972 to 2016, a total of 18 patients were clinically diagnosed as having hepatocellular carcinoma in the follow-up period after the Kasai portoenterostomy (Tables 42.3a and 42.3b). Eleven of these 18 patients were diagnosed before the teenage, suggesting malignant development in the earlier phase of the disease process. It is noteworthy that hepatocellular carcinoma developed less than ten years of age in eight (Table 42.3a, patients no. 1 to 8) of 18 patients after Kasai portoenterostomy. Nor the age of Kasai portoenterostomy or the outcome of jaundice were associated with malignant development. Tumor size at diagnosis varies from 10 mm at the smallest detected by an ultrasound examination. All the patients before the teenager received a liver transplant except the one (Table 42.3a, patient no. 4) who declined the surgical therapy. However, over 16 years of age, four out of seven patients underwent alternative treatments other than liver transplant surgery, suggesting that older patients may have a progressive change of HCC development in the cirrhotic liver. Posttransplant prognosis is relatively good in patients who are early diagnosed as having a tumor of the liver during the follow-up period after the Kasai portoenterostomy.

## 42.4 Cholangiocarcinoma

Cholangiocarcinomas arise from the epithelial cells of the bile ducts. Cholangiocarcinoma was found in seven biliary atresia patients (Table 42.4). Cholangiocarcinoma may develop in older patients of age, compared with hepatocellular carcinoma. Two patients (Table 42.4, patients no. 1 and 2) before the era of the Kasai portoenterostomy were diagnosed as having cholangiocarcinoma at an earlier age than the patients undergoing the Kasai portoenterostomy. Four patients (Table 42.4, patients no. 3 to 7) had cholangiocarcinoma after the Kasai portoenterostomy. Cholangiocarcinomas were found in the explanted liver on the liver transplantation in the two patients (Table 42.4, patients no. 4 and 5) and discovered during their follow-up in the rest two patients (Table 42.4, patients no. 5 and 7). The prognosis of cholangiocarcinoma is worse than that of hepatocellular carcinoma. All the patients except one patient did not survive despite aggressive adjuvant chemotherapy for recurrent and metastatic disease.

## 42.5 Hepatoblastoma

Hepatoblastomas were found in four biliary atresia patients (Table 42.5). The relationship between hepatoblastoma and biliary atresia remains unknown. All the patients were diagnosed as having hepatoblastoma before five years of age. The Kasai portoenterostomy was not successful in the three patients (Table 42.5, patients no. 1 to 3). Hepatoblastomas were found in the explanted liver on the liver transplantation in two patients (Table 42.5, patients no. 1 and 3), and found clinically during the follow-up period in the rest two patients (Table 42.5, patients no. 2 and 4). Serum alpha-fetoprotein may sensitively elevate, but not specific for hepatoblastoma developing in biliary atresia [26]. Three patients (Table 42.5, patients no. 1, 3, and 4) underwent liver transplantation with good results.

**Table 42.2** Hepatocellular carcinoma incidentally diagnosed in the explanted liver for transplantation

| No. | 1 [4] | 2 [5] | 3 [6] | 4 [7] | 5 [8] | 6 [9] | 7 [10] | 8 [11] | 9 [7] |
|---|---|---|---|---|---|---|---|---|---|
| Publication year | 2011 | 2012 | 2007 | 2011 | 1994 | 2015 | 1972 | 2009 | 2011 |
| Age at hepatic tumor diagnosis | 0.7 years | 8 months | 8 months | 2 years | 11 years | 25 years | 4 years incidental explanted liver | 10 months incidental explanted liver | 1 year incidental explanted liver |
| Gender | F | F | M | F | n/a | M | F | M | M |
| Age at Kasai op | n/a | 3 months | 56 days | 71 days | n/a | 40 days | No Kasai op | No Kasai op | No Kasai op |
| Outcome of jaundice | n/a | Persistent | Persistent | Persistent | n/a | Cleared | Unchanged | Unchanged | Unchanged |
| Tumor size | 6 mm | 9 mm solitary | 5 mm | 11 + 9 mm | 15 mm | 25 + 12 mm | 180 mm | 7 mm | 6 mm |
| Location | n/a | Left lobe | Several small foci of HCC in the regenerative nodule of the right lobe | Left lobe | n/a | S7 | n/a | n/a | Left lobe |
| Histologic subtype of HCC | Moderately-differentiated | Nodular type, Edmondson grade I with no microvascular invasion | n/a | n/a | n/a | Well-differentiated | n/a | n/a | n/a |
| Treatment | LT | LRLT | LT | LT | LT | LT | LT | LT | LRLT |
| Survival period after LT | 1.6 years | 4 months | 12 months | 4.1 years | 44 months | 2 months | 18 months | 4 months | 2 years |
| Outcome | Alive | Alive | Alive | Alive | Alive | Alive | Alive | Alive | Alive |

n/a, not available

*HCC* Hepatocellular carcinoma, *CCC* Cholangiocellular carcinoma, *LT* Liver transplantation, *LRLT* Living-related liver transplantation

**Table 42.3a** Hepatocellular carcinoma clinically diagnosed during follow-up period after the Kasai portoenterostomy

| No. | 1 [12] | 2 [7] | 3 [4] | 4 [13] | 5 [7] | 6 [9] | 7 [14] | 8 [4] | 9 14] | 10 [10] | 11 [15] |
|---|---|---|---|---|---|---|---|---|---|---|---|
| Publication year | 2014 | 2011 | 2011 | 1995 | 2011 | 2015 | 2001 | 2011 | 2002 | 1972 | 1996 |
| Age at hepatic tumor diagnosis | 7 months | 1 years | 3.6 years | 4 years | 4 years | 4 years | 8 years | 8 years | 10 years | 12 years | 12 years |
| Gender | F | F | F | F | M | M | M | M | F | F | n/a |
| Age at Kasai op | 1 month | 68 days | n/a | 2 months | 66 days | n/a | 66 days | n/a | 70 days | n/a | n/a |
| Outcome of jaundice | n/a | Cleared | n/a | Persistent | Cleared | n/a | n/a | n/a | n/a | Cleared | Cleared |
| Mode of diagnosis | US | One by CT and the other incidental explanted liver | US | US and biopsy | CT | MRI and biopsy | CT | US | CT | Hepatic arteriogram | US and biopsy |
| Tumor size | 10 mm | 19 + 25 mm | 25 mm | 10 mm | 54 mm | 38 + 20 mm | 60 + 13 mm | 30 mm | 50 mm | 100 mm | n/a |
| Location | S3 | Right lobe | n/a | S4 | Right lobe | S2, 3 | Lateral segment and S7 | n/a | Lateral segment | Right lobe | Left lobe |
| Histologic subtype of HCC | n/a | n/a | Poorly-differentiated | n/a | Well-diferentiated | Well-differentiated | Moderately differentiated | Well-differentiated | Well-differentiated | Well-differentiated | n/a |
| Treatment | LT | LT | LT | PEITx7 | LT | LT | LT | LT | LT | LT | LT |
| Follow-up period from the diagnosis of liver tumor | 20 months | 2.5 years | 4.0 years[a] | 17 months | 2.5 years | 12 months[a] | 5 years | n/a | 33 months | 2 months | 36 months[a] |
| Outcome | Alive | Alive | Alive | Dead (bleeding due to tumor rupture) | Alive | Alive | Alive | Dead | Alive | Dead | Alive |

n/a, not available

*US* Ultrasonography, *HCC* Hepatocellular carcinoma, *LT* Liver transplantation, *PEIT* Percutaneous ethanol injection therapy

[a]Survival period after treatment

**Table 42.3b** Hepatocellular carcinoma clinically diagnosed during follow-up period after the Kasai portoenterostomy

| No. | 12 [16] | 13 [12] | 14 [7] | 15 [17] | 16 [18] | 17 [19] | 18 [20] | 7 |
|---|---|---|---|---|---|---|---|---|
| Publication year | 1993 | 2014 | 2011 | 2008 | 2003 | 2012 | 2016 | 2004 |
| Age at hepatic tumor diagnosis | 16 years | 16 years | 17 years | 19 years | 20 years | 23 years | 39 years | 7 years |
| Gender | F | F | F | M | M | F | M | M |
| Age at Kasai op | 140 days (hepaticojejuno-stomy) | 2 m/0 | 49 days | n/a | 115 days | 3 months | 60 days | 84 days |
| Outcome of jaundice | Cleared | n/a | n/a | n/a | Cleared | Cleared | Cleared | Icteric |
| Mode of diagnosis | CT | MRI | US | US, MRI and CT | CT and biopsy | CT and biopsy | US | CT and biopsy |
| Tumor size | 70 mm | 15 mm | 105 mm | 100 mm | Multiple masses | 30 mm | 60 mm | 10 + 19 + 39 mm |
| Location | Lateral segment | S6 | Right lobe | Right liver | Entire liver | Right lobe | S1 | S5, 7 |
| Histologic subtype of HCC | Well-differentiated | n/a | n/a | Well-differentiated, without vascular invasion | n/a | n/a | CCC + HCC | n/a |
| Treatment | Planned for hepatectomy | RFA | LT | LT | TAE | On the waiting list for LT | TACE(CDDP EPI MMC)gem | LRLT |
| Follow-up period from the diagnosis of liver tumor | 2 months | 15 months | 5.7 years | 72 months | 6 months | n/a | 8 months* | 84 months |
| Outcome | Dead (intracranial bleeding) before treatment | Alive | Alive | Alive | Dead (hepatic failure) | Alive | Dead (hepatic failure) | Dead |

n/a, not available

*US* Ultrasonography, *HCC* Hepatocellular carcinoma, *CCC* Cholangiocellular carcinoma, *LT* Liver transplantation, *LRLT* Living-related liver transplantation, *PEIT* Percutaneous ethanol injection therapy, *RFA* Radiofrequency ablation, *TACE* Transcatheter arterial chemoembolization

[a]Survival period after Treatment

**Table 42.4** Cholangiocarcinoma developed in biliary atresia

| No. | 1 [21] | 2 [22] | 3 [12] | 4 [23] | 5 [24] | 6 [20] | 7 [25] |
|---|---|---|---|---|---|---|---|
| Publication year | 1968 | 1977 | 2014 | 2012 | 2013 | 2016 | 2019 |
| Age at hepatic tumor diagnosis | 3 years | 11 years | 13 years | 16 years | 30 years | 39 years | 62 years |
| Gender | M | F | F | F | F | M | F |
| Age at Kasai op | No Kasai op | No Kasai op | 3 months | 109 days | 105 days | 60 days | 3 months |
| Outcome of jaundice | – | – | n/a | Cleared | n.a. | Persistent | Cleared |
| Mode of diagnosis | Autopsy | Biopsy and autopsy | US CT | Incidental explanted liver | Incidental explanted liver | US | CT |
| Tumor size | n/a | 5 to 35 mm | 35 mm | 2x3 mm | 40 mm | 60 mm | n/a |
| Location | n/a | n/a | S6 | n/a | At HPE anastomosis | S1 | Porta hepatis |
| Treatment | n/a | None | LT | LT | LT | TACE(CDDP EPI MMC) gem | Chemotherapy |
| Metastasis and recurrence | n/a | No metastasis | Recurrence in the graft liver and mesenteric lymph nodes at 7 months after LT | Extensive bone metastasis 6 months after LT | Recurrence of mesenteric lymph nodes, graft liver, lung at 3 months after LT | n/a | n/a |
| Adjuvant treatments | n/a | None | None | Extensive resection of the costal metastasis. *chemotherapy radiotherapy | Chemotherapy(cisplatin and gemcitabine) for metastasis of graft liver and lung | n/a | Gemcitabine |
| Follow-up period from the diagnosis of liver tumor (years) | n/a | 1 week | 11 months | 33 months | 7 months | 8 months | 4 months |
| Outcome | Dead | Dead | Dead | Alive | Dead | Dead (hepatic failure) | Dead |

n/a, not available
*LT* Liver transplantation, *TACE* Transcatheter arterial chemoembolization
[a]Gemcitabine and oxaliplatin (GEMOX), sirolimus, and mycophenolate mofetilfor

**Table 42.5** Hepatoblastoma developed in biliary atresia

| No. | 1 [26] | 2 [27] | 3 [26] | 4 [14] |
|---|---|---|---|---|
| Publication year | 2016 | 2004 | 2016 | 2001 |
| Age at hepatic tumor diagnosis | 17 months | 32 months | 38 months | 53 months |
| Gender | M | F | M | F |
| Age at Kasai op. | 268 days | 7 weeks | 197 days | 47 days |
| Outcome of jaundice | Persistent | Decreased | Persistent | n/a |
| Mode of diagnosis | US(FNH), explanted liver | Biopsy | Incidental explanted liver | CT |
| Serum AFP level (μg/L) | 9131 | 116 | 1038 | 12,924 |
| Tumor size | 30 mm | 60 + 65 mm(at autopsy) | 12 mm | 30 + 8 mm |
| Location | S4b | S4 + 8 | S1 | S1 + 8 |
| Histologic type of hepatic tumor | Mixed mesenchymal/ epithelial | Embryonic | Fetal/embryonic | Poorly differentiated/ embryonic |
| Treatment | LRLT | Chemotherapy (cisplatin, carboplatin, doxorubicin) | LT (cadaveric) | LRLT |
| Adjuvant treatments | None | None | None | Pirarubicin and paraplatin |
| Follow-up period from the diagnosis of liver tumor (years) | 20 months | n/a | 6.8 years | 39 days |
| Outcome | Alive | Dead due to bleeding from tumor rupture(autopsy) | Alive | Alive |

n/a, not available
*FNH* Focal nodular hyperplasia, *AFP* Alpha-fetoprotein, *US* Ultrasonography, *LT* Liver transplantation, *LRLT* Living-related liver transplantation

## References


1. Okuyama K. Primary liver cell carcinoma associated with biliary cirrhosis due to congenital bile duct atresia. J Pediatr. 1965;67:89–93. https://doi.org/10.1016/s0022-3476(65)80308-0.
2. Fish JC, McCary RG. Primary cancer of the liver in childhood. Arch Surg. 1966;93(2):355–9. https://doi.org/10.1001/archsurg.1966.01330020147025.
3. Deoras MP, Dicus W. Hepatocarcinoma associated with biliary cirrhosis. A case due to congenital bile duct atresia. Arch Pathol. 1968;86(3):338–41.
4. Romano F, Stroppa P, Bravi M, Casotti V, Lucianetti A, Guizzetti M, et al. Favorable outcome of primary liver transplantation in children with cirrhosis and hepatocellular carcinoma. Pediatr Transplant. 2011;15(6):573–9. https://doi.org/10.1111/j.1399-3046.2011.01528.x.
5. Kim JM, Lee SK, Kwon CH, Joh JW, Choe YH, Park CK. Hepatocellular carcinoma in an infant with biliary atresia younger than 1 year. J Pediatr Surg. 2012;47(4):819–21. https://doi.org/10.1016/j.jpedsurg.2012.01.020.
6. Brunati A, Feruzi Z, Sokal E, Smets F, Fervaille C, Gosseye S, et al. Early occurrence of hepatocellular carcinoma in biliary atresia treated by liver transplantation. Pediatr Transplant. 2007;11(1):117–9. https://doi.org/10.1111/j.1399-3046.2006.00623.x.
7. Hadzic N, Quaglia A, Portmann B, Paramalingam S, Heaton ND, Rela M, et al. Hepatocellular carcinoma in biliary atresia: King's college hospital experience. J Pediatr. 2011;159(4):617–22. e1. https://doi.org/10.1016/j.jpeds.2011.03.004.
8. Esquivel CO, Gutierrez C, Cox KL, Garcia-Kennedy R, Berquist W, Concepcion W. Hepatocellular carcinoma and liver cell dysplasia in children with chronic liver disease. J Pediatr Surg. 1994;29(11):1465–9. https://doi.org/10.1016/0022-3468(94)90145-7.
9. Hirzel AC, Madrazo B, Rojas CP. Two rare cases of hepatocellular carcinoma after Kasai procedure for biliary atresia: a recommendation for close follow-up. Case Rep Pathol. 2015;2015:982679. https://doi.org/10.1155/2015/982679.
10. Van Wyk J, Halgrimson CG, Giles G, Lilly J, Martineau G, Starzl TE. Liver transplantation in biliary atresia with concomitant hepatoma. S Afr Med J. 1972;46(26):885–9.
11. Iida T, Zendejas IR, Kayler LK, Magliocca JF, Kim RD, Hemming AW, et al. Hepatocellular carcinoma in a 10-month-old biliary atresia child. Pediatr Transplant. 2009;13(8):1048–9. https://doi.org/10.1111/j.1399-3046.2008.01094.x.
12. Yoon HJ, Jeon TY, Yoo SY, Kim JH, Eo H, Lee SK, et al. Hepatic tumours in children with biliary atresia: single-centre experience in 13 cases and review of the literature. Clin Radiol. 2014;69(3):e113–9. https://doi.org/10.1016/j.crad.2013.10.017.
13. Kohno M, Kitatani H, Wada H, Kajimoto T, Matuno H, Tanino M, et al. Hepatocellular carcinoma complicating biliary cirrhosis caused by biliary atresia: report of a case. J Pediatr Surg. 1995;30(12):1713–6. https://doi.org/10.1016/0022-3468(95)90461-1.
14. Tatekawa Y, Asonuma K, Uemoto S, Inomata Y, Tanaka K. Liver transplantation for biliary atresia associated with malignant hepatic tumors. J Pediatr Surg. 2001;36(3):436–9. https://doi.org/10.1053/jpsu.2001.21600.
15. Superina R, Bilik R. Results of liver transplantation in children with unresectable liver tumors. J Pediatr Surg. 1996;31(6):835–9. https://doi.org/10.1016/s0022-3468(96)90147-5.
16. Tamura M, Hata Y, Sasaki F, Takahashi H, Hamada H, Uchino J, et al. A case of biliary atresia ssociated with hepatocellular carcinoma (in Japanese). Journal of the Japanese Society of Pediatric Surgeons. 1992;29(1):131–5.
17. Hol L, van den Bos IC, Hussain SM, Zondervan PE, de Man RA. Hepatocellular carcinoma complicating biliary atresia after Kasai portoenterostomy. Eur J Gastroenterol Hepatol. 2008;20(3):227–31. https://doi.org/10.1097/MEG.0b013e3282cfb716.
18. Azuhata T, Koshinaga T, Tanaka M, Ikeda T, Hagiwara N, Takekawa M, et al. Hepatocellular carcinoma complicating biliary atresia caused by HCV infection: a case report (in Japanese). Journal of the Japanese Society of Pediatric Surgeons. 2003;39(6):765–70.

19. Aggarwal S, Vadada D, Sharma V. A rare complication in an adult patient after Kasai portoenterostomy for biliary atresia. Arab J Gastroenterol. 2012;13(3):148–9. https://doi.org/10.1016/j.ajg.2012.08.010.
20. Arai Y, Kubota M, Kobayashi T, Ohyama T, Yokota N. A case of synchronous combined with intrahepaticcholangiocarcinoma and hepatocellular carcinoma 39 years after operation for biliary atresia (in Japanese). Journal of the Japanese Society of Pediatric Surgeons. 2016;52(7):1303–8.
21. Fraumeni JF Jr, Miller RW, Hill JA. Primary carcinoma of the liver in childhood: an epidemiologic study. J Natl Cancer Inst. 1968;40(5):1087–99.
22. Kulkarni PB, Beatty E Jr. Cholangiocarcinoma associated with biliary cirrhosis due to congenital biliary atresia. Am J Dis Child. 1977;131(4):442–4. https://doi.org/10.1001/archpedi.1977.02120170068013.
23. Vera A, Villaveces D, Lopez R. Orthotopic liver transplantation for biliary atresia complicated by incidental cholangiocarcinoma. J Pediatr Gastroenterol Nutr. 2012;55(3):336–7. https://doi.org/10.1097/MPG.0b013e318233ff17.
24. Fukuda A, Sakamoto S, Kanazawa H, Shigeta T, Karaki C, Hamano I, et al. Incidentally detected cholangiocarcinoma in an explanted liver with biliary atresia after Kasai operation. Pediatr Transplant. 2013;17(2):E62–6. https://doi.org/10.1111/petr.12036.
25. Nio M, Wada M, Sasaki H, Tanaka H, Hashimoto M, Nakajima Y. Correctable biliary atresia and cholangiocarcinoma: a case report of a 63-year-old patient. Surg Case Rep. 2019;5(1):185. https://doi.org/10.1186/s40792-019-0748-9.
26. Amir AZ, Sharma A, Cutz E, Avitzur Y, Shaikh F, Kamath BM, et al. Hepatoblastoma in explanted livers of patients with biliary atresia. J Pediatr Gastroenterol Nutr. 2016;63(2):188–94. https://doi.org/10.1097/MPG.0000000000001167.
27. Taat F, Bosman DK, Aronson DC. Hepatoblastoma in a girl with biliary atresia: coincidence or co-incidence. Pediatr Blood Cancer. 2004;43(5):603–5. https://doi.org/10.1002/pbc.20115.

# Transition in Biliary Atresia

# 43

Miwako Nakano

## 43.1 Adult Survivors with Biliary Atresia in Japan

Due to the advances in medical care, most pediatric surgical patients have survived into adulthood, are living a normal life, and have reached old age. Among various conditions, biliary atresia (BA) has been recognized as a disease for which many patients have survived into adulthood but have continuously required healthcare.

By the recent report from The Japanese Biliary Atresia Registry (JBAR), the 20-year and 25-year native-liver survival rates are 42.5% and 39.4%, respectively. In these 25-year survivors, 29.6% of patients have episodes of cholangitis, 20–30% developed portal hypertension, such as esophageal varices and hypersplenism, and nearly half of the patients show low serum cholinesterase levels [1]. These results and decreasing survival rate by years apparently indicate the difficulties of medical care in BA. We must continue to seek appropriate management for this condition.

## 43.2 Definition of Transition

"Transition"was defined by the Adolescent Health Society in 1933 as the "purposeful, planned process that addresses the medical, psychosocial, and educational/vocational needs of adolescents and young adults with chronic physical and medical conditions from child-centered to adult-oriented health care systems." Meanwhile, it was defined by the American Academy of Pediatrics in 2002as follows: "The goal of transition in health care for young adults with special health care needs is to maximize lifelong functioning and potential through the provision of high-quality developmentally appropriate health care services that continue uninterrupted as the individual moves from adolescence to adulthood" [2].

## 43.3 Transitional Care in Europe and US

In Europe and the United States (US), transitional care is discussed jointly in the context of childhood liver disease or pediatric-onset chronic liver disease, and reports showed positive outcomes of transition programs.

Timing of transition: According to Vajro [3], the timing is "specific for each person" but should be at age 15–20 years or at the time of completion of schooling. They also mentioned the opinion of the American Academy of Pediatrics and Family Physicians along with the American College of Physicians, who stated that the age of 18–21 years is the appropriate timing of the transition. Furthermore, Joshi et al. recommended that the introduction of the concept of transition should be started early in puberty and that according to the development of the patient, they should become more independent from their parents/caregivers [4]. Most clinics and wards prefer to carry out the patient's transition at the age 14–18 years; however, they stated that age should not only be considered when conducting the transition, but it should be carried out according to the individual circumstances and in a more flexible way, such as when symptoms have stabilized.

Transition program: The content of patient education for the promotion of independence should include an understanding of the illness, associated symptoms, and the corresponding treatments; methods of contacting the healthcare team; how to contact the healthcare team in the event of an emergency; providing explanations, keeping patients' records, and providing referral/clinic letters explaining the patient's medical history; how to make appointments for consultation and to talk with the healthcare team without

M. Nakano (✉)
Department of Pediatric Surgery, Saitama City Hospital, Saitama, Japan
e-mail: m.nakano@kap.ac.jp


M. Nio (ed.), *Introduction to Biliary Atresia*, https://doi.org/10.1007/978-981-16-2160-4_43

parents/caregivers; how to explain one's medications and to request for prescriptions; and how to ask questions according to a checklist.

According to Joshi et al., a transition team consists of a nurse coordinator, pediatric, and adult hepatologists, a social worker, and a clinical psychologist, and the use of a multidisciplinary approach is imperative [4]. Vajro et al. also stated that transition should proceed with the assistance of a joint team of pediatric and adult staff, but a coordinator (mainly a nurse) will facilitate this process [3].

Transition services: Joshi et al. stated that in a national survey of pediatric and adult transition liver services focusing on secondary and tertiary liver centers in the United Kingdom (UK) in 2017–2018, nine out of eighteen centers had a dedicated transition service and twelve were affiliated with a pediatric center. In the UK, 61% of centers had a formal transition program, while 22% had no transition strategy; during the transition period, young adult clients were reported to have adequate knowledge about their condition, patients showed better adherence to treatment, and the pediatric patient or family showed less dependence on the healthcare provider [5]. During the post-transplant period, in a national survey of adult transplant hepatologists in the US in 2015, only 16% of the centers had a formal transition program, while 32% had no transition strategy [6].

## 43.4 Transitional Care in Japan

The Japan Pediatric Society's "Working Group on Transitional Patients" defined transition as "a series of processes required to meet the needs of individuals as they grow from children into adults," and transitional care as "the transition from childhood to adult medical care appropriate for each individual for ongoing care for a chronic childhood condition." Therefore, the transition is different from a simple transfer from a pediatric clinical department to an adult clinical department [7].

This Working group made proposals about the concrete plan for transition. They suggest three ways of transition, (1) Complete transition to the adult team, (2) Patient sees both the pediatric and adult teams, (3) Patient sees the pediatric team continuously with adult healthcare model, relying on autonomous skills for personal care [8].

The Japanese Society of Pediatric Surgeons (JSPS) also established the Transition Review Committee and, in 2016, compiled the Guidebook on Adult Transition of Children with Surgical Diseases, which also addresses BA [9]. However, the medical care system, which is the basis for transition, is hardly mentioned in this guide.

The Ministry of Health, Labor, and Welfare made suggestions for the Transitional care support plan through the council for intractable diseases and requested the local government to construct the system. However, this system is in its early stages. The National Center for Child Health and Development and Tokyo Metropolitan Children's Medical center has already started the transition program with the transition team including nurse coordinators and clinics for transitional care [10]. Now, these programs are mainly for pediatric internal medicine, surgical diseases, including BA survivors have not received limited benefits so far. Several University Hospitals and General Hospitals are also preparing for building the system.

## 43.5 Transitional Care for BA

### 43.5.1 Current Status in Japan

In patients with BA, even if the Kasai procedure is successfully performed in early infancy and jaundice has resolved, the patient's liver will not completely return to normal, with varying degrees of liver fibrosis remaining. In fortunate patients, they may have an average life expectancy; however, at some point in their life, they will likely experience the sequelae and complications of liver damage. Depending on their course, liver transplantation may be indicated. The quality of life of some patients may not be extremely impaired despite the occurrence of hepatic disorders. This and other physical, social, mental, and economic issues that occur in various life stages are discussed in other chapters of the book.

Here, we will review the current status of the medical care system and transition of patients with BA who survived into adulthood in Japan.

Originally in Japan, there are no nationally concentrated hepatic centers such as those in the UK; hence, advanced hepatic disease medical treatment is possible in university or its affiliated hospitals and in many the regional hospitals. Patients have free access to any health facility; as healthcare is covered by public insurance in Japan, the patient can choose a medical facility. In theory, the pediatric surgeon can treat the patient even when they reach adulthood; if desired, the patient can visit the pediatric surgeon for consultation any time they want throughout their lifetime. However, in reality, children's hospitals usually have no adult wards for patients who require hospitalization and many facilities have restrictions on the outpatient treatment of adults.

At the time of this report, there are no transition centers for BA or other pediatric liver diseases in Japanese university hospitals and other tertiary care centers. Only a few facilities have formal transition programs or aforementioned transition strategies available in clinical practice. In Japan, pediatric surgeons continue outpatient and inpatient care in regional hospitals with adult gastroenterology or hepatology departments, even if the patients have already reached adulthood. Therefore, pediatric surgeons play a central role in the long-term management of BA after the Kasai procedure and sometimes act as coordinators while consulting and receiving assistance from gastroenterologists, hepatologists, radiologists, and psychiatrists psychotherapists if needed. In other words, pediatric surgeons themselves take on the mission as an "individualized" transition center. In instances where specialized treatments from gastroenterologists or hepatologists are required, the adult team will be in charge, and the patient may transit to the adult team thereafter.

If a liver transplantation is indicated, the patient will move from a pediatric surgery department to a facility offering liver transplants. The patient will gradually transit to the adult transplant team. Occasionally the transplant surgeon is also a pediatric surgeon, and he/she can take care of the patient continuously.

Regarding the age of transition, there are no standardized regulations in Japan it is likely that the transition will start around the age of 15as in Europe and North America, and that the transition will be completed either around the age of 20, which is the age of adulthood in Japan, or around the age of 22, when a patient has graduated from college and has become a fully-fledged member of the society. Once a young adult becomes a member of society, he/she is expected to behave like an adult who can manage themselves socially, mentally, and financially, which most of the patients manage to do so in several years.

The benefit of not transferring a patient to the adult team is that patients can be treated consistently, and adherence is maintained. For example, the transition will not be carried out automatically in adolescents or young adults who have various medical problems; instead, they are transferred to adult departments on a case-by-case basis, when there is a greater need for treatment in adult care departments, or when the patient is willing to be transferred. Some patients may visit the pediatric clinics for longer duration compared to others, regardless of their self-management skills. The period of transition remains rather ambiguous in Japan, a country with a lot of peer pressure.

### 43.5.2 Issues Discussed at the 30th Fall Symposium of the Japanese Society of Pediatric Surgeons

The author was the chairperson of the 30th Fall Symposium of the JSPS, held in 2016, and the theme of this symposium was transition. BA was also discussed as part of the 36th Symposium for the Japanese Society for Pediatric Endoscopic Surgery and Surgical Procedures within the meeting, and the current status of Japan was reported. It was confirmed that there were still inadequacies related to the recognition of the need for transfer to the adult team and for building a consistent system to support the transfer. In the symposium, the difficulties of transferring patients from children's hospitals were primarily discussed. This was due to the fact that many children's hospitals in Japan are independent organizations and have no connection with university hospitals or tertiary care centers at each region. In addition, although many university hospitals and general hospitals with pediatric surgery departments have adult teams that can provide advanced treatment, only a few patients have actually been tranferred. When transferred other pediatric surgery departments or pediatric medical specialist facilities, the patient was referred to a pediatric surgery department rather than to an adult medical department. The most concerning issue was that follow-up was discontinued in some cases; hence, the transplantation team at Kyoto University requested that BA patients who are transferred should be treated by the adult team as well as the pediatric team. The reasons for the interruption of care in the transferred hospitals are termination of care due to "good clinical course" as assessed by the physician in charge, or the patient has chosen not to undergo follow-up. In some cases, the physician was no longer working at the hospital due to career promotion, etc. Moreover, it was difficult to find a hospital or center that the patient can be referred to when an obstetrical or gynecological event occurred, or the patient was referred to another specialized center due to the occurrence of rare complications [11]. There is a lot of room for improvement to facilitate the transition process for BA patients.

### 43.5.3 Special Considerations

1. First, adult teams are less knowledgeable about BA itself, regardless of whether they are internal medicine specialists or surgeons in the gastrointestinal or hepatobiliary field. Liver disease is recognized as a national disease in Japan, and over 400,000–500,000 patients have liver cirrhosis. In Japan, 61% of the liver cirrhosis are due to viral hepatitis, with increasing number of alcoholic liver disease and non-alcoholic steatohepatitis [12]. Generally speaking, Japanese hepatologists are often preoccupied with managing a number of patients with liver disorders. In the Evidence-based Clinical Practice Guidelines for Liver Cirrhosis for Physicians in 2015 (2nd Edition), published by the Japanese Society of Gastroenterology, on September 1, 2015, and in a public health guide titled "Understanding liver disease" (published on April 1, 2020), planning and editing by The Japan Society of Hepatology: Project and

Advertising Committee, although other hereditary liver diseases that are rarer than BA have been pointed out, BA was not mentioned at all. Therefore, BA is not on the radar of adult hepatologists and gastroenterologists. In BA, the management of cholangitis is specific, in addition to the management of cirrhosis, so it takes a long time for the adult teams to understand take care of BA patients. In addition, adult teams also seem to feel uncomfortable with the intimate patient-family-physician relationship that was established from their childhood.

2. Healthcare in adults and that in children are demonstrably different. In the pediatric field, parents/caregivers receive explanations about, and consent to, the course of treatment and take responsibility for adherence to treatment. In adults, the patient/client themselves are the focus and are the ones who make the decisions and take responsibility for his or her own treatment. The same thing happens in the management of any adult illnesses that may develop. First of all, education is needed for the patients to have a clearer understanding of their illness and to encourage them to self-manage the different aspects of their physical health.
3. The transition period, which is the puberty and young adult years, is the most susceptible and delicate period for these individuals; it is the period when amidst the multitude of problems they experience, major changes are happening in their healthcare. In BA, in addition to Kasai procedure in early infancy, both patients and parents may continue to experience physical and mental burdens, which tends to enhance the interdependence of the parent and child. Problems arise when liver transplantation has to be considered. In Japan, the vast majority of liver transplants are preformed using living donors from family members. This can become an immense burden for the patient, and the dependent relationship that the patient has established with the donor can become even more complex. Hence, psychosocial support is essential to develop a patient's independence.

## 43.6 Future Perspectives

Japanese Biliary Atresia Society (JBAS) has published the Clinical Guidelines on BA and published in 2018 in order to standardize the management of BA. Strategy for transition is not included in this guideline, however, the guidelines already pointed out existing problems including comprehensive management for long-term complications, and establishment of an optimal lifelong follow-up system including transitional care. JBAS is planning to revise the guidelines every five years. The next version is expected to make recommendations for appropriate transition.

The Japanese government has designated BA as an intractable disease to support BA adult survivors socially and economically, discussed in a separate chapter of the social support system of this guidelines. Furthermore, the government is moving forward to establish a standardized transitional care system as one of the main initiatives of health and welfare policy.

At present, successful transition mainly relies on the level of awareness of each pediatric surgeon or the surgical team. It is desirable to consider providing team-based care and having a non-physician coordinator so that the patient-family-physician relationship is not too entrenched. Building transition programs and checklists to enhance the process is urgently needed and are suggested to be included in the next revision of clinical guidelines. Close collaboration with adult care departments where patients are likely to make transition should continue, both at individual patient and community levels. It would takes a long time to establish an ideal transition center which was mentioned by Taguchi mentioned [13], but technological advances may enable centralized care of each patient based on online, lifetime electronic. A national transition center for BA patients is warranted in the future.

In conclusion, establishing patient's self-management is the critical component of transition. It is the responsibility of pediatric surgeons to educate and support the long-term survivors of BA. Pediatric surgeons are required to continue to work together with patients and their caregivers to further improve patients' lives.

## References

1. Japanese Biliary Atresia Society. Results of Japanese biliary atresia registry 2018. J Jpn Pediatr Surg Soc. 2020;56:219–25.
2. American Academy of Pediatrics AAoFP. American Academy of Physicians—American Society of Internal Medicine. A consensus statement on health care transitions for young adults with special health care needs. Pediatrics. 2002;110:1304–6.
3. Vajro P, Ferrante Lenta S, et al. Management of adults with pediatric-onset chronic liver disease: Strategic issues for transitional care. Dig Liver Dis. 2014;46:295–301.
4. Joshi D, Gupta N, Deheragoda M, et al. The management of childhood liver diseases in adulthood. J Hepatol. 2017;66:631–44.
5. Joshi D, Dyson J, Hudson M, et al. Pediatric to adult liver transition services: the state of play in the UK. Clin Med. 2019;19:425–6.
6. Heldman MR, Sohn MW, Gordon EJ, et al. National survey of adult transplant hepatologists on the pediatric-to-adult care transition after liver transplantation. Liver Transpl. 2015;21:213–23.

7. Mizuguchi M. Transitional issues and pediatric society initiatives. Jpn J Pediatr. 2016;52:489–94.
8. Working group on transitional patients, Japan Pediatric Society. Proposal for transitional care of patient with pediatric-onset chronic disease. J Jpn Pediatr Soc. 2014;118:98–106.
9. Review committee for transitional care, JSPS. The guidebook on adult transition of children with pediatric-onset surgical diseases. 2016.
10. Research group for transitional care, subsidized by Scientific research projects of Ministry of Health, Labor and Welfare. Core guide on health care transition. 2020.
11. Records of 36th Japanese endoscopic surgery.
12. Liver Cancer White Paper 2015 and the 2011 Patient Survey (MHLW), the Japan Society of Hepatology.
13. Taguchi T, Maeda K, Nino M. The transition from pediatric surgery to adult medicine. Diagn Treat. 2013;101:1785–91.

# Social Support System for Biliary Atresia in Japan

44

Hiromu Tanaka and Masaki Nio

**Abstract**

Public subsidies and allowances available to patients with biliary atresia and their families in Japan include the national medical insurance system as well as independence support services, pediatric chronic specific diseases, designated intractable diseases, physical disability certificate system, disability pensions, special child-rearing allowance, and welfare allowance for disability. Each system has different purposes and subsidy standards; thus, patients with biliary atresia in various situations can take advantage of multiple such systems with a wide range of subsidies. Such a broad spectrum of support systems seems to play a major role in boosting the outcome of treatment for biliary atresia in Japan.

**Keywords**

Biliary atresia · Social support system · Insurance
Public subsidy · Allowance · Pension

## 44.1 General Information on the Social Support System in Japan

Many patients have been rescued because of the improved outcomes of Kasai portoenterostomy and liver transplantation, and the number of long-term survivors is steadily increasing. Lifelong follow-up is essential for both native-liver and post-transplant survivors, as many cases require treatment with various complications.

While a national health insurance system exists in Japan, the postoperative medical expenses for this disease, which is chronic, would impose a significant burden on the household budget of the patient's family. As the monetary liability would high, various public subsidy programs are currently available.

Biliary atresia was once regarded as a childhood disease and was covered by subsidy programs for pediatric diseases; however, patients were excluded from these support programs when they reached adulthood. With the increase in the number of patients afflicted with this disease subject to the transition from childhood to adulthood medical care, the need to reduce the burden of medical expenses for adult patients has become apparent. Since 2016, when biliary atresia was recognized as a nationally designated intractable disease (mentioned later), patients have become eligible for public subsidies for their entire lifetime.

This chapter introduces the social support system in Japan for patients with biliary atresia and their families. It includes the national medical insurance system, independence support service, pediatric chronic specific diseases, designated intractable diseases, disability certificate system, disability pensions, special child-rearing allowance, and welfare allowance for disability.

## 44.2 National Medical Insurance System

In Japan, all citizens are obligated to sign up for one of the public medical insurances, which includes occupational insurance and regional insurance. Occupational insurance comprises health insurance for general salaried workers and mutual aid associations for government workers. Regional insurance includes national health insurance that is organized for each municipality. When people receive medical care under medical insurance, the system allows them to receive treatment by paying only a part of the medical expenses. Currently, the burden for the people is 30% of the

H. Tanaka (✉)
Department of Pediatric Surgery, Showa University Northern Yokohama Hospital, Yokohama, Japan
e-mail: tanaka@ped-surg.med.tohoku.ac.jp

M. Nio
Department of Pediatric Surgery, Tohoku University Graduate School of Medicine, Sendai, Japan


M. Nio (ed.), *Introduction to Biliary Atresia*, https://doi.org/10.1007/978-981-16-2160-4_44

total medical expenses (20% before compulsory education, 20% for those aged 70 to 75 years [30% for active-income earners]), and the remaining 70–80% of medical expenses are paid by public medical insurances. In addition, when medical expenses become high due to hospitalization or surgery, a system exists (high-cost medical treatment system) that publicly supports the amount of expenses exceeding the monthly standard amount, which is determined according to the income level [1].

## 44.3 Independence Support Services

### 44.3.1 Medical Rehabilitation Service

The medical rehabilitation service is a publicly funded medical system that helps reduce the payment of medical expenses for patients over the age of 18 years. These services are provided to a patient with a physical disability certificate (mentioned later) that requires treatment such as surgery. In this system, the burden for the patient is 10% of the total medical expenses. Furthermore, in the case of low-income earners, the maximum amount of payment is set in stages from 0 to 5000 yen, depending on the income situation of the household. High-income earners are not eligible for this subsidy.

### 44.3.2 Medical Aid for Children with a Potential Disability

This is a publicly funded medical system that seeks to reduce the payment of medical expenses for patients under the age of 18. Patients who require treatment such as surgery are eligible for this subsidy. In this system, the burden for the patient is 10% of the total medical expenses. Furthermore, in the case of low-income households, the maximum monthly payment is set in stages from 0 to 10,000 yen, depending on the income situation. High-income households are not eligible for this subsidy.

## 44.4 Pediatric Chronic Specific Diseases

### 44.4.1 Requirements for Subsidy

The prerequisite conditions for availing of a subsidy under the pediatric chronic specific diseases include that the disease:

1. Is chronic and life-threatening
2. Deteriorates the quality of life for a long period; and
3. Continues to entail a high medical cost for a long period

### 44.4.2 Details of Subsidy

Children under the age of 18 who meet all of the above requirements for diseases specified by the Ministry of Health, Labor, and Welfare are eligible for this subsidy. However, those who are under the age of 20 are also eligible if they still require treatment after reaching the age of 18. As of October 2020, 762 diseases, including biliary atresia, have been designated as pediatric chronic specific diseases. Depending on the household income level, the upper limit of out-of-pocket expenses per month is divided into six levels—from 0 to 15,000 yen—and the medical expenses are reduced further for severe cases requiring high-cost medical care. In addition, food expenses during hospitalization are reduced to half.

## 44.5 Designated Intractable Diseases

### 44.5.1 Eligibility for Public Subsidy of Designated Intractable Disease

If a patient is diagnosed with a designated intractable disease showing severe symptoms/findings, the patient is eligible for the subsidy for medical expenses. As of October 2020, 333 diseases, including biliary atresia, have been designated as intractable diseases. The subsidy is divided into six levels according to the income level—from full subsidy to the monthly maximum burden of 30,000 yen for the patients. In biliary atresia, patients with severity 2 or higher, based on the following severity classification, are eligible for this subsidy.

### 44.5.2 Severity Classification

Relief: No symptoms or findings are evident due to biliary atresia, and no treatment is required.

Severity 1: Symptoms/findings caused by biliary atresia and treatment are required, but physical activity is not restricted, or nursing care is not required.

Severity 2: Symptoms/findings caused by biliary atresia that require treatment, restriction of physical activity, and nursing care, but the condition is reversible, or its progression is slow, and liver transplantation is not urgent or needed.

Severity 3: Symptoms/findings or severe sequelae caused by biliary atresia that are life-threatening or require early liver transplantation.

### 44.5.3 Severity Judgment

Severity is judged by the degree of six conditions, namely, cholestasis, cholangitis, portal hypertension, related disorders, liver dysfunction, and performance status (PS), and the

**Table 44.1** Items for severity judgment

| | Normal | Mild | Moderate | Severe |
|---|---|---|---|---|
| Cholestasis | – | 1+ | * | * |
| Cholangitis | – | 1+ | 2+ | 3+ |
| Portal hypertension | – | 1+ | 2+ | 3+ |
| Related disorder | – | 1+ | 2+ | 3+ |
| Liver dysfunction | – | 1+ | 2+ | 3+ |
| Performance status | – | 1+ | 2+ | 3+ |

degree of the most severe item is regarded as the relevant severity degree (Table 44.1).

### 44.5.4 Severity Criteria for Each Judgment Item

#### 44.5.4.1 Cholestasis

1+. Persistent jaundice

If cholestasis is present, the severity is 1 or higher. The degree of cholestasis alone is not a factor that determines the severity of 2 or higher.

#### 44.5.4.2 Cholangitis

1+. Cholangitis needs hospitalization at least once and for less than one month in a year.
2+. Cholangitis needs hospitalization for more than one month and less than six months in a year.
3+. Cholangitis needs hospitalization for more than six months in a year, or cholangitis complicated with severe sepsis.

#### 44.5.4.3 Portal Hypertension

**Esophageal/Gastric/Ectopic Varices**

1+. Varices without the risk of bleeding
2+. Varices with the risk of bleeding or controllable variceal bleeding
3+. Uncontrollable variceal bleeding

**Hepatopulmonary Syndrome**

1+. Partial Pressure of Oxygen in Arterial Blood (PaO2): 70–80 mmHg in indoor air
2+. PaO2: 50–70 mmHg in indoor air
3+. PaO2: < 50 mmHg in indoor air

**Table 44.2** Level of itchy skin

| Level | Severity | Daytime | Night |
|---|---|---|---|
| 0 | No | No | No |
| 1 | Mild 1 | Itching requiring no scratch | Itching with good sleep requiring no scratch |
| 2 | Mild 2 | Itching requiring scratch | Itching with good sleep requiring scratch |
| 3 | Moderate | Constantly itching scratch | Waking up with itching/ itching while sleeping |
| 4 | Severe | Unbearable itching | Insomnia due to itching |

**Portal Vein Pulmonary Hypertension**

1+. Mean pulmonary arterial pressure 25–35 mmHg
2+. Mean pulmonary arterial pressure >35 mmHg

**Symptoms**

1+. One or more symptoms among bleeding tendency, splenomegaly, and anemia, but no treatment is required.
2+. One or more of the symptoms among bleeding tendency, splenomegaly, and anemia that require treatment.

#### 44.5.4.4 Related Disorders

**Itchy Skin** (Table 44.2)

1+. Level 1
2+. Level 2 or 3
3+. Level 4

**Failure to Thrive**

1+. Height standard deviation (SD) score < −1.5 SD
2+. Height SD score < −2 SD
3+. Height SD score < −2.5 SD

#### 44.5.4.5 Liver Dysfunction

**Liver Function Test Results**

1+. Two or more highly abnormal values (Table 44.3)
2+. Child–Pugh score 7–9 (Table 44.4)
3+. Child–Pugh score >9 (Table 44.4)

#### 44.5.4.6 Performance Status (Table 44.5)

1+. PS 1
2+. PS 2 or 3
3+. PS 4

**Table 44.3** Highly abnormal values

| | | |
|---|---|---|
| 1 | Albumin | >2.8 g/dl |
| 2 | Bilirubin (Total) | >5.0 mg/dl |
| 3 | Aspartate aminotransferase | >200 IU/L |
| 4 | Alanine aminotransferase | >200 IU/L |
| 5 | Gamma-glutamyl transpeptidase | >200 IU/L |

**Table 44.4** Child–Pugh score

| Score | 1 | 2 | 3 |
|---|---|---|---|
| Bilirubin (Total) | <2 mg/dL | 2–3 mg/dL | >3 mg/dL |
| Albumin | >3.5 g/dL | 2.8–3.5 g/dL | <2.8 g/dL |
| Prothrombin time | >70% | 40–70% | <40% |
| Ascites | Absent | Slight | Moderate |
| Encephalopathy | No | Grade 1–2 | Grade 3–4 |

**Table 44.5** Grade of performance status

| Grade | PS |
|---|---|
| 0 | Asymptomatic (fully active, able to carry on all pre-disease activities without restriction) |
| 1 | Symptomatic but completely ambulatory (restricted in physically strenuous activity but ambulatory and able to carry out work of a light or sedentary nature. For example, light housework, office work) |
| 2 | Symptomatic, <50% in bed during the day (ambulatory and capable of all self-care but unable to carry out any work activities; up and about more than 50% of waking hours) |
| 3 | Symptomatic, >50% in bed, but not bedbound (capable of only limited self-care, confined to a bed or chair for 50% or more of waking hours) |
| 4 | Bedbound (completely disabled; unable to carry on any self-care; totally confined to a bed or chair) |

## 44.6 Physical Disability Certificate System

The physical disability certificate is issued when the patient is associated with severe physical dysfunction. Various public support services are available with this certificate, including medical subsidies, tax exemptions, transportation, and discounts on utility charges. In the case of biliary atresia, if liver dysfunction significantly disturbs daily living activities, the patient is eligible for this subsidy. The content of support varies depending on the local government.

## 44.7 Disability Pensions

### 44.7.1 Public Pension and Disability Pension

In Japan, all citizens between the ages of 20 and 60 are required to join a public pension [2], which includes the national pension and the welfare pension. The national pension covers all citizens, while the welfare pension is for those employed by organizations such as company employees to join together with the national pension. The disability pension is paid to support people's lives when those who are enrolled in the public pension become disabled due to illness or injury. Depending on the type of public pensions enrolled in, the insured person of the national pension is paid the "basic disability pension" and the insured person of the welfare pension is paid the "disability welfare pension." Given that the insured person of the welfare pension is also the insured person of the national pension automatically, if the disability grade is level 1 or 2, the disability basic pension is also paid to the insured person of the welfare pension.

### 44.7.2 Disability Grade

Level 1: A state of disability that makes daily life almost impossible without the assistance of others.

Level 2: A state of disability that makes daily life extremely difficult, which makes it impossible to earn income from labor.

Level 3: Not listed

### 44.7.3 Disability Basic Pension (National Pension)

The annual amount of disability basic pension is 975,125 yen for level 1 disability and 780,100 yen for level 2 disability. If the insured has children, a fixed amount (224,500 yen per child for up to two children and 74,800 yen per child for the third and subsequent children) is added and paid according to the number of children.

### 44.7.4 Disability Welfare Pension (Welfare Pension)

The pension amount of the disability welfare pension is calculated based on the income before the disability and the enrollment period. A sum of 1.25 times and equal to the pension amount proportional to income are paid as disability welfare pensions for the first- and second-class disabilities, respectively. If the insured has a spouse under the age of 65, 224,500 yen is additionally paid.

## 44.8 Special Child-Rearing Allowance

The national government provides this allowance to promote the welfare of children with physical and mental disabilities. This allowance is provided to parents who have children under the age of 20 years with severe disabilities at home. The amount of payment is 52,500 yen or 34,970 yen per month, depending on the severity of the disability. High-income earners are not eligible for this allowance.

## 44.9 Welfare Allowance for Disability

### 44.9.1 Welfare Allowance for Children with Disabilities

A monthly subsidy of 14,880 yen is provided to persons under the age of 20 years who are at home and have severe physical disabilities, and require constant care in their daily lives. High-income households are not eligible for this subsidy.

### 44.9.2 Special Disability Allowance

A monthly subsidy of 27,350 yen is provided to patients aged 20 years and over in the same situation as mentioned above. High-income households are not eligible for this allowance.

## 44.10 Current Role and Future Tasks of the Social Support System in Biliary Atresia in Japan

Japan has many patient support systems, and each system has different purposes and subsidy standards. The availability of multiple such systems is a great advantage because it leads to a wide range of subsidies for patients in various situations. However, the operation of each system has ample room for improvement as the procedures for receiving subsidies/allowances are complicated, and patients may not always fully understand each system. It may be necessary to simplify the procedures for each system, change the system itself to a more understandable form, and build a system to educate patients about the various support programs. According to the data from the Japanese Biliary Atresia Registry, 27% and 29% of patients were associated with esophageal varices and hypersplenism, respectively, at the 20th-year follow-up registry. The 20-year-native-liver and overall survival rates were less than 50% and less than 90%, respectively [3]. Furthermore, it is expected that cases in which the disease progresses or new symptoms appear will increase in number over time, even during adulthood [4]. Biliary atresia requires proper management throughout life, for which comprehensive and collaborative efforts by medical personnel, the government, and the community are important. One such effort is the appropriate operation and optimization of the public subsidy system.

Various social support programs for patients with biliary atresia and their families have been introduced in Japan, as described above. Although these programs for biliary atresia patients differ depending on the disease severity and the amount of household income, all patients generally to receive equally high-quality medical services at a very low cost. Therefore, it seems that these systems play a major role in boosting the short- and long-term treatment outcomes of biliary atresia in Japan.

**Acknowledgments** We would like to thank Editage (www.editage.com) for English language editing.

## References

1. Ministry of Health, Labour and Welfare. An outline of the Japanese Medical System. 2012. https://www.mhlw.go.jp/bunya/iryouhoken/iryouhoken01/dl/01_eng.pdf. Accessed 29 Sept 2020.
2. Japanese Pension Service. Japanese National Pension System. 2020. https://www.nenkin.go.jp/service/pamphlet/kaigai/kokunen-seido.files/2English.pdf. Accessed 1 Oct 2020.
3. Nio M. Japanese biliary atresia registry. Pediatr Surg Int. 2017;33:1319–25.
4. Kelay A, Davenport M. Long-term outlook in biliary atresia. Semin Pediatr Surg. 2017;26:295–300.

# The Society of the Children with Biliary Atresia and Their Families

45

Koichi Takeuchi

**Abstract**

The Society of the Children with Biliary Atresia and Their Families (SCBAF) is a membership society of patients with biliary atresia, their parents, individuals, and organizations that agree with the spirit of the society. The SCBAF works to support patients and their families. As of 2020, approximately 900 members comprise the SCBAF, which is a voluntary organization run on membership fees and donations.

**Keywords**

Biliary atresia · Family society · Early diagnosis · Liver transplantation · Social support systems

## Abbreviations

| | |
|---|---|
| APS: | Adult Patient Section |
| JBAS: | Japanese Biliary Atresia Society |
| MCHH: | Maternal and Child Health Handbook |
| MHLW: | Ministry of Health, Labour and Welfare |
| SCBAF: | Society of the Children with Biliary Atresia and Their Families |
| USBA: | Urinary Sulfated Bile Acid |

## 45.1 History of the SCBAF

The SCBAF originated through support activities by Pastor Fujiwara of The Tokyo Sugamo Church to save an 8-month-old girl with biliary atresia, who came to Japan from the United States in 1973 to undergo Kasai portoenterostomy. Unfortunately, she passed away, but after that, the founding members of SCBAF noticed that many children in Japan were suffering from biliary atresia; thus, the SCBAF was launched as a support group for the families of patients with biliary atresia. Prof. Keijiro Suruga (Juntendo University) attended the first meeting of the SCBAF and continued to support the SCBAF as an advisor. In 1974, Prof. Morio Kasai (Tohoku University) launched the Japanese Biliary Atresia Society (JBAS), an academic organization of biliary atresia that includes physicians and researchers involved in biliary atresia. With the aid of the JBAS, the SCBAF continues to offer member services to exchange information, provide advice, and make efforts to improve the health care and social security systems to improve the quality of life of patients with biliary atresia and their families.

## 45.2 Member Services of the SCBAF

### 45.2.1 Response to Consultations from Patients and Their Families

One of the major activities of the SCBAF is providing consultations to patients and their families, who often have great anxiety regarding biliary atresia and require information on this rare disease. The SCBAF provides information to members and helps them address concerns regarding childcare for children with biliary atresia. The SCBAF quickly responds to more than 50 consultation requests from members every year.

### 45.2.2 Distribution of the SCBAF Bulletin

The SCBAF has periodically issued the society bulletin, *Biliary Atresia News*, since 1973 when the SCBAF was launched (Latest issue No. 188). The bulletin provides members with information on medical care and welfare systems as well as the current status of patients and their families.

K. Takeuchi (✉)
Representative of the Society of the Children with Biliary Atresia and Their Families, Saitama, Japan
e-mail: koichi1717@jcom.home.ne.jp


M. Nio (ed.), *Introduction to Biliary Atresia*, https://doi.org/10.1007/978-981-16-2160-4_45

### 45.2.3 Activities of the Adult Patient Section

In 2001, the SCBAF launched the Adult Patient Section (APS) of the society, which consists of adult patients with biliary atresia. Initially, social gatherings were the main activities of the APS; however, but regular section meetings began in 2011. The APS can now independently try to solve disease-related problems. In 2012, the APS conducted surveys of adult patients with biliary atresia to analyze their challenges.

## 45.3 Enlightenment Activities Related to Biliary Atresia

### 45.3.1 Learning and Educational Activities

SCBAF members continue to participate in JBAS scientific meetings every year to better understand the disease. New information received from these meetings is utilized in daily advising activities.

In addition, the SCBAF has invited doctors treating biliary atresia as speakers of the annual SCBAF meetings and local branch meetings. Members can learn about biliary atresia through invited lectures and discussions with doctors.

Many member patients require liver transplantation; thus, the SCBAF holds an annual workshop for members to talk with transplant surgeons and to continue learning about transplantation medicine.

### 45.3.2 Publishing Books on Biliary Atresia

In 1986, the SCBAF contributed a portion of the donations from its 10th-anniversary fundraiser to the JBAS as an incentive to publish a book on biliary atresia for medical professionals; however, the JBAS instead proposed publishing and editing a guidebook for patients and their families. This guidebook was published under the title "Everything About Biliary Atresia." Following three revisions, the SCBAF and JBAS published "The New Edition of Everything About Biliary Atresia" in 2013. This book helps members to better understand the illness and is a tool that can enlighten Japanese society regarding biliary atresia.

## 45.4 Achievements of the SCBAF

### 45.4.1 Promotion of the Early Diagnosis of Biliary Atresia

#### 45.4.1.1 Revision of the Maternal and Child Health Handbook and the Stool Color Card

Since 1974, the SCBAF had proposed that the Ministry of Health, Labour and Welfare (MHLW) in Japan revise the Maternal and Child Health Handbook (MCHH) to include the description of infantile jaundice and pale-colored stools as symptoms of biliary atresia for the early diagnosis of this disease.

The revised MCHH in 1987 included descriptions of jaundice and pale-colored stools at the 1-month health check of the infant. Mothers carried the MCHH describing these conditions and their babies underwent 1-month health checks. However, this revision did not increase the early diagnosis of biliary atresia as expected.

In 1994, Prof. Akira Matsui (Jichi Medical University/Tsukuba University/National Center for Child Health and Development) devised a prototype and verified the usefulness of the stool color card that was the model for the cards later utilized in Taiwan and other countries. In addition, he organized the MHLW research group to further revise the stool color card and verified it in Kanagawa and Miyagi prefectures. During this time, the SCBAF requested that the MHLW and local governments use the stool color card and add pages including this card to the MCHH. In 2012, the MCHH was finally revised to include these new pages card. This was the moment when Dr. Matsui's enthusiasm and enthusiastic parents' voices reached the Japanese government.

#### 45.4.1.2 Promotion of a New Screening System Using Urinary Sulfated Bile Acid

The analysis of USBA was developed by Prof. Shigeaki Baba (Kobe University) in 1992. Prof. Yuichiro Yamashiro (Juntendo University) and Dr. Toshihiro Muraji (Kobe Children's Hospital/Ibaraki Children's Hospital) suggested Urinary Sulfated Bile Acid (USBA) as a potentially useful screening method for the early diagnosis of biliary atresia and proposed organizing the Study Group for Early Diagnosis of Biliary Atresia (SGEDBA) to study and discuss the usefulness of USBA. The first SGEDBA meeting was held in 2004. Since then, the SCBAF and SGEDBA have held the Forum for Early Diagnosis of Biliary Atresia promoting USBA across Japan. USBA is currently used in some regions in Japan as a screening modality for biliary atresia.

We plan to continue promoting activities toward the establishment of a newborn screening system, for instance, combining the stool color card and USBA analysis.

### 45.4.2 Promotion of Liver Transplantation

#### 45.4.2.1 Background on the Promotion Activities Regarding Deceased-Donor Liver Transplantation in Japan

In 1986, when liver transplantation was practically unavailable in Japan, a Japanese girl went to the United States to undergo this medical procedure. In 1987, a SCBAF member underwent the first deceased-donor liver transplantation in Australia, followed by other patients with biliary atresia.

The SCBAF raised money to save the hospital during the financial problems at the Royal Children's Hospital in Brisbane, Australia to express our gratitude for its having saved the lives of many SCBAF member patients. Many Japanese people including business leaders, professional athletes, and celebrities donated a total amount exceeding 500 million yen, which helped the hospital overcome its financial crisis.

However, with the increasing number of patients requiring liver transplantation, there were limitations to accepting patients as recipients in countries where transplantation was performed. Moreover, the high medical costs of transplantation were another serious issue for patients and their families.

In 1989, a 1-year-old boy, Yuya Sugimoto, underwent living-donor liver transplantation in Shimane Medical University; this was the first case of living-donor liver transplantation in Japan. Subsequently, living-donor liver transplantation has finally become a general medical practice in Japan.

However, living-donor transplantation has ethical problems regarding the harvest of grafts from healthy donors; thus, patients unable to find a living donor had to travel abroad and undergo transplantation or give up on survival.

To solve this problem, deceased-donor transplantation had to be implemented in Japan; however, at that time, the law to recognize brain death as a human death was not in place even in cases of transplantation.

#### 45.4.2.2 The Symposium to Enlighten on Deceased-Donor Transplantation and the Signature Movement

To achieve deceased-donor transplantation in Japan, the SCBAF held symposiums educating on deceased-donor transplantation across Japan between 1994 and 1997. Simultaneously, the SCBAF repeatedly submitted petitions to the MHLW, the National Diet, and lawmakers and strengthened efforts to legislate deceased-donor transplantation.

#### 45.4.2.3 Enactment of the Organ Transplantation Law

The transplantation promotion liaison committee was organized by groups of patients and families of patients with intractable diseases including biliary atresia to more actively promote legislature on organ transplantation law. The deceased-donor transplantation law was eventually enacted in 1997. However, organ donation required written informed consent from the donors and donors under 15 years of age were not allowed.

#### 45.4.2.4 Amendment of the Organ Transplantation Law

To enable transplantation of children, an amendment to organ transplantation law was needed to permit organ donation from pediatric donors by confirming the will of the family. Groups of patients, the families of patients with diseases requiring organ transplantation, and the Japan Society for Transplantation worked together to facilitate the amendment of the organ transplantation law, persistently appealing for the need for deceased-donor transplantation from pediatric donors. The amendment was implemented in 2009, paving the way for organ donation from deceased donors under 15 years of age.

### 45.4.3 Activities to Improve the Quality of Life of Patients and Their Families

#### 45.4.3.1 Activities to Establish a Public Support System for Medical Expenses

As biliary atresia requires long-term treatment, considerable medical expenses are borne by the families of these patients; thus, a public support system to reduce this burden was a keen issue.

The grant-in-aid program for chronic diseases in childhood became a public support system for medical expenses only for congenital metabolic disorders in 1968. This system gradually expanded to cover other diseases, and biliary atresia was certified in this system in 1983. The SCBAF continued to petition the Diet and MHLW and gathered more than 35,000 signatures supporting the petition.

The burden of medical expenses for patients' families has consequently been greatly reduced.

#### 45.4.3.2 The Legislature of the Grant-in-Aid Program for Chronic Diseases in Childhood

The grant-in-aid program for chronic diseases in childhood was an unstable system because it was an optional work of the MHLW; thus, the SCBAF worked with many groups of patients and their families to negotiate with the MHLW to amend the Child Welfare Law Child Welfare Act in 2004 to establish a stable system.

#### 45.4.3.3 Public Grant System for Adult Patients

The grant-in-aid program for chronic diseases in childhood covered pediatric patients until 20 years of age and there was previously no support system for medical expenses for adult patients with biliary atresia. Currently, disability certificate and designated intractable disease support systems cover adult patients.

The Disability Certificate was launched in 1949 to encourage and support the independence and social activities of people with physical disabilities, as defined by the Welfare Law for the Disabled. However, this system targeted only five disabilities: vision impairment, language dysfunction, central nervous dysfunction, hearing impairment, and physical disability. Organ failures such as cardiac failure, respiratory failure, and liver failure were not previously covered by this system.

The designated intractable disease support system started in 1974 in the form of intractable disease research and the reduction of the burden of medical expenses for patients. However, only eight diseases were initially covered and only one or two diseases were added annually.

While the SCBAF requested each year that the MHLW apply these systems to biliary atresia, the medical expenses of biliary atresia were not covered by either system for a long time.

However, the persistent efforts eventually paid off and in 2010, first-grade Disability Certificates were first issued to liver transplant recipients taking immunosuppressive agents. While this certificate is not issued to native-liver survivors, the burden of medical expenses is significantly improved for patients and families following liver transplantation.

With regard to designated intractable diseases, the MHLW has been considering a new intractable disease support system since 2010 to allow more patients with intractable diseases to receive coverage for medical expenses as well as welfare support. In cooperation with academic organizations and many groups of patients and families including the SCBAF, negotiations were made with the MHLW to appeal to the government to implement fair and equitable support systems for patients with intractable diseases.

A new Intractable Disease Law was legislated in May 2015 in which biliary atresia was finally approved as a designated intractable disease.

The nomination of biliary atresia as a designated intractable disease required significant documentations with objective information. Data from the Japanese Biliary Atresia Registry and scientific and clinical products (diagnostic standards, medical guidance, severity classification, etc.) played a major role in this effort. The vigorous research of the MHLW research group under the leadership of Prof. Tomoaki Taguchi (Kyushu University) and Prof. Masaki Nio (Tohoku University) greatly contributed to the nomination. The accreditation of biliary atresia as a designated intractable disease has been a great step forward in improving patient welfare.

## 45.5 Ongoing Activities of the SCBAF

### 45.5.1 Improving the Availability of the Disability Pension for Biliary Atresia Patients

Some adult patients cannot work at all due to illness. In this situation, the basic pension for disabled people is prepared. This is one of the social security systems in Japan. However, most patients are not eligible to receive this pension due to the high hurdle of payment criteria.

The SCBAF needs to survey the actual status of adult patients who cannot work to enlighten the government regarding the conditions of survivors and to seek to revise the standards for payment criteria for disability pensions.

### 45.5.2 Achieving Stable Employment for Biliary Atresia Patients

The APS is currently conducting a survey regarding the employment of patients with biliary atresia. The serious situation of the employment of patients with biliary atresia is gradually becoming apparent. Although there are employment support systems in Japan, these systems currently do not work very well.

It is necessary to eliminate social constraints and make efforts to realize a truly barrier-free society. The SCBAF is seeking a system in which companies equally accept patients with biliary atresia so that they can play an active role in the same way as do healthy people.

## 45.6 Problems in the SCBAF and Future Perspectives

Maintaining and managing an organization for a long time requires a generational change of members and executives.

However, successors responsible for the activities of the society are not increasing in number and the executives and active members are aging.

In addition, as young members are likely to think that membership fees are paid for information, there is a decreasing trend in the rate of payment of membership fees; thus, the SCBAF is encountering financial difficulties.

In this situation, the role of SCBAF remains the same and we believe that the SCBAF must continue its activities to assess what is needed and what can be done for patients and their families until biliary atresia is fully overcome.

## 45.7 Conclusions

The achievements of the SCBAF in terms of its significance and benefits to a group of patients and their families are as follows:

By supporting patients and their families and sharing information, we have maintained motivation for the treatment of diseases and brought peace of mind and hope to our members.

We have identified the problems of the welfare and health care systems of patients and families and solved them through the power of the organization.

We have contributed to the progress of treatment and welfare through cooperation with medical staff, researchers, and the government.

The significantly improved outcomes of both Kasai portoenterostomy and liver transplantation have markedly increased the number of patients reaching adulthood. We sincerely appreciate the efforts of doctors, other medical staff, and researchers involved in biliary atresia. To our regret, the cause of the disease has not yet been clarified. We ask for further efforts to investigate the cause and to develop definitive therapeutic modalities based on this etiology.

# 46 International Collaboration in Biliary Atresia

Toshiharu Matsuura, Koichiro Yoshimaru,
and Tomoaki Taguchi

**Abstract**

Pediatric liver surgery in developing countries is generally inadequately managed and many lives that can be survived in the developed countries are lost. We have initiated surgical volunteerism and operative collaboration for pediatric hepatobiliary diseases in Southeast Asian countries since 2016. We aimed to contribute to provide our routine management and techniques in Japan and organ transplant surgery to the developing countries where it is currently out of reach. We herein report our successful experiences of starting our international collaboration program in biliary atresia.

**Keywords**

Biliary atresia · Liver transplantation · International collaboration · Developing country · Southeast Asia

## 46.1 Introduction

Surgical care, especially for children, is desperately needed in developing countries. Surgical volunteerism can provide advanced surgical techniques and medical information to patients in developing countries where medical care is still inadequate.[1] In addition, collaborative operations with host surgeons in developing countries can also provide mentorship and training to supplement the base of training for host surgeons. Interest in global surgery is increasing, and many surgeons in high-income countries are interested in contributing to surgical care in developing countries, but may not be aware of ways to begin. We herein report our experiences collaborating pediatric hepatobiliary surgery and launching pediatric liver transplantation program in Southeast Asia where have never had a pediatric liver transplant.

T. Matsuura (✉) · K. Yoshimaru
Department of Pediatric Surgery, Graduate School of Medical Sciences, Kyushu University, Fukuoka, Japan
e-mail: matsuura@pedsurg.med.kyushu-u.ac.jp

T. Taguchi
Fukuoka College of Health Sciences, Fukuoka, Japan

## 46.2 Demographics of Developing Countries in Southeast Asia

The number of birth in Japan had already decreased to less than one million babies per year and the government of Japan estimates that it will continue to decrease in future to half a million babies per year in 2060. The fertility rate in Japan is 1.41 births per woman, which is far below the population replacement of 2.1. The total population of Japan has been declining since 2009. A peak population was over 128 million in 2009 and it is expected to fall below 100 million by 2058. On the other hand, according to the data of the Ministry of Labour, Immigration and Population in Myanmar, current Myanmar's population is 54.0 million and is growing at a rate of about 0.67%. The government of Myanmar estimates that Myanmar's population will increase to 65 million in 2055. The fertility rate in Myanmar is 2.13 births per woman, which is high enough for population replacement. Currently, Vietnam's population is 96.5 million people, a number expected to hit 100 million by the end of 2024. Vietnam's population is increasing by about 1% each year, adding about one million people per year. Vietnam's fertility rate in 1980 was 5 births per woman, which has decreased to 2.0 births per woman. This is the result of the government's "two-child policy" that limits births by issuing contraception. The percentage of child population under 15 years old is higher in Myanmar and Vietnam compared with Japan and the USA (26.4 and 23.2% vs 12.7 and 18.7%). Neonatal, infant, and child mortality rate is also much higher in Myanmar and Vietnam compared with Japan and the USA (Table 46.1). That indicates the level of medical care and public health for children is not fully established.

Developing countries are defined according to their Gross National Income (GNI) per capita per year. Countries with a


M. Nio (ed.), *Introduction to Biliary Atresia*, https://doi.org/10.1007/978-981-16-2160-4_46

**Table 46.1** Overview of demographics in developing and developed countries

| Demographics | | | | |
|---|---|---|---|---|
| Population (millions) | 54.0 | 96.5 | 126.3 | 328.2 |
| Child population < 15 y.o. (%) | 26.4 | 23.2 | 12.7 | 18.7 |
| Mortality rate (deaths per 1000 live births) | | | | |
| Neonate | 23.0 | 10.7 | 0.9 | 3.8 |
| Infant | 37.0 | 16.3 | 1.8 | 5.6 |
| Child | 46.4 | 20.4 | 2.5 | 6.6 |
| GDP per capita (US$) | 1408 | 2715 | 40,247 | 65,118 |
| Govt expenditure on health % GDP | 4.7 | 5.5 | 10.9 | 17.1 |
| Biliary atresia registry | No | No | Yes | Yes |
| Liver transplant registry | No | No | Yes | Yes |

This data is based on the following site: *statista.com* accessed September 2020

per capita GNI of US$ 12,235 and less are defined as developing countries. GNI per capita of Japan and the USA are US$ 45,470 and US$ 63,080, but that of Myanmar and Vietnam are US$ 5830 and US$ 6450, respectively. Government health expenditure accounted for 4.7% and 5.5% of GDP in Myanmar and Vietnam, respectively, which are much lower than that in developed countries (Table 46.1). These data represented that when compared to developed nations, it is a lot more challenging to deliver care for children with intractable diseases in developing countries. Both in Myanmar and Vietnam, there is no nationwide registries concerning biliary atresia nor liver transplantation.

## 46.3 Biliary Atresia in Southeast Asia

According to the World Health Organization, 11% of the global burden of disease is treatable by operative intervention. Biliary atresia (BA) is regarded as a disease with a high surgical burden, because BA is the most common cause of operative jaundice in newborns and of chronic end-stage liver disease in children and is the leading indicator for liver transplantation. Furthermore, the long-term outcome after Kasai procedure is limited to some extent and a transplant-free survival at 5 years even in developed countries has not improved over the last 50 years.

The incidence of BA has been reported to be higher in Asian countries compared to Western countries and according to the Japanese Biliary Atresia Registry (JBAR) it is supposed to be about 1.03-1.37: 10,000 in Japan. However, based on the previous review about the worldwide incidence of BA, there was no detailed data from both Myanmar and Vietnam. In developed countries including Japan, almost all BA patients receive surgical treatment with Kasai portoenterostomy, which is accepted worldwide as the first-line therapy for BA. However, the outcomes for BA in developing countries including Myanmar and Vietnam are poorly understood. According to the only previous report from Hanoi, Vietnam, there was a total of 287 consecutive BA patients for three years and surprisingly, 52% of them (149 patients) did not undergo a Kasai procedure even though a median age at hospital presentation of non-Kasai patients was 2.4 months which was not too late (Fig. 46.1a).[2] One- and 2-year transplant-free survival after Kasai procedure was 84% and 71%, respectively (Fig. 46.1b), which is comparable to the outcome reported from some developed countries. Despite such similar favorable outcomes, the family decision against Kasai procedure appears to be rooted in cultural or economic attitudes, as well as poor education about the benefits of Kasai procedure. The incidence, age of presentation of BA, surgery rate of Kasai procedure, and the outcomes are unknown at all in Myanmar. Of course, the screening system using stool color card is not established both in Vietnam and Myanmar. Different from Japan, because there are quite limited centers for pediatric surgery in Vietnam and Myanmar, the annual number of new BA cases per hospital is estimated around 50–60 cases, which is 10–15 times of number in Japan. In the respect of surgical skill training, this intensification of patients is considered to be advantageous.

## 46.4 Liver Transplantation Around the World

Up to two-thirds of BA patients will need to undergo liver transplantation at some stage in their lives, including children who had an initial successful Kasai operation.

According to a data by the *Global Observatory on Donation and Transplantation*, in the year 2017,[3] Croatia had the largest number of liver transplants in the world. The data states that the liver transplant rate stood at 33.57 per million population (pmp) in Croatia. That of the USA and Japan was 23.2 pmp and 3.59 pmp, respectively. In Vietnam, that was 0.09, but there was no data of Myanmar (Fig. 46.2). Japan has a cultural proscription on deceased donation, but recent changes in Japanese law have begun to change in this respect. The revised Organ Transplant Law in 2010 allows organ procurement from deceased donors. The absolute number of deceased donor liver transplantation (DDLT) remains low, approximately 50–60 cases each year or 10% of the total number of yearly liver transplants.

In developing countries without organ transplant programs, there is no way to survive for patients with organ failure other than organ transplants overseas. However, it is a sensitive issue because of the possibility of organ trafficking and transplant tourism. In the Istanbul Declaration, "trans-

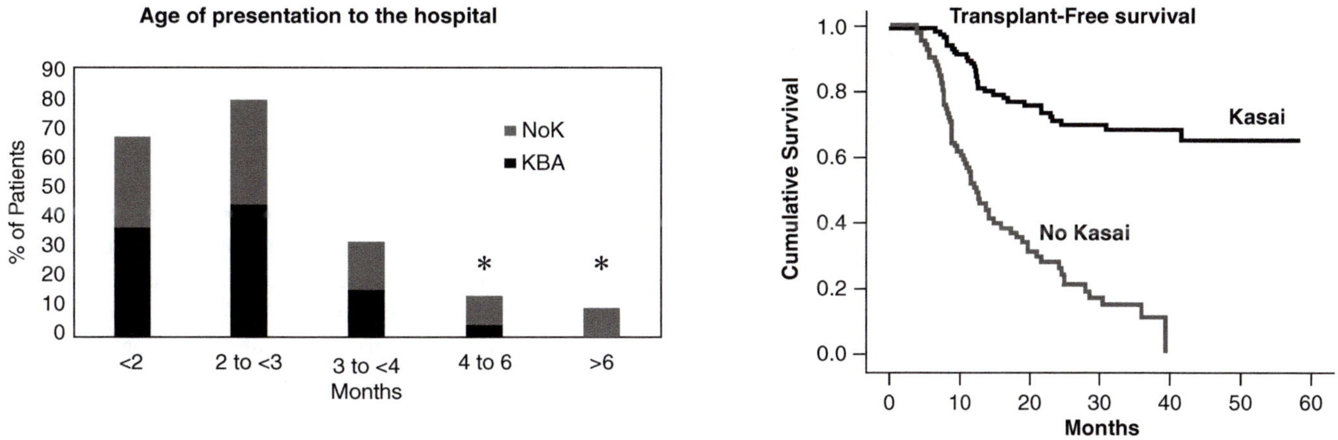


**Fig. 46.1** (**a**) Age of biliary atresia children in months at presentation to the hospital. (**b**) Kaplan–Meier survival curve by months of age for NoK and KBA. NoK: without Kasai procedure, KBA: with Kasai procedure. Both figures are cited from Ref. [2]

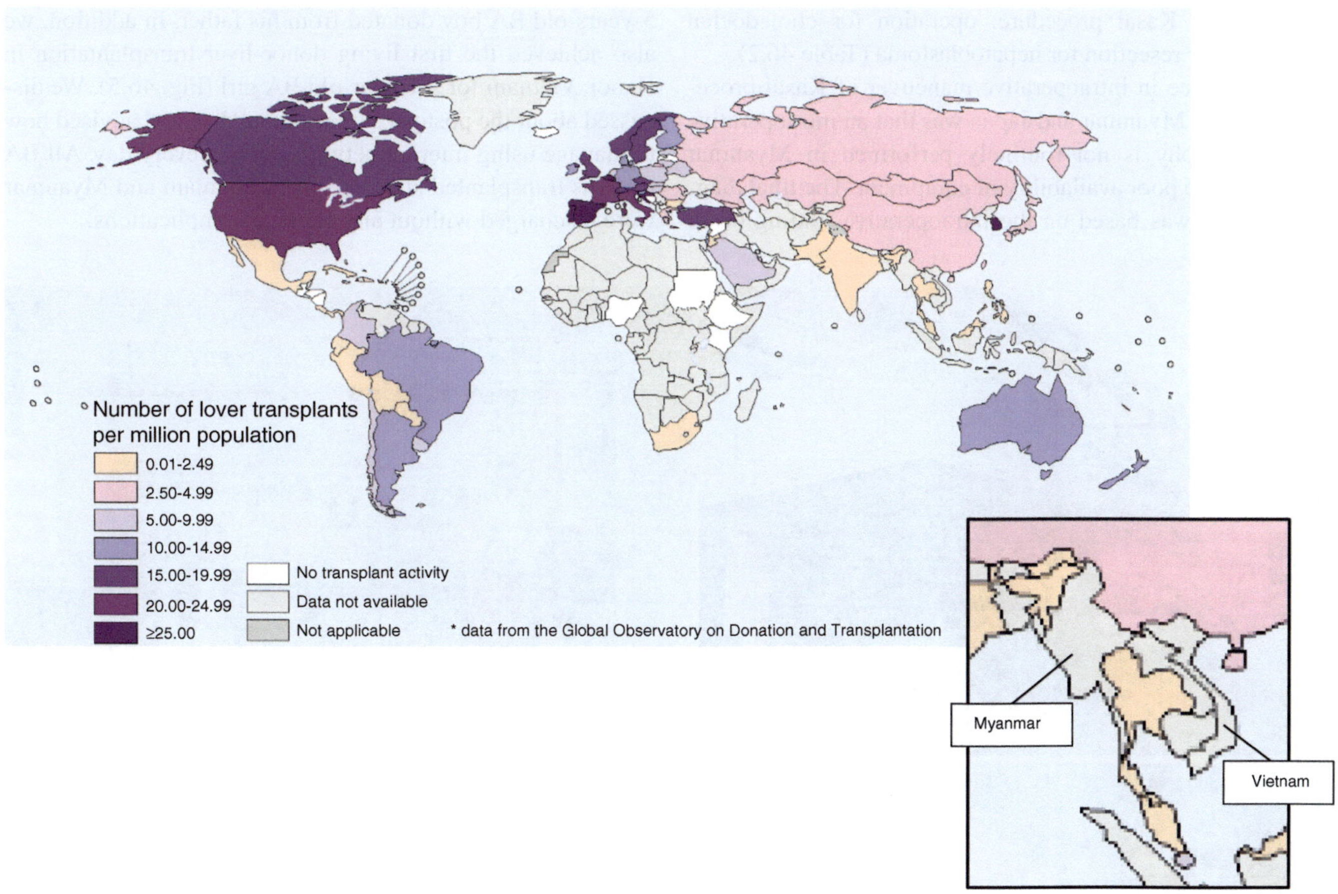


**Fig. 46.2** Number of liver transplants (per million population) around the world. There is no data both in Vietnam and in Myanmar

plant tourism" was differentiated from "travel for transplantation." Although "transplant tourism" has all the negative connotations, "travel for transplantation" was defined as the movement of organs, donors, recipients, or transplant professionals across jurisdictional borders for transplantation purposes.[4] Travel abroad for transplantation can save a child, but on return home, follow-up was less secure and many of these children fell to late complications of poor adherence and rejection or infectious complications.[5] To establish an organ transplant program in developing countries, "full-set" medical and social care for organ transplantation is indispensable.

## 46.5 Collaboration Project for Pediatric Hepatobiliary and Transplant Surgery

We have started our collaboration project for pediatric hepatobiliary surgery since 2016 in Yangon Children's Hospital (YCH), Myanmar. This project was greatly supported by International Medical Volunteers Japan Heart (Tokyo, Japan). Japan Heart was founded by Dr. Hideto Yoshioka in 2004 as a volunteer-based international health care organization. It initially began offering services in Myanmar and has since expanded into Cambodia and Laos. Their goal is to contribute to providing medical care to areas where it is currently out of reach, wherever that may be. Our volunteer team was composed of two fixed board-certified instructors of the Japanese Society of Pediatric Surgeons with some young pediatric surgeons (Fig. 46.3). Our missions have been completed eight times so far and performed a total of 45 hepatobiliary surgeries including Kasai procedure, operation for choledochal cyst, and liver resection for hepatoblastoma (Table 46.2).

A difference in intraoperative maneuver of Kasai procedure between Myanmar and Japan was that an intraoperative cholangiography is not routinely performed in Myanmar because of the poor availability of equipment. The final diagnosis of BA was based on the intraoperative finding of an atrophic gallbladder and the nodular and fibrotic appearance of the liver surface. In addition, they confirmed that they could not push a connected syringe to the cannula inserted into the atrophic gallbladder occluding the proximal and the distal side of the fibrotic bile duct structural tissue. An anatomical type of BA is not classified in Myanmar.

One of our important goals is to start and establishing pediatric liver transplantation program in Vietnam and Myanmar. For this spectacular project, we have discussed many times with all medical staffs whatever necessary to perform successful pediatric liver transplantation, including operative equipment, medicine, and pre- and post-operative care for donors and recipients. In YCH, they drastically redesigned their intensive care unit (ICU) to manage the recipients intensively. After a total of 2–3 years of preparation, we have finally achieved the first case of pediatric liver transplantation in Myanmar (Fig. 46.4). The first case was a 5-years-old BA boy donated from his father. In addition, we also achieved the first living donor liver transplantation in Hanoi, Vietnam for a 1-year-old BA girl (Fig. 46.5). We discussed about the postoperative clinical data and advised how to manage using internet network service every day. All BA patients transplanted successfully in Vietnam and Myanmar were discharged without any surgical complications.

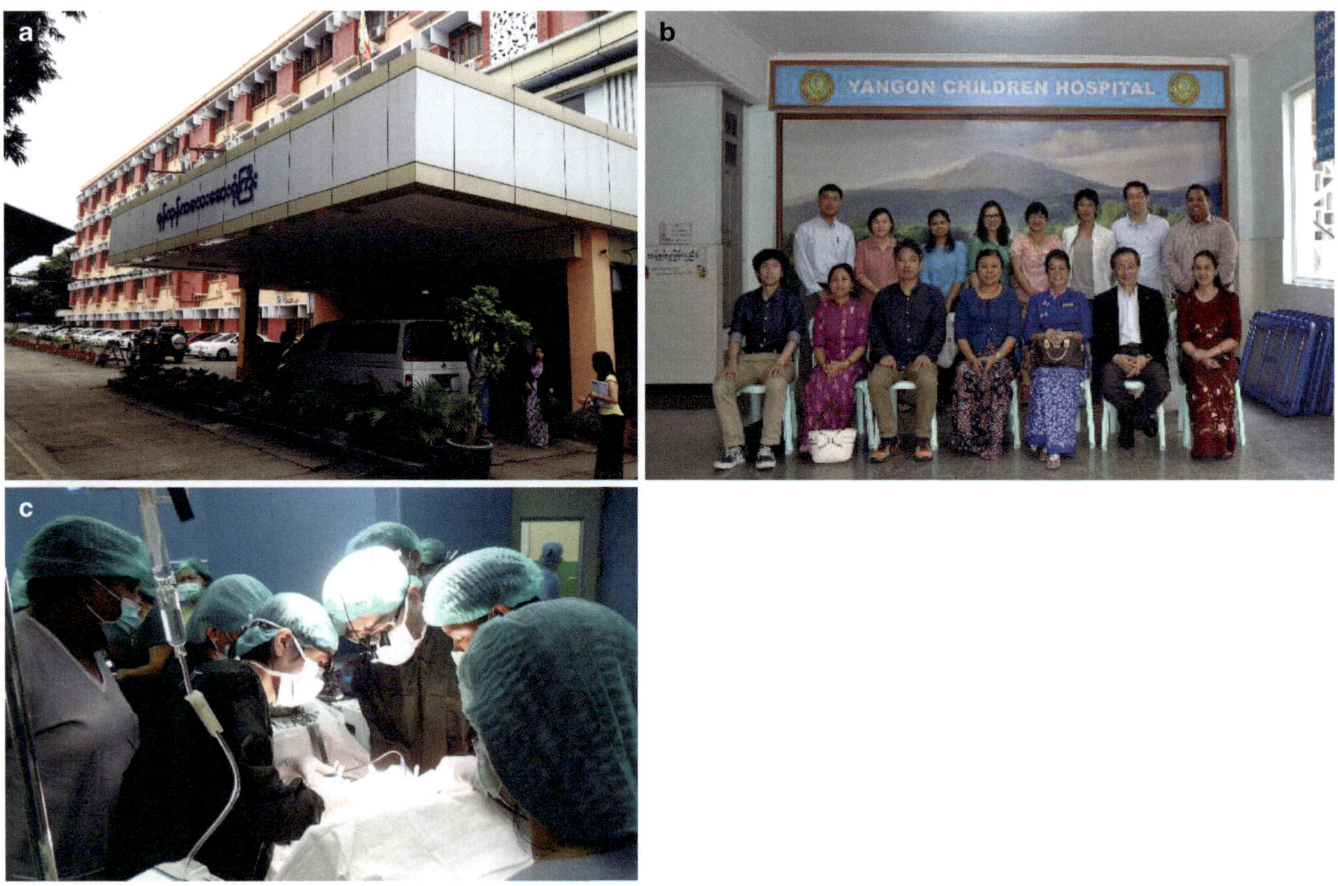


**Fig. 46.3** (**a**) Yangon Children's Hospital. (**b**) Collaboration team of YCH and Kyushu University. (**c**) Collaborative Kasai procedure for BA in YCH

**Table 46.2** Surgical case number collaborated in Myanmar

| Mission number of times | | 1 | 2 | 3 | 4 | | 5 | 6 | 7 | | 8 | Total |
|---|---|---|---|---|---|---|---|---|---|---|---|---|
| Hospital | | YCH | YCH | YCH | MCH | YCH | YCH | YCH | MCH | YCH | YCH | |
| Hepato-biliary | Biliary atresia | 3 | 4 | | 3 | | 1 | | 2 | | 1 | 14 |
| | Choledochal cyst | 6 | 5 | 2 | 3 | 1 | | | 2 | 2 | | 21 |
| | Hepatoblastoma | 1 | 1 | 2 | | 2 | | 1 | | | 1 | 8 |
| | HCC | | | | | 1 | | | | | | 1 |
| | Cholecystectomy for Cholelithiasis | 1 | | | | | | | | | | 1 |
| Total | | | | | | | | | | | | 45 |

*YCH* Yangon Children's Hospital, *MCH* Mandalay Children's Hospital

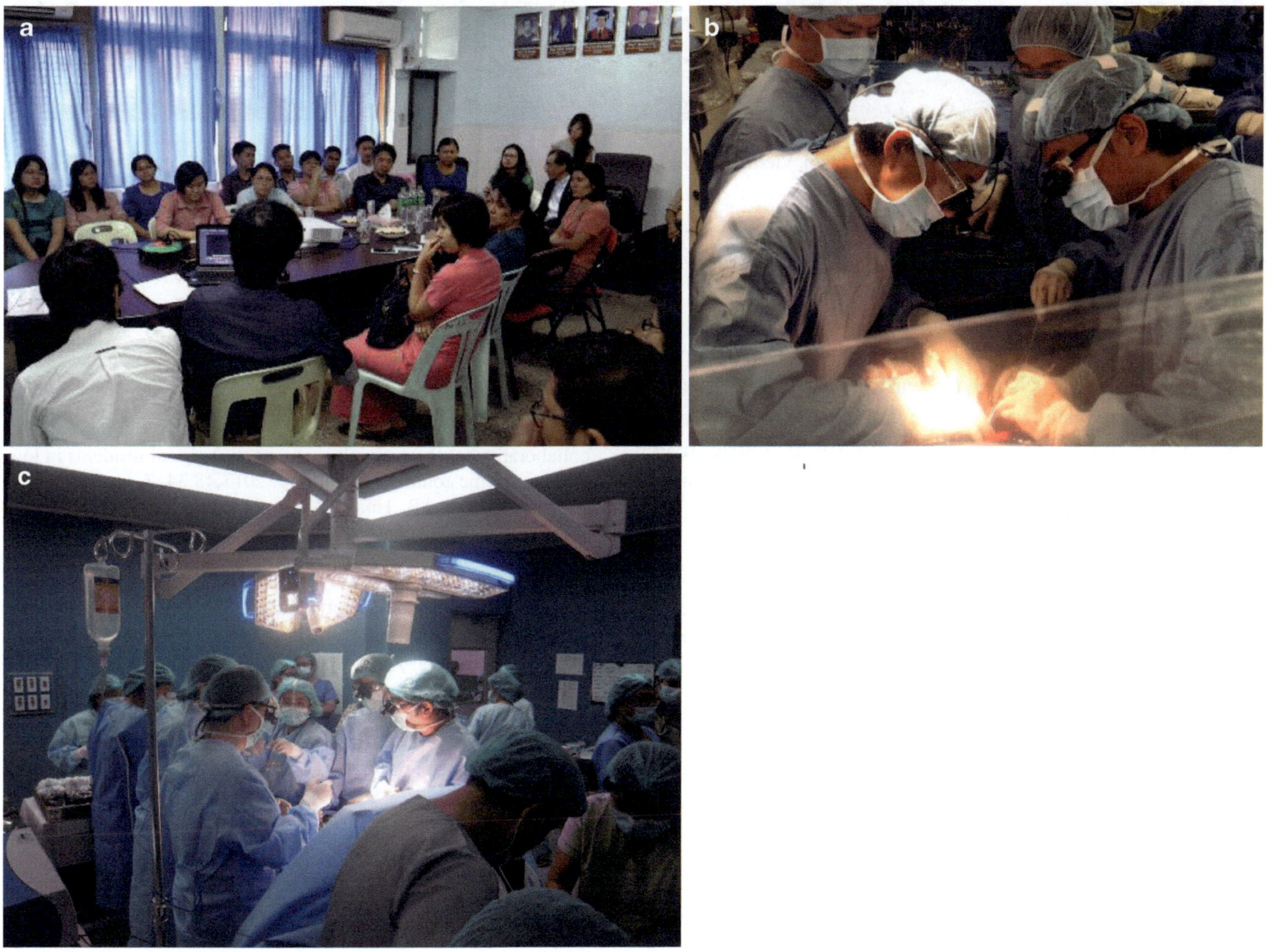

**Fig. 46.4** (**a**) Preparation meeting and lecture for starting pediatric liver transplantation in YCH. (**b**), (**c**) First successful pediatric liver transplantation for BA patient in Myanmar

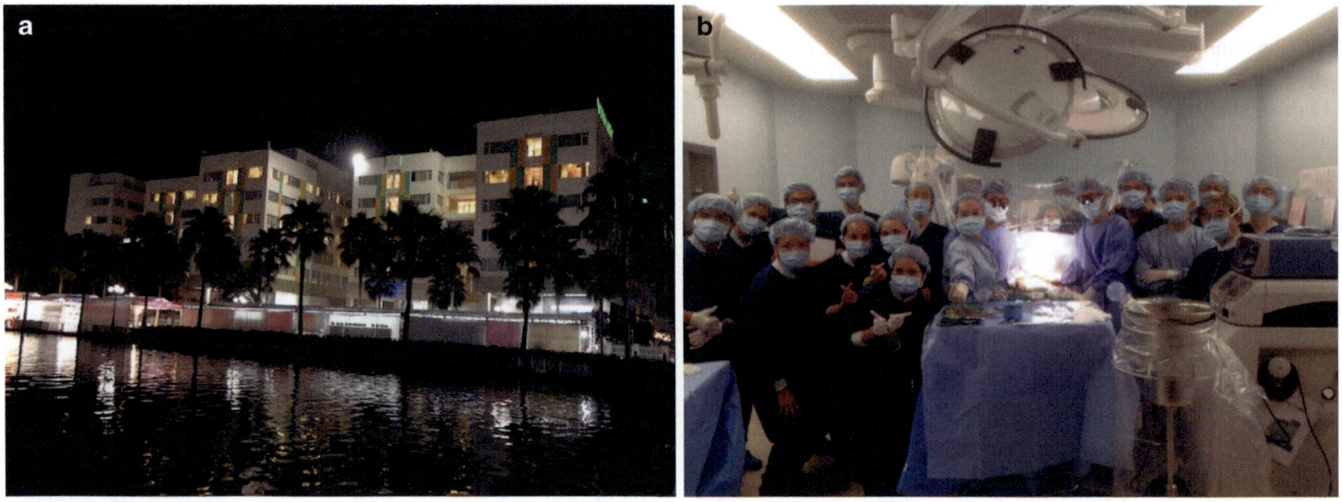


Fig. 46.5 (**a**) Vinmec International Hospital in Hanoi, Vietnam. (**b**) First successful pediatric liver transplantation for BA infant patient in Vietnam

## 46.6 Future Project

To save BA children in developing countries, we have to continue our collaboration project. We can suggest and help to establish a screening system for early detection of BA and close follow-up system and nationwide registry after Kasai operation in developing countries. As for pediatric liver transplantation, we can help the training of the transplant surgery technically and perioperative management. Because the lifelong follow-up is mandatory for long-term success after liver transplantation, the national health insurance system should give more support to the families. We have to emphasize that social activities in developing countries should focus on increasing public awareness and understanding of organ transplantation.

**Acknowledgment** This project was greatly supported by International Medical Volunteers Japan Heart (Tokyo, Japan).

## References

1. Hayton RA, Donley DK, Fekadu A, et al. Surgical volunteerism as a collaborative teaching activity can benefit surgical residents in low-middle income countries. Int J Surg. 2017;48:34–7.
2. Liu MB, Huong TB, Hoang X, et al. Biliary atresia in Vietnam: management and the burden of disease. Surgery. 2017;161:533–7.
3. WHO. Global Observatory on Donation and Transplantation. Available at: http://www.transplant-observatory.org/Pages/Data-Reports.aspx (accessed September 2020).
4. Delmonico FL. The implications of Istanbul declaration on organ trafficking and transplant tourism. Curr Opin Organ Transplant. 2009;14:116.
5. Millar AJW, Hamza AF. Liver transplantation in an African setting. Semin Pediatr Surg. 2012;21:164–71.

# Future Prospects of Biliary Atresia

# 47

Tomoaki Taguchi, Satoko Kijima, Madoka Kuroki, Ayako Ishii, Koichiro Yoshimaru, and Toshiharu Matsuura

**Abstracts**

Biliary atresia (BA) is one of the most stimulating and exciting pathological conditions for pediatric surgeons, pediatric physicians, and transplant surgeons. We, pediatric surgeons, have been covering almost all aspects of BA, including diagnosis, Kasai operation (KO), postoperative medical management, re-operation, long-term follow-up, liver transplantation (LT) (pre- and postoperational management, operative procedure), and transition to adult. From our experiences in Japan as well as in developing countries, we may propose the following issues as future prospect. (1) Screening and Early diagnosis in Developing countries, (2) Optimal timing of KO, (3) Primary LT, (4) Oral Care for BA patients, (5) Regenerative Medicine. BA will provide us lots of interesting aspects now and in the future and will contribute further development of medicine. Communication, Collaboration, and Cooperation (3C) in multidisciplinary team are important for further advance of BA.

**Keywords**

Kasai operation · Primary liver transplantation Developing country · Screening · Cost-effectiveness Oral care · Pigmentation · Dental pulp · Regenerative medicine · Mesenchymal stem cell

T. Taguchi (✉) · S. Kijima · M. Kuroki · A. Ishii
Fukuoka College of Health Sciences, Fukuoka, Japan
e-mail: taguchi@pedsurg.med.kyushu-u.ac.jp; satoko@college.fdcnet.ac.jp; madokak@college.fdcnet.ac.jp; amatsu@college.fdcnet.ac.jp

K. Yoshimaru · T. Matsuura
Department of Pediatric Surgery, Graduate School of Medical Sciences, Kyushu University, Fukuoka, Japan
e-mail: yosimaru@pedsurg.med.kyushu-u.ac.jp; matsuura@pedsurg.med.kyushu-u.ac.jp

## 47.1 Introduction

We have experienced and learned lots of interesting things from biliary atresia (BA) patients. BA is one of the most stimulating and exciting pathological conditions for pediatric surgeons, pediatric physicians, and transplant surgeons. We, pediatric surgeons, are covering almost all aspects of BA, including diagnosis, Kasai operation (KO), postoperative medical management, re-operation, long-term follow-up, liver transplantation (LT) (pre- and postoperational management, operative procedure), and transition to adult.

Currently, we have been establishing the international collaboration system with Asian developing countries (Myanmar, Cambodia, and Vietnam) for hepatobiliary surgery, including liver transplantation, and have realized that oral care is quite important in BA patients. Because, the candidate of LT in Myanmar showed that all 20 of his primary teeth were caries. Then we removed all teeth of him prior to LT. Education of oral care is very important in Japan as well as in such developing countries. Furthermore, we have been challenging the experimental regenerating medicine, using SHED (stem cells from human exfoliated dental pulp). From these exciting experiences, we may propose the following issues as future prospects.

1. Screening and Early diagnosis in Developing countries
2. Optimal timing of Kasai Operation
3. Primary Liver Transplantation
4. Oral Care for BA patients
5. Regenerative Medicine

### 47.1.1 Screening and Early Diagnosis in Developing Countries

In the current 3 years, we operated around 16 KO in Yangon and Mandalay children's hospital in Myanmar. The mean age at operation was 115.5 ± 33.3 days. Most of the cases showed severely fibrotic liver and atrophic gall bladder.



M. Nio (ed.), *Introduction to Biliary Atresia*, https://doi.org/10.1007/978-981-16-2160-4_47

Therefore, in developing countries, the establishment of simple and economical screening system and simple, definitive diagnostic tool for BA is called for. Education for parents that BA is a correctable disease is also important.

#### 47.1.1.1 Stool Color Card (SCC): Screening

Matsui developed Stool Color Card (SCC) for screening of BA. Screening with SCC has been implemented in Tochigi Prefecture, Japan, since 1994 and showed regional effectiveness in Japan [1]. The concept of SCC screening was introduced from Japan and resulted in nationwide screening with SCC for the first time in Taiwan in 2004 [2]. The sensitivity of detecting BA using stool cards before 60 days of age was 72.5% in 2004, which improved to 97.1% in 2005. The rate of the KP before 60 days of age increased from 60% in 2004 to 74.3% in 2005. The jaundice-clearance rate (<2 mg/dL) at 3 months after the Kasai operation among infants with BA in 2004–2005 was 59.5% (44 of 74), significantly higher than the historical data of 37.0% in 1976–2000 before the stool card screening program ($P = 0.002$) [2]. In 2009, a national screening pilot program for BA was started in Switzerland using a similar SCC. The Swiss SCC is available in German, French, Italian, and English [3]. Home-based screening using SCC is easy and cost-effective.

Two cost-effectiveness analyses of BA screening with SCC have been published so far. Schreiber et al. demonstrated that the increase in cost for passive screening, compared with no screening, was $213,584 and the gain in life years was 9.7 ($22,000 per life-year gained) for the Canadian population [4]. Mogul et al. developed a Markov model to simulate the natural history, and transplant-related outcomes of patients with BA in a US cohort studied for 20 years. They found that there was a >97% probability that screening with SCC would be cost-saving and associated with an increase in life-year gained in the USA [5].

Introduction of SCC at one-month health check-up may contribute to avoid late diagnosis >90 days in developing countries. Nio et al. reported the 5- and 10-year survival rates of 735 patients after the Kasai operation and found that the impact of age at operation was not significant until 90 days of life [6]. Therefore, the timing of Kasai's operation before 90 days is acceptable.

#### 47.1.1.2 GGTP: Laboratory Test

We published an effective laboratory parameter for the diagnosis of biliary atresia on 2017 in Pediatrics International [7]. We compared several clinical characteristics and preoperative imaging between BA patients and non-BA patients showing an obstructive jaundice. There were no significant differences in acholic stool, hepatobiliary scintigraphy, duodenal fluid aspiration or splenomegaly. We also compared clinical and laboratory characteristics. There were significant differences in birth weight, gestational age, and GGTP. As shown in this figure, there was a significant difference in GGTP between BA and non-BA ($P = 0.015$). Preoperative GGTP, however, was 585.3–356.1 IU/L in the BA group, which was significantly higher than the 249.1–167.6 IU/L in the non-BA group ($P = 0.015$). Furthermore, no non-BA group patients had serum GGTP >500 IU/L (Fig. 47.1). The area under the curve was 0.82 for a GGTP cut-off of 500 IU/L. Therefore, GGTP is considered as a useful parameter for the diagnosis of biliary atresia, differentiating from other cholestatic diseases.

#### 47.1.1.3 Abdominal Ultrasonography: Imaging

Another relatively easy and economical diagnostic tool is abdominal ultrasonography. Ultrasonographic findings, such as triangular cord sign and atrophic gall bladder, are useful for the diagnosis of BA (Fig. 47.2) [8–10].

We are going to propose the simple algorithm for the early diagnosis of biliary atresia in developing countries (Fig. 47.3). So far, SCC at 1month health check-up is considered simple and cost-effective for screening. And then, GGTP and ultrasonography are the second step. Education about biliary atresia is also very important for parents as well as medical professionals, including pediatricians, obstetricians, nursing staff, and general practitioners. Further research about simple, cost-effective, and accurate diagnostic systems for biliary atresia is urgently called for. This kind of system will also be beneficial for the advanced country.

### 47.1.2 Optimal Timing of Kasai Operation (KO)

Kasai et al. [11] emphasized the importance of the early operation, concluding from their 1971–1977 series that 60 days of age was the critical time for operation, and a 10-day

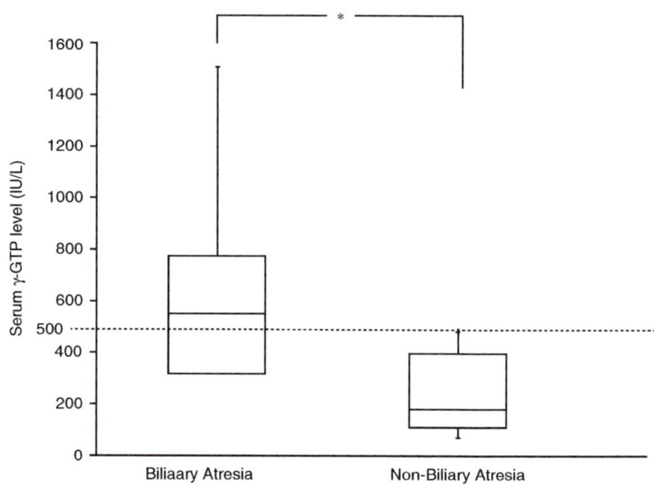


Fig. 47.1 Preoperative GGTP in the biliary atresia and non-BA group. (Modified and cited from Ref. [7])

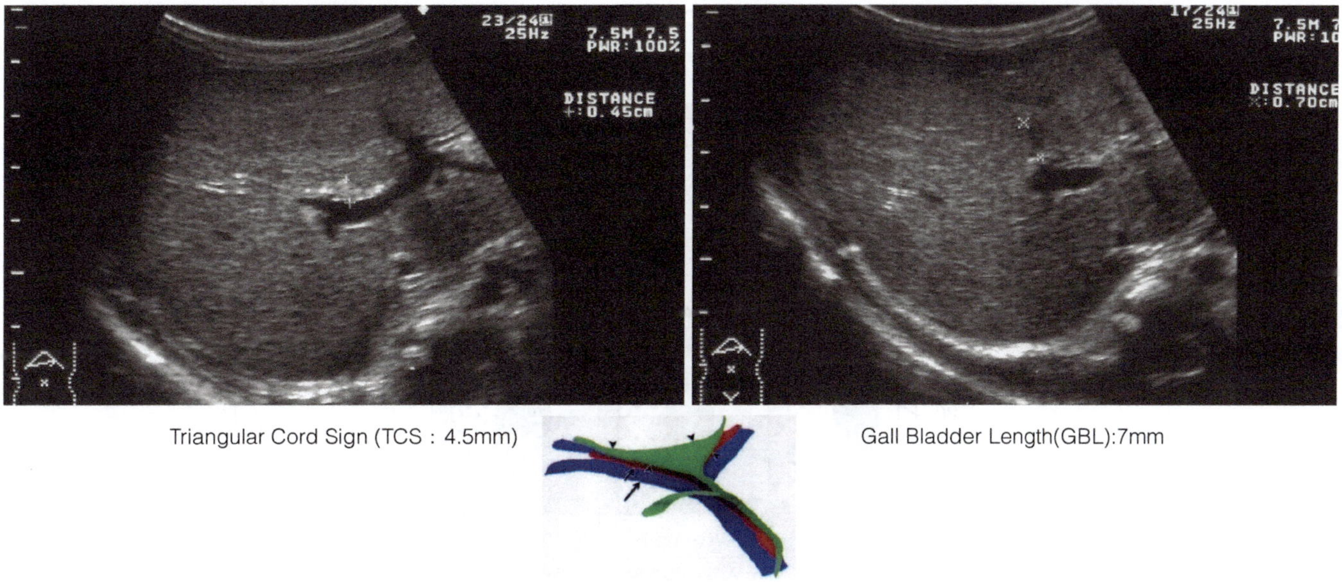


**Fig. 47.2** Abdominal Ultrasonography (33 day, girl, personal experience). Criteria for BA (Ref. [10]): TCS > 3 mm (thickness of TCS), GBL < 15 mm (length of GB) in Ref. [10]

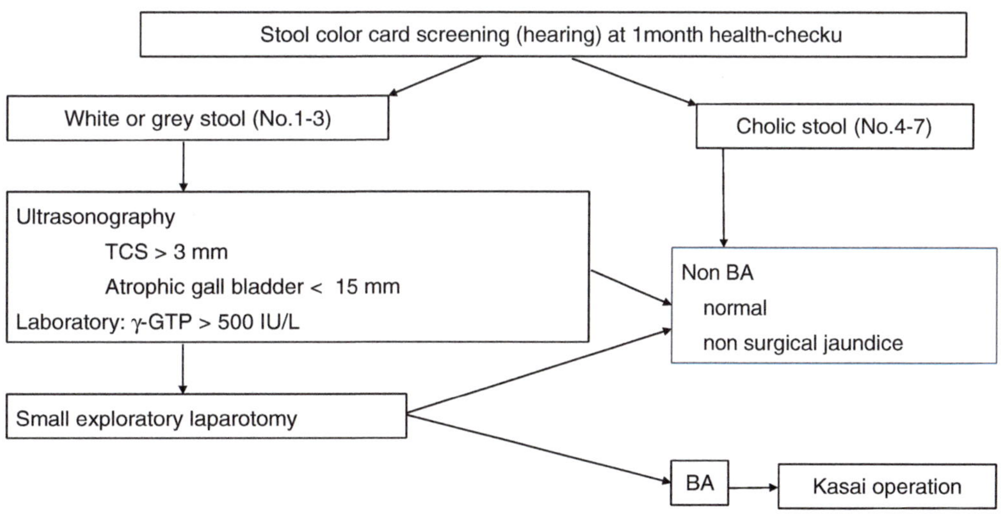


**Fig. 47.3** Proposal of simple algorithm for early diagnosis of biliary atresia in developing countries

delay resulted in a decrease in success rate by half. Mieli-Vergani et al. [12] reported good bile flow in 86% of infants treated by KO before 8 weeks of age, compared with 36% in older infants. The rally for early surgery for BA continued into the 1990s [13]. Subsequently, Altman et al. [14] concluded from their multivariate analysis that operation on or before 49 days could achieve the best result, whereas operation beyond 70 days led to the highest failure rate. This was substantiated by a recent review by the Swiss National Study, concluding that operation after 75 days was associated with a success rate of 11.3% [15]. Serinet et al. reported that earlier KO did impact the better outcome in the native liver survival rates [16].

Nonetheless, some recent studies have questioned the conventional wisdom of early surgery. Nio et al. reported the 5- and 10-year survival rates of 735 patients after the Kasai operation and found that the impact of age at operation was not significant until 90 days of life [6]. Davenport et al. [17] reported that looking at the degree of liver fibrosis and cirrhosis, there was no difference histologically between patients who had surgery before 60 days and those between 61 and 80 days, with little or no progression to cirrhosis until at least beyond 100 days of life.

Wong et al. reported that the best postoperative outcome was found in the patients who underwent KO between 61 and 80 days after birth (Fig. 47.4) [18]. These patients also had the lowest mean postoperative bilirubin level. Therefore, they suggest that the optimal age for performing the KO should be between 61 and 80 days. They postulate that 1 possible reason may be attributable to a better portal anat-

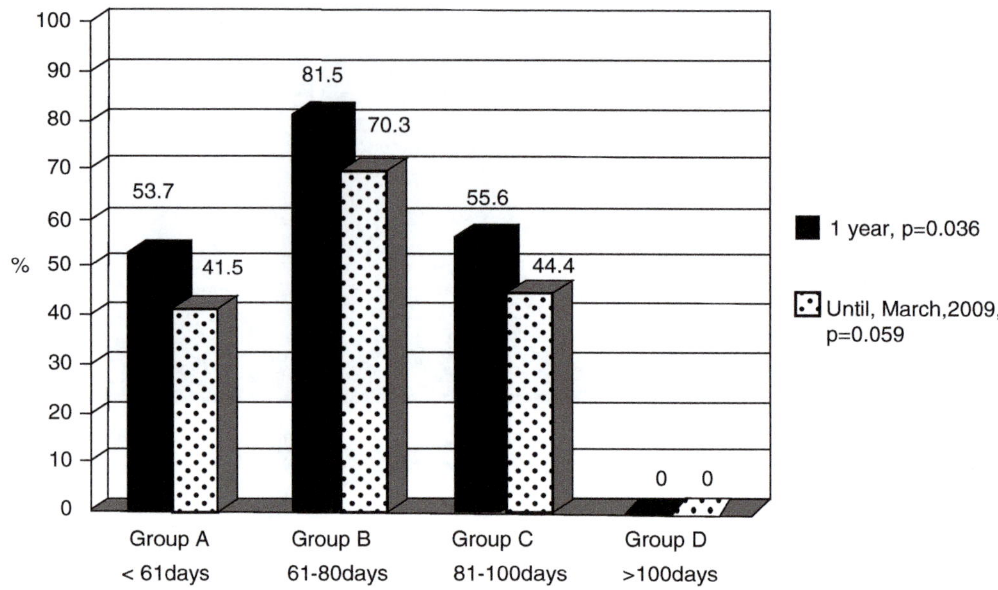


**Fig. 47.4** The percentage of patients in each group (classified by age at Kasai operation) who had survived native livers at 1 year after the operation and at the end of follow-up (March 2009) (cited from Ref. [18]). Group A < 61 days, Group B 61–80 days, Group C 81–100 days, Group D > 100 days

omy with the formation of a fibrous cord for dissection in this age group. This would also allow better anastomosis of the portoenterostomy, resulting, in theory, in better bile drainage.

Current review from Japan showed an early KO, when performed before 30 days of age, significantly improves the native liver survival rate [19]. Nowadays, according to the recent Japanese Biliary Atresia Registry, about 40% of BA patients were operated on at <60 days of age. Now we may be able to re-evaluate the optimal timing of Kasai's operation.

### 47.1.3 Primary Liver Transplantation

Primary transplantation is rarely done despite the excellent outcome. Deaths on the waiting list also have improved with the routine use of split and live donor transplantation. The Kasai operation has the highest failure rate in its stated objective than any other operation in pediatric surgery. Failure to achieve any improvement in jaundice occurs in over 30% of all cases, even in the best of hands, and transplantation or listing for transplantation occurs in over half the children with type II and III BA by one year of age in countries where liver transplantation is readily available.

In Japan, where KO originated, KO is the preferred procedure and is performed more often than in Western countries. In fact, the outcome of KO tends to be good in terms of native liver survival [20, 21]. Limited access to deceased donor liver transplantation (LT) was another reason for the priority of KO in Japan, where living-donor LT (LDLT) accounts for more than 95% of all LTs. In Japan Biliary Atresia Registry, of 2895 patients registered (1989–2013), primary LT ($n$ = 15) or exploratory laparotomy (EL) followed by LT ($n$ = 9) without KP was performed in 24 cases (0.8%). The main reason for primary LT was late diagnosis, and for EL followed by LT, lack of fibrous tissue at the porta hepatis (o-type). The prognoses of LT without KO were good [22]. Intraoperative diagnosis of o-type is sometimes difficult, because the very thin hilar structure of the patients with Alagille syndrome shows a similar appearance of o-type biliary atresia. Intraoperative real-time evaluation of biliary flow using near-infrared fluorescent cholangiography with Indocyanine green (ICG) fluorescent examination will be helpful for a definitive diagnosis of o-type [23]. Liver stiffness measurement using Fibroscan can be used to assess the grade of liver cirrhosis and predict the difficulty in dissecting fibrous portal plate be helpful for preoperative diagnosis for liver cirrhosis. If the patient shows liver cirrhosis and difficulty of Kasai operation, primary liver transplantation is recommended [24].

According to the etiological homogeneity, patients who belong to developmental BA, including biliary atresia splenic malformation (syndromic BA) and cystic BA [25], may be of a different category from the majority with isolated BA and have a different prognosis [6, 17]. Syndromic BA showed very poor outcomes by native liver, therefore, this category is considered as a candidate for primary liver transplantation. Cystic BA with hilar cyst showed a favorable outcome by cyst-jejunostomy [25].

Wong KKY reported that Regarding patients who underwent the operation beyond 100 days, we believe that by that time, irreversible liver damage has already occurred. It would be better, therefore, to refer these patients directly for LT without attempting the Kasai operation [18].

LeeVan E et al. compared the survival of patients with BA initially treated with KO with patients who underwent primary LT in 1252 patients with biliary atresia in California

[26]. Although patients who underwent primary LT had a higher mortality rate within the first 3 months after the procedure, they had a reduced risk of long-term mortality compared with patients initially managed with Kasai operation. Patients requiring salvage liver transplants had a substantially higher risk of mortality than patients who received primary liver transplantation. They concluded that patients who underwent primary liver transplantation experienced superior long-term survival compared with patients who underwent Kasai operation.

However, meta-analysis, including 1560 patients out of 14 studies, did not reveal significant differences in either patient survival rate or graft survival rate over a 5-year follow-up between BA patients with and without a portoenterostomy procedure prior to liver transplantation: patients who received a prior portoenterostomy procedure had a higher risk of postoperative infection [27].

Ng et al. demonstrated that patients with BA surviving with native livers after the Kasai operation were at increased risk for neurodevelopmental delays (ND) at 12 and 24 months of age. Those with unsuccessful Kasai operations were over four times more likely to have neurodevelopmental impairment compared with those with successful Kasai operations. Therefore, early liver transplantation is recommended. Infancy and early childhood is a time of critical brain development, and an important period for ND surveillance, especially in children with chronic illnesses. Infants diagnosed with BA are potentially more vulnerable given the absence of alternative treatments and the need for timely surgical intervention (KO) requiring prolonged general anesthesia (GA) within the first month of life [28]. However, a recent study examining 336 infants found few significant effects of GA in the first year of life on ND outcomes compared with controls [29]. Additionally, interim results from two long-term studies—one a randomized trial comparing

GA with regional anesthesia [30], and another looking at sibling pairs [31]—noted no significant effect of GA on ND outcomes using standardized testing after a single GA exposure. Given the essential role of GA for surgical procedures (like the HPE) to be performed safely in infants, concern for GA on the developing brain should not result in a delay in the timely completion of the KO, as it is likely that the ND issues are related to the primary conditions and comorbidities, and not to the use of GA [30, 31]. Therefore, we should choose a single GA exposure, KO, or primary liver transplantation, during the infant period. If the success rate of KO is not high, primary liver transplantation should be selected.

In the future, it is postulated that a prospective trial in children predicted to have a poor prognosis after KO based on age at KO, anatomic pattern, liver histology, and presence of associated anomalies would yield improved care, spare some infants needless surgery, and quite possibly result in diminished morbidity and mortality following a liver transplant. Even though it is a very limited possibility, a consensus must be reached regarding the criteria for the selection of a primary LT other than KO as the initial procedure for BA.

### 47.1.4 Oral Care for BA Patients

The patients with BA show poor absorptions of fat-absorbable Vitamins, including Vitamin D, and influence the development of teeth. Therefore, in general, the patients with BA have fragile teeth and dental caries. Previously, before the liver transplantation era, about half of the patients became endstage liver disease and showed (1) gross caries of most primary teeth, (2) pigmentation of remnant teeth, (3) severe generalized gingival hyperplasia and edema [32]. For survivors with native liver, including candidates of liver transplantation, oral care is quite important. Caries and periodontal infection should be controlled, because bacteria in oral cavity may cause systemic infection and sepsis. Especially, candidates of liver transplantation should be completely free from infection, because immunosuppressive agents are administered after transplantation. In order to avoid gross caries, regular check-up of teeth and oral cavity and education of oral care by the professional special team for oral care, composed of dentist, dental hygienist, dietitian, pharmacist, nurse, and pediatric surgeon or gastroenterologist.

LT in younger age has overcome the developmental problem of teeth. Yamaza H, et al. showed that bilirubin-induced impairments in odontogenic stem cells were reversible when bilirubin stimulation is interrupted after liver transplantation [33]. However, after transplantation, the same professional team is also required to continue regular check-up of oral care and appropriate education. Oral infection is one of the focuses of bacterial infection under immunosuppression.

There are several reports about adolescent patients who underwent liver transplantation as children. They are suffering from some problems, such as green teeth, gingival enlargement, and chronic sinusitis with calcification [34] in adolescents. Green teeth continiues long period after liver transplantation, and gingival hyperplasia and vesiculobullous lesions are found due to adverse effects of cyclosporin. Abscess, periodontal inflammation, and Herpes infection are sometimes encountered [35]. Conversion of cyclosporin to tacrolimus, nonsurgical as well as surgical treatment for the mandible, and mask by composite restorations for green coloration are choices of treatment (Fig. 47.5) [36].

The establishment of oral care program including education for patient and parents by special team is called for after Kasai operation as well as after liver transplantation to achieve a good quality of life in patients with biliary atresia.

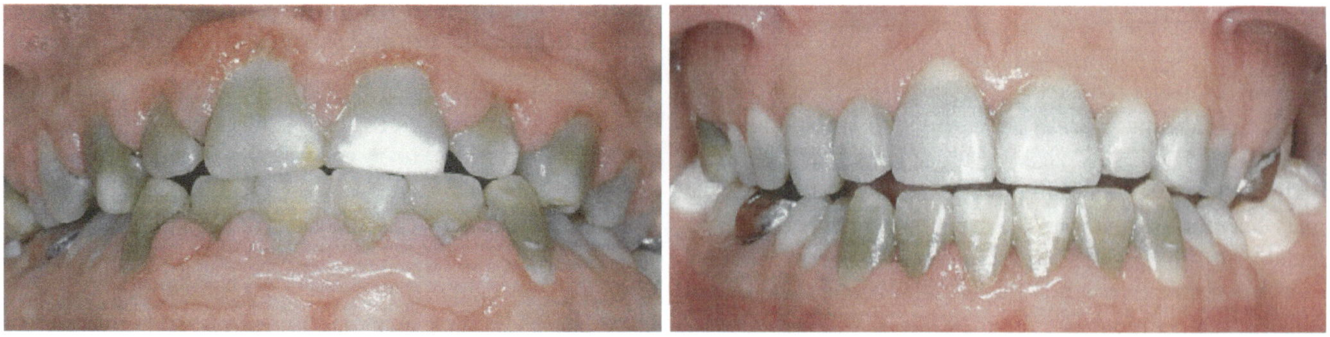

Fig. 47.5 Effect of conservative and surgical treatment for adolescent BA patients (cited from Ref. [16]). Left: Before treatment. Green teeth and gingival enlargement are evident. Right: After restorative and periodontal treatment (conservative and surgical)

### 47.1.5 Regenerative Medicine

BA achieved a dramatical improvement of survival rate by living-donor liver transplantation. However, the shortage of cadaveric donors and several long-term complications after transplantation are problems resolved. Living-donor liver transplantation should be avoided in the future, to stop the surgical procedures of healthy donor. BA has been designated as an official intractable disease and the medical cost is almost covered completely by the Japanese government. Thus, there is an urgent need for the development of new radical therapy instead of living-donor liver transplantation.

#### 47.1.5.1 Stem Cells from Human Exfoliated Deciduous Teeth (SHED)

Mesenchymal stem cells (MSCs) exhibit self-renewal and multipotency into a variety of mature cells and have been identified in a variety of human tissues, including bone marrow, adipose tissue, umbilical cord blood, amniotic fluid, and dental pulp tissue. Recent studies also evaluate the immunomodulatory effects of MSCs. MSCs are therefore considered a feasible cell source for tissue engineering and regenerative medicine.

SHED have been discovered in remnant dental pulp tissues of human exfoliated deciduous teeth and share MSCs characteristics, including fibroblastic features, clonogenicity, cell surface antigen expression, cell proliferative capacity, and multi-differentiation potency [37]. SHED also modulate regulatory T cells (Tregs), and dendritic cells, moreover, SHED showed a significant inhibiting effect in reducing interleukin-17 levels when compared to bone marrow mesenchymal stem cells [38].

#### 47.1.5.2 Hepatocyte Transplantation

There have been several reports about mature hepatocyte transplantation in clinical trials [39]. However, the effect of mature hepatocyte transplantation continued in 3 months and only worked as a bridge to liver transplantation. Due to their potential to differentiate into a variety of mature cells, stem cells are considered feasible cell sources for liver regeneration. SHED exhibit hepatogenic capability in vitro.

There is accumulating evidence that a variety of human MSCs is capable of differentiating into hepatocyte-like cells in vivo in animal models of hepatic failure. Advanced tissue engineering techniques accelerate a trans-differentiation ability of human MSCs into hepatocytes. In comparison with other human tissues, exfoliated deciduous teeth offer significant advantages of less ethical controversies and readily accessible source, easy and minimally invasive collection, and retain high stem cell potentials such as cell proliferation, multipotency, and immunomodulatory functions [40], even after cryopreservation (Fig. 47.6) [41].

We investigated in vivo capabilities of homing and hepatocyte differentiation and therapeutic efficacy for liver disorders in carbon tetrachloride ($CCl_4$)-induced liver fibrosis model mice [42]. We transplanted SHED into CCl4-induced liver fibrosis model mice through the spleen and analyzed the in vivo homing and therapeutic effects by optical, biochemical, histological, immunological, and molecular biological assays (Fig. 47.7). We then sorted human leukocyte antigen-ABC (HLA-ABC)-positive cells from primary CCl4-damaged recipient livers and analyzed their fusogenicity and hepatic characteristics by flow cytometric, genomic DNA, hepatocyte-specific gene assays. Furthermore, we examined the treatment effects of HLA-positive cells to a hepatic dysfunction by a secondary transplantation into $CCl_4$-treated mice [42].

Transplanted SHED homed to recipient's livers and expressed HLA-ABC, human hepatocyte-specific antigen hepatocyte paraffin 1 and human albumin. SHED transplantation markedly recovered liver dysfunction and led to antifibrotic and anti-inflammatory effects in the recipient's livers. SHED-derived HLA-ABC-positive cells that were sorted from the primary recipient liver tissues with CCl4 damage did not fuse with the host mouse liver cells. Sorted HLA-positive cells not only expressed human hepatocyte-specific genes including albumin, cytochrome P450 1A1, fumarylacetoacetase, tyrosine aminotransferase, uridine

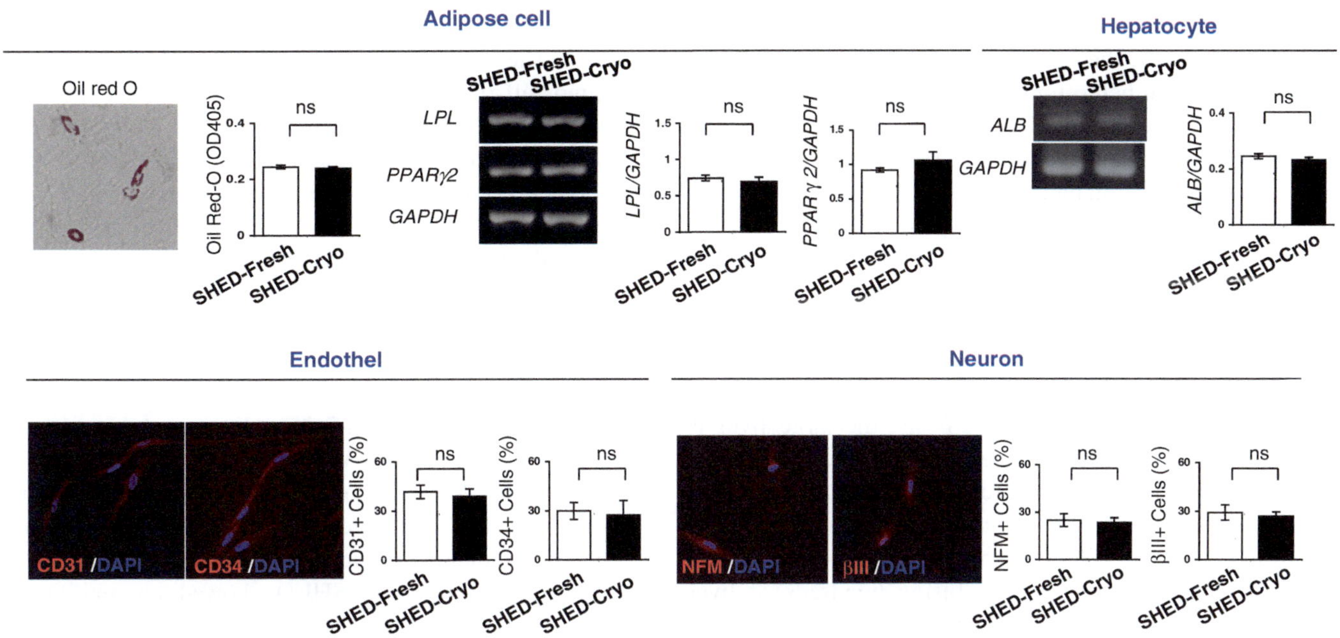


**Fig. 47.6** Pulripotentiality of SHED after 2 years frozen preservation. (Modified from Ref. [40])

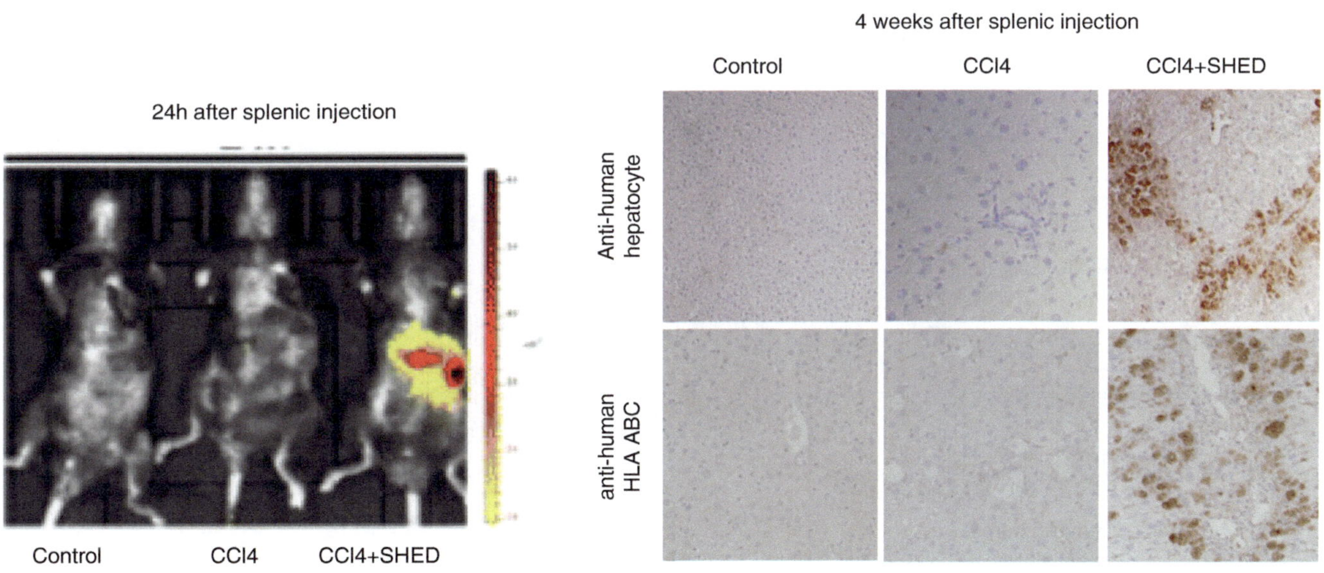


**Fig. 47.7** The liver-homing capacity of SHED after splenic injection. (Modified from Ref. [42])

5′-diphospho-glucuronosyltransferase, transferrin, and transthyretin but also secreted human albumin, urea, and blood urea nitrogen. Furthermore, SHED-derived HLA-ABC-positive cells were secondary transplanted into CCl4-treated mice. The donor cells were homed into secondary recipient livers and expressed hepatocyte paraffin 1 and human albumin, as well as HLA-ABC. The secondary transplantation recovered a liver dysfunction in secondary recipients [42].

This study indicates that transplanted SHED improved hepatic dysfunction and directly transform into hepatocytes without cell fusion in CCl4-treated mice, suggesting that SHED may provide a feasible cell source for liver regeneration.

#### 47.1.5.3 Creation of Mini Liver

Cell-based therapy has been proposed as an alternative to orthotopic liver transplantation. The novel transplantation of an in vitro-generated liver bud might have therapeutic potential. In vivo and ex vivo methods for growing a liver bud are essential for paving the way for the clinical translation of liver bud transplantation. Takebe et al. co-cultured liver-like cells derived from iPS, endothelial cells, and MSC. As a result, they created "Liver bud" and successfully transplanted heterotopically [43]. Sakai et al. created "Liver sheet" composed of hepatocyte and fibroblast and successfully transplanted subcutaneously [44]. We reported a novel transplantation method for liver buds that are grown in vivo involving orthotopic transplantation on the transected parenchyma of the liver, which showed long engraftment and marked growth in comparison to heterotopic transplantation [45].

#### 47.1.5.4 Creation of Large Liver

For radical treatment of liver cirrhosis, the large liver is necessary. At least 40% of the standard liver volume is required. One method is the creation of the decellularized liver scaffold. And this scaffold is recellularized by iPS cells [46]. We are developing a method for rapidly fabricating scalable liver-like tissue by fusing hundreds of liver bud-like spheroids using a 3D bioprinter (Fig. 47.8). Its system to fix the shape of the 3D tissue with the needle-array system enabled the fabrication of elaborate geometry and the immediate execution of culture circulation after 3D printing—thereby avoiding an ischemic environment ex vivo. The ex vivo fabricated human liver-like tissue exhibited self-tissue organization, which showed endothelial network and biliary duct formation (Fig. 47.9), and also exhibited engraftment on the liver of nude rats. These achievements conclusively show both in vivo and ex vivo methods for growing in vitro-generated liver buds [45]. These methods provide a new approach for in vitro-generated liver organoids transplantation. The creation of scaffold-free 3D organ will be able to be achieved by this unique technique (Fig. 47.10) [47].

#### 47.1.5.5 Summary and Future Prospects of Regenerative Medicine

SHEDs are an ideal cell source for regenerative medicine with minimal risk of oncogenesis, high proliferative capacity, high multipotency, and immunosuppressive ability. Stem cell transplantation using SHED showed an antifibrotic effect in liver fibrosis in mice. Liver and diaphragm were able to be created using Bio 3D printer in scaffold-free manner. SHED transplantation and Bio 3D printer will provide us new innovative treatment modality for intractable pediatric

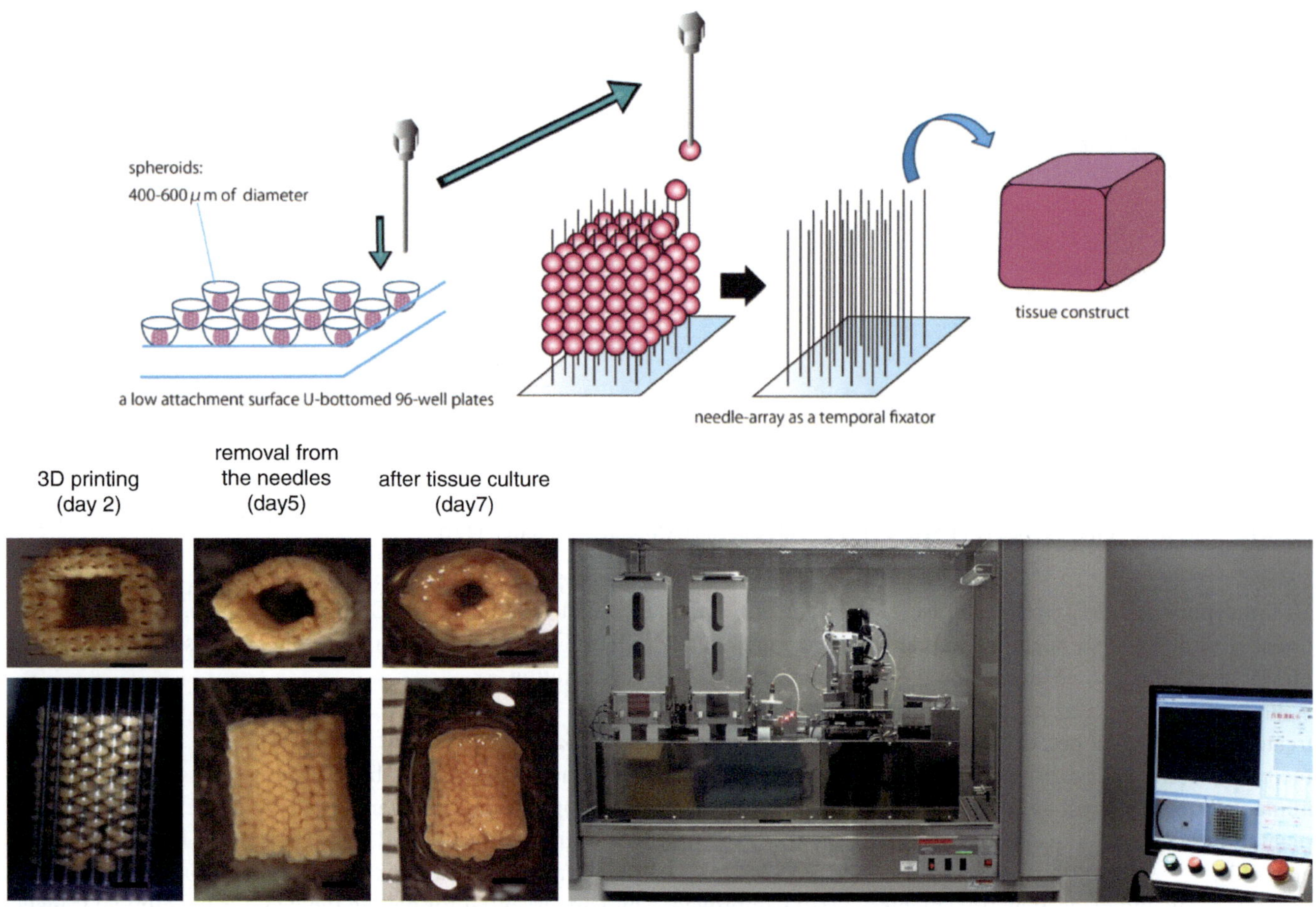


Fig. 47.8 Ex vivo fabrication of scalable human liver-like tissue using a bio-3D printing technology

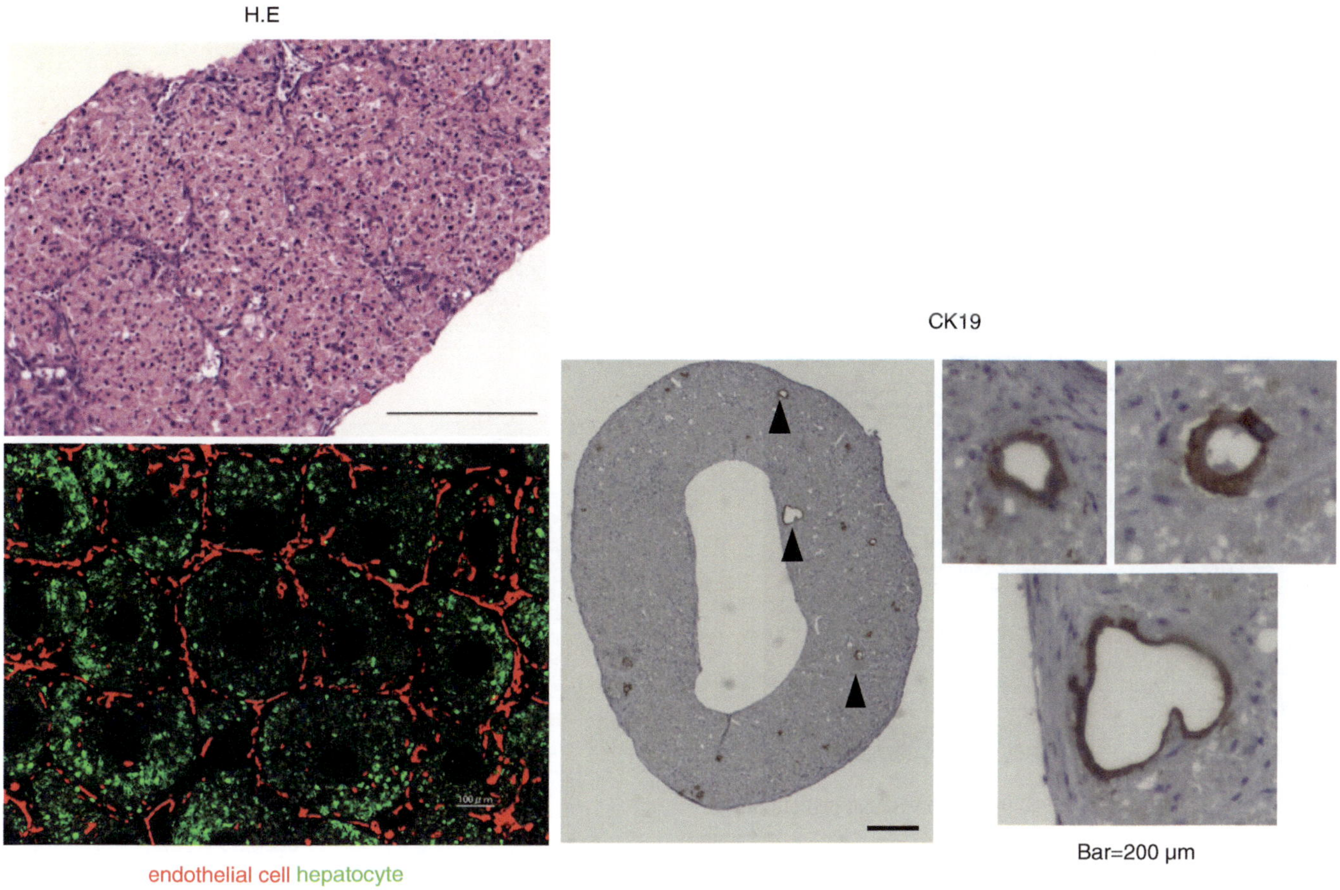


Fig. 47.9 Artificial liver tissue fabricated by 3D bioprinter

surgical diseases, like biliary atresia and diaphragmatic hernia. Aiming to the clinical trial of SHED, there are two possibilities for design, autotransplantation, and allotransplantation. Looking for HLA-homo donors and creating an SHED bank will be helpful for SHED allotransplantation. Dental pulp stem cells can also be created by the wisdom tooth or supernumerary tooth of the adult. Regenerative medicine using stem cells from dental pulp will provide new aspects for surgical treatment in the child as well as the adult.

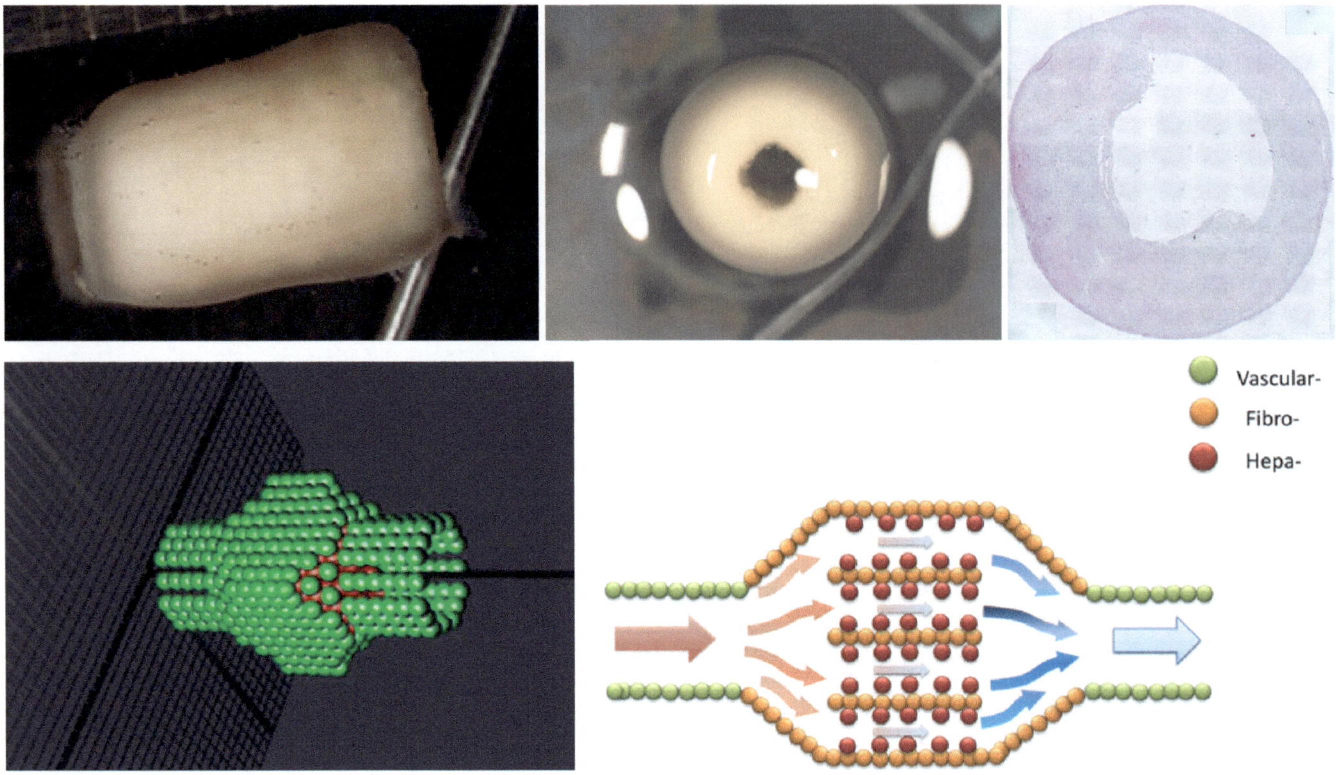


**Fig. 47.10** Scaffold-free artificial liver with vascular pedicle (image)

## References


1. Matsui A, Sasaki N, Arakawa Y, Ishikawa T, Momoya T, Kasano Y, Yanagisawa M, Tsukagoshi N, Kawai T. Neonatal mass screening for biliary atresia. Screening. 1993;2:201–9.
2. Hsiao CH, Chang MH, Chen HL, Lee HC, Wu TC, Lin CC, Yang YJ, Chen AC, Tiao MM, Lau BH, et al. Universal screening for biliary atresia using an infant stool color card in Taiwan. Hepatology. 2008;47:1233–40.
3. Wildhaber BE. Screening for biliary atresia: Swiss stool color card. Hepatology. 2011;54:367–8.
4. Schreiber RA, Masucci L, Kaczorowski J, Collet JP, Lutley P, Espinosa V, Bryan S. Home-based screening for biliary atresia using infant stool colour cards: a large-scale prospective cohort study and cost-effectiveness analysis. J Med Screen. 2014;21:126–32.
5. Mogul D, Zhou M, Intihar P, Schwarz K, Frick K. Costeffective analysis of screening for biliary atresia with the stool color card. J Pediatr Gastroenterol Nutr. 2015;60:91–8.
6. Nio M, Ohi R, Miyano T, et al. Five- and 10-year survival rates after surgery for biliary atresia: a report from the Japanese biliary atresia registry. J Pediatr Surg. 2003;38:997–1000.
7. Hayashida M, Matsuura T, Kinoshita Y, Esumi G, Yoshimaru K, Yanagi Y, Takahashi Y, Taguchi T. Parameters that help to differentiate biliary atresia from other diseases. Pediatr Int. 2017;59:1261–5.
8. Choi SO, Park WH, Lee HJ, et al. 'Triangular cord': a sonographic finding applicable in the diagnosis of biliary atresia. J Pediatr Surg. 1996;31:363–6.
9. Mittal V, Saxena AK, Sodhi KS, Thapa BR, Rao KL, Das A, Khandelwal N. Role of abdominal sonography in the preoperative diagnosis of extrahepatic biliary atresia in infants younger than 90 days. AJR. 2011;196:w438–45.
10. Takamizawa S, Zaima A, Muraji T, Kanegawa K, Akasaka Y, Satoh S, Nishijima E. Can biliary atresia be diagnosed by ultrasonography alone? J Pediatr Surg. 2007;42:2093–6.
11. Kasai M, Suzuki H, Ohashi E, et al. Technique and results of operative management of biliary atresia. World J Surg. 1978;2:571–80.
12. Mieli-Vergani G, Howard ER, Portman B, et al. Late referral for biliary atresia-missed opportunities for effective surgery. Lancet. 1989;16:421–3.
13. Mowat AP, Davidson LL, Dick MC. Screening for biliary atresia. Lancet. 1993;342:1234–5.
14. Altman RP, Lilly JR, Greenfeld J, et al. A multivariable risk factor analysis of the portoenterostomy (Kasai) procedure for biliary atresia. Ann Surg. 1997;226:348–55.
15. Wildhaber BE, Majino P, Mayr J, et al. Biliary atresia: Swiss National Study, 1994–2004. J Paediatr Gastroenterol Nutr. 2008;46:299–307.
16. Serinet MO, Wildhaber BE, Broue´ P, et al. Impact of age at Kasai operation on its results in late childhood and adolescence: a rational basis for biliary atresia screening. Pediatrics. 2009;123:1280–6.
17. Davenport M, Caponcelli E, Livesey E, et al. Surgical outcome in biliary atresia: etiology affects the influence of age at surgery. Ann Surg. 2008;247:694–8.
18. Wong KKY, Chung PHY, Chan IHY, Lan LCL, Tam PKH. Performing Kasai Portoenterostomy Beyond 60 Days of life is not necessarily associated with a worse outcome. J Pediatr Gastroenterol Nutr. 2010;51:631–4.
19. Nio M, Wada M, Sasaki M, Tanaka H. Effects of age at Kasai portoenterostomy on the surgical outcome: a review of the literature. Surg Today. 2015;45:813–8.
20. Shinkai M, Ohhama Y, Take H, Kitagawa N, Kudo H, Mochizuki K, Hatata T. Long term outcome of children with biliary atresia who were not transplanted after the Kasai operation. 20-year

experience at a children's hospital. J Pediatr Gastroenterol Nutr. 2009;48:443–50.
21. Nio M. Japanese biliary atresia registry. Pediatr Surg Int. 2017;33:1319–25.
22. Uto K, Inomata Y, Sakamoto S, Hibi T, Sasaki H, Nio M. A multicenter study of primary liver transplantation for biliary atresia. Pediatr Surg Int. 2019;35:1223–9.
23. Yanagi Y, Yoshimaru K, Matsuura T, Shibui Y, Kohashi K, Takahashi Y, Obata S, Sozaki R, Izaki T, Taguchi T. The outcome of real-time evaluation of biliary flow using near-infrared fluorescence cholangiography with indocyanine green in biliary atresia surgery. J Pediatr Surg. 2019;54:2574–8.
24. Shen Q, Chen Y, Peng C, Pang W, Wang Z, Wu D, Wang K, Huang X. Liver stiffness measurement predicts the difficulty of Kasai procedure in biliary atresia: a single center retrospective analysis of 199 patients. BMC Pediatr. 2019;19:465.
25. Takahashi Y, Matsuura T, Saeki I, Zaizen Y, Taguchi T. Excellent long-term outcome of hepaticojejunostomy for biliary atresia with a hilar cyst. J Pediatr Surg. 2009;44:2312–5.
26. LeeVan E, Matsuoka L, Cao S, Groshen S, Alexopoulos S. Biliary-enteric drainage vs primary liver transplant as initial treatment for children with biliary atresia. JAMA Surg. 2019;154:26–32.
27. Wang P, Xun P, He K, Cai W. Comparison of liver transplantation outcomes in biliary atresia patients with and without prior portoenterostomy: a meta-analysis. Dig Liver Dis. 2016;48:347–52.
28. Ng V, Sorensen LG, Alonso EM, Fredericks EM, Ye W, Moore J, et al. Neurovevelopmental outcome of young children with biliary atresia and native liver: results from the ChiLDReN study. J Pediatr. 2018;196:139–147.e3.
29. Nestor KA, Zeidan M, Boncore E, Richardson A, Alex G, Weiss M, et al. Neurovdevelopmental outcomes in infants indergoing general anesthesia. J Pediatr Surg. 2017;52:895–900.
30. Davidson AJ, Disma N, deGraff JC, Withington DE, Dorris L, Bell G, et al. Neurodevelopmental outcome at 2 years of age after genweal anaesthesia and awake-regional anaesthesia in infancy (GAS): an internatinal multicentre, randomised controlled trial. Lancet. 2016;387:239–50.
31. Sun LS, Li G, Miller TL, Salorio C, Byrne MW, Bellinger DC, et al. Association between a single general anesthesia exposure before age 36 months and neurocognitive outcomes in laterchildhood. JAMA. 2016;315:2312–20.
32. Majewski RF, Hess J, Kabani S, Ramanathan G. Dental findings in a patient with biliary atresia. J Clin Pediatr Dent. 1993;18:33–7.
33. Yamaza H, Tomoda E, Sonoda S, Nonaka K, Kukita T, Yamaza T. Bilirubin reversibly affects cell death and odontogenic capacity in stem cells from human exfoliated deciduous teeth. Oral Dis. 2018;24:809–19.
34. Macedo AF, Costa C, Matta Mattar RHG, Azevedo RA. Dystrophic calcification of maxillary sinus in pediatric patients with liver transplantation and pigmentation of dental organ. Rev Paul Pediatr. 2018;36:117–20.
35. Zaia AA, Graner E, Almeida OP, Scully C. Oral changes associated with biliary atresia and liver transplantation. J Clin Pediatr Dent. 1993;18:39–42.
36. Range H, Camy S, Cohen J, Colon P, Bouchard P. Dental treatment of an adult patient with a histry of biliary atresia. Quintessence Int. 2012;43:337–41.
37. Miura M, Gronthos S, Zhao M, Lu B, Fisher LW, Robey PG, et al. SHED. Stem cells from human exfoliated deciduous teeth. PNAS. 2003;100:5807–12.
38. Yamaza T, Akiyama K, Chen C, Liu Y, Shi Y, Gronthos S, et al. Immunomodulatory properties of stem cells from human exfoliated deciduous teeth. Stem Cell Res Ther. 2010;1:5.
39. Liu Y, Chen C, Liu S, Liu D, Xu X, Chen X, Shi S, et al. Acetylsalicylic acid treatment improves differentiation and immunomodulation of SHED. J Dent Res. 2015;94:209–18.
40. Ma L, Makno Y, Yamaza H, Akiyama K, Hoshino Y, Song G, et al. Cryopreserved dental pulp tissues of exfoliated deciduous teeth is a feasible stem cell resource for regenerative medicine. PLoS One. 2012;7:e51777.
41. Enosawa S, Horikawa R, Yamamoto A, Sakamoto S, Shigeta T, Nosaka S, et al. Hepatocyte transplantation using a living donor reduced graft in a baby with ornithine transcarbamylase deficiency: a novel source of hepatocytes. Liver Transpl. 2014;20:391–3.
42. Yamaza T, Alatas FS, Yuniartha R, Yamaza H, Fujiyoshi JK, Yanagi Y, et al. In vivo hepatogenic capacity and therapeutic potential of stem cells from human exfoliated deciduous teeth in liver fibrosis in mice. Stem Cell Res Ther. 2015;6:171.
43. Takebe T, Sekine K, Enomura W, Koike H, Kimura M, Ogaeri T, et al. Vascularized and functional human liver from an iPSC-derived organ bud transplantation. Nature. 2013;499:481–4.
44. Sakai Y, Yamanouchi K, Ohashi K, Koike M, Utoh R, Hasegawa H, et al. Vascularized subcutaneous human liver tissue from engineered hepatocyte/fibroblast sheets in mice. Biomaterials. 2015;65: 66–75.
45. Yanagi Y, Nakayama K, Taguchi T, Enosawa S, Tamura T, Yoshimaru K, et al. In vivo and ex vivo methods of growing a liver bud through tissue connection. Sci Rep. 2017;7:14085.
46. Uygun BE, Soto-Gutierrez A, Yagi H, Izamis ML, Guzzardi MA, Shulman C, et al. Organ reengineering through development of a transplantable recellularized liver graft using decellularized liver matrix. Nat Med. 2010;16:814–20.
47. Taguchi T, Yanagi Y, Yoshimaru K, Zhang X-Y, Matsuura T, Nakayama K, Kobayashi E, Yamaza H, Nonaka K, Ohga S, Yamaza T. Regenerative medicine using stem cells from human exfoliated deciduous teeth (SHED): a promising new treatment in pediatric surgery. Surg Today. 2019;49:316–22.

# Clinical Practice Guidelines for Biliary Atresia

48

Hisami Ando, Yukihiro Inomata, Tadashi Iwanaka, Tatsuo Kuroda, Masaki Nio, Akira Matsui, Masahiro Yoshida, and The Japanese Biliary Atresia Society

**Abstract**

The Japanese Biliary Atresia Society (JBAS) prepared for clinical practice guidelines for biliary atresia (BA) according to the Medical Information Network Distribution Service (MINDS) Handbook 2014. Twenty-five clinical questions (CQs) essential for daily clinical practice for BA were grouped into diagnosis, treatment, complications, and prognosis. Systematic literature search performed by the review members and medical evidence was extracted from articles published until July 2014 on PubMed and the Japan medical abstracts society. To reach the guideline consensus, a majority (>70%) adoption was made by the guidelines drafting members according to Delphi procedures. Recommendations for 21 CQs were appropriately provided. However, for 4 CQs (stool color cord, postoperative steroid administration, timing for liver transplantation, and primary liver transplantation), recommendations could not be determined due to a scarcity of evidence. This guideline is the first clinical practice guideline for biliary atresia created by such procedures.

**Keywords**

Biliary atresia · Kasai procedure · Liver transplantation Jaundice · Guidelines

H. Ando (✉)
Aichi Developmental Disability Center, Kasugai, Japan
e-mail: hando@med.nagoya-u.ac.jp

Y. Inomata
Prof. Emeritus, Department of Pediatric Surgery and Transplantation, Kumamoto University, Director, Kumamoto Rosai Hospital, Yatsushiro, Japan

T. Iwanaka
Department of Pediatric Surgery, Faculty of Medicine, The University of Tokyo, Tokyo, Japan

T. Kuroda
Department of Pediatric Surgery, Keio University, School of Medicine, Tokyo, Japan

M. Nio · The Japanese Biliary Atresia Society
Department of Pediatric Surgery, Tohoku University Graduate School of Medicine, Sendai, Japan

A. Matsui
College of Nursing, St Luke's International University, Tokyo, Japan

M. Yoshida
Department of Surgery, International University of Health and Welfare Ichikawa Hospital, Chiba, Japan

The first successful surgery for non-correctable type of biliary atresia (BA) was reported by Morio Kasai and Suzuki [1] in 1959. Since then, hepatic portoenterostomy (Kasai procedure) has enabled the long-term survival of many patients and has become accepted around the world. On the other hand, in 1963, the world's first liver transplant was performed by Thomas Starzl et al. [2], and due to advances in immunosuppressive therapy, it became indispensable for the treatment of this disease. In particular, the development of living donor liver transplantation in Japan has greatly contributed to the improvement of treatment results for BA. In addition, in 1989, the Japanese Biliary Atresia Society (JBAS) started the national BA registration system and the total number of registered 3483 cases in 2019 [3]. However, according to the JBAS aggregate results, the jaundice disappearance rate and autologous liver survival rate have been leveled off in recent years. Because BA is a rare disease, medical personnel do not have sufficient experience with this disease, and delays in diagnosis and treatment, and the lack of unified treatment, etc., are thought to be the factors that cause treatment results to reach a peak.

In this background, the JBAS executive committee made a proposal in 2013 to develop clinical practice guidelines for BA according to the Medical Information Network Distribution Service (MINDS) Handbook 2014. Immediately, the guidelines executive committee was formed and started to create the scope. The guideline committee has consisted of a guideline drafting team, a systematic review team, litera-


M. Nio (ed.), *Introduction to Biliary Atresia*, https://doi.org/10.1007/978-981-16-2160-4_48

ture evaluation selection team, an external evaluation committee. The guideline drafting group consisted of pediatric surgeons, pediatricians, transplant surgeons, and pediatric radiologists, all of whom are specialists in the treatment of biliary atresia in Japan. The guidelines were developed using the MINDS Handbook for Clinical Practice Guideline Development 2014. The guidelines were formulated according to the following four steps: (1) CQ development, (2) systematic review, (3) evaluation of the quality of evidence, and (4) determination of recommendations. The guideline drafting group determined 25 CQs essential for daily clinical practice. These CQs were grouped into the following four major categories: diagnosis, treatment, complications, and prognosis. To reach a consensus on the recommendations and the strength of each recommendation, majority voting (>70%) of the panel of the guideline drafting group was adopted according to the Delphi technique. If a consensus was not reached during the first vote, votes were taken twice or thrice until >70% approval was obtained. If a consensus was not reached after the third vote, the strength of the recommendation was determined as "none," and no recommendation was presented. Systematic literature search was performed by the review team, and medical evidence was extracted from articles published up to and including July 2014 on PubMed and the Japan Medical Abstracts Society. Medical evidence was critically evaluated and divided into four levels, A–D, covering estimated effects with higher reliability (A) to those that were mere speculations (D).

Below are CQs and their recommendations, including those that failed to get recommendations.

## 48.1 Clinical Questions and Recommendations

### 48.1.1 Diagnosis

**CQ 1: Is screening for biliary atresia useful?**

Recommendation: Screening with a stool color card reportedly increases the incidence of early diagnosis and improves the native liver survival rate; therefore, an examination to screen for BA is proposed.

Strength of recommendation 2: Weakly recommended (agreement rate=90%).

Strength of evidence: C (weak).

**Commentary**

The possible candidate indicators for mass screening for BA include bile acid, direct bilirubin and other blood components, urinary sulfated bile acid, and stool color. While several of these have been tested, screening with a stool color card was the only one to be proven to increase the incidence of early diagnosis.

When the stool color card was first introduced to Taiwan in 2002 and was expanded nationwide in 2004, Lien et al. [4] found that the number of cases that underwent the Kasai procedure less than 60 days after birth increased significantly from 49.4% to 65.7% and the jaundice-free native liver survival rate also increased significantly.

Gu et al. [5] screened 313,230 neonates in Japan's Tochigi Prefecture over 19 years and reported that the dates (50.3 days) when the screening group underwent the Kasai procedure were significantly earlier than those before the start of screening (70.3 days).

**CQ 2: Is examination for biliary atresia useful in neonates and infants with stool color card No. 4?**

Recommendation: At this time, screening for BA may be considered in neonates and infants of scoring No.4 on the stool color card [6]. However, as there is insufficient scientific evidence to support this, no recommendation could be made. Strength of recommendation: "none"—explicit recommendation impossible (prevailing opinion: weakly recommended, agreement rate = 52%)

Strength of recommendation "none": Explicit recommendation impossible (Prevailing opinion: Weakly recommended (agreement rate = 52%).

Strength of evidence: D (very weak).

**Commentary**

The stool color card is divided by stool color into numbers 1 to 7. The timing for checking the stool color is 2 and 4 weeks after birth, as well as 1 to 4 months; visiting a medical institution is recommended if the stool color is any number between 1 and 3, and even No. 4 is believed to require checking if the stool color becomes lighter. In a 2016 [7] Report from the JBAS registry office, out of 77 cases of BA in which the stool color could be checked before surgery, 13 cases had shown stool color No.4 at 1 month. Cases diagnosed with BA after the stool color was deemed normal even using the stool color cards have been reported, cases of even with stool color No. 4 need to be handled carefully [8–10].

If the stool color is clearly white, testing under the suspicion of BA is considered very useful. Examination with the stool color card is easy, is not detrimental to the subject, and has little economic burden on subjects and guardians. However, stool color No.4 needs to be handled carefully. Although there have been no reports, the Japanese Society of Pediatric Surgeons noted in a 2015 publication that about 60% of mothers decided that their child's stool color was No. 4 2 weeks after birth. Therefore, careful examinations for stool color No. 4 may impose an excessive burden on many healthy children.

One reported method whereby a specialist determines the stool color is to send them a photograph showing the stool and a stool color card side by side [11]. In the future, applications for use on mobile terminal devices allowing of analyzing the stool color optically and other innovations have the potential to enable the early detection of BA.

**CQ 3: Is examination for biliary atresia useful in patients with prolonged jaundice and hepatomegaly?**

Recommendation: If a patient with prolonged jaundice is found to have hepatomegaly, an abnormal stool color, or brown urine, the recommendation is to collect blood, evaluate their direct bilirubin levels, and examine them for a differential diagnosis of BA if cholestasis is suspected.

Strength of recommendation 1: Strongly recommended (agreement rate = 72%).

Strength of evidence: B (medium).

**Commentary**

It cannot be overemphasized that a checkup 1 month after birth is a golden opportunity to diagnose BA. However, as many neonates and infants present physiological jaundice (up to around 2 weeks after birth in full-term neonates and up to around 3 weeks in pre-term neonates [12]), breast milk jaundice (up to 2–3 months after birth), and other aspects of high indirect bilirubin, there is a risk that pathological direct hyperbilirubinemia may go unnoticed. Moreover, even if prolonged jaundice is observed at the 1-month checkup, blood collection involving direct bilirubin is not easy to perform in all cases. Therefore, the above CQ was drafted by handling hepatomegaly as a symptom suggestive of BA, in addition to an abnormal stool color and brown urine.

The National Institute for Health and Care Excellence (NICE) guidelines [13] recommend that patients with prolonged jaundice after full-term birth be checked for stool color abnormalities and brown urine and examined for bilirubin, including direct bilirubin. The American Academy of Pediatrics guidelines [14] recommend performing a cost/benefit analysis before collecting bilirubin, including direct bilirubin, in order to search for cholestasis in patients with prolonged jaundice and performing further examinations when signs of cholestasis are found.

In a prospective cohort study by Lee and Chai [15], it was stated that 95% of patients with obstructive jaundice also had hepatomegaly, and the other case reports [16, 17] also mention that all cases of BA exhibited hepatomegaly. This suggests that although the strength of evidence is low, hepatomegaly may be an important finding for the detection of BA.

**CQ 4: Is intraoperative cholangiography useful for the diagnosis and treatment of biliary atresia?**

Recommendation: As intraoperative cholangiography is used to exclude diseases other than BA and to classify the type of BA, which correlates with prognosis, the recommendation is to perform intraoperative cholangiography.

Strength of recommendation 1: Strongly recommended (agreement rate = 87%).

Strength of evidence: C (weak).

**Commentary**

BA cases in which intraoperative cholangiography was possible were classified by intrahepatic/extrahepatic cholangiography findings, and the prognosis predictions (i.e., native liver survival) were investigated according to this classification. Chiba et al. [18] classified the type I intrahepatic bile ducts into hazy (cloudy), small cystic signs, and mixed, and showed that the small cystic type was associated with more cases of persistent jaundice and worse prognoses. Nio et al. [19] studied the transplantation-free survival rate and overall survival rate in types I and II/III and showed that they were statistically significantly higher in type I. The transplantation or survival rates were shown with type I subdivided into 3 groups—a cloudy type, tree-like type, and mixed type (50%, 100%, and 97%, respectively). The extrahepatic cholangiography findings were also investigated by Karrer et al. [20], who classified them into gallbladder/distal common bile duct patency, extrahepatic bile duct obstruction, and proximal bile duct patency (the so-called correctable type), calculated the 5-year survival rate and found it to be 72% for proximal bile duct patency, 62% for gallbladder/distal common bile duct patency, and 38% for extrahepatic bile duct obstruction. In other words, cholangiography is needed to determine the disease type and is regarded as useful in predicting prognostic factors such as native liver survival.

In BA, native liver survival cannot be predicted by the type of bile duct obstruction alone, and it is susceptible to be influenced by a large number of factors, including postoperative cholangitis, portal hypertension, and other complications. However, intraoperative cholangiography is a basic procedure to exclude BA or to make a diagnosis, including of the disease type, and it is also minimally invasive when performed carefully. Therefore, this leads to the conclusion that it should be recommended.

**CQ 5: Is liver biopsy useful for the preoperative diagnosis of biliary atresia?**

Recommendation: Diagnosis by liver biopsy is highly specific and sensitive. Therefore, it is deemed useful for preoperative diagnosis. However, percutaneous needle biopsy techniques have the potential to cause serious complications and even death. Moreover, performing a liver biopsy also delays radical surgery. Therefore, it is suggested that liver biopsies should not be performed.

Strength of recommendation 2: Weakly recommended (agreement rate = 70%).

Strength of evidence: C (weak).

**Commentary**

BA is definitively diagnosed by intraoperative cholangiography and surgical findings. Although preoperative liver biopsy has a high diagnostic power, it is not absolute, and if the age at which it is performed for this disease is at the neonatal or infant stage, a high risk of complications can be expected. Moreover, the number of days from biopsy to tissue diagnosis is longer in Japan than in the West. Therefore, the performance of preoperative liver biopsy delays the performance of radical surgery, thereby hindering early treatment, which is the most important thing in the treatment of this disease. On that basis, the proposal is that it should not be performed in Japan.

**CQ 6: Is pathological examination of tissue specimens useful for the diagnosis and treatment of biliary atresia?**

Recommendation: The histopathological findings of specimens collected during the Kasai procedure are useful for the prediction of native liver survival. The recommendation is to histopathological findings when determining the treatment strategy.

Strength of recommendation 1: Strongly recommended (agreement rate = 82%).

Strength of evidence: C (weak).

**Commentary**

Many of the extracted texts were not adjusted for the age at surgery, the type, and the follow-up period. Moreover, as the timing of the outcome assessment also varied from paper to paper, there was a high bias risk in the meta-analysis. Future relevant large-scale studies should be conducted in order to reassess this item. This recommendation was written in consideration of the fact that in the clinical field, there are many scenarios in which postoperative steroid administration, repeat corrective surgery or liver transplantation indications should be considered based on the histopathological findings from the liver and hepatic portal region connective tissue.

### 48.1.2 Treatment

**CQ 7: Is preoperative administration of vitamin K useful?**

Recommendation: In patients with obstructive jaundice and suspected BA, attention must be paid to bleeding diathesis caused by vitamin K deficiency. Furthermore, to reduce the risk of hemorrhagic complications during surgery, the recommendation is to administer vitamin K intravenously prior to surgery.

Strength of recommendation 1: Strongly recommended (agreement rate = 78%).

Strength of evidence: D (very weak).

**CQ 8: Should the Kasai procedure be performed within the first 30 days after birth?**

Recommendation: It is recommended that the Kasai procedure should be performed within the first 30 days after birth, considering the native liver survival rate for BA.

Strength of recommendation 2: Weakly recommended (agreement rate = 94%).

Strength of evidence: C (weak).

**Commentary**

The jaundice resolution rates by age (days) over 10 years (from 2005 to 2014) derived from data of the JBAS were 73.1% for surgery within 30 days, 66.5% for surgery within 60 days, 59.5% for surgery within 90 days, 57.4% for surgery within 120 days, and 19.6% for surgery at 121 days or older [21]. Thus, the jaundice resolution rate from the performance of the Kasai procedure within 30 days showed a significant difference ($p < 0.0001$) in improvement as compared with the surgery at 30 days or later, suggesting that early surgery is useful, although the relationship with the native liver survival rate was not studied.

**CQ 9: Is postoperative steroid administration useful?**

Recommendation: The evidence collected to date has not shown that steroid administration to have a significant reduces jaundice long-term or improves the native liver survival rate. As it depends on the experts' previous therapeutic experience and on the results of the consensus meeting, no recommendation could be made on whether the administration of steroids improves the jaundice-free native liver survival rate.

Strength of recommendation "none": Explicit recommendation impossible (agreement rate = 58%).

Strength of evidence: B (medium).

**CQ 10: Is long-term postoperative intravenous administration of antimicrobials effective?**

Recommendation: Taking the onset of cholangitis and improvements in the jaundice-free native liver survival rate into account, the recommendation is to administer intravenous antibiotics for 2–4 weeks after BA surgery and then administer oral antibiotics.

Strength of recommendation 2: Weakly recommended (agreement rate = 74%).

Strength of evidence: D (very weak).

**Commentary**

In BA, as there are no normal bile ducts in the hepatic portal region and little bile is excreted, cholangitis is likely to occur after surgery. According to the aggregated results from the 2014 nationwide registry of the JBAS, the incidence of postoperative cholangitis is 39.7% [7]. Although it is common to see increased jaundice or a worsened hepatic function after the onset of cholangitis, no document has directly stated that the administration of antimicrobials lowers the incidence of cholangitis, and there have been no high-quality comparison of different durations of antimicrobial administration. Regarding the prophylactic administration of oral antibiotics, as well, there is little evidence about the types of antibiotics or about the administration duration.

Concerns about the appearance of resistant microbes and the emergence of fungal infections from antimicrobial usage have been suggested. However, the treatment of postoperative cholangitis poses a major burden on patients from hospitalization and the like, and few reports have addressed the harms from antimicrobials; in consideration of this, it is proposed to administer antibiotics intravenously for 2–4 weeks after surgery and to then continue with oral antibiotics.

**CQ 11: Is postoperative ursodeoxycholic acid administration useful?**

Recommendation: Taking improvements in the jaundice-free native liver survival rate after BA surgery into account, the recommendation is to administer ursodeoxycholic acid (UDCA) postoperatively.

Strength of recommendation 2: Weakly recommended (agreement rate = 78%).

Strength of evidence: D (very weak).

**Commentary**

After BA surgery, cholestasis and the reduced bile acid production in the hepatocytes cause too little bile acid to be secreted in the intestines. This impairs the absorption of fat and fat-soluble vitamins, suppresses the intestinal bacterial growth in the small intestine, impairs the enterohepatic circulation of the bile acid, and so forth [21]. Therefore, in patients with BA, it is inferred that the administration of UDCA to replenish the bile acid improves the absorption of fat and fat-soluble vitamins. The damaging effect on the hepatocytes can be reduced by increasing the proportion of UDCA, which causes little tissue damage, instead of the bile acids such as chenodeoxycholic acid, deoxycholic acid, or lithocholic acid, which cause more tissue damage, in the enterohepatic circulation of bile acid. The amount of bile acid produced is increased, and the incidence of cholangitis from cholestasis is reduced. These and similar effects have been expected from the administration of UDCA [22–25].

Many specialist facilities in Japan administer UDCA to patients after BA surgery on account of the observed improvement in hepatic function and bile outflow. Although there has been no assessment of the improvement in the jaundice-free native liver survival rate, UDCA has potential benefits in the promotion of bile acid secretion, the mitigation of impaired absorption, and the protection of hepatocytes. In addition, as no serious harm has been reported, its administration after BA surgery is recommended.

**CQ 12: Is a repeat Kasai procedure useful for patients who experience a temporary disappearance of jaundice after biliary atresia surgery?**

Recommendation: Taking the improvements in the native liver survival rate and total survival rate into account, it is recommended that a repeat Kasai procedure is performed in patients who experience a temporary resolution of jaundice or temporary improvement in biliary excretion after BA surgery.

Strength of recommendation 2: Weakly recommended (agreement rate = 76%).

Strength of evidence: C (weak).

**Commentary**

Among the retrospective studies on the repeat, Kasai procedure with relatively large sample sizes had a jaundice resolution rate of 31–55.6% after the repeat Kasai procedures. Regarding the indications for the repeat Kasai procedures, Ando et al. [26] reported that the latter were effective in cases in which jaundice had shown a tendency to resolve after the first surgery or had resolved temporarily and then resurged. Saeki et al. [27] reported that cases that had exhibited a sudden stop in the bile outflow after the first surgery tended to have a higher jaundice resolution rate (50%). Nio et al. [28] stated that the repeat Kasai procedure was effective in patients who had exhibited temporarily favorable biliary excretion after the first surgery but had experienced a sudden stoppage of their biliary excretion.

### 48.1.3 Complications

**CQ 13: Is the prophylactic administration of antibiotics for cholangitis useful?**

Recommendation: The recommendation is to consider administering antimicrobials such as trimethoprim/sulfamethoxazole to prevent cholangitis after BA surgery.

Strength of recommendation 1: Strongly recommended (agreement rate = 78%).

Strength of evidence: C (weak).

**Commentary**

Despite the relatively weak evidence, in light of the observational studies and case reports, it was concluded that it is valid to recommend the administration of postoperative prophylactic antimicrobials. This decision was based on the suggestion by several reports that they are effective in the prevention of cholangitis; however, it must always be kept in mind that antimicrobial usage generates resistant bacteria.

**CQ 14: Is it useful to administer drugs for cholangitis?**

Recommendation: The recommendation is to initially treat cholangitis with broad-spectrum antimicrobials and to later administer antimicrobials specific to isolated strains identified via bacteriological analysis.

Strength of recommendation 2: Weakly recommended (agreement rate = 81%).

Strength of evidence: C (weak).

**Commentary**

At the time of first treatment after the onset of cholangitis, it is worth consulting the revised Updated Tokyo Guidelines (TG13) [29], which are international clinical practice guidelines for biliary tract infections. The guidelines select the antimicrobials deemed to be appropriate for use in the initial treatment (empiric therapy) until a bacteriological diagnosis is reached, in accordance with the severity of the biliary tract infection and for different municipalities and medical institutions. The variation in the causative organisms to be treated is similar to that in BA, and the guidelines can be consulted as a reference for initial treatment, provided that the differences between pediatric and adult patients are understood and that the special aspects that follow hepatoportojejunostomy are known.

There were no papers reporting serious side effects. Thus, the administration of antimicrobials with favorable bile migration and sensitivity to isolated strains is effective against cholangitis in BA. For treatment, it is both reasonable and useful to perform tests to identify the pathogenic organism and to select antimicrobials based on the results.

On the other hand, it was not possible to find documents providing evidence for the effectiveness of the administration of steroids or cholagogues in the treatment of cholangitis.

**CQ 15: Is percutaneous transhepatic biliary drainage effective against intrahepatic bile duct cystic dilatation in patients who have undergone biliary atresia surgery?**

Recommendation: After BA surgery, percutaneous transhepatic biliary drainage (PTBD) for intrahepatic bile duct cystic dilatation is recommended as a short-term, intermediate palliative treatment for the control of cholangitis.

Strength of recommendation 2: Weakly recommended (agreement rate = 84%).

Strength of evidence: D (very weak).

**Commentary**

Intrahepatic bile duct cysts represent a pathology that involves many factors, and the context of the pathology and the criteria for the indication of PTBD are not standardized. The meta-analysis showed no reports demonstrating that PTBD has an effect on the lowering of the cholangitis frequency or the improvement of the native liver survival rate. Some observational studies and case reports have shown a cholangitis control effect. Although there have been no reports of complications, the recommendation was drafted by emphasizing the stress of catheter insertion/placement on the patients and by comprehensively considering the balance between the effects and disadvantages for the patients.

**CQ 16: What treatments are useful for gastroesophageal variceal bleeding after biliary atresia surgery?**

Recommendation: It is recommended that prompt endoscopic therapy (variceal ligation or, if this is too difficult, sclerotherapy) be administered as an acute-stage treatment after taking measures to counteract hemorrhagic shock, including vascular agonists administration.

Strength of recommendation 1: Strongly recommended (agreement rate = 71%).

Strength of evidence: C (weak).

**Commentary**

Gastroesophageal variceal bleeding is a life-threatening adverse event, and the life-saving effects are regarded as the most important. The search results showed that the relevant guidelines and literature containing strong evidence in the adult field and the like should be considered and used, and even pediatric or BA surgery reports with weak evidence should be considered. At this time, the recommendation does not include treatments that are performed infrequently on pediatric patients.

**CQ 17: Is outpatient monitoring of oxygen saturation (SpO2) useful for the early diagnosis of hepatopulmonary syndrome?**

Recommendation: The recommendation is to measure SpO2 overtime for the early detection of hepatopulmonary syndrome after BA surgery.

Strength of recommendation 2: Weakly recommended (agreement rate = 87%).

Strength of evidence: D (very weak).

**Commentary**

Hepatopulmonary syndrome is one of the postoperative complications of BA. This condition is a form of hypoxemia caused by a right/left shunt due to dilated vessels or new vessels in the liver and is alleviated by oxygen administration. However, liver transplantation is required as a radical treatment, and early detection is important as the progression of hypoxemia affects the outcome of liver transplantation [30].

There has been shown to be a higher likelihood of hepatopulmonary syndrome when the SpO2 measurement over time showed a downward trend [31]. However, SpO2 measurement is significant in that it is non-invasive and easy, although the reliability is not high enough. Therefore, although measurement of the SpO2 over time cannot be described as having high diagnostic sensitivity or specificity for the early detection of hepatopulmonary syndrome, it is nonetheless recommended since it is non-invasive and simple.

**CQ 18: Is echocardiography useful for the early diagnosis of pulmonary hypertension?**

Recommendation: It is recommended that echocardiography is performed in cases presenting with portal hypertension, while taking into consideration the possibility of latent pulmonary hypertension.
Strength of recommendation 1: Strongly recommended (agreement rate = 84%).
Strength of evidence: B (medium).

**Commentary**
Pulmonary hypertension is an important complication of BA that is relevant to the decision of whether transplantation is indicated and is defined as a mean pulmonary arterial pressure (mean PAP) of 25 mmHg or higher, as measured by right heart catheterization at rest [32]. If pulmonary hypertension is suspected, echocardiography is essential, and it is useful for the non-invasive estimation of the pulmonary arterial pressure, thus offering a useful testing method to screen for pulmonary hypertension [33]. However, although the risk associated with right heart catheterization is not high in an experienced facility, about 1% of adverse events were reported, and fatal complications were also observed [34]. In addition, the risk of catheterization in children was higher than that in adults, and 5.7% (4/70) of cardiac massages were performed under general anesthesia in children with pulmonary hypertension [35].

### 48.1.4 Prognosis

**CQ 19: Is liver transplantation useful for native liver subjects with biliary atresia involving growth/developmental disorders?**

Recommendation: Liver transplantation is recommended as a useful way to mitigate growth-developmental disorders in native liver subjects with BA, especially if performed relatively early, for example, at 1-t years of age.
Strength of recommendation 2: Weakly recommended (agreement rate = 74%).
Strength of evidence: C (weak).

**Commentary**
Regarding the usefulness of living-donor liver transplantation for the mitigation of impaired growth/development, it has been reported that impaired growth had improved significantly, both in terms of height and weight, 1 year after liver transplantation [36]. The performance of living-donor liver transplantation on children under 1 year and under 5 years was also shown to be effective in the improvement of the patients' impaired growth and development [37, 38]. Hoshino et al. [39] stated that although patients who had undergone liver transplantation at 8 years or younger showed poor development before transplantation, they had caught up better after transplantation than children who had undergone it at age 8 or older. On the other hand, steroid administration after transplantation is reportedly a risk factor of impaired growth and development if prolonged [38, 40]. It is also reported that 25% of adult native liver survival patients experience anxiety, worry, and depression; as it is necessary, early transplantation should also be recommended in this regard [41].

**CQ 20: Is multidisciplinary management necessary for pregnancy/birth in biliary atresia patients living with their native liver?**

Recommendation: Multidisciplinary management is recommended for pregnancy/birth in BA patients with their native liver to prepare for deterioration in health status or worsening of liver function during pregnancy.
Strength of recommendation 1: Strongly recommended (agreement rate = 77%).
Strength of evidence: C (weak).

**Commentary**
For pregnancy and childbirth in patients who have undergone the Kasai procedure, complications during the course require careful attention even if the hepatic function is stable, and stricter pregnancy management than normal is considered to be needed [42]. In terms of complications, attention must be paid to the worsening of the hepatic dysfunction or of portal hypertension (varices), and to ascending cholangitis; these complications may even cause miscarriage or hepatic failure [43–45]. However, this is not to say that pregnancy is contraindicated but that strict management has enabled safe pregnancy and delivery.

**CQ21: Should regular imaging studies be performed?**

Recommendation: Regular imaging studies are strongly recommended as they are useful for the early detection of impairment. If radiation exposure is involved, the "as low as reasonably achievable" principle should be followed.
Strength of recommendation 1: Strongly recommended (agreement rate = 74%)
Strength of evidence: C (weak)

**Commentary**

As regular imaging reportedly makes it possible to ascertain early-stage impairment of the native liver in patients who have undergone the Kasai procedure, it is believed that it can contribute to the improvement of the native liver survival rate by enabling the early detection and treatment of complications.

**CQ 22: Is prophylactic varicose vein therapy useful for the treatment of gastroesophageal varices?**

Recommendation: Prophylactic varicose vein therapy is recommended for the treatment of gastroesophageal varices as a useful way to improve the native liver survival rate and to lower the risk of bleeding.

Strength of recommendation 2: Weakly recommended (agreement rate 74%).

Strength of evidence: C (weak).

**Commentary**

Regarding the improvement of the native liver survival rate from prophylactic therapy against varices, prophylactically treated patients reportedly had a higher native liver survival rate for 3 years after treatment than those who were treated for hemorrhaging (45% versus 30%) [46]. In a report from Duché et al. [47], the patients who underwent prophylactic therapy for varices had a native liver survival rate of 23.1% (3 cases of native liver survival, 2 deaths, and 8 liver transplantations out of 13 cases), while it was 29.4% in a report from Nishi et al. [48] (5 cases of native liver survival, 2 deaths, and 10 liver transplantations out of 17 cases).

Meanwhile, serious complications associated with this treatment are uncommon, and no reports limited to pediatric BA have mentioned instances of portal thrombosis becoming problematic in adulthood. However, even after treatment, the rebleeding rate is not low, and follow-up observation is required. Moreover, if a certain length of time after treatment is stipulated, the native liver survival rate during that time could be described as having improved, but there has been no report to state that the ultimate native liver survival rate had improved.

The recommendation decision for prophylactic treatment against varices was made in light of the many reports stating that the harm was outweighed by the contribution to native liver survival from the prevention of bleeding and the consequent prevention of a rapid decrease in the hepatic function associated with bleeding.

**CQ 23: Is hypersplenism therapy useful?**

Recommendation: Hypersplenism therapy is recommended.

Strength of recommendation 1: Strongly recommended (agreement rate: 76%).

Strength of evidence: D (very weak).

**Commentary**

In all reports, the platelets improved significantly after surgery. Meanwhile, the coagulation system, including the PT and APTT, did not change before and after surgery [49]. The embolization of 70% or more of the spleen is needed to obtain an effective increase in platelets has been reported [50].

Clinically, there have been statements that no symptoms of a decreased immune function [51] were observed and that surgery was not followed by serious infections [52]. However, partial splenic embolization (PSE) brought about abdominal pain, fever, intestinal paralysis, or splenic abscess are reported. In a comparison of the 34 patients who underwent splenectomy before transplantation and the 87 patients who did not, a higher risk of infection was reported in the patients who had undergone splenectomy (21/34, 61.7% versus 22/87, 25.3%) [53].

**CQ 24: What is the recommended timing for liver transplantation after the Kasai procedure? (Is early transplantation recommended?)**

Recommendation: There is insufficient evidence to allow us to make an explicit recommendation with regards to the age at which liver transplantation should be performed.

Strength of recommendation 2: Weakly recommended (agreement rate 71%).

Strength of evidence: D (very weak).

**Commentary**

Although the absolute indication for liver transplantation is an unavoidable hepatic failure, there is currently a wide range of relevant symptoms and findings, which often makes it difficult to decide on the appropriate time for each individual patient. The aggregated results from the Japanese Liver Transplantation Society showed that the post-transplantation survival rate differs between the period from infancy to 10 years and at later ages. This may represent weak evidence for the recommendation of early transplantation. However, the elevated risk of infection and the tendency to develop secondary cancer from post-transplantation immunosuppression are consequences that may undermine the benefits of transplantation. In light of this, there is no evidence to explicitly recommend the age at which liver transplant is indicated, and it is considered that timing recommendations for age should not be provided.

**CQ 25: Is primary liver transplantation useful for biliary atresia patients with a pediatric end-stage liver disease score of 10 or higher?**

Recommendation: A recommendations could not be given.

Strength of recommendation 1: Strongly recommended (agreement rate 90%).

Strength of evidence: D (very weak).

**Commentary**

Although the evidence is weak as they had a small sample size and were designed as case control studies, the results of their meta-analysis showed that primary liver transplantation and liver transplantation after the Kasai procedure did not differ significantly in their 1-year survival rate (risk ratio: 0.99 (95%), confidence interval: 0.74–1.33, $p$ = 0.96). A report from Wang et al. [54] showed no significant difference in the PELD score, although primary liver transplantation patients were deemed to exhibit a worsening of their condition, and future examination of the background factors was thought to be needed. The latest meta-analysis also suggested that the performance or non-performance of the Kasai procedure before transplantation does not affect the patient survival rate or the transplanted liver survival rate [55].

At the current time, there are too few opportunities to study primary liver transplantation, as it is seldom needed in Japan, and there is no evidence at all for it. In these circumstances, the recommendation was determined by keeping voting about whether or not it was valid not to vote on the usefulness of primary transplantation.

## 48.2 Addition

The Japanese version of the clinical practice guidelines for BA was completed at the end of 2018 [56] and can be accessed using the following URL: https://minds.jcqhc.or.jp/n/med/4/med0362/G0001073. The English version of summaries of CQs was released at the Journal of Hepato-Biliary-Pancreatic Sciences in 2021 [57]. It will be expected that these guidelines will be used worldwide and that standardization of treatment for BA will improve treatment outcomes.

## References


1. Kasai M, Suzuki S. New surgical procedure for so-called "inoperable" cases of congenital biliary obstruction: hepatoportoenterostomy. Surgery. 1959;13:733–9.
2. Starzl TE, Marchioro TL, Von Kaulla KN, Hermann G, Brittain RS, Waddell WR. Homotransplantation of the liver in humans. Surg Gynecol Obstet. 1963;117:659–76.
3. Japanese Biliary Atresia Society. Japanese Biliary Atresia Registry. https://jbas.net/en/national-registration/.
4. Lien TH, Chang MH, Wu JF, Chen HL, Lee HC, Chen AC, et al. Effects of the infant stool color card screening program on 5-year outcome of biliary atresia in Taiwan. Hepatology. 2011;53:202–8.
5. Gu YH, Yokoyama K, Mizuta K, Tsuchioka T, Kudo T, Sasaki H, et al. Stool color card screening for early detection of biliary atresia and long-term native liver survival: a 19-year cohort study in Japan. J Pediatr. 2015;166:897–902.
6. Matsui A. Screening for biliary atresia. Pediatr Surg Int. 2017;33:1305–13.
7. Japanese Biliary Atresia Society. Office of the Japanese Biliary Atresia Registry, Japanese Biliary Atresia Registry 2014 summary results. J Jpn Soc Pediatr Surg. 2016;52:291–7.
8. Chen SM, Chang MH, Du JC, et al. Screening for biliary atresia by infant stool color card in Taiwan. Pediatrics. 2006;117:1147–54.
9. Takakura M, Yoshinaga M, Hanai J. Status of biliary atresia screening, 2001–2011. Sapporo City Inst Public Health Annu Rep. 2012;39:41–7.
10. Ohama K, Shimotake T, Ishikawa N. Introducing the 'Stool color check card' for early detection of biliary atresia: an attempt in Ishikawa Prefecture. Jpn J Pediatr. 2010;63:1735–41.
11. Watayo H, Muraji T, Yanai T. Screening for biliary atresia with the stool color card using email on mobile phones. J Jpn Soc Pediatr Surg. 2014;50:1017–21.
12. McKiernan P. Neonatal jaundice. Clin Res Hepatol Gastroenterol. 2012;36:253–6.
13. NICE clinical guideline 98. Neonatal jaundice. National Institute for Health and Clinical Excellence; 2010.
14. American Academy of Pediatrics Subcommittee on Hyperbilirubinemia. Management of hyperbilirubinemia in the newborn infant 35 or more weeks of gestation. Pediatrics. 2004;114:297–316.
15. Lee WS, Chai PF. Clinical features differentiating biliary atresia from other causes of neonatal cholestasis. Ann Acad Med Singap. 2010;39:648–54.
16. Li SX, Zhang Y, Sun M, et al. Ultrasonic diagnosis of biliary atresia: a retrospective analysis of 20 patients. World J Gastroenterol. 2008;14:3579–82.
17. Kimura S, Nakacho M, Ida S. Two cases of biliary atresia discovered due to elevated direct bilirubin despite yellow stool in neonates. J Osaka Med Cent Res Inst Matern Child Health. 2007;23:58–62.
18. Chiba Y, Oi R, Mochizuki I. Extrahepatic and intrahepatic bile ducts in congenital biliary atresia. J Jpn Soc Pediatr Radiol. 1986;2:16–9.
19. Nio M, Sano N, Ishii T, et al. Long-term outcome in type I biliary atresia. J Pediatr Surg. 2006;41:1973–5.
20. Karrer FM, Lilly JR, Stewart BA, et al. Biliary atresia registry, 1976 to 1989. J Pediatr Surg. 1990;25:1076–80.
21. Iinuma Y. Study on inhibited bile acid metabolism after biliary atresia surgery using an oral ursodeoxycholic acid loading test. J Jpn Soc Pediatr Surg. 1994;30:76–84.
22. Ando T, Oi R, Ohkohchi N, et al. Effects of enteral administration of conjugated UDCA added to intravenous fat emulsion for biliary atresia. Dig Absorpt. 1993;16:103–8.
23. Mohanty MK, Gupta SD, Bhatnagar V. Surgical outcome in relation to duct size at the porta hepatis and the use of cholagogues in patients with biliary atresia. Trop Gastroenterol. 2010;31:184–9.
24. Yamashiro Y, Ohtsuka Y, Shimizu T, et al. Effects of ursodeoxycholic acid treatment on essential fatty acid deficiency in patients with biliary atresia. J Pediatr Surg. 1994;29:425–8.
25. Nittono H, Tokita A, Hayashi M, et al. Ursodeoxycholic acid therapy in the treatment of biliary atresia. Bimed Pharmacother. 1989;43:37–41.
26. Ando H, Kaneko K, Ono Y, Tainaka T, Sumida W. Value of the reoperation after Kasai`s portoenterostomy going against the current of the times of the liver transplantation for biliary atresia. Jpn Soc Pediatr Surg. 2008;40:119–22.
27. Saeki M, Nakano M, Kuroda T. [Biliary atresia] Repeat surgery for hepatoportoenterostomy: Study on biliary atresia cases with repeat surgery. Jpn Soc Pediatr Surg. 1997;29:972–6.
28. Nio M, Sasaki H, Tanaka H, Okamura A. Redo surgery for biliary atresia. Pediatr Surg Int. 2013;29:989–93.
29. Gomi H, Solomkin JS, Takada T, et al. TG13 antimicrobial therapy for acute cholangitis and cholecystitis. J Hepatobiliary Pancreat Sci. 2013;20:60–70.

30. Swanson KL, Wiesner RH, Krowka MJ. Natural history of hepatopulmonary syndrome: Impact of liver transplantation. Hepatology. 2005;41:1122–9.
31. Kochar R, Tanikella R, Fallon MB. Serial pulse oximetry in hepatopulmonary syndrome. Dig Dis Sci. 2011;56:1862–8.
32. Galie N, Hoeper MM, Humbert M, Torbicki A, Vachiery JL, Barbera JA, et al. Guidelines for the diagnosis and treatment of pulmonary hypertension: The task force for the diagnosis and treatment of pulmonary hypertension of the European Society of Cardiology (ESC) and the European Respiratory Society (ERS), endorsed by the International Society of Heart and Lung Transplantation (ISHLT). Eur Heart J. 2009;30:2493–537.
33. Nakanishi N, Ando M, Ueda H, et al. Guidelines for treatment of pulmonary hypertension. 2012 rev. ed. Pulmonary Hypertension Guidelines; 2012. p. 7–12.
34. Hoeper MM, Lee SH, Voswinckel R, Palazzini M, Jais X, Marinelli A, et al. Complications of right heart catheterization procedures in patients with pulmonary hypertension in experienced centers. J Am Coll Cardiol. 2006;48:2546–52.
35. Taylor CJ, Derrick G, McEwan A, Haworth SG, Sury MRJ. Risk of cardiac catheterization under anaesthesia in children with pulmonary hypertension. Br J Anaesth. 2007;98:657–61.
36. Beath S, Pearmain G, Kelly D, et al. Liver transplantation in babies and children with extrahepatic biliary atresia. J Pediatr Surg. 1993;28:1044–7.
37. Alonso G, Duca P, Pasqualini T, et al. Evaluation of catch-up growth after liver transplantation in children with biliary atresia. Pediatr Transplant. 2004;8:255–9.
38. Orii T, Ohkohchi N, Koyamada N, et al. Growth of pediatric patients with biliary atresia after liver transplantation: influence of age at transplantation and steroid administration. Transplant Proc. 2000;32:2210–2.
39. Hoshino K, Yamada Y, Ono N, Shimojima N, Fumoto Y, Morikawa Y. [Biliary atresia: Forefront of diagnosis, treatment, and research] Timing and effects of liver transplantation as seen from growth and development. Jpn Soc Pediatr Surg. 2008;40:123–7.
40. Saito T, Mizuta K, Hishikawa S, et al. Growth curves of pediatric patients with biliary atresia following living donor liver transplantation: factors that influence post-transplantation growth. Pediatr Transplant. 2007;11:764–70.
41. Lind RC, de Vries W, Keyzer-Dekker CM, et al. Health status and quality of life in adult biliary atresia patients surviving with the native livers. Eur J Pediatr Surg. 2015;25:60–5.
42. Shimaoka S, Ohi R, Saeki M, et al. Problems during and after pregnancy of former biliary atresia patients treated successfully by the Kasai procedure. J Pediatr Surg. 2001;36:349–51.
43. Kuroda T, Saeki M, Morikawa N, et al. Management of adult biliary atresia patients: should hard work and pregnancy be discouraged? J Pediatr Surg. 2007;42:2106–9.
44. Sasaki H, Nio M, Hayashi Y, et al. Problems during and after pregnancy in female patients with biliary atresia. J Pediatr Surg. 2007;42:1329–32.
45. Watanabe N, Tanemoto T, Shin'ya M, et al. Study on 13 pregnancies in 10 patients after congenital biliary atresia surgery. Kanto J Obstet Gynecol. 2006;43:353–7.
46. Duché M, Ducot B, Ackermann O, et al. Experience with endoscopic management of high-risk gastroesophageal varices, with and without bleeding, in children with biliary atresia. Gastroenterology. 2013;145:801–7.
47. Duché M, Habes D, Roulleau P, et al. Prophylactic endoscopic sclerotherapy of large esophagogastric varices in infants with biliary atresia. Gastrointest Endosc. 2008;67:732–7.
48. Nishi A, Yamamoto H, Toki F, et al. [Pediatric gastrointestinal endoscopy: The frontier in diagnosis and treatment] Endoscopic therapy for esophageal varices after biliary atresia surgery. Jpn J Pediatr Surg. 2012;44:254–8.
49. Otsuka T, Okada T, Yoshida H, Matsunaga M, Kochi K, Onuma N. Study on partial splenic embolization for hypersplenism after biliary atresia surgery in our department. J Jpn Soc Pediatr Surg. 2002;38:1057–63.
50. Sasaki S, Yano H, Fujito Y. [Portal hypertension after congenital biliary atresia surgery] Treatments for portal hypertension after congenital biliary atresia surgery, in particular partial splenic embolization. Jpn J Pediatr Surg. 1988;20:183–8.
51. Hinoki A, Shinkai M, Ohama Y, Take H, Fukuzato Y, Murakami T, Nishi T. Study on effects and long-term prognosis of PSE in hypersplenism after biliary atresia surgery. Kanagawa Child Med Cent J. 2002;31:137–43.
52. Ando H, Ito T, Nagaya M. Partial splenic embolization decreases the serum bilirubin level in patients with hypersplenism following the Kasai procedure for biliary atresia. J Am Coll Surg. 1996;182:206–10.
53. Lüsebrink R, Blumhardt G, Lohmann R, Bachmann S, Knoop M, Lemmens HP, Neuhaus P. Does concomitant splenectomy raise the mortality of liver transplant recipients? Transpl Int. 1994;7(Suppl 1):S634–6.
54. Wang Q, Yan LN, Zhang MM, et al. The pre-Kasai procedure in living donor liver transplantation for children with biliary atresia. Hepatobiliary Pancreatic Dis Int. 2013;12:47–53.
55. Wang P, Xun P, He K, et al. Comparison of liver transplantation outcomes in biliary atresia patients with and without prior portoenterostomy: A meta-analysis. Dig Live. 2016;48:347–52.
56. Japanese Biliary Atresia Society edition. Clinical practice guidelines for biliary atresia. Tokyo: Herusu Shuppan; 2018.
57. Ando H, Inomata Y, Iwanaka T, Kuroda T, Nio M, Matsui A, et al. Clinical practice guidelines for biliary atresia in Japan. J Hepatobiliary Pancreat Sci. 2021;28:55–61.

GPSR Compliance

*The European Union's (EU) General Product Safety Regulation (GPSR) is a set of rules that requires consumer products to be safe and our obligations to ensure this.*

*If you have any concerns about our products, you can contact us on ProductSafety@springernature.com*

In case Publisher is established outside the EU, the EU authorized representative is:

Springer Nature Customer Service Center GmbH
Europaplatz 3
69115 Heidelberg, Germany

**Batch number: 10731528**

Printed by Printforce, the Netherlands